WELLNESS
Guidelines For A Healthy Lifestyle

2nd Edition

Brent Q. Hafen
Brigham Young University

Werner W. K. Hoeger
Boise State University

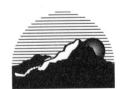

Morton Publishing Company
925 W. Kenyon Avenue, Unit 12
Englewood, Colorado 80110

Publisher	Douglas N. Morton
Managing Editor	Ruth Horton
Designer	Joanne Saliger
Copy Editor	Carolyn Acheson
Illustrator	Jennifer Johnson George Hazelwood
Cover Design	Bob Schram, Bookends
Typography	Ash Street Typecrafters, Inc.
Software Developer	Sharon A. Hoeger

Chapter 8 Opening Photo © Fitness & Wellness, Inc.

Printed in the United States of America
by Morton Publishing Company
925 W. Kenyon Ave., Unit 12
Englewood, CO 80110
http://www.morton-pub.com
1-800-348-3777

9 8 7 6 5 4 3 2

ISBN: 0-89582-397-7

Preface

Contemporary knowledge and ethical considerations suggest a broad approach to health behavior, involving the social, emotional, mental and spiritual natures and consequences. Ignorance of these aspects breeds myth, misconceptions, and exploitation, all of which are avoidable through better understanding. Few books have explained, with support from the scientific literature, how each dimension contributes to wellness. In the pages that follow, you will learn what the research literature has to say about traditional health-related topics, as well as what we know about how emotions impact health and wellness. You'll see how nurturing negative attitudes, emotions, and relationships can hurt, and positive attitudes, emotions, and relationships, when nurtured, can enhance wellness, and even help to heal. What is written here will help you appreciate what we know about the mind/body connection and the tremendous healing power of your mind and heart.

Wellness – Guidelines for a Healthy Lifestyle is not a book about disease, but, rather, one that provides guidelines for preventing disease and enhancing health and wellness. Self-responsibility is emphasized throughout the book, with the realization that enhancing wellness requires personal decision making and realistic goal setting, with positive and optimistic follow through. The responsibility of enhancing health and wellness and developing a healthy lifestyle rests primarily with the individual. According to research literature, improving happiness, quality of life, and longevity is a matter of personal choice. The purpose of this book is not only to increase readers' understanding about health and wellness but also to help assess their own personal attitudes and behavior and, where necessary, to make appropriate changes. The book places a strong emphasis on fitness, because the scientific evidence has shown clearly that one of the most effective ways to enhance wellness and longevity is to increase one's level of physical activity and fitness.

WHAT'S NEW IN THIS EDITION

All chapters in the second edition of *Wellness – Guidelines for a Healthy Lifestyle* have been revised and updated to conform with advances and recommendations made since the first edition was published.

The most significant changes in this new edition are:

- Key terms appear in boldface type and, together with their definitions, appear in boxes within the text. The terms are also combined in a glossary at the end of the book.

- The 1996 U.S. Surgeon General's Report on Physical Activity and Health has been reviewed and information from this report has been included in this second edition.

- Each chapter is studded with tips for putting health principles into practice — providing practical, easy-to-use guidelines that will make this book a valued handbook toward a healthier life.

- Each chapter includes comprehensive self-assessments that let the student determine his or her own level of wellness. Based on these assessments, the student can then use any of a variety of behavior-change guidelines included here to design a personalized, powerful program for a healthy lifestyle.

- New and essential information on motivation and behavior modification to help students implement a lifetime wellness program are included in Chapter 7.

- As a result of several reports regarding the validity and reliability of the abdominal crunch test and the large number of requests and concerns expressed by instructors throughout the country, the Bent-leg Curl-up test has again been incorporated into the Muscular Strength and Endurance and the Muscular Endurance Tests in Chapter 6. The Abdominal Crunch Test has been left as an alternative for use by individuals who are at risk for low back injury.

- Chapter 8, on nutrition, also has been extensively revised and contains an update on recent information released on antioxidant nutrients, phytochemicals, and the recent 1995 Dietary Guidelines for North Americans. The list of nutrients in Appendix A has also been expanded to 514 food items. Most of the new additions to this list are commercially prepared meals.

- Based on the latest research reports, the importance of physical activity as a major factor, if not the most important one, in preventing obesity and maintaining recommended body weight has been enhanced in Chapter 10, on weight control. Further, evidence showing that lack of physical activity, and not excessive weight itself, as the cause of premature death rates associated with obesity is presented in this chapter. This finding is significant because it seems that aerobically fit/overweight men have a lower risk of death than unfit men of normal weight and as low a risk of death as fit men of normal weight.

- The prescription of flexibility exercise conforms with the new 1995 guidelines for exercise testing and prescription by the American College of Sports Medicine (ACSM).
- Chapter 11, on preventing cardiovascular disease, has been updated to conform with recent developments in this area.
- New color photography and many new graphs have been added throughout the book.

ANCILLARIES

The following ancillaries are provided free of charge to all qualified *Wellness – Guidelines for a Healthy Lifestyle* adopters:

- Profile Plus for Windows, a nutrient analysis computer software package. This software package helps provide a more meaningful experience to all participants and greatly decreases the workload of course instructors.
- Microtest, a Fitness and Wellness Computerized Testbank contains the following options: (a) more than 600 questions, (b) capability to add/or edit test questions, previously generated tests can be recalled — creating new exam versions because

multiple choice answers can be rotated with each new test generated, and (d) capability to generate tests using a LaserJet printer.

- More than 70 color overhead transparency acetates.
- A comprehensive instructor's manual.

Student Supplement for the World Wide Web

The World Wide Web has emerged as a valuable educational resource. Visiting cyberspace can make for a unique teaching and learning experience. The problem is: How do students identify sites that are academically appropriate and begin to use WWW sites in an educational context?

To make use of the resources of the World Wide Web in a practical way, *JumpStart with WebLinks: A Guidebook for Fitness/Wellness/Personal Health* is a suggested supplement. Edited by Professor Eileen L. Daniel, Ph.D., this spiral-bound guidebook contains 36 topics on fitness, wellness, and personal health. For each topic (e.g., cardiovascular endurance, eating disorders), a topic introduction orients students to the topic and concludes with a mix of personal assessment and content-related questions.

Following the topic introduction is a directory of WebLinks: the addresses (URLs) of four to six relevant WWW sites, appropriate for students and faculty alike. Each site has been fully verified and approved by a WebAdvisory Board made up of academics from colleges and universities throughout the United States and Canada. A brief Instructor's Resource Guide provides general information on how to incorporate *JumpStart with Weblinks* into any classroom setting.

The authors wish to express gratitude to Charles Scheer for his continued support in making this work possible. Special thanks to Debbie Thompson, Kaselah Crockett, Louise Cashmere, Josh Schkrohowsky, Merikarol Welch, Scott and Jamie Whiles, Amber Hoeger, Angela Hoeger, Christina Kleiss, Erin C. Caskey, and David T. Aschenbrener for their kind help with the photography in this new edition.

A special thanks to Joanne Saliger, Carolyn Acheson, Stacey Hosier, and Ruth Horton for their skillful work in editing, formatting, typesetting, and other phases of production.

Thanks to all our many users of the first edition, especially David Moates and Mike Perrine for their valuable input into this edition.

And, finally, we express thanks to Kathryn J. Frandsen for her help in organizing and writing this edition and thanks to Sharon Hoeger for her many hours developing the software.

Contents

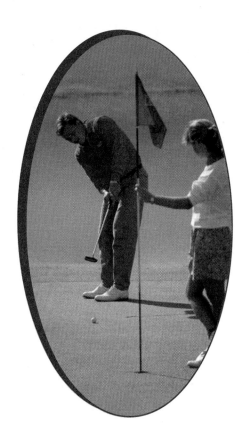

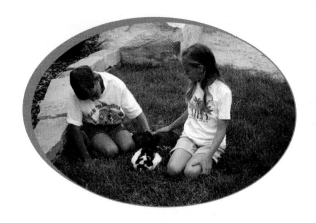

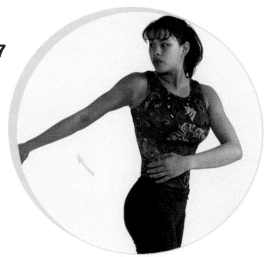

8 Nutrition and Wellness   197

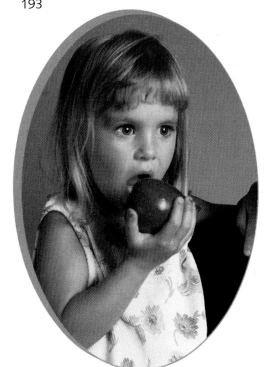

9 Body Composition Assessment   239

10 Weight Management, Eating Disorders, and Wellness   259

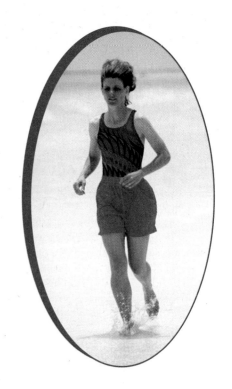

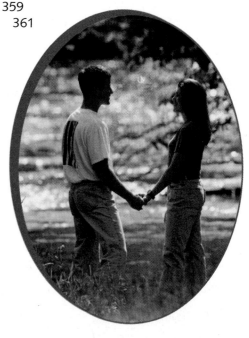

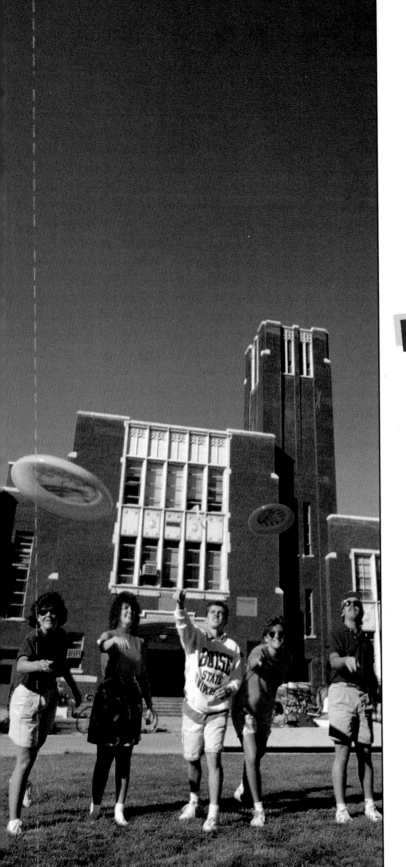

Introduction to Wellness

OBJECTIVES

- Identify five of the leading health problems in the United States.
- Identify the characteristics of wellness.
- Identify and describe the dimensions of wellness.
- Identify six risk factors that compromise wellness.
- List the three main goals of the *Year 2000 National Health Objectives*.
- Discuss at least four things you can do as part of a personalized approach to health and wellness.

The silvered bulb of a thermometer is poked under a tongue, and the mercury inches its way along a measured scale. The cold metal of the stethoscope probes for a faintly distinguishable rhythm. A drop of crimson blood is smeared beneath the powerful gaze of a microscope. Using medical tools such as these, we can draw a line of demarcation between health and disease. Or is it that easy? In reality, health and wellness are not easy to define. Clutching at an elusive definition, the World Health Organization earmarks health as "a state of complete physical, mental, and social well-being, and not merely the absence of disease or infirmity." The key word in that definition is possibly *well-being*, and true health actually may denote a condition in which we are able to avoid illness even if we are predisposed to it.

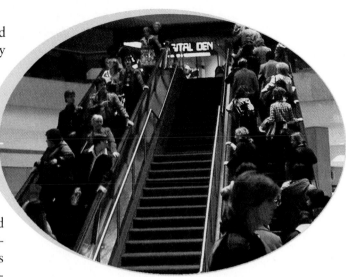

Modern technology has contributed to a sedentary lifestyle and accompanying health problems.

At the turn of the 20th century, the most common health problems in the United States were infectious diseases such as influenza, diphtheria, polio, and tuberculosis. Scientific advances enabled us to wipe out many of those diseases or, at the least, to reduce dramatically the deaths they caused. Those same scientific advances, however, heralded an age of convenience chronicled by a sedentary lifestyle, more alcohol consumption, and a diet permeated by fats and sugars. The result is America's *new* health problem, **chronic diseases**, such as heart disease, cancer, diabetes, emphysema, and cirrhosis of the liver.

The focus at the turn of the 20th century was treatment. Researchers confronted with infectious diseases searched for a cure and often met with success. Our focus on the eve of the 21st century, however, must be on prevention. The health problems that face the population are, in large measure, the result of lifestyle decisions. Emphatic statements released year after year by the U.S. Surgeon General's Office point out that the leading causes of premature death and illness in the United States could be prevented through positive lifestyle habits. The solution to those health problems, then, is largely within our control.

Until recently the American health-care system has not addressed prevention. We have instead a sickness-care system. About $750 billion — more than a twelfth of the gross national product — is

> " *You, the individual, can do more for your health and well-being than any doctor, any hospital, any drug, any exotic medical device.* "
>
> Joseph A. Califano
> (former Secretary of Health, Education, and Welfare)

spent on the nation's health care, encompassing hospitals, doctors, health maintenance organizations, pharmaceuticals, and other related companies. As a nation, the United States spends more per capita on health care than any other country in the world. People in England, who spend a third what the United States does per person on health care, outlive us by an average of 3 years.

Further, Americans have a higher age-adjusted mortality rate and a higher infant mortality rate than a number of nations. Of 20 countries that researchers at Northwestern University Medical School in Chicago studied, the typical American diet was highest of all in the percentage of fat. Only a few nations ranked higher in the amount of artery-clogging cholesterol consumed. The typical American diet also is the lowest in dietary fiber. As a result, the United States is one of the fattest nations in the world. Approximately two-thirds of middle-aged men in the United States are overweight, compared to only 3% of the middle-aged men in Japan.

As if that isn't enough, the United States has the highest rate of heart disease of the developed nations of the world. The country also has some of the highest rates in the world of cancer of the colon, rectum, breast, and lung.

Considering how much the nation spends on medical care, it should outshine the world in health and wellness, but it doesn't, because it has failed to make prevention a top priority. Critical to a focus on prevention, say health-care experts, is a change in attitude by patients and health-care providers alike. Patients have to stop demanding medication for every ailment and hospitalization or surgery for every illness. In turn, physicians have to be more conservative in their approach to disease. According to Joseph A. Califano, former Secretary of Health, Education and Welfare, America's doctors need to be "more skeptical in resorting to surgery and less promiscuous in dispensing pills."

The problem, in essence, lies with us, not with the medical establishment. Of all the people who die in the United States every year, only 10% die because of inadequate health care. Only 20% die because of environmental or biological factors. The rest die as a direct result of an unhealthy lifestyle (see Figure 1.1).

Health and wellness include physical, emotional, social, intellectual, and spiritual dimensions.

LEADING HEALTH PROBLEMS IN THE UNITED STATES

About 83% of all deaths before age 65 in the United States could have been prevented. Almost half of all deaths among people of all ages is attributable to lifestyle factors. An additional 16% is caused by environmental factors. More than half of all disease is what researchers call "self-controlled"; we can influence it through lifestyle changes and other preventive methods.

At the beginning of this century, almost one-third of all deaths in the United States resulted from tuberculosis, influenza, and pneumonia. Millions died of influenza in a 1918 epidemic. Fewer than 5% died from cancer, and only about 10% died of cardiovascular disease. Today, virtually no one dies of tuberculosis. Only 4% or 5% die from influenza and pneumonia. According to statistics for 1994, more than 60% of all deaths in the United States are from heart disease (including stroke) and cancer (see Figure 1.2). Nearly 80% of those deaths could have been prevented by making lifestyle changes — things as basic as eating a diet lower in fat, getting regular exercise, and quitting smoking.

The other top two causes of death — bronchitis/emphysema, called chronic obstructive pulmonary disease (COPD), and injuries — also are largely preventable. Most cases of chronic and obstructive pulmonary disease are caused by cigarette smoking. Many fatal accidents are the result of alcohol abuse, drug abuse, or failure to use seatbelts. And, though our modern-day "epidemic," AIDS, cannot be cured, it can be prevented by lifestyle choices.

According to the American Council on Science and Health, four of the five leading causes of death are related directly to cigarette smoking. Smoking is responsible for an estimated 30% of all cancer deaths, 30% of all heart disease fatalities, and 85% of all deaths from chronic bronchitis and emphysema. It also is an "unquantifiable risk factor" for cerebrovascular disease.

According to the Council, infant and fetal mortality also could be reduced substantially by less cigarette smoking. Smoking is responsible for higher rates of spontaneous abortion and stillbirth and accounts for up to 14% of all premature births in the United States.

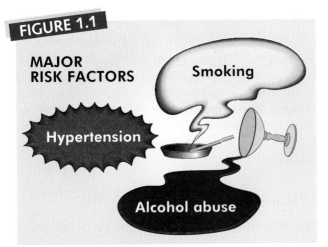

FIGURE 1.1

MAJOR RISK FACTORS

Smoking

Hypertension

Alcohol abuse

Three major risk factors for five of the leading causes of death in the United States.

Chronic diseases Illnesses that linger over time and may get progressively worse.

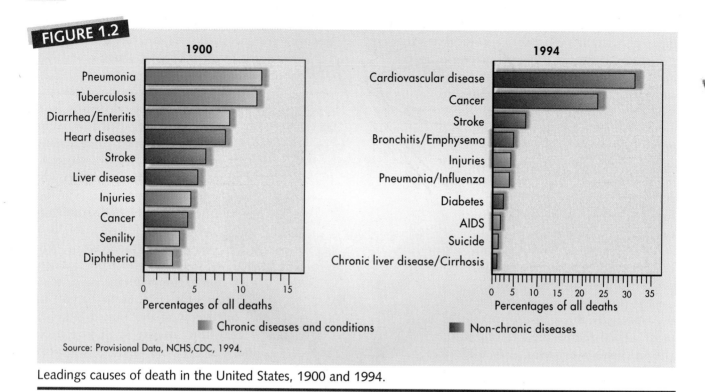

FIGURE 1.2

Leadings causes of death in the United States, 1900 and 1994.

The official position of the World Health Organization on smoking is clear: "The control of cigarette smoking could do more to improve health and prolong life in developed countries than any other single action in the whole field of preventive medicine."[1] And, according to former U.S. Surgeon General C. Everett Koop, cigarette smoking is the number-one preventable cause of death and disease in the United States and the most important health issue of our time.[2]

WHAT ARE HEALTH AND WELLNESS?

More than five decades ago health-care education pioneer Jesse Williams proclaimed that health is a condition that allows one to do the most constructive work, render the best possible service to the world, and experience the highest possible enjoyment of life. "Health as freedom from disease is a standard of mediocrity," he wrote. "Health as a quality of life is a standard of inspiration and increasing achievements."[3]

Williams was ahead of his time. Most Americans have taken decades to catch on to his vision. A series of Gallup polls finally hinted at his much broader scope of health and wellness. In increasing numbers,

Americans now are defining health as "the energy to do the things we care about."

Health

The word **health** is derived from the Old English "hal," which means *whole*. Researchers on the cutting edge consider health to be a continuum, a perpetual but ever-changing balance of the various dimensions that make us whole: physical, mental, emotional, social, and spiritual.

Everything with which you interact — the place you live, the air you breathe, the food you eat, the job you have, the people you associate with — affects your position on the health continuum. The same series of Gallup polls shows that Americans are beginning to understand the influence of interactive factors. When ranking their "health priorities," their top concern was staying free of disease, but the third highest was "living in an environment with clean air and water."

Wellness

Wellness combines physical, mental, emotional, social, and spiritual well-being into a quality way of living. It is the ability to live life to the fullest, to have a zest for life, to maximize personal potential in a variety of dimensions. Illness and health are opposite states, but you can be ill and still enjoy wellness if you have a purpose in life, a deep appreciation for living, a sense of joy.

People who are bound by the strictures of traditionally defined physical health wait until some disease has crept up on them, then consult a professional to evaluate their condition and prescribe treatment. Simply put, they turn over their physical health to someone else. Wellness, on the other hand, places responsibility on the individual. Wellness becomes a matter of self-evaluation and self-assessment. You continually work on learning and on making changes that will enhance your state of wellness. *You* take the reins. Rather than delegating your physical health to someone else, you make a deep personal commitment to wellness.

Whereas physical health is a fairly simple concept, wellness is multifaceted and involves much more than simple physical condition. Physical health is something that is not available to everyone. On the other hand, everyone can enjoy wellness — despite physical limitations, disease, and handicap. Wellness fully integrates physical, mental, emotional, social, and spiritual well-being — a complex interaction of the factors that lead to a quality life. It is not something that is "achieved" once; it is a horizon that we move toward throughout life. We move along a continuum, and the important factor is the direction in which we are moving. Finally, wellness affects not only the individual but also can encompass the family and society as a whole.

If we are to accept a definition of wellness that goes beyond mere freedom from disease, we also must accept a notion that calls for a dramatic change in the way we deal with health. For centuries our emphasis has been on identifying bacteria, classifying viruses, and waging a determined war on devastating diseases. We have concentrated on treatment. If we are to redefine health to reflect a condition of wellness, however, we also must redefine the ultimate goal of our health efforts: *to concentrate on a way of preventing disease.* Inherent in that challenge is the recognition that behavior — physical, mental, emotional, social, and spiritual — plays a key role in the development of disease and also in our ability to resist disease and maintain optimum health.

Embodied in the definition of wellness and behavioral health is a philosophy calling for consideration of the whole person, not a segmented fractionalization into separate parts. We need to consider ourselves as we interact in our environment, not as separate complaints or body parts in a sterile laboratory or the unnatural environs of a physician's examining room. It stresses a conscious and active commitment by the individual, refusing to admit that optimum health is something that just happens. Most significantly, it calls for concentration on the factors that precede illness instead of concern solely with the anatomy of disease once it strikes.

THE DIMENSIONS OF WELLNESS

Writing in *The History and Future of Wellness*, author Donald Ardell[4] points out that living by the principles of wellness is considered a richer way to be alive. Optimum wellness balances five basic dimensions: physical, mental, emotional, social, and spiritual. These are depicted in Figure 1.3.

Signs of Wellness

- Persistent presence of support network.
- Chronic positive expectations; tendency to frame events in a constructive light.
- Episodic peak experiences.
- Sense of spiritual involvement.
- Increased sensitivity.
- Tendency to adapt to changing conditions.
- Rapid response and recovery of adrenaline system as a result of repeated challenges.
- Appetite for physical activity.
- Tendency to identify and communicate feelings.
- Repeated episodes of gratitude, generosity, or related emotions.
- Compulsion to contribute to society.
- Persistent sense of humor.

If five or more of these indicators are present, you may be at risk for full-blown wellness.

Adapted from "Commentary," in *Brain/Mind* (March, 1993), P.O. Box 42211, Los Angeles, CA 90042. Reprinted by permission.

Health A state of complete well-being, and not just the absence of disease or infirmity.

Wellness Full integration of physical, mental, emotional, social, and spiritual well-being into a quality life.

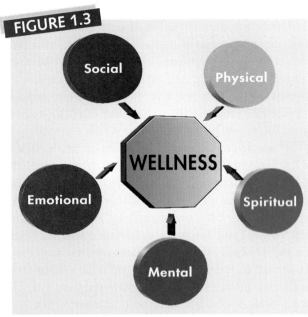

FIGURE 1.3

The dimensions of wellness.

Physical Dimension

Physical wellness is the kind most commonly associated with being healthy. A person who is physically well eats a well-balanced diet, gets plenty of physical activity and exercise, maintains proper weight, gets enough sleep, avoids risky sexual behavior, tries to limit exposure to environmental contaminants, and restricts intake of harmful substances such as alcohol, tobacco, caffeine, and drugs. Physical wellness is characterized by good cardiorespiratory endurance, muscular strength and flexibility, proper body composition, and the ability to carry out daily tasks.

To remain well requires that you take steps to protect your physical health: do self-exams and get regular, thorough physical examinations, including appropriate screening tests, from a physician. It also involves taking effective measures if you do become sick, such as seeking medical care and using medications conservatively.

Physical wellness entails confidence and optimism about one's ability to take care of health problems. These conditions need not prevent one from enjoying life. Physical wellness brings with it a remarkable resistance to disease. The right combination of nutrition, exercise, and sleep renders healthy people capable of resisting the common colds and influenza that wipe out others.

People who enjoy physical wellness are intelligent about their health. When they *do* develop an unusual or irritating symptom, they do what is necessary to relieve it. If symptoms persist, they check with a doctor.

Irrespective of whether healthy individuals are muscular, they usually are physically powerful. Exercise attunes their muscles and endows them with a high level of physical coordination and self-confidence. Instead of shying away from physical challenge, they accept it with enthusiasm, confident they can make their body work for them. Reaction time is good, strength is obvious, and endurance is high.

People characterized by physical wellness have an active lifestyle. They like to be outdoors. They enjoy a fast-paced bicycle ride along a roadside choked with apple blossoms or a vigorous game of touch football on a crisp autumn afternoon. They have the energy they need to do the things they enjoy, as well as the energy they need to complete demanding tasks at work, breeze through final exams on a wink of sleep, or clear out all the debris from last year's vegetable garden.

People who are physically well respect and like their own body. They have a natural grace and ease. You can see their health in the way they move. Beauty in the traditional sense of the word has little to do with it. People with physical wellness make the most of their body, and they delight in it.

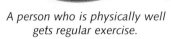

A person who is physically well gets regular exercise.

Mental Dimension

Just as the physical dimension of wellness embodies much more than the mere absence of disease, so, too, **mental wellness** is characterized by signs of wellness. Pioneers in the field of psychoneuroimmunology are proving scientifically what philosophers such as Homer, Plato, and Aristotle speculated more than 5,000 years ago: The mind has a striking influence on the body (and, therefore, on health and wellness).

Education shouldn't stop with commencement exercises. A sound mental dimension of wellness involves unbridled curiosity and ongoing learning. This dimension of wellness implies that you can apply the things you have learned (whether at home or on the job), that you create opportunities to learn more, and that you engage your mind in lively interaction with the world around you.

People who are mentally well can think clearly, are quick to pick up new concepts, and catch on rapidly to new ideas. Instead of being intimidated by facts and figures with which they

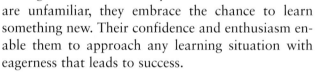

Mental wellness involves curiosity and ongoing learning.

are unfamiliar, they embrace the chance to learn something new. Their confidence and enthusiasm enable them to approach any learning situation with eagerness that leads to success.

Mental wellness breeds creativity. In contrast to people who seem burdened with the task of getting a job done, mentally well people are able to approach the same task in a new way. They don't seem restricted by what they always have done before. They are willing to tackle the chore from a different angle, one that lets them exercise creativity and initiative.

Logic is a basic attribute of mental wellness. People who are confronted suddenly with an unfamiliar situation tend to experience mild panic. Mental wellness brings with it common sense and logic that enable those who are mentally well to reason their way through.

A genuine sense of curiosity leads mentally well people into a world that is always new and challenging. Whereas others accept what life has to offer with quiet resolve, mentally well people grasp each aspect of life with a desire to understand. They are the people who know why the surface of a lake is so blue, how a newspaper is printed, how a robin can tell that spring has arrived. They know the answers because they ask the questions. Some people pass a flowering hedge and notice that it is beautiful. Healthier people want to know why the blooms are pink, what kind of hedge it is, how they can grow one like it.

Along with alertness and brightness, mental wellness brings with it stimulation and capability. Mentally well people have a good memory and use it to their greatest advantage. They are skilled in their chosen area of expertise, and they are open to new ideas and suggestions. They relish the chance to improve themselves and to learn something new.

Mental wellness brings with it vision and promise. More than anything else, mentally well people are open-minded and accepting of others. Instead of being threatened by those who are different from themselves, they show respect and curiosity without feeling they have to conform. They are faithful to their own ideas and philosophies and allow others the same privilege. Their self-confidence guarantees that they can take their place among others in the world without having to give up part of themselves and without requiring others to do the same.

Emotional Dimension

Emotions involve both the mind and the body, and, as a result, they can bridge the gap between the mind and the body. Emotions are a contributing factor in a number of diseases, such as rheumatoid arthritis, bronchial asthma, peptic ulcer, ulcerative colitis, hypertension, and dermatitis.

What constitutes **emotional wellness?** Foremost is probably the ability to understand your own feelings, to accept your limitations, and to achieve emotional stability. It also involves being comfortable with your emotions. Understanding and accepting your own feelings helps you understand and accept the emotions of others, which leads to the ability to maintain intimate relationships with other people. Emotional wellness also implies the ability to express emotions appropriately, adjust to change, cope with stress in a healthy way, and enjoy life despite its occasional disappointments and frustrations.

The hallmark of emotional wellness is a deep and abiding happiness — not a happiness that depends

Physical wellness   Flexibility, endurance, strength, and optimism about your ability to take care of health problems.

Mental wellness   A state in which your mind is engaged in lively interaction with the world around you.

Emotional wellness   The ability to understand your own feelings, accept your limitations, and achieve emotional stability.

on some frail set of circumstances but, rather, a happiness that stems from a powerful inner contentment. Instead of being dependent on a certain income or status in life, the happiness that signals real wellness is an emotional anchor that gives meaning and joy to life.

In penning the Declaration of Independence, Thomas Jefferson promised three things to all Americans: the rights to life, liberty, and the pursuit of happiness. He did not promise happiness itself, because he knew that the government could not deliver it. Happiness is not a fleeting emotion tied to a single event. It is a long-term state of mind that permeates the various facets of life and influences our outlook. We can experience true happiness and temporary unhappiness at the same time. Happiness may seem to vanish temporarily, giving way to bursts of depression or disappointment, but it returns. As Harry Emerson Fosdick stated:

> One who expects to completely escape low moods is asking the impossible. Like the weather, life is essentially variable, and a healthy person believes in the validity of his high hours even when he is having a low one.[5]

No one has ever come up with a simple recipe for producing happiness, but researchers agree that certain ingredients seem universal among those who have the kind of true, abiding happiness characteristic of emotional wellness. Those who are happy usually are part of a family. They are partners, parents,

> **❝ *Happiness is a long-term state of mind that permeates the various facets of life and influences our outlook.* ❞**

or children. They love others, and they feel loved themselves. Healthy, happy people enjoy friends, work hard at something fulfilling, get plenty of exercise, and enjoy play and leisure time. They know how to laugh, and they laugh often. They give of themselves freely to others and seem to have found deep meaning to life.

An attitude of true happiness signals freedom from the tension and depression that many people endure. Emotional wellness obviously is subject to the same kinds of depression and unhappiness that

plague all of us once in a while, but the difference lies in the ability to bounce back. Well people take minor setbacks in stride and have the uncanny ability to enjoy life despite it all. When something unhappy happens, they put it behind them. They don't waste energy or time recounting the situation, wondering how they could have changed it, or dwelling on the past.

The spirit of optimism basic to healthy, happy individuals enables them to focus their energy on the present. They recognize that the past can hold powerful lessons, but they do not let it control the here and now. Instead of worrying about what they should have done differently back then,

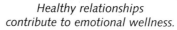
Healthy relationships contribute to emotional wellness.

they concentrate with enthusiasm and energy on what they can do today.

In addition to avoiding the pitfalls of the past, they avoid the temptation to pin all their hopes and dreams on the future. They are goal-oriented and ambitious, and at the same time are able to enjoy themselves today. They aren't waiting until they graduate from college, until they get married, until they pay off their home, or until they are the president of a company. Instead, they are happy today in the circumstances they are in. They may aspire to graduate with honors, marry their sweetheart, pay off the mortgage, or gain the top spot at the firm, but they are happy regardless. They know that happiness is not related to some *thing* but instead is a *condition*.

Part and parcel of happiness is acceptance of self. Healthy people value themselves as having something to contribute and being worthwhile. Healthy people enjoy a sense of success — not as measured traditionally by the world but as measured against their own standards. They know what is important to them, and they are confident they can achieve it. They are in touch with self to the point that they have a clear definition of their own needs.

Emotional wellness brings with it a certain stability, an ability to look both success and failure squarely in the face and to keep moving along a predetermined course. When success is evident, the emotionally well person radiates the expected joy and confidence. When failure seems evident, the emotionally well person responds by making the best of circumstances and moving beyond the failure. Wellness enables us to move ahead with optimism and energy instead of spending time and talent worrying about failure. We learn from it, identify ways to avoid it in the future, and then go on with the business at hand.

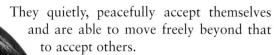

Emotional wellness also embodies the ability to get in touch with your own feelings. Because healthy people have a good self-image, they do not worry about showing their feelings or sharing them with others. They are not concerned with what others think of them. They do not feel the need to prove themselves to others, nor do they feel they have to force others to accept their point of view.

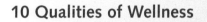

A good sense of humor is an important part of wellness.

They quietly, peacefully accept themselves and are able to move freely beyond that to accept others.

Sensitive, yet independent, emotionally well people accept themselves to an extent that they are extremely insightful about themselves and others. Emotional wellness brings with it a necessary frame of mind that allows involvement with other people. A truly healthy person is one who enjoys others and who is not threatened by what other people might do or say.

Emotional wellness also brings with it a maturity that allows the individual to forgive others. Emotionally well people accept responsibility for their own happiness instead of blaming others when they are unhappy. They are free from anger and resentment because they recognize that anger is almost always destructive. By accepting responsibility for their own emotional well-being, they free themselves to achieve it.

More than dictating happiness and optimism, emotions play a profound part in physical health and avoiding disease. Biobehavioralist Norman Cousins maintained that what you think, what you believe, and how you react to experiences can impair or aid the workings of the body's immune system.

Studies of terminally ill cancer patients reveal that those who survive have one characteristic in common: their utter refusal to give up hope. Cousins said:

> Nothing is more wondrous about the fifteen billion neurons in the human brain than their ability to convert thoughts, hopes, ideas, and attitudes into chemical substances. Every emotion, negative or positive, makes its registrations on the body's systems. . . . The most important thing I have learned about the power of belief is that an individual patient's attitude toward serious illness can be as important as medical help. It would be a serious mistake to bypass or minimize the need for scientific treatment, but that treatment will be far more effective if people put their creative hopes, their faith, and their confidence fully to work in behalf of their recovery.[6]

Harvard-trained surgeon Bernie Siegel, who has spent his medical career working with cancer victims, remarked:

> I can say from my own experience that patients who have given up, who have come to me feeling defeated

10 Qualities of Wellness

1 Deeply committed to a cause outside oneself.

2 Physically able to do whatever one wants with intensity and great energy; seldom sick.

3 Caring and loving; a person others can lean on in a crisis.

4 In tune with the spiritual, having a clear sense of purpose and direction.

5 Intellectually sharp, able to handle information, possessing an ever-curious mind and a good sense of humor.

6 Well organized and able to accomplish plenty of work.

7 Able to live in and enjoy the present rather than focusing on the past or looking toward the future.

8 Comfortable with experiencing the full range of human emotions.

9 Accepting of one's limitations, handicaps, and mistakes.

10 Able and willing to take charge of one's life, to practice positive self-care, and to be assertive when necessary.

and desperate, feeling that nothing can possibly help them, have often made their own predictions come true. The fighter-type patients who are willing to try anything that has a chance to help them, who have real faith in their survival, always do better.[7]

Social Dimension

Social wellness, with its accompanying self-image, endows us with the ease and confidence to be outgoing, friendly, and affectionate toward others. Social wellness involves not only a concern for the individual, but also an interest in humanity and the environment as a whole.

One of the hallmarks of social wellness is the ability to relate to others, to reach out to other people, both within the family unit and outside it. Healthy people are honest and loyal. Their own balance and sense of self allow them to extend respect and tolerance to others. They are confident of themselves and don't feel threatened by opening up to others.

People who are socially healthy are able to develop and maintain intimacy but are not promiscuous. They organize themselves in family groups and are loyal and faithful to family members. They are trustworthy and loyal to those outside the family unit and have the ability to make and keep friends. They treat others with fairness and respect.

Social wellness goes hand in hand with social graces. Socially healthy people are affectionate, polite, and helpful toward others; can handle conflict without exploding; and are true to their ideals and beliefs while allowing others to be true to theirs. They do not interpret a difference of opinion as the basis for destruction. Instead, they are tolerant, respectful, and secure. They can say "no" when they should and are sensitive in responding to others' needs without sacrificing their own.

Socially well people love themselves. This is not a vain, self-centered kind of love that causes them to develop an over-inflated image of themselves. Instead, it is the kind of love that enables individuals to feel secure enough, confident enough, and good enough about themselves to reach

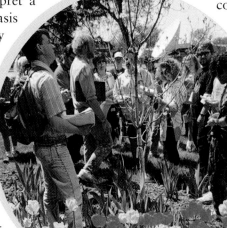
Group activities enhance social wellness.

out to others. Before you can love others, you must be able to love yourself.

The socially well person relishes touch, especially hugging, as a vital, irreplaceable means of communicating caring and concern for others. Long-term research by experts in a variety of disciplines has confirmed that touch is critical to well-being. San Diego psychologist James Hardison wrote:

> It is through touching that we are able to fulfill a large share of our human needs and, in doing so, to attain happiness. By touching someone, we can affirm our friendship or approval, communicate important messages, promote health, and bring about love.[8]

Unfortunately, Hardison continues, too many people put up barriers to the language of touch, equating touching "with either sex or violence. Consequently many people avoid the simple acts of touching — pats on the back, heartfelt handshakes, cordial hugs — that affirm goodwill."

Benefits of Wellness

Wellness reaps benefits not only to the physical body but to the "soul" as well. Achieving a high level of wellness helps you:

- Delay the aging process.
- Reduce your risk of chronic illness.
- Be self-confident.
- Boost your muscle strength, endurance, and flexibility.
- Identify and meet your needs.
- Function better.
- Increase your energy.
- Do better at school, on the job, and in everyday living.
- Maintain optimism and hope.
- Get good nutrition.
- Look better.
- Stay stimulated intellectually.
- Bounce back faster after illness or injury.
- Raise your level of cardiovascular health.
- Look at problems as challenges, not stumbling blocks.

Socially well people — whether at home, in the classroom, or at work — develop a spirit of teamwork with those around them. They do not view others with suspicion, jealousy, or contempt. They find no satisfaction in the thought of outdoing, putting down, or getting ahead of others. They find great joy in cooperation, mutual support, and working together to accomplish something of lasting value for all.

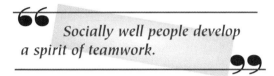

> *Socially well people develop a spirit of teamwork.*

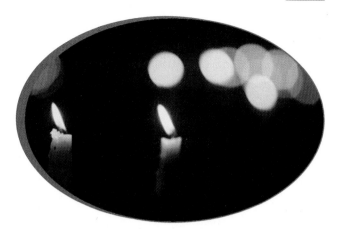

Spiritual wellness recognizes a power higher than oneself.

Spiritual Dimension

Spiritual wellness — comprising the ethics, values, and morals that guide us — gives meaning and direction to life. Every human being needs the sense that life is meaningful, that life has purpose and direction, and that some power (nature, science, religion, or some higher power) brings all of humanity together. In essence, spiritual wellness entails a search for greater value in life.

Spiritual wellness embodies commitment to a worthwhile purpose, faith, and peace, and an undaunted comfort with life and its outcome. It is characterized by faith and optimism, by a hope that sustains through whatever life has to offer. It entails developing the inner self and identifying a purpose to life. Optimum spiritual wellness occurs when you are able to discover, articulate, and *act* on that purpose.

Spiritually well people have the unique ability to see beyond the isolated event, to envision the whole picture. A spiritually well person sets realistic goals and goes about reaching them with hope, enthusiasm, and determination. Those goals are never the end result. They are part of the whole, cogs in the larger machine in life. Spiritually healthy people are enthused about what lies ahead, not merely content with what they have accomplished in the past.

That's not to say that spiritually well people never experience disappointment. Spiritually healthy people, however, are able to bridge the gap from one success to another, able to develop the fortitude necessary to keep going. Spiritually healthy individuals don't dwell on discouragement. They mobilize their inner resources to reach the next pinnacle. Instead of envisioning disappointments or setbacks as craggy stone walls, spiritually well people see them as smooth stepping stones, inviting them to keep going, inviting them to make their way, carefully but securely, to the other side.

Occupational Dimension

Some models also consider a sixth dimension of wellness: occupational wellness. Occupational wellness is not tied to high salary, prestigious position, or extravagant working conditions. *Any* job can bring occupational wellness if it provides rewards that are important to the individual. Salary might be the

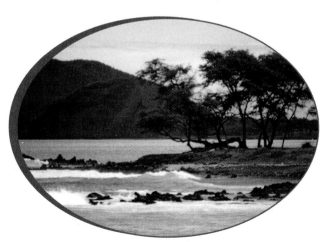

Spiritual wellness includes enjoying the wonder and beauty of nature.

Social wellness   The ability to relate well to others, both within and outside the family unit.

Spiritual wellness   The sense that life is meaningful, that life has purpose, and that some power brings all humanity together; the ethics, values, and morals that guide us and give meaning and direction to life.

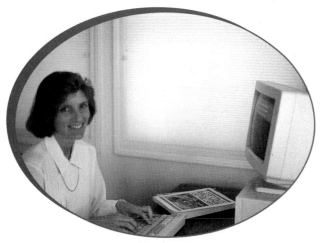

Occupational wellness occurs when a job provides important personal rewards.

most important factor to one person, whereas another might place a much greater value on creativity.

People with occupational wellness face demands on the job, and they also have some say over demands that are placed on them. Any job has routine demands but occupational wellness means that routine demands are mixed with new, unpredictable challenges that keep a job exciting. Occupationally well people are able to maximize their skills, and they have the opportunity to broaden existing skills or gain new ones. There is opportunity for advancement and recognition for achievement.

Occupational wellness also brings some sense of control. People are given the chance to participate in long-term planning and are able to determine some corporate policies, including policies on discipline. People with occupational wellness control the machines they work with, not the other way around. There is ready access to feedback from both customers and management.

Occupational wellness encourages collaboration among co-workers, fostering a sense of teamwork and support. There is good interaction. When problems arise, democratic procedures are used to solve them; those with a grievance have an accepted and effective way to solve it.

A workplace free from physical stressors promotes occupational wellness. Among the many things in the workplace that can cause stress are noise, poor temperature control, crowding, poor arrangement of space, lack of privacy, and problems with lighting (lights are too bright, too dim, too glaring, or flickering). Occupational wellness also implies freedom from safety hazards on the job, such as dangerous machinery, toxic chemicals, air pollution, or the threat of nuclear accidents.

People with occupational wellness consistently work toward a satisfying balance between the time and energy spent at work and the time and energy spent in family and leisure activities. At a healthy job, people share responsibilities so everyone has time (and energy) left for activities away from work.

BEHAVIORAL HEALTH

Behavioral health brings with it solutions that seem simple in comparison to the array of scientific tests, the complex chemical formulas, the powerful lens of the microscope, and the elaborate array of available treatments. Researchers have found that the following simple lifestyle habits can add significantly to longevity:

1. Eat a well-rounded diet low in fats and cholesterol and high in dietary fiber, and make sure you eat a good breakfast every day.

2. Maintain recommended weight.

3. Get at least 30 minutes of moderate exercise at least three times a week.

4. Get a good night's sleep.

5. Surround yourself with a supportive network of friends and family.

6. Implement personal safety measures — things as simple as wearing seatbelts.

7. Stay informed about the environment, and avoid potential contaminants whenever you can.

8. Take any medication your doctor prescribes, and follow directions precisely.

9. Limit your intake of alcohol.

10. If you smoke, quit.

WELLNESS CHALLENGES FOR THE NEXT CENTURY

With the landmark 1979 publication of *Healthy People,* the U.S. Surgeon General's report on health promotion and disease prevention, the government embarked on a plan to establish broad national goals intended to promote wellness among all Americans. Those goals were converted into specific health objectives a year later, with a precise list of measurable goals we hoped to attain by the year 1990.

Americans were successful at some; we failed at others. After assessing what had been achieved and what still had to be done, the U.S. Public Health Service in 1987 began to conduct hearings across the nation with health professionals from a variety of settings. The result is the *Year 2000 National Health Objectives*, a set of goals aimed at taking Americans into the 21st century with a higher level of health and wellness. The health objectives have three main goals:

1. To increase the span of healthy life for all Americans

2. To reduce health disparities among Americans

3. To achieve access to preventive health services for all Americans.

Priorities for health protection, promotion, and prevention are given in Table 1.1. These objectives are classified according to three goals: protection, promotion, and prevention. The table lists examples of each.

Furthermore, a major report on the influence of regular physical activity on health was released by the U.S. Surgeon General in 1996. The report states that regular moderate physical activity provides substantial benefits in health and well-being for the vast majority of Americans who are not physically active. This report has become a call to nationwide action.

TABLE 1.1	**Goals of Healthy People 2000**
Classification	**Goals/Programs**
Health protection	Improve food and drug safety
	Protect environmental health
	Improve oral health
	Boost occupational safety and health
	Reduce incidence of unintentional injuries
Health promotion	Develop nutrition programs
	Offer physical fitness activities
	Provide family planning
	Develop programs addressing violent and abusive behavior
	Develop mental health programs
	Provide tobacco, alcohol, and other drug rehabilitation programs
Health prevention	Reduce maternal and infant mortality
	Prevent chronic diseases:
	• heart disease and strokes
	• cancer
	• diabetes
	Reduce HIV infection
	Reduce sexually transmitted diseases
	Provide immunization services
	Prevent infectious diseases

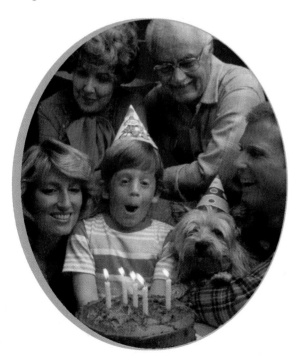

Objectives for enhancing health and wellness are aimed at protection, promotion, and prevention.

According to the Surgeon General, improving health through physical activity is a serious public health challenge that we must meet head on at once. More than 60% of adults do not achieve the recommended amount of physical activity, and 25% are not physically active at all. Benefits of leading a moderately active lifestyle include a significant reduction in the risk of developing or dying from heart disease, diabetes, colon cancer, and high blood pressure. Regular physical activity also helps to maintain a high quality of life into old age. Additional information on this report is given in Chapter 6.

Experts who were instrumental in formulating the national objectives and the report on physical activity and health point to the commitment of the government toward achieving wellness goals. They also invite the commitment and involvement of each American in accepting responsibility for health and wellness.

Behavioral health   The role of lifestyle in health.

Health Objectives for the Year 2000

I. Physical Activity and Fitness
1. Increase the proportion of people who engage regularly, preferably daily, in *light* to *moderate* physical activity for at least 30 minutes per day.
2. Increase the proportion of people who engage in *vigorous* physical activity that promotes the development and maintenance of cardiorespiratory fitness 3 or more days per week for 20 or more minutes per occasion.
3. Increase the proportion of people who regularly perform physical activities that enhance and maintain muscular strength, muscular endurance, and flexibility.
4. Reduce the proportion of people who engage in no leisure-time physical activity.
5. Reduce overweight to a prevalence of no more than 20% among people aged 20 and older and no more than 15% among adolescents aged 12 through 19.
6. Increase to at least 50% the proportion of overweight people aged 12 and older who have adopted sound dietary practices combined with regular physical activity to attain an appropriate body weight.

II. Nutrition
1. Reduce dietary fat intake to an average of 30% of calories or less and average saturated fat intake to less than 10% of calories among people aged 2 and older.
2. Increase complex carbohydrate and fiber-containing foods in the diets of adults to 5 or more daily servings for vegetables and fruits, and to 6 or more daily servings for grain products.
3. Increase calcium consumption in the diet.
4. Reduce iron deficiency among children 1 through 4 and women of childbearing age.
5. Decrease salt and sodium intake in the diet.
6. Increase to at least 85% the proportion of people aged 18 and older who use food labels to make nutritious selections.

III. Chronic Diseases
1. Increase years of healthy life to at least 65 years.
2. Reduce coronary heart disease deaths.
3. Reduce the mean serum cholesterol level among adults to no more than 200 mg/dL.
4. Increase the proportion of adults with high blood cholesterol who are aware of their condition and are taking action to reduce their blood cholesterol to recommended levels.
5. Increase the proportion of people with high blood pressure whose blood pressure is under control.
6. Increase the proportion of people with high blood pressure who are taking action to help control their blood pressure.
7. Reverse the rise in cancer deaths.
8. Slow the rise in lung cancer deaths.
9. Reduce the rate of breast cancer deaths.
10. Reduce colorectal cancer deaths.
11. Reduce diabetes-related deaths.
12. Reduce the proportion of people with asthma who experience activity limitation.
13. Reduce deaths from cirrhosis of the liver.
14. Reduce hip fractures among older adults.
15. Reduce activity limitation due to chronic back conditions.
16. Reduce the proportion of people who experience a limitation in major activity due to chronic conditions.

IV. Mental Health and Disorders
1. Reduce the prevalence of mental disorders.
2. Reduce the suicide rate.
3. Reduce the proportion of people who experience adverse health effects from stress.
4. Decrease the proportion of people who experience stress who do not take steps to reduce or control their stress.

V. Tobacco
1. Reduce the incidence of cigarette smoking.
2. Reduce the initiation of cigarette smoking by children and youth.
3. Reduce the proportion of children who are regularly exposed to tobacco smoke at home.
4. Reduce smokeless tobacco use.
5. Increase the proportion of worksites with a formal smoking policy that prohibits or severely restricts smoking at the workplace.

VI. Alcohol and Other Drugs
1. Reduce the proportion of young people who have used alcohol, marijuana, and cocaine.
2. Reduce the proportion of high school seniors and college students engaging in recent occasions of heavy drinking of alcoholic beverages.
3. Reduce alcohol consumption by people aged 14 and older to an annual average of no more than 2 gallons of ethanol per person.
4. Increase the proportion of high school seniors who associate risk of physical or psychological harm with the heavy use of alcohol, occasional use of marijuana, and experimentation with cocaine.
5. Reduce the proportion of male high school seniors who use anabolic steroids.
6. Reduce deaths caused by alcohol-related motor vehicle crashes.
7. Reduce drug-related deaths.
8. Increase the proportion of all intravenous drug abusers who are in drug abuse treatment programs.
9. Increase the proportion of intravenous drug abusers not in treatment who use only uncontaminated drug paraphernalia ("works").

VII. AIDS, HIV Infection, and Sexually Transmitted Diseases
1. Confine annual incidence of diagnosed AIDS cases to no more than 98,000 cases.
2. Confine the prevalence of HIV infection to no more than 800 per 100,000 people.
3. Increase the proportion of sexually active, unmarried people who used a condom at last sexual intercourse.
4. Reduce the incidence of gonorrhea.
5. Reduce the incidence of Chlamydia.
6. Reduce the incidence of primary and secondary syphilis.
7. Reduce the incidence of genital herpes and genital warts.
8. Reduce the incidence of pelvic inflammatory disease.
9. Reduce the incidence of sexually transmitted hepatitis B infection.

VIII. Family Planning
1. Reduce the number of pregnancies that are unintended.
2. Reduce the proportion of adolescents who have engaged in sexual intercourse.
3. Increase the proportion of sexually active, unmarried people aged 19 and younger who use contraception, especially combined method contraception that both effectively prevents pregnancy and provides barrier protection against disease.

IX. Unintentional Injuries
1. Reduce deaths caused by unintentional injuries.
2. Increase use of occupant protection systems, such as safety belts, inflatable safety restraints, and child safety seats among motor vehicle occupants.
3. Increase use of helmets among motorcyclists and bicyclists.

Source: Adapted from the U.S. Department of Health and Human Services, Public Health Service. *Healthy People 2000: National Health Promotion and Disease Prevention Objectives.* Boston, Jones and Bartlett Publishers, 1992. Refer to this publication for further information on these objectives.

A PERSONALIZED APPROACH TO HEALTH AND WELLNESS

Vital to achieving health and wellness is your willingness to take personal responsibility for your behaviors and choices. We know enough about disease and premature death that we can formulate a set of goals that applies to the nation as a whole. How you achieve those goals, however, requires a personal decision. It entails careful, intelligent planning. How you apply the principles you'll learn in this book has to be highly personalized. What will work for someone else won't necessarily work for you.

As you study the information in this book on achieving wellness, the following personalized approach may be helpful:

- If you're smoking now, determine how you are going to stop. Find out what community resources are available to help you. If you need to, talk to your doctor. Outline a specific course of action that will work for you.

- If you have a drinking problem or a drug dependency, find out specifically where you can get help. Make an appointment. Follow through. Start by figuring out *why* you started using drugs or alcohol to begin with. Your personal motives have a lot to do with your ability to kick the habit.

- If you have a weight problem, get help. With guidance from your doctor or another health-care professional, outline specifically how you are going to change your eating and exercise habits so you can lose weight safely and permanently.

- Increase your level of physical activity. Before you do, however, take a critical look at your situation and determine whether you need a doctor's okay. If you do, schedule an appointment for a thorough physical examination, discuss your objectives with your physician, and get the go-ahead for a safe, effective fitness program. Then design a program that works for you, based on your situation and preferences. If you hate running, try bicycling or swimming instead. If you can't afford the fees at the racquetball court, challenge a group of friends to an equally demanding but less expensive competition a couple of times a week.

- Pinpoint your individual sources of stress. You probably can eliminate some of them. You can

Some Physical Activities

Here are some examples of moderate activity going from less to more vigorous:

- Washing and waxing a car for 45–60 minutes.
- Playing volleyball for 45 minutes.
- Playing touch football for 30–45 minutes.
- Gardening for 30–45 minutes.
- Wheeling self in wheelchair for 30–40 minutes.
- Walking 1¾ miles in 35 minutes (20-minute mile).
- Basketball (shooting baskets) for 30 minutes.
- Bicycling 5 miles in 30 minutes.
- Dancing fast for 30 minutes.
- Pushing a stroller 1½ miles in 30 minutes.
- Raking leaves for 30 minutes.
- Walking 2 miles in 30 minutes.
- Doing water aerobics for 30 minutes.
- Swimming laps for 20 minutes.
- Playing basketball for 15–20 minutes.
- Jumping rope for 15 minutes.
- Running 1½ miles in 15 minutes.
- Shoveling snow for 15 minutes.
- Stairwalking for 15 minutes.

Source: *Physical Activity and Health: A Report of the Surgeon General.*

respond to others differently. If you have a particularly difficult class, for example, get on top of things by scheduling an extra hour every day to study that subject or talk to the professor about getting individualized help from a teaching assistant. Stress has a major impact on disease. A wellness plan demands that you handle stress with determination and commitment.

At the center of wellness is self-responsibility. No one else can make you eat better, exercise more regularly, stop smoking, use alcohol in moderation, or cope with stress. Accepting the challenge to achieve wellness implies that you are willing to make lifelong lifestyle changes. Wellness doesn't happen in a day. It involves an ongoing process of healthy choices throughout the rest of your life.

NOTES

1. World Health Organization, Ch-1211 Geneva 27, Switzerland.
2. U.S. Dept. of Health and Human Services, Office on Smoking and Health, *The Health Consequences of Smoking* (Rockville, MD: DHHS (PHS) 84-50205, 1984), p. xii.
3. Jesse Williams.
4. Ardell, Donald, *The History and Future of Wellness* (IA: Kendall Hunt, 1985).
5. Miller, Robert Moats, *Preacher, Pastor, Prophet* (NY: Oxford University Press, 1988).
6. Cousins, Norman, *Head First: The Biology of Hope* (NY: E. P. Dutton, 1989).
7. Siegel, Bernie, *The Complete Book of Cancer Prevention* (Emmaus, PA: Rodale Press, 1986).
8. Hardison, James, *Let's Touch: How and Why To Do It* (NJ: Prentice Hall, 1980).

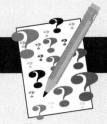

ASSESSMENT 1-1

Health Assessment

Name _____ Date _____ Grade _____

Instructor _____ Course _____ Section _____

Assessing mental health and stress is a complex task and difficult to do in limited space. The following assessment instruments represent a sampling of stress and mental-health indicators.

Self-Esteem Assessment

For each item write *a* in front of each statement that describes you and *b* in front of each statement that does not describe you.

_____ 1. People generally like me.
_____ 2. I am comfortable talking in class.
_____ 3. I like to do new things.
_____ 4. I give in easily.
_____ 5. I'm a failure.
_____ 6. I'm shy.
_____ 7. I have trouble making up my mind.
_____ 8. I'm popular with people at school.
_____ 9. My life is all mixed up.
_____ 10. I often feel upset at my home, room, or apartment.
_____ 11. I often wish I were like someone else.
_____ 12. I often worry.
_____ 13. I can be depended on.
_____ 14. I often express my views.
_____ 15. I think I am doing okay with my life.
_____ 16. I feel good about what I have accomplished recently.

Scoring/Interpretation

Determine how many matches you have with the following key. Total that number.

1. a	5. b	9. b	13. a
2. a	6. b	10. b	14. a
3. a	7. b	11. b	15. a
4. b	8. a	12. b	16. a

From the total number of matched, interpret as follows:

12-16 high self-esteem
8-11 moderately high self-esteem
4-7 moderately low self-esteem
0-3 low self-esteem

Depression Assessment

Indicate which of the following reflect what you do or how you feel. Indicate by marking an *X* in the space provided if it is like you.

_____ 1. I use drugs to relax or have fun.
_____ 2. I need to see a professional about how sad I feel.
_____ 3. I have trouble making it to class.
_____ 4. I think I would be better off dead.
_____ 5. My life seems hopeless.
_____ 6. I have thought through how I would kill myself.
_____ 7. People around me would be better off if I were gone.
_____ 8. I change my moods often.
_____ 9. I'm not interested in much anymore.
_____ 10. I can't seem to concentrate.
_____ 11. I feel unloved and unwanted.
_____ 12. I have a quick temper.
_____ 13. I feel guilty.

_____ 14. I take things too hard.
_____ 15. I have been thinking a lot about death lately.

Scoring/Interpretation

If you have marked number 2, 4, 5, 6, 7, or 11, you should talk with someone right away about your feelings and needs. You may want to talk to your instructor about where to go for help.

If you have marked any of the other responses (number 1, 3, or 8-13) in conjunction with number 15, then you should also talk with someone about how you feel.

If you have marked three or more of the remaining statements (number 1, 3, or 8-13), you also may want to seek help.

Assertiveness Assessment

Indicate what you would do in the following situations by circling *a*, *b*, or *c*.

1. A professor gives you a grade that is lower than you had expected.
   a. Ask the professor to recalculate the grade because you feel he or she is in error.
   b. Complain to the professor but accept the grade.
   c. Say nothing.
2. In a cafeteria line after waiting some time to get something to eat, a group of people recognize the person in front of you and crowd in line.
   a. Ask them to please move to the back of the line and wait like everyone else.
   b. Make a comment but not ask them to move back.
   c. Say nothing.
3. Someone near you is smoking in a nonsmoking section.
   a. Ask him or her to notice the no smoking sign and please put out the cigarette.
   b. Make a comment like, "Can't you read?" but don't ask him or her to put it out.
   c. Say nothing.
4. You have waited for ten minutes at a department secretary's office to get course information, and she is obviously making a personal call.
   a. Get her attention and say, "Can you help me?"
   b. Sigh heavily and give frustrated looks.
   c. Wait patiently.

Scoring/Interpretation

Assign the following number of points to each of your answers. Total your points.

a = 4   b = 2   c = 0

Interpret as follows:

12-16 assertive
6-11 moderately assertive
0-6 unassertive

Stress Index

To identify the types and degrees of stress you are experiencing, complete the following index. Circle the number that corresponds to your reaction to each statement. Total the numbers in each column and add them to arrive at a subtotal for each section

	Always	Often	Sometimes	Rarely	Never
1. I get upset when I have to wait in lines.	5	4	3	2	1
2. I work by the clock to see how much I can get done in a short time.	5	4	3	2	1
3. I get upset if something takes too long.	5	4	3	2	1
4. I make almost every activity I do competitive with myself or others.	5	4	3	2	1
5. I feel guilty when I'm not working on something.	5	4	3	2	1

Section subtotal _____

	Always	Often	Sometimes	Rarely	Never
6. I get upset when I can't do something my way.					
7. I get upset when my accomplishments depend on others' actions.	5	4	3	2	1
8. I get anxious when my plans become disrupted.	5	4	3	2	1
9. All good things are worth waiting for.	1	2	3	4	5
10. When I set a goal I can't reach, I simply alter it.	1	2	3	4	5

Section subtotal _____

	Always	Often	Sometimes	Rarely	Never
11. I have been given too much responsibility.	5	4	3	2	1
12. I get depressed when I think of everything I have to do.	5	4	3	2	1
13. People demand too much of me.	5	4	3	2	1
14. I often find myself without enough time to complete my work.	5	4	3	2	1
15. Sometimes I feel that my head is spinning, or I get confused because so much is happening.	5	4	3	2	1

Section subtotal _____

	Always	Often	Sometimes	Rarely	Never
16. I succeed in most things and try even when the task is difficult.	1	2	3	4	5
17. I am comfortable being with members of the opposite sex.	1	2	3	4	5
18. I am generally comfortable around teachers, bosses, and other superiors.	1	2	3	4	5
19. I prefer that others make decisions for me.	5	4	3	2	1
20. I don't think I have too much going for me.	5	4	3	2	1
21. I'm most relaxed when I'm busy.	5	4	3	2	1
22. I throw away old clothes, toys, and other mementos.	1	2	3	4	5
23. I enjoy being alone.	1	2	3	4	5
24. I feel the need to belong to a social group.	5	4	3	2	1
25. I get homesick easily.	5	4	3	2	1

Section subtotal _____

	Always	Often	Sometimes	Rarely	Never
26. I often feel my stomach knotting, my mouth getting dry, and my heart pounding when I get nervous.	5	4	3	2	1
27. When I get nervous, I can feel my muscles tense, my hands and fingers shake, and my voice become unsteady.	5	4	3	2	1
28. After a crisis I relive the experience over and over in my mind, even though it is resolved.	5	4	3	2	1
29. I know I must resolve a crisis or it will bother me for a long time.	5	4	3	2	1
30. When I'm nervous, I imagine the worst possible outcomes of the original crisis.	5	4	3	2	1

Section subtotal = _____

TOTAL = _____

Scoring/Interpretation

By summing all the subtotals on the index, you estimate your overall susceptibility to stress based on social situation and personality. Interpret your score as follows:

100 or higher – High stress   **50–99** – Moderate stress   **49 or below** – You are doing well for now; keep it up

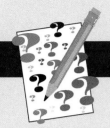

ASSESSMENT 1-2

The Wellness and Longevity Potential Test

Name _____ Date _____ Grade _____

Instructor _____ Course _____ Section _____

CHANGEABLE LIFE-STYLE FACTORS

1. Tobacco

(1 pipe = 2 cigarettes, 1 cigar = 3 cigarettes)

Never smoked	**+20**
Quit smoking	**+10**
Smoke up to one pack per day	**–10**
Smoke one to two packs per day	**–20**
Smoke more than two packs per day	**–30**

Pack-years smoked (number of packs smoked per day, times number of years smoked):

7-15	**–5**
16-25	**–10**
Over 25	**–20**

2. Alcohol

(1 beer or 1 glass of wine = 1.25 oz. alcohol)

1.25 oz. per day or less	**+10**
Between 1.25 and 2.5 oz. per day	**–4**
–1 more for each additional 1.25 oz. per day	**–___**

3. Exercise

(20 min. or more moderate aerobic exercise)

3 or more times per week	**+20**
2 times per week	**+10**
No regular aerobic activity	**–10**
Work requires regular physical exertion or at least 2 miles walking per day	**+3**
+1 more for each additional mile walked per day	**+___**

4. Weight

Maintain ideal weight for height	**+5**
5-10 lbs. over ideal	**–1**
11-20 lbs. over ideal	**–2**
21-30 lbs. over ideal	**–3**
–1 more for each additional 10 lbs.	**–___**
Yo-yo dieting	**–10**

5. Nutrition

Eat a well-balanced diet	**+3**
Do not eat a well-balanced diet	**–3**
Regularly eat meals at consistent times	**+2**
Do not regularly eat meals at consistent times	**–2**
Snack or eat meals late at night	**–2**
Eat a balanced breakfast	**+2**
Eat fish or poultry as primary protein source (totally replacing red meat)	**+5**
Do not eat grains and fish as primary protein source	**–2**
Eat at least 5 servings of green leafy vegetables per week	**+3**
Eat at least 5 servings of fresh fruit or juice	**+3**
Try to avoid fats	**+5**
Do not try to avoid fats	**–5**

For each of the following foods eaten 2 or more times per week:

Beef, veal or pork	**–1**
Bacon or sausage	**–1**
Luncheon meat or hot dogs	**–1**
Fast food	**–1**
Fried food	**–1**
Processed food/TV dinners	**–1**
Eggs	**–1**
Cheese	**–1**
Butter	**–1**
Whole milk or cream	**–1**
Pastries, doughnuts, muffins	**–1**
Candy, chocolate	**–1**
Pretzels, potato chips	**–1**
Ice cream	**–1**

Eat some food every day that is high in fiber (whole-grain bread, fresh fruits and vegetables)	**+3**
Do not eat some food every day that is high in fiber	**–3**
Take a daily multivitamin/mineral supplement	**+10**
Women: Take a calcium supplement	**+5**
Subscribe to health-related periodicals	**+2**

Subtotal:	___	___
	A	**G**

This test was developed for the average healthy person. If you already have a serious health condition, such as heart disease, diabetes, cancer or kidney disease, ask your physician for a health-risk assessment designed especially for you.

FIXED FACTORS

1. Gender

Male	–5
Female	+10

2. Heredity

Any grandparent lived to be over 80	+5
Average age all four grandparents lived to:	
60-70	+5
71-80	+10
Over 80	+20

3. Family history

Either parent had stroke or heart attack before age 50	–10

–5 for each family member (grandparent, parent, sibling) who prior to age 65 has had any of the following:

Hypertension	–___
Cancer	–___
Heart disease	–___
Stroke	–___
Diabetes	–___
Other genetic diseases	–___

Subtotal B: ___ +___

PARTIALLY FIXED FACTORS

1. Family income

0-$5,000	–10
$5,001-$14,000	–5
$14,001-$20,000	+1
+1 for each additional $10,000, up to $200,000	+___

2. Education

Some high school (or less)	–7
High school graduate	+2
College graduate	+5
Postgraduate or professional degree	+7

3. Occupation

Professional	+5
Self-employed	+6
In the health-care field	+3
Over 65 and still working	+5
Clerical or support	–3
Shift work	–5
Unemployed	–7
Possibility for career advancement	+5
Regularly in direct contact with pollutants, toxic waste, chemicals, radiation	–10

4. Where you live

Large urban area	–5
Near an industrial center	–7
Rural or farm area	+5
Area with air-pollution alerts	–5
Area where air pollution has curtailed normal daily activities	–7
High crime area	–3
Little or no crime area	+3
Home has tested positive for radon	–7
Total commuting time to and from work:	
0-1/2 hour	+3
1/2 hour-1 hour	+0
–1 for each 1/2 hour over 1 hour	–___
Within 30 miles of major medical/trauma center	+3
No major medical/trauma center in area	–3

Subtotal C: ___ +___

CHANGEABLE HEALTH STATUS AND MAINTENANCE FACTORS

1. Health status

■ Present overall physical health:

Excellent	+15
Good	+12
Fair	+5
Poor	–10

■ Normal or low blood pressure +5

High blood pressure	–10
Don't know	–5

■ Low cholesterol (under 200) +10

Moderate cholesterol (200-240)	+5
High cholesterol (over 240)	–10
Don't know	–5

■ HDL cholesterol 29 or less –25

30-36	–20
37-40	–5
41-45	+5
Over 45	+10
Don't know	–5

■ Have medical insurance coverage	+10
Able to use physicians of your choice	+5

2. Preventive and therapeutic measures

Physical exams (every 3 to 4 years before age 50, every 1 to 2 years over 50)	+3

Women:

Yearly gynecological exam and Pap smear	+2
Monthly self breast exam	+2
Mammogram (35-50, every 3 years; over 50, every year)	+2

Smoke and use oral contraceptives −5

Men:

Genital self-exam every 3 months +2

Rectal or prostate exam
(yearly after age 30) +2

All:

Current on mumps, measles, rubella,
diphtheria and tetanus immunizations +2

Tested for hidden blood in stool
(over 40, every 2 years; over 50,
every year) +2

If over age 50:

Yearly sigmoidoscopy of the
lower bowel +2

All:

Regularly use sunscreen and avoid
excessive sun +2

Actively involved in a life-extension,
prevention, or comprehensive
wellness program +10

3. Accident control

Always wear seat belt as driver and
passenger +7

Do not always wear seat belt as driver
and passenger −5

Never drink and drive or ride with a driver
who has been drinking +2

−10 for each arrest for drinking while
under the influence of alcohol in the
past 5 years −___

−2 for every speeding ticket or accident in
the past year −___

For each 10,000 miles per year driven
over 10,000 (national average) −1

Primary car weighs more than 3,500 lbs. +10

Subcompact −5

Motorcycle −10

−2 for every fight or attack you were
involved in, or witness to, in the
past year −___

Smoke alarms in home +1

Subtotal D: ___ +___

CHANGEABLE PSYCHOSOCIAL FACTORS

Married or in long-term committed
relationship +5

Satisfying sex life +3

Children under 18 living at home +3

For each 5-year period living alone −1

No close friends −10

+1 for each close friend (up to 5) +___

+2 for each active membership in a
religious community or volunteer
organization (up to 4) +___

Have a pet +2

Regular daily routine +10

No regular daily routine −10

Hours of uninterrupted sleep per night:

Less than 5 hours −5

5-8 hours +5

8-10 hours −7

−1 for each additional hour over 10 −___

Not consistent −7

Regular work routine +5

No regular work routine −5

−2 for every 5 hours worked over
40 in a week −___

Take a yearly vacation from work
(at least 6 days) +5

Regularly use a stress-management
technique (yoga, meditation, music, etc.) +3

Subtotal E: ___+ ___

CHANGEABLE EMOTIONAL STRESS FACTORS

N = Never   R = Rarely   S = Sometimes
A = Always (or as much as possible)

	N	R	S	A
Generally happy	−2	−1	+1	+2
Have and enjoy time with family and friends	−2	−1	+1	+2
Feel in control of personal life and career	−2	−1	+1	+2
	N	R	S	A
Live within financial means	−2	−1	+1	+2
Set goals and look for new challenges	−2	−1	+1	+2
Participate in creative outlet or hobby	−2	−1	+1	+2
Have and enjoy leisure time	−2	−1	+1	+2
Express feelings easily	−2	−1	+1	+2
Laugh easily	−2	−1	+1	+2
Expect good things to happen	−2	−1	+1	+2
	A	S	R	N
Anger easily	−2	−1	+1	+2
Critical of self	−2	−1	+1	+2
Critical of others	−2	−1	+1	+2
Lonely, even with others	−2	−1	+1	+2
Worry about things out of your control	−2	−1	+1	+2
Regret sacrifices made in life	−2	−1	+1	+2

Subtotal F: ___ +___ +___ +___

SCORING

A+B+C+D+E+F = _____ (Subtotal, up to 200*)

Subtotal + G = Total

Divide total by 2. This gives your chance (in %) of living to or beyond average life expectancy of a person your age.

Total: _____ ÷ 2 = _____ %

If you scored 100%, congratulations. But don't rest on your laurels. Keep looking for ways to improve your good health. And if you didn't score as well as you would have liked, it's never too late to begin improving your longevity potential.

*If this number is higher than 200, use 200 as your subtotal. Maintain those healthy habits that allowed you to score much higher than the average person (around 50%), and try to turn any of the negatives in section G (e.g., smoking) into positives. You have the very best chance of living a long and healthy life, because these factors are totally in your control. — *Linda Addlespurger*

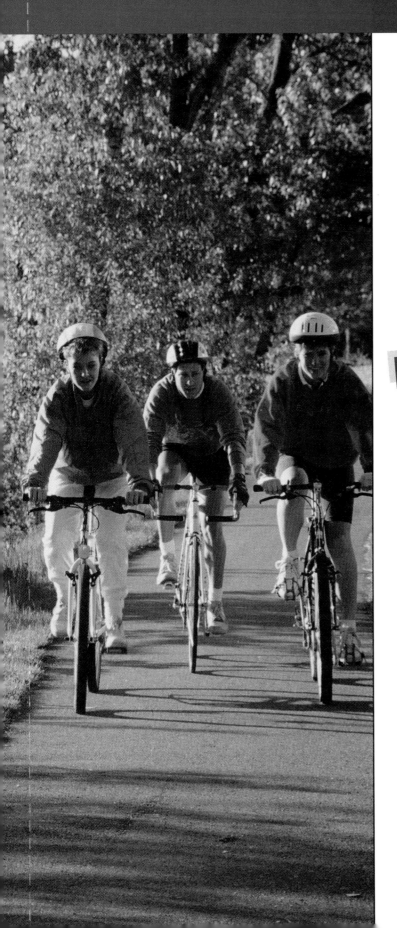

2

The Mind-Body Connection

OBJECTIVES

■ Understand the physiological manifestations of specific emotions.

■ Define psychoneuroimmunology and its emphasis on links between the mind, the brain, and the immune system.

■ Identify the connection between disease and personality.

■ Learn the characteristics of the Type A personality and the coronary-prone personality.

■ Become acquainted with the Type B and Type C personalities.

■ Understand the differences between anger and hostility and the health effects of each.

■ Understand the health effects of depression.

■ Identify the disease-resistant personality.

Agrowing body of evidence indicates that virtually every illness known to modern humanity — from arthritis to migraine headaches, from the common cold to cancer — is influenced for good or bad by our emotions. Illnesses don't just happen. Many are caused by bacteria, viruses, fungi, and other microbes. Certain factors, however, determine whether we will become ill when we are confronted by these microscopic troublemakers.

To a profound extent, emotions impact our susceptibility and our **immunity.** The American Medical Association has estimated that half of all disease is preventable. At least half of the leading causes of death among Americans (see Chapter 1) are related to behavioral factors. The way we react to what comes along in life can determine in great measure how we will react to the disease-causing organisms that we face. The way we emote — the feelings we have and the way we express them — can either boost our immune system or weaken it.

>
> *What's really starting to be understood and documented about the mind-body connection is that there is a physiological effect for all our thoughts and feelings.*
> — Mark Liponis, MD

There's a physiological reason why emotions can influence health. Certain parts of the brain are associated with specific emotions and specific hormone patterns. The release of certain hormones is associated with various emotional responses, and those hormones affect health. The *inability* to express emotions may be an even greater cause of disease. Loyola University Medical Center professor of psychiatry Domeena Renshaw maintains that emotions have to be expressed somewhere, somehow. If they are suppressed repeatedly, and there is conflict about controlling them, they often reveal themselves through physical symptoms. Research bears out her theory: In a series of studies, breast cancer patients who showed little emotion were the ones to die early on. The survivors were the ones who felt and openly expressed emotions.[1]

One of the reasons strong emotions can cause illness — even infectious disease — is that they may weaken the immune system over time. A growing body of evidence suggests that emotions send chemical messages to the brain that alter involuntary physiologic responses. This may affect the way the brain responds to messages from the immune system in the presence of disease. Emotions have been linked to a wide variety of conditions, including allergies, asthma, angina, heart disease, high blood pressure, arthritis, back pain, cancer, dental cavities, diabetes, gastric ulcers, insomnia, irritable bowel syndrome, and a variety of skin problems.

A number of scientists agree that it's not the emotion itself but, rather, the way we react to it that can help determine health. In an address to the Institute for the Advancement of Health, Rachel Naomi Remen advised that perhaps there is a positive way to feel *all* emotions. Perhaps it is not so much the emotions themselves as the way we deal with them that is or is not life affirming.[2]

THE SCIENCE OF PSYCHONEUROIMMUNOLOGY

The scientific investigation of how the brain affects the body's immune cells and how the immune system can be affected by behavior is called **psychoneuroimmunology,** a term coined in 1964 by Dr. Robert Ader, director of the division of behavioral and psychosocial medicine at New York's University of Rochester. In 1975, Ader published his findings,[3] reporting that the immune system could be "trained" to react in certain ways. This breakthrough occurred at a time when scientists thought the brain was the only part of the body that could "learn."[4] The resulting study of psychoneuroimmunology (PNI)

The late Norman Cousins, former editor of the *Saturday Review* and member of the UCLA medical faculty, twice intrigued the medical community and the public alike by overcoming usually fatal conditions — once a massive heart attack, and once an advanced case of ankylosing spondylitis (a degenerative spinal disease). Cousins followed his physicians' regimen each time and also infused himself with vast doses of positive emotions and laughter. According to Cousins himself, he was healed not only by the miracle of modern medicine but also by the healing emotions of love, hope, faith, confidence, and a tremendous will to live.

focuses on the links between the mind, the brain, and the immune system. As a science, it has received the endorsement of the National Institutes of Health.

Although controversy and some skepticism still surround the science itself and the concepts behind it, PNI researchers are proving that the way we think and feel influences our immune system. One report hails PNI as "the hottest and most promising area of medical research today."[5] A glance at a few recent and ongoing research studies shows that mind-body medicine is moving from the fringes to the mainstream:[6]

- The Institute of HeartMath is studying how positive emotions can help protect the heart.

- Duke University studies of people with existing heart disease show that pessimism is deadly but a healthy outlook is healing.

- A Harvard Medical School study of heart attack survivors finds that remaining calm during emotional conflict reduces the risk of heart attack.

- A study at the Montreal Heart Institute found that anxiety and suppressed anger tripled the risk of premature death; depression boosted the risk of premature death eight times.

The theories behind PNI aren't new. Chinese physicians noted more than 4,000 years ago that physical illness often followed episodes of frustration. Some of the world's greatest physicians and philosophers — including Hippocrates, Galen, and Descartes — believed in a fundamental link between the body and the mind. Only in the 1980s, however, did immunologists finally begin to consider seriously the possibility of anatomical links between the brain, the nervous system, and the immune system. Based on overwhelming evidence, they found that the brain literally "talks" to the cells of the immune system. Many researchers believe that the body's various anatomical systems communicate routinely with each other, and that the mind and the body converse continually using a "vocabulary" of chemicals produced in the body.

Today, brain research is booming. Even though psychoneuroimmunology is still considered to be in its infancy, a number of medical schools already have integrated it into their curricula. Almost every important conference on immunology now includes at least one seminar on the relationship between the brain and the immune system, and an increasing number of physicians acknowledge that the way a patient thinks and feels can be a powerful determinant of physical health.

The Brain

The brain is a privileged organ. The heart supplies it with blood; the lungs supply it with oxygen; the intestines supply it with nutrients; and the kidneys remove poisons from its environment. It is the most important part of the nervous system. For the body to survive, the brain must be maintained. All other organs sacrifice to keep the brain alive and functioning when the entire body is under severe stress.

The brain masterminds nerve impulses that are carried throughout the body. It controls voluntary processes, such as the direction, strength, and coordination of muscle movements; the processes involved in smelling, touching, and seeing; and voluntary functions over which you have conscious control. The brain controls many automatic, vital functions in the body, such as breathing, heart rate, digestion, control of the bowels and bladder, blood pressure, and release of hormones. These functions are illustrated in Figure 2.1.

The brain is the cognitive center of the body, the place where ideas are generated, memory is stored, and emotions are experienced. The brain has a powerful influence over the body in its link to the emotions and the immune system. That link is extremely complex. One California neuroscientist summed up the process by comparing the manufacture of emotion to a television set. It has individual tubes, each of them with a specific function, and if you take out even one tube, the television doesn't work.[7]

The emotions the brain produces are a mixture of feelings and physical responses. Every time the brain

> *When [people] become seriously ill, they often "forget" what it is like to be physically healthy, and can no longer access a psychophysiological state of wellbeing.*
> — Psychologist Joan Klagsbrun

Immunity The body function that guards the body from invaders, both internal and external.

Psychoneuroimmunology (PNI) The scientific investigation of how the brain affects the body's immune cells and how the immune system can be affected by behavior.

FIGURE 2.1

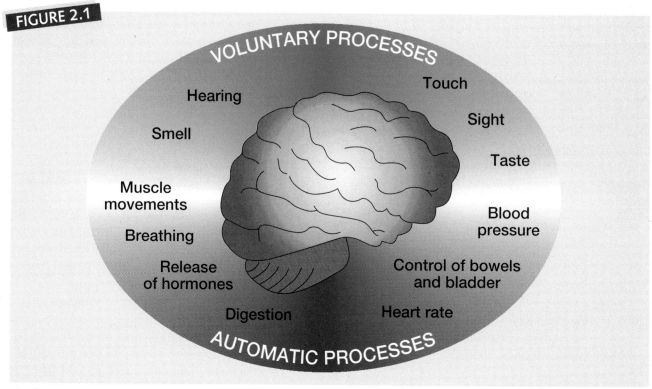

The brain controls voluntary and automatic processes throughout the body.

manufactures an emotion, physical reactions accompany it. The brain's natural chemicals, such as endorphins and peptides, form literal communication links between the brain, its thought processes, and the cells of the body, including those of the immune system.

The Immune System

The immune system patrols and guards the body against attackers, both from without and from within. This system consists of about a trillion cells called **lymphocytes** and about a hundred million trillion molecules called **antibodies**. The brain and the immune system are closely linked in a connection that allows the mind to influence both susceptibility and resistance to disease. A number of immune system cells — including those in the thymus gland, spleen, bone marrow, and lymph nodes — are laced with extensive networks of nervous system cells.

Further, the cells of the immune system seem to be equipped to respond to chemical signals from the central nervous system. For example, the surface of the lymphocytes contains receptors for a variety of central nervous system chemical messengers, such as catecholamines, prostaglandins, serotonin, endorphins, sex hormones, the thyroid hormone, and the growth hormone. National Institute of Mental Health researchers discovered that certain white blood cells are equipped with the molecular equivalent of

Linking Feelings with Immunity

According to Leonard A. Wisneski, M.D., clinical professor of medicine at The George Washington University School of Medicine and Health Sciences, these important links affect our immunity:

- Nerve fibers extend into the organs that produce immune cells, including the thymus, bone marrow, spleen, and lymph nodes.
- Immune system cells have specific receptors for hormones and neuropeptides.
- Immune cells are able to penetrate the blood/brain barrier and take up residence in the brain.
- The cascade of hormones produced by the hypothalamus, pituitary gland, and adrenal glands all impact immune cells.

antennas tuned specifically to receive messages from the brain.

Because of these receptors on the lymphocytes, physical and psychological stress alters the immune system. Chapter 3 addresses the topic of stress. Suffice it to say here that stress causes the body to release several powerful neurohormones that bind with the receptors on the lymphocytes and alter immune function. Corticosteroids, for example, have been found to have such powerful influence in suppressing the immune system that they are used widely as drugs in the treatment of allergic conditions (such as asthma and hayfever) and autoimmune disorders (such as rheumatoid arthritis and rejection of transplanted organs). These corticosteroids and other brain chemicals unleashed by the hypothalamus have profound effects on the immune system.

The link between the mind and the immune system has gained a new dimension with the growing evidence that psychosocial factors directly affect immune function and, thus, potentially influence a wide range of disorders. As one practitioner put it, "The human body can be conceived of as a five-million-year-old healer, with an internal pharmacopoeia of neuropeptides, neuroendocrine secretions, and immunological restoratives that maintain and enhance health."[8]

PERSONALITY AND HEALTH

Howard S. Friedman, psychologist and clinical professor of community medicine at the University of California, wrote, "I have never seen a death certificate marked, 'Death due to unhealthy personality.' But maybe pathologists and coroners should be instructed to take into account the latest scientific findings on the role of personality in health."[9]

Personality is the whole of your personal characteristics, the group of behavioral and emotional tendencies that make you up. It is the way your habits, attitudes, and traits combine to make the person that is uniquely you. Because of your personality, you act in a similar way from one day to the next, and when you are placed in various situations, you still tend to act in a generally consistent way. Your personality, in essence, is the pattern of behavior that distinguishes you from everybody else. Personality depends partly on biology and genetics (the unique set of genes you inherited from your parents) but also is shaped heavily by the family you grow up in, the environment that surrounds you, and the culture and subcultures that influence you.

The theory that personality impacts health is, as world-renowned psychologist Hans Eysenck put it, a theory based on centuries of observations made by keen-eyed physicians.[10] The notion that a certain personality type leads to heart disease dates back

---

Do You Have an Immune-Competent Personality?

Consider the following questions as a probe to help you determine whether you have the elements of an immune-competent personality. Questions to which you answer "no" represent areas that need your attention, except for the last two, which need attention if you answer "yes." The questions are based on Dr. George Solomon's research and ideas about the effects of personality, coping, and emotions on our immune systems.

1. Do I have a sense of meaning in my work, daily activities, family, and relationships?
2. Am I able to express anger appropriately in defense of myself?
3. Am I able to ask friends and family for support when I am feeling lonely or troubled?
4. Am I able to ask friends or family for favors when I need them?
5. Am I able to say no to someone who asks for a favor if I can't or don't feel like doing it?
6. Do I engage in health-related behaviors (exercise, diet, meditation, etc.) based on my own self-defined needs instead of someone else's prescriptions or ideas?
7. Do I have enough play in my life?
8. Do I find myself depressed for long periods, during which time I feel hopeless about ever changing the conditions that cause me to be depressed?
9. Am I dutifully filling a prescribed role in my life (that is, wife, husband, parent, boss, nice guy) to the detriment of my own needs?

Reprinted with permission from Natural Health, 17 Station St., Box 1200, Brookline Village, MA 02147.

Lymphocytes Specialized immune system cells.

Antibodies Substances produced by the white blood cells in response to an invading agent.

Personality The whole of a person's characteristics.

more than 2,000 years to Hippocrates, and the belief that a certain personality is associated with cancer goes back several centuries. What *is* new is the flood of scientific data that now seems to be substantiating those notions.

We should not assume that people always bring illness on themselves. This viewpoint may lead to inhumanity and a lack of compassion for people who need it the most. On the other hand, we can do a great deal to protect and preserve our health. It won't work all of the time for all of the people in all circumstances, but we can help ourselves stay healthy a fair share of the time. And a fair share of those who become ill can help themselves recover.

Research suggests that personality may play a role in health and wellness.

Most people associate certain personalities with certain illnesses: Workaholics have heart attacks. Worriers get ulcers. People who get too uptight have asthma attacks. In reality, can these be so neatly categorized? No. Yet, researchers have made tremendous strides in proving that personality *does* have an impact on health. They have found that the way we look at things, as determined by our personality, may contribute to illness or help keep us well.

Numerous studies show a link between personality and health. In one, University of California psychologists Howard Friedman and Stephanie Booth-Kewley analyzed 101 studies that had been conducted over the four decades from 1945 to 1984. They concluded that strong links exist between personality and health.[11] Based on their analysis of the studies, they are not sure there is a specific "personality" for individual diseases, but they are convinced of a "generic disease-prone personality." Personality may function much like nutrition: Imbalances may predispose a person to all sorts of diseases.

Researchers have been able to ascribe certain personality traits to specific illnesses. Dr. Arnold Levy, vice-president of the American Digestive Disease Society, says that young women who are characteristically self-demanding and high achievers are the most likely candidates for irritable bowel syndrome.[12]

Personality Types

Some researchers believe a specific combination of personality traits may make a person susceptible to a general classification of disease conditions, not just a specific disease. The most prominent in research has been the **coronary-prone personality**, characterized by a hard-driving and competitive person who is also hostile, angry, and suspicious. Sometimes called the **Type A personality**, it is opposite from the Type B personality. The **Type B personality** is characterized as relaxed, easygoing, noncompetitive, and laid-back. Type B people have no hostility. They have high self-esteem, a sense of humor, a healthy sense of independence and humility, and a realistic balance between goals and achievements. People generally are not exclusively one type but instead fluctuate between the traits of both personalities.

Some of the longest-standing research in this area has been conducted by Caroline Bedell Thomas and her co-workers at the Johns Hopkins School of Medicine. Based on her extensive research beginning in 1947, she categorizes people into three broad personality types — Type A, Type B, and Type C — that can determine whether a person is most apt to become ill or stay healthy.[13] The **Type C personality** also has been called the *cancer-prone personality*. These people show little emotion, are ambivalent toward self and others, and have not developed a close attachment with their parents.

Based on their study of 194 different groups of people who had taken the well-respected Minnesota Multiphasic Personality Inventory (MMPI), Georgia State University researchers Douglas Stanwyck and Carol Anson identified five clusters of personalities. The clusters range from people who are most apt to stay well (those who scored closest to "normal" on the MMPI) to those most apt to get sick (those characterized by depression, indecision, hopelessness, chronic fatigue, physical weakness, and severely low self-esteem).[14]

The Coronary-Prone Personality

In a summary of research, a writer editorialized,

> By treating the heart as an unfeeling pump, surgeons have been able to create pacemakers and work their way up to the ultimate in high-tech medicine: the

A Debate

Marcia Angell, pathologist and senior deputy editor of the *New England Journal of Medicine*, editorialized in 1985 that too much credit is given to personality and emotions in relationship to physical health, saying that "our belief in disease as a direct reflection of mental state is largely folklore." The journal was flooded with letters from physicians and former cancer patients, disputing the editorial's claims. The 60,000-member American Psychological Association (APA) issued a statement attacking Angell's piece as "inaccurate and unfortunate." In the succeeding years, the debate has continued to rage.

Source: "Disease as a Reflection of the Psyche," *New England Journal of Medicine*, 312 (1985), 1570–1572.

artificial heart. But even as Barney Clark and other courageous patients were testing the electronic pumps, scientists were using chemistry, psychology, and hard data to discover that trouble in the heart may come in part from sickness of the soul."[15]

The idea of a "sickness of the soul" began three decades ago as a notion called the Type A personality. Today it has evolved into a more broad-based concept that entails not so much a distinct personality as a behavior pattern. For ease of discussion, however, we will refer to that pattern by the name most researchers prefer: the Type A personality.

The Type A personality does not equate with stress, cautions cardiologist Ray Rosenman — who, with colleague Meyer Friedman, originated the theory of Type A personality three decades ago. The Type A behavior pattern, he says, does not imply a stressful situation or distressed response. The Type A person is not necessarily anxious, depressed, worried, fearful, or neurotic. Type A refers to the behaviors of an individual who reacts to the environment with characteristic gestures, facial expressions, fast pace, and the perception of daily events and stresses as challenges, all leading to an aggressive, time-urgent, impatient, and more hostile style of living.[16]

One researcher estimated conservatively that 40% of all Americans are Type A.[17] Though original research focused on men, more recent studies show that women and children also can be Type A's. Although the Type A personality can result from a

number of influences, including genetic and environmental factors; most prominent is a hostile, angry, nonsupportive family environment.

Type A has been dubbed the "hurry sickness." Type A personalities never seem to slow down. They

— try to do two or more things simultaneously;
— have a sense of time-urgency;
— are extremely competitive and tend to keep score of even trivial situations;
— are aggressive;
— make forceful, rapid, or "staccato" gestures;
— are insecure about their status;
— sometimes harbor an unconscious drive to self-destruct.

Friedman says these traits add up to "joyless striving."

According to prominent Duke University researcher Redford B. Williams, the Type A personality is in a chronic state of "vigilant observation."[18] The hormones that are released continually (particularly epinephrine and cortisol) cause an increase in serum cholesterol and fat levels, leaching of blood platelets, overworking of the heart and arteries, excessive insulin secretion, and suppression of the immune system. The result is a higher risk for heart disease.

In one long-term study, researchers found that Type A personalities were more than twice as likely to develop heart disease; among those aged 39 to 49, the risk leaps to six times as high.[19] If Type A personality exists along with two other risk factors for heart disease (such as cigarette smoking or high blood pressure), the risk for developing coronary heart disease is eight times greater.[20]

Coronary-prone personality A classification that describes a hard-driving, competitive person who is also hostile, angry, and suspicious and is at increased risk for heart attack; sometimes referred to as Type A personality.

Type A personality Sometimes referred to as "hurry sickness," a classification that describes a person who is hard-driving and competitive and also is hostile, angry, and suspicious; sometimes referred to as coronary-prone behavior.

Type B personality A classification that describes a person who is easy-going and generally free of hostility, anger, and suspicion.

Type C personality A classification that describes an emotionally nonexpressive person who demonstrates ambivalence and is at increased risk for cancer; sometimes referred to as cancer-prone personality.

Researchers have been able to pinpoint who is most likely to be hostile. Many studies suggest that the risk factors for hostility are the same as those for heart disease: being male, Black, older, of low socioeconomic level, or of low socioeconomic status.[21]

One of the components of hostility — anger — has been shown to be a particular risk factor for heart disease. The Type A personality is increasingly

being defined as a person who can't manage anger. Anger speeds up the heart and sends blood pressure soaring. Suppressed anger is even more dangerous; the more anger is suppressed, the higher is the blood pressure.

The traits that are most detrimental to health, the most predictive of coronary disease, are the harmful Type A traits, a **toxic core** characterized by anger,

Changing a Type A Personality

- Make a contract with yourself to slow down and take it easy. Put it in writing. Post it in a conspicuous spot, then stick to the terms you set up. Be specific. Abstracts ("I'm going to be less uptight") don't work.

- Work on only one or two things at a time. Wait until you change one habit before you tackle the next one.

- Eat more slowly, and eat only when you are relaxed and sitting down.

- If you smoke, quit.

- Cut down on your caffeine intake, as it increases the tendency to become irritated and agitated.

- Take regular breaks throughout the day, even as brief as 5 or 10 minutes, when you totally change what you're doing. Get up, stretch, get a drink of cool water, walk around for a few minutes.

- Work on fighting your impatience. If you're standing in line at the grocery store, study the interesting things people have in their carts instead of getting upset.

- Work on controlling hostility. Keep a written log. When do you flare up? What causes it? How do you feel at the time? What preceded it? Look for patterns, and figure out what sets you off. Then do something about it. Either avoid the situations that cause you hostility or practice reacting to them in different ways.

- Plan some activities just for the fun of it. Load a picnic basket in the car and drive to the country with a friend. After a stressful physics class, stop at a theater and see a good comedy.

- Choose a role model, someone you know and admire who does not have a Type A personality. Observe the person carefully, then try out some techniques the person demonstrates.

- Simplify your life so you can learn to relax a little bit. Figure out which activities or commitments you can eliminate right now, then get rid of them.

- If morning is a problem time for you and you get too hurried, set your alarm clock half an hour earlier.

- Take time out during even the most hectic day to do something truly relaxing. Because you won't be used to it, you may have to work at it at first. Begin by listing things you'd really enjoy that would calm you. Include some things that take only a few minutes: Watch a sunset, lie out on the lawn at night and look at the stars, call an old friend and catch up on news, take a nap, sauté a pan of mushrooms and savor them slowly.

- If you're under a deadline, take short breaks. Stop and talk to someone for 5 minutes, take a short walk, or lie down with a cool cloth over your eyes for 10 minutes.

- Pay attention to what your own body clock is saying. You've probably noticed that every 90 minutes or so, you lose the ability to concentrate, get a little sleepy, and have a tendency to daydream. Instead of fighting the urge, put down your work and let your mind wander for a few minutes. Use the time to imagine and let your creativity run wild.

- Learn to treasure unplanned surprises: a friend dropping by unannounced, a hummingbird outside your window, a child's tightly clutched bouquet of wildflowers.

- Savor your relationships. Think about the people in your life. Relax with them and give yourself to them. Give up trying to control others, and resist the urge to end relationships that don't always go as you'd like them to.

cynicism, suspiciousness, and excessive self-involvement. Probably the most detrimental trait of the toxic core is free-floating **hostility**, a permanent, deep-seated anger that hovers quietly until some trivial incident causes it to erupt.

Apparently a person can have many of the characteristics typically associated with Type A personality — such as competitive drive, an aggressive personality, and impatience — without running the risks of a heart attack *as long as the person is not hostile.* The hostility component is more accurate in predicting coronary heart disease than the more general notion of Type A behavior.

As Williams points out, not all components of the Type A personality are harmful to health. People do not have to slow down, he says, as long as they are not driven by hostility. Those who have many of the Type A traits without the toxic core that harms health are "driven by a positive, enthusiastic approach to the world" — a characteristic that can be protective, not harmful.[22]

The Cancer-Prone Personality

One of the most controversial notions is the **cancer-prone personality**, a set of personality traits that dispose a person to cancer. The exact effect of personality on cancer is difficult to assess. People can be exposed unwittingly to carcinogens that may be a factor. Nonetheless, more and more physicians believe in a link between personality and cancer.

Researchers became keenly interested in the possibility of a cancer-prone personality during the 1950s, when psychologist Eugene Blumberg began noticing a "trademark" personality among cancer patients in a Long Beach, California, veterans' hospital. He wrote: "We were impressed by the polite, apologetic, almost painful acquiescence of the patients with rapidly progressing disease as contrasted with the most expressive and sometimes bizarre personalities of those who responded brilliantly to therapy with remissions and long survival."[23]

To figure out whether there was any connection, Blumberg administered psychological tests to the cancer patients. He found that the patients with the fastest-growing tumors were consistently serious, overly cooperative, overly nice, overanxious, painfully sensitive, passive, and apologetic. Furthermore, they had been that way all their lives. The patients with the slow-growing tumors, on the other hand, had developed a way of coping with life's stresses.

At about the same time, physicians at San Francisco's Malignant Melanoma Clinic were gaining interest in the same thing. They had noticed a disturbing pattern in the personalities of patients with melanoma, a particularly virulent form of skin cancer. These patients were nice — too nice. They were passive about everything, including their cancer.[24]

Mindful that these traits could be a coincidence, the physicians asked University of California School of Medicine psychologist Lydia Temoshok to talk to the patients and determine whether a personality pattern emerged. After talking in detail to 150 of the clinic's melanoma patients, Temoshok declared that a distinct pattern was present. The cancer patients were, indeed, very, very nice. They never seemed to express any negative emotion — not fear, or sadness, or anger, or denial, or any of the other emotions common to a patient struggling with a terminal disease. The researchers characterized these patients as the rock of stability for their families. Even in the face of cancer, they maintained this composure. When one of them was diagnosed, she might say, "I'm doing fine, but I'm really worried about my husband. He takes things so hard."[25]

The results of this and other research led Temoshok to coin the term Type C personality, and other researchers have looked at the same thing. One of the scientists most prominent in the study of a cancer personality is psychologist Lawrence LeShan, who interviewed 250 patients hospitalized for cancer and compared them with interviews of patients hospitalized for other diseases.[26] Based on his study, LeShan identified specific life events that seemed common to the cancer patients:

1. They had a "bleak" childhood characterized by a tense or hostile relationship with one or both parents and feelings of loneliness and isolation.

2. As young adults, they made a strong, central emotional commitment to someone or something, and then something happened to remove

Toxic core   Type A personality traits most detrimental to health; anger, cynicism, suspiciousness, and excessive self-involvement.

Hostility   An ongoing accumulation of anger and irritation; a permanent, deep-seated type of anger that hovers quietly until some trivial incident causes it to erupt.

Cancer-prone personality   A classification that describes an emotionally nonexpressive person who demonstrates ambivalence and is at increased risk for cancer; sometimes called Type C personality.

the source of the emotional investment. Six to 8 months later, these people were diagnosed with cancer.

The hallmark of the cancer personality is the *nonexpression of emotion.* Even when these people are experiencing tremendous despair, they characteristically bottle it up. Although other people often describe cancer patients as kind, sweet, and benign, this sweetness is really a mask they wear to conceal their feelings of anger, hurt, and hostility. Other personality traits that seem common in cancer victims are loneliness (in one study, "loners" developed cancer 16 times more often) and an attitude of helplessness and hopelessness (those who have this attitude usually fare the worst).

In this area, as in almost all other areas of medical research, the findings are inconsistent. Not every study finds a link between cancer and personality, and a few have found no relationship at all between the two. Others find that personality may play a role in either — but not both — developing cancer or its progression once the disease is established. Even with these inconsistencies, however, leading researchers believe that enough evidence of a link between cancer and personality is present for them to take a hard look at the possibility.

As a caveat, Harvard psychologist Joan Borysenko cautions that the very presence of cancer can create physiological changes that could affect personality,[27] such as attacking the central nervous system or skewing the delicate internal balance of hormones. Certain tumors are known to secrete hormones, some of which alter behavior or moods.

Personality and Rheumatoid Arthritis

Of all the forms of arthritis, rheumatoid arthritis clearly is the most crippling and most devastating. It is an **autoimmune disease**, in which the immune system begins attacking the collagen, the connective tissues in the joints.

Could rheumatoid arthritis be associated with a set of characteristic personality traits? One of the most convincing studies began in the 1960s when a team of researchers from the University of Rochester studied eight pairs of female identical twins, only one of whom had rheumatoid arthritis. Using identical twins for the study eliminated the possibility of a genetic factor.[28]

A distinct pattern emerged. The women with arthritis actually seemed to seek out stress. The healthy twins felt free to express criticism and argue. They also described their marriages as happy, whereas the arthritic twins spoke poorly of their husbands and apparently put up with considerable abuse in their marriage. The healthy women described themselves as people who liked people; they said they were easy to get acquainted with, active, constantly busy, productive workers, and enjoyed life in general. The self-image of the arthritic twins was just the opposite. They described themselves as moody and easily upset, nervous, tense, worried, depressed, and high-strung.

Other research has shown similar findings. One researcher who studied more than 5,000 rheumatoid arthritis patients found that, in a high percentage of cases, the patients suffered from worry, work pressures, marital disharmony, and concerns about relatives immediately prior to the onset of disease.[29]

Still other researchers have found that people with rheumatoid arthritis are more likely to have emotional disturbance and that they tend to be perfectionistic, chronically anxious, depressed, hostile, and introverted. The disease seems to become the most severe when the arthritic person exhibits the following traits: self-sacrificing, masochistic, conforming, self-conscious, shy, inhibited, perfectionistic, interested in sports, nervous, tense, worried, moody, depressed, and fearful of marital rejection.[30] Those with the poorest prognosis are more anxious and depressed, more isolated, introverted, alienated, and least able to suppress anger over time.

Personality and Ulcers

People with stomach ulcers secrete too much gastric acid. Among the factors identified as causing an increase in gastric acid are tobacco, alcohol, caffeine, and aspirin, as well as certain emotions such as frustration, hostility, and resentment.

An "ulcer personality" has been identified that either may cause ulcers or may determine how severe existing ulcers become. This personality is characterized by excessive dependence on others, far less social support than normal, excessive worry, annoyance, and fear of common situations or circumstances, as well as frequent crises. Ulcer patients show a fairly consistent quality: Whereas other people are able to "bend" with stress, ulcer patients tend to "break." Ulcer patients may have the same number of stressful situations as people who don't have ulcers, but the ulcer patients *perceive* the situations as being far more negative than do other people.[31]

Specific Personality Traits

Anger

Anger is a temporary emotion that combines physiological and emotional arousal. It can range in severity all the way from intense rage to "cool" anger that doesn't really involve arousal at all (and might be defined more accurately as an "attitude," such as resentment). Although the terms *anger* and *hostility* are often used interchangeably, they are not the same. Unlike anger, hostility is not a temporary emotion but, rather, an attitude expressed in aggressive behavior motivated by animosity and hatefulness.

> 66 *Expressing anger is healthy only if the expression itself is healthy.* 99

To be healthy, people need to express anger. We need to confront the things that are making us angry and to work through the anger. Problems arise when anger is misdirected, when anger is expressed through miscommunication, emotional distancing, escalation of conflicts, endless rehearsal of grievances, assuming a hostile disposition, acquiring angry habits, making a bad situation worse, loss of self-esteem, and loss of the respect of others. Misdirected anger buries the real problem and creates more problems along the way.

> The purpose of anger is to make a grievance known, and if the grievance is not confronted, it will not matter whether the anger is kept in, let out, or wrapped in red ribbons and dropped in the Erie Canal.[32]

Even more serious problems derive from suppressed anger. Bottling up anger can lead to many health consequences — among them heart disease, cancer, rheumatoid arthritis, hives, acne, psoriasis, peptic ulcer, epilepsy, migraine, Raynaud's disease, and high blood pressure. Expressing anger is healthy only if the expression itself is healthy.

> Ventilating is cathartic only when it restores our sense of control, reducing both the rush of adrenaline that accompanies an unfamiliar and threatening situation and the belief that you are helpless and powerless.[33]

Physiological Reactions Accompanying Anger

changes in muscle tension	teeth clenching
scowling	neck or jaw pain
grinding of teeth	ringing in the ears
glaring	lower skin temperature
clenching of fists	excessive sweating
flushing	skin redness
goosebumps	hives
chills/shudders	acne
prickly sensations	itching
numbness	tension headache
choking	migraine headache
twitching	belching
sweating	hiccupping
losing self-control	peptic ulcers
feeling hot or cold	chronic indigestion
fatigue	diarrhea
loss of appetite	constipation
frequent colds	intestinal cramping

And

No matter how many times you work out at the gym or how careful you are to eat correctly, you're putting yourself at risk if you don't manage your anger effectively.[34]

Chronic repression of anger has physical effects similar to those of chronic stress (see Chapter 3). One of the major physiological effects is the release of chemicals and hormones, principally adrenaline and noradrenaline, which impact proper heart functioning and the amount of constriction or dilation of the arteries. This situation is chiefly responsible for the development of arterial diseases.[35]

Mismanaged anger is perhaps the principal factor involved in

A person who is unable to manage anger is at particular risk for disease.

Autoimmune disease   A condition in which the immune system attacks the body.

Anger   A temporary emotion that combines physiological and emotional arousal.

predicting cardiovascular disease.[36] In addition to heart attack, anger carries a much higher risk of high blood pressure.

Studies conducted as long ago as the 1950s show a link between anger and cancer. Researchers who studied the life patterns of approximately 400 cancer patients found that many seemed unable to express anger or hostility in defense of themselves. The same patients could get angry in the defense of others or even in the defense of a cause, but not in defense of themselves.[37]

Researchers have found a big difference in the way cancer victims express anger. Women with normal health tend to get angry and then forget about it. Those with benign disease tend to get angry and stay angry. Those with cancer get angry but either don't express it or apologize for it, even when they are in the right.[38]

The effect of anger on cancer may result from its effect on the immune system. In one study, volunteers were divided into two groups. One of the groups did exercises and watched videos that produced feelings of caring and compassion; the other experienced the emotions of anger and frustration.

When their saliva was tested for signs of immune system activity, the people who had felt compassionate and caring had an *increase* in immunity. Those who had felt angry and frustrated had a drop in immunity that lasted for as long as 5 hours.[39] The angry, frustrated group also reported a variety of symptoms, including headache, indigestion, muscle pain, and fatigue. The only symptom reported by the caring group was relaxation.

Hostility

Hostility comes from the Latin word *hostis*, which means "enemy." Enemies seem to abound. They are everywhere: in the classroom, in the elevator, in checkout lines, on the freeway. Further, because of the health-damaging effects of hostility, hostile people become their own enemies.

Simply stated, hostility is an ongoing accumulation of anger and irritation. It is a permanent kind of anger that shows itself with ever greater frequency in response to increasingly trivial happenings.[40] Carol Tavris says that "into each life come real problems that people should be angry about. But hostile personality types get equally angry about cold soup and racial injustice. They're walking around in a state of wrath."[41] Redford Williams — whose research on hostility is making medical history — claims that hostility is a basic lack of trust in human nature, in human motives; it's a belief that people are more bad than good, and that they will mistreat you.[42] Generally, a hostile person has an orientation toward hurting other people, either physically or verbally.

Victims of free-floating, generalized hostility typically have the following characteristics:

- Even when they're smiling, they look uptight and tense; they appear ready to jump into a fight at a second's notice.

- They have an intense need to win in sports and in games, even when other people are playing just for relaxation or fun.

- They are extremely sensitive to any perceived criticism against them and at the same time are loudly critical of others and of themselves.

- They argue incessantly, even over trivial issues. Every conversation gets turned into an angry debate, and they refuse to lose an argument.

Although almost everyone exhibits one or more of these traits occasionally, victims of free-floating hostility demonstrate them continuously. Life has

Blowing Off Anger the Healthy Way

- Recognize the anger for what it is. Don't be afraid of it or try to suppress it.

- Figure out what made you so angry, then decide whether it's worth being so upset. Chances are that it's really a minor irritation or hassle.

- Stop before you act. Calm down first. Count to 10, take a deep breath, mentally recite the words to a favorite verse, or initiate some other distracting and relaxing activity. *Then* get ready to deal with the anger.

- If you're ticked off at somebody else, use calm tact to say why, without ripping into the other person. Tell him or her how *you're* feeling, and try to negotiate some things.

- Be generous with the other person. Maybe he just failed an exam. Maybe she just heard bad news from home. Maybe he's having a rotten day. Listen carefully to her side of things, and try as much as you can to understand.

- When all else fails, forgive the other person. Everyone makes mistakes. Carrying a grudge will hurt *you* worse than it hurts the other person.

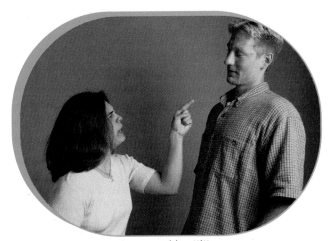

*Anger and hostility
can be a health risk factor.*

become a sordid battle for them, and they charge into the fray armed with anger and irritation.

Through his research, Redford Williams has isolated what he believes are the most harmful traits associated with hostility. These include cynical beliefs that others are inherently bad, selfish, mean, and not to be trusted; frequent angry feelings when these negative expectations are fulfilled; and overtly expressing those angry feelings in aggressive acts directed toward others.[43]

The effects of hostility are especially devastating to the body for two reasons:

1. Hostility causes the constant, unending release of hormones that destroy health in a variety of ways.

2. Hostility weakens the branch of the nervous system designed to calm down the body after an emergency.

In essence, a hostile person goes throughout the entire day in a stressed condition. Many hostile people don't even get relief at night while sleeping. Stress hormones are secreted throughout the night and are eliminated in the urine around the clock.

To begin with, hostility causes the body to release corticotropin-releasing factor, which kicks into gear the whole sequence of stress hormones. The body secretes, among other hormones, epinephrine, norepinephrine, cortisol, prolactin, and testosterone. Blood pressure increases, the heart beats harder and faster, blood volume increases, blood moves from the skin and organs to the brain and muscles, the liver releases stored sugar, and breathing speeds up. Those reactions in themselves wouldn't be so bad if they were to happen only occasionally and if the body

were to have ways to physically overcome the reaction. With hostility, neither is the case.

The autonomic nervous system has two main branches:

1. the "emergency branch," which pumps out hormones and prepares the body to respond in case of emergency; and

12 Steps to a Trusting Heart

The following behavior modification program will help you develop a more trusting, less hostile heart.

1 **Monitor your destructive thoughts**. Keep a log of incidents that trigger your anger so you learn to recognize and arrest them.

2 **Share your hostility problem with someone**. Let your spouse, or a close friend, know that you recognize you have a problem with hostility, and that you hope he or she will support your efforts to change.

3 **Stop those hostile thoughts**. As soon as you realize you are having cynical thoughts, say loudly to yourself, "STOP!" Those thoughts will stop, and the anger may cease also.

4 **Reason with yourself**. Because you are a rational being, try to reason with yourself.

5 **Put yourself in the other person's shoes**. Empathy and anger are incompatible.

6 **Learn to laugh at yourself**. Humor is an excellent strategy to deflect cynical mistrust and defuse your anger.

7 **Learn to relax**. [The relaxation techniques presented in Chapter 3 may be helpful.]

8 **Practice trust**. Trusting others makes them feel good about you and in turn allows you to feel good about them.

9 **Learn to listen**. By not interrupting others, you will learn to value their opinion, and they, in turn, will value you and your ideas.

10 **Learn to be assertive**. A measured response to injustice is more effective than a hostile one.

11 **Pretend today is your last**. Which would you rather be remembered for — angry feelings and aggressive acts, or joyful feelings and acts of kindness?

12 **Practice forgiving**. By letting go of resentment, you may find the weight of anger lifting, helping you to forget the wrong.

Executive Health Report, Vol. 26, No. 5, February, 1990, p. 5. Developed by Dr. Redford B. Williams. Used by permission.

2. the "calming branch" (the parasympathetic branch), which switches off the hormones when the emergency is over. The calming branch soothes the body, preventing it from remaining in an aroused state too long, which can result in disease.

Hostility weakens the parasympathetic branch of the nervous system. The body can't bounce back from the surge of stress hormones, no calming takes place, and the body remains in a state of prolonged arousal.

One of the most pronounced effects of hostility is heart disease. Hostility now is known to be an independent risk factor for coronary heart disease. Heart-harming hostility is characterized by proneness to anger, resentment, and suspicion. It also is marked by explosive and vigorous vocal mannerisms, competitiveness, impatience, and irritability.

A study of more than 400 patients at Duke Medical Center showed that more than 80% of the men who were classified as Type A and who *also* measured high in hostility had seriously diseased coronary arteries; only half of the other men did. The risk for women was even more significant.[44]

Hostility has been shown to cause coronary blockages, coronary heart disease, and coronary death; to contribute significantly to a second heart attack; and to lead to the premature death of people with existing heart disease. In one study spearheaded by Redford Williams and his colleagues, more than 2,280 Duke University Medical Center patients were studied for signs of Type A behavior and for the trait of hostility. The researchers found that they could predict which patients would be diagnosed with coronary heart disease simply by pinpointing which ones were hostile, and that hostility served as well as or better than Type A as a predictor.[45]

In a smaller but still convincing study, more than 250 physicians were tested for personality traits and then followed for 25 years. The death rate from heart disease and from all causes in general was six

Tips For Action

Beating Hostility

Hostility can be overcome. Here are some ways to do it.

- This may sound too simple, but when you realize you're feeling hostile, tell yourself to *stop*. You might have to shout it aloud at first. Later, as you get better at it, you can change to a silent command.

- Talk to yourself about how you're feeling. Evaluate the situation. Figure out why you're so upset. Decide whether your anger and hostility are justified. If they aren't, give them up. If they *are* (and in many cases they are), figure out another way to respond to the situation — one that won't fuel your fire.

- Don't let yourself get trampled. If your anger is justified, deal with it calmly and rationally, but deal with it. Stand up for yourself. Work to correct a wrong. If a classmate fails to recognize your contribution on an important project, for example, don't just blow up and seethe with hostility. Talk to the professor, set the record straight, and spell out what you did toward the project. Then confront your classmate *calmly*, and express your feelings. Ask for a specific commitment (that he or she will explain to the professor what you did to help).

- Learn to trust other people. This might be hard at first, and, strange as it sounds, you might have to practice. Start with a minor situation in which you usually take control. Then let someone else be in charge. As you learn that others can do it, too, you gradually can learn to trust what other people can do.

- Be tolerant and nonjudgmental of others. The source of anger and hostility is often our response to someone else. Put yourself in the other's shoes. Consider the situation from the other's point of view. Even if you still think you're right, you might gain empathy for that person that will allow you to deal with the situation free of hostility.

- Cut down on things that speed up your system, cause your body to churn out hormones, and lead to physical stress. These include sugar, caffeine, and nicotine, and the hidden sources of caffeine such as soft drinks, chocolate, and many over-the-counter and prescription drugs.

- If all else fails, distract yourself. If you're caught in traffic, turn on the radio. Start singing. Visualize the last concert you went to. Do something to take your thoughts off the situation that is getting you riled up.

times greater for the physicians who measured high in hostility.[46]

Researchers with the Recurrent Coronary Prevention Project in San Francisco found that hostility is a significant factor in determining which heart attack patients will have a second heart attack. In addition, people who want to get back at others are much more likely to have another heart attack than hostile people who are less retributional.[47]

Hostility contributes to premature death from many causes, including cancer. In one study, students in law school were given a battery of psychological tests intended to measure hostility. In a 25-year follow-up, only 4% of the non-hostile lawyers had died from any cause, but 20% of the hostile attorneys had died during the 25-year period.[48]

WORRY, ANXIETY, AND FEAR

According to clinical psychologist Thomas Pruzinsky of the University of Virginia, **worry** is a state in which we dwell on something so much it causes us to become apprehensive. It differs from the far stronger emotion of **fear**, which causes physical changes such as a racing pulse and fast breathing. Worry is the thinking part of **anxiety**.[49]

When people convert emotions such as worry, anxiety, or fear into physical complaints, they actually *feel* something. These physical changes can impair the immune system and result in physical illness. Worry has been shown to affect the heart and the circulatory system as a whole, causing arrhythmia (irregular heartbeat), high blood pressure, and various abnormalities involving the arteries. Worry also causes the body to produce the chemical acetylcholine, which causes the airways to contract and can result in asthma.

One specific kind of worry, *uncertainty*, has been shown to create a particularly devastating kind of stress. Uncertainty keeps a person in a constant state of semiarousal, putting an extreme burden on the body's adaptive resources and resistance systems. The result is often disease, particularly gastrointestinal disease.

When worry escalates, the outcome is fear. Fear causes the heart to race, the head to spin, the palms

Worry may trigger or increase the stress response.

to sweat, the knees to buckle, and breathing to become labored. The human body can't withstand it indefinitely. Fear causes the body to secrete epinephrine, or adrenaline, which has a powerful effect on the heart. Both the rate and strength of contractions increase, and blood pressure soars. The body is stimulated in turn to release other hormones. If the fear is intense enough, all systems can be overloaded fatally.

The emotion of fear has a lot to do with context and experience, as illustrated by Dr. Leonard Wineski, clinical professor of medicine at the George Washington University School of Medicine and Health Sciences.

Take, for example, the ocean. If you know how to swim, and have countless fond memories of family vacations at the seashore, a trip to the beach is probably an experience that

---

Tips For Action — Beating Fear

The following is a simple strategy for overcoming fear.

- First, admit you're afraid. List the things that cause you fear. As you mentally re-create those fears, try to imagine them *without* the emotion of fear. It takes some practice, but you can do it.
- Next, confront your fear. Do whatever it is you're so afraid of. *Realize that your fear will intensify as you face it*, but do it anyway. Go back to your mental pictures, and try to imagine that the situation is not fearful.
- Do at least three times whatever it is that you're so afraid of. Chances are, you'll be less afraid each time. Chances are even better that you were afraid because you were *unsure*.
- As you confront your fear, call it something else — excitement or a thrill, for example.

Worry   A state in which we dwell on something so much that we become apprehensive.

Fear   A state of escalated worry and apprehension that causes distinct physical and emotional reactions.

Anxiety   A state of intense worry that is not grounded in reality.

summons up feelings of pleasure and enjoyment, certainly not fear. But if you're not really a strong swimmer and your sole experience of the ocean is the movie *Jaws*, a seaside excursion might be fraught with peril. In both cases, the stimulus is the same: the ocean. But in one case, owing to the memories through which it is filtered, that stimulus produces joy, and in another instance, fear.[50]

The physical effects of fear are the same whether the fear is understandable or illogical.

The messages from the brain to the body are the same whether you're teetering on the edge of a cliff, about to fall, or standing safely at the foot of a mountain, fearful of climbing to the top.[51]

DEPRESSION

Depression is much more than an occasional sad mood. A depressed person does less and less, loses interest in people, abandons hobbies, and gives up in school or work. Depression is evasive. Steven Paul, chief of clinical neuroscience at the National Institute of Mental Health, says depression is "like a fever, in that it's often an unspecific response to an internal or external insult. Like fever, it has a number of origins and treatments."[52]

An estimated 10 to 14 million Americans suffer from depression at any given time. One study says the percentage of teenagers with clinical depression has increased more than fivefold over the past 40 years.[53]

Depression often is caused by the loss of something valued or someone important. It might set in with death of a loved one, divorce, aging, diagnosis of serious illness, automobile accident, termination of employment, retirement, or children leaving home. Under those circumstances, feeling sad or discouraged is normal. In some cases, though, depression is caused by biological factors — a chemical imbalance in the brain, a physical illness, a disturbance in the nervous system or neurotransmitters, or an injury involving brain tissue.

Frederick Goodwin, scientific director of the National Institute of Mental Health, says that depression is the richest, most striking example in psychiatry — and possibly in all of medicine — of the relationship between the mind and the body.[54] Some

A depressed person lacks energy and interest in life.

of its effects on the body are obvious. In many cases, a depressed person does not have the physical energy to get out of bed in the morning.

> **❝** *Women are twice as likely as men to develop depression.*
>
> — *John Rush, M.D.* **❞**

Other characteristics of depression may not be as obvious but can have even more profound effects. During depression the body undergoes hormonal and chemical changes similar to those of stress. According to National Institute of Mental Health psychiatrist Phillip Gold, this is because the mechanisms that normally regulate the stress response fail in depressed people.[55] In addition to having high levels of the hormones usually associated with stress, depressed people have significantly lower levels of three important brain chemicals — norepinephrine, dopamine, and serotonin, the chemicals that make us feel good.

Depression can increase mortality in some obvious ways. Severe depression, for example, can lead to suicide. Depression also can worsen the plight of people who are physically ill already. They tend to become sicker, need more medication, and spend more days in the hospital. Depression can actually shorten life.

Studies of depressed people show that people who are depressed have significantly higher mortality rates than people who are not depressed. One study following 1,593 patients hospitalized for depression at a care facility in Iowa showed that, when compared to a control group, death rates for the depressed patients soared for the first 2 years following hospitalization and remained higher than average throughout the 14 years of the study.[56]

Depression can become a potent risk factor in determining whether a person will die sooner than expected, either of natural causes or of underlying disease. Depression also becomes a significant risk factor for mortality among elderly people, people with health impairments, those who have pre-existing immune system problems, and people who have been exposed to an infectious agent or a carcinogen.

Depression and the Immune System

Depression has a significant impact on the immune system in a variety of ways, one of the most significant being the impact on the natural killer cells — the immune cells that assist the body in its surveillance against tumors and its resistance to viral disease. Natural killer cell activity is lower in people who are depressed, and the more severe the depression, the greater is the impairment in natural killer cell activity.

Other components of the immune system are crippled by depression as well. Depression causes a striking reduction in white blood cells, an upset in the ratio of helper and suppressor cells, a reduction in the number of T cells, and overall suppression of immune function.

Depression and the Heart

The hormones triggered by depression — especially cortisol and norepinephrine — have significant damaging effects on the heart. Norepinephrine speeds up heart rate, encourages blood clotting (which can lead to heart attack), increases the level of harmful cholesterol in the blood, and impairs the heart's ability to adapt when demands increase. The cortisol that is produced during depression leads to a particularly dangerous kind of irregular heartbeat and encourages fat storage around the abdomen (a not-yet-understood risk factor in heart disease).

Perhaps some of the most profound influences of depression are on people who already have coronary artery disease or other cardiac problems. Three studies show how depression affects patients with heart disease:[57]

■ A study of 222 heart attack survivors looked at how many later died of heart problems. According to the *Journal of the American Heart Association*, 17% of the people who had been depressed in the hospital died of cardiac problems

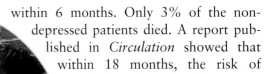

Depression can range from a mild form of the blues to severe clinical depression.

within 6 months. Only 3% of the nondepressed patients died. A report published in *Circulation* showed that within 18 months, the risk of death from heart problems was 14% higher among patients who were depressed.

■ A study published in the *American Journal of Cardiology* followed 1,250 heart attack survivors for 10 years after their initial hospitalization. Slightly more than half of the people who had been depressed in the hospital died of cardiovascular problems during the study. Only 35% of the nondepressed patients died.

■ A 27-year Danish study of more than 700 people found that depressed heart disease patients were 70% more likely to have a heart attack. The study, published in *Circulation*, also found that the depressed patients were 60% more likely to die than those who were not depressed.

A study published in the *British Medical Journal* demonstrated the importance of depression and

Heart Disease and Depression

Each year in the United States, mild or major depression affects 50% of the people who survive a heart attack, and up to 40% of the nation's 350,000 heart-bypass patients.

Until recently, few doctors treated their patients' minds after they treated their hearts. It's now known that patients who *aren't* treated for depression are at far greater risk for a second heart attack and death.

At highest risk for post-cardiac depression are women (who often out-live their husbands and have to face illness alone), people with a history of depression, and people who are socially isolated or recently bereaved.

Memory loss — a common but temporary side effect of heart surgery — also can trigger depression. Symptoms to watch for include lethargy, sleeplessness, and weight changes.

Source: National Institutes of Health, Hope Heart Institute.

attitude on recovery from heart attack. The survivors who believed their heart condition would *not* be incapacitating helped their own predictions come true. They returned to work much more quickly than people who believed their heart attack would cause permanent disability. The patient's belief

---

How to Relieve Depression

If your depression is caused by biological factors, you need medical help. If your depression is mild or your physician rules out biological factors, try these coping measures:

- Start by admitting you are depressed, then try to figure out why. Once you have identified a cause, you might be able to eliminate it.

- As much as you can, stick to your normal routine. Change, even positive change, is a source of stress and can intensify depression.

- If you can, plan some quiet times each day when you can relax, pamper yourself, do something you enjoy, or just get away from stresses you might feel. If you've been feeling depressed for a while, you might start by actually making a list of things you'd like to do: Read the newest book on the best-selling list, take a watercolor class, travel to a new area.

- Find a confidant, someone you can talk to about your feelings. If you're lucky, you'll find someone who will listen without judging or giving advice. Whatever you do, don't choose another depressed person as your confidant. You'll only end up dragging each other down.

- Do something you're good at: Write an essay for a literary magazine, enter a local bicycle race, volunteer to play the piano at a local retirement center, ask your landlord if you can plant flowers around your apartment building. You'll get an immediate boost.

- Get regular exercise. Studies have shown that exercise is one of the best ways to conquer depression. Exercise causes the body to produce endorphins, natural painkillers that result in a "high" for people who exercise longer than 30 minutes. Plan an activity you enjoy, something you can do regardless of the weather, and something for which you have the equipment.

- Whatever you do, don't try to get rid of depression by using alcohol or drugs. They only make things worse.

---

seemed to be the determining factor and was more powerful than the severity of the disease in predicting which ones had the best recovery.[58]

> *Over the past decade, depression has emerged as one of the most common complications of heart disease.*

People who are depressed tend to magnify their medical problems. They are apt to have multiple chronic medical illnesses, as well as more aches and pains. They may not do as well in surgery either. Depressed elderly women who had hip fractures did much more poorly following surgery than did the same type of patients who were not depressed.[59]

HARDINESS

Too often we ask ourselves why someone got ill instead of how someone managed to stay well. Howard Friedman noted that tendency when he wrote, "Each week the prestigious *New England Journal of Medicine* publishes a 'Case Record of the Massachusetts General Hospital,' detailing the pathology of an unusual or informative patient's case. There is no corresponding 'Case History of a Person Who Remained Well Throughout a Long Life.'"[60]

> *Two big causes of stress are unrealistic expectations we place on ourselves and unrealistic expectations we place on others.*

Certain groups of people enjoy remarkably good health and longevity. Among them are "Mormons, nuns, symphony conductors, and women who are listed in *Who's Who*. This suggests that something in the way these people live, possibly even such abstractions as faith, pride of accomplishment, or productivity, plays a role."[61]

One of the most important concepts in staying well is hardiness. Suzanne Ouellette Kobasa, who teaches psychology in the City University of New York's graduate school and is the acknowledged pioneer of the hardiness concept, defines the personality traits of **hardiness** as the "three Cs": commitment, control, and challenge.

Commitment

Commitment entails a commitment to yourself, your work, your family, and the other important values in your life. This is not a fleeting involvement. It is a deep and abiding interest. People who are committed are greatly involved with their work and their families, have a deep sense of meaning, and have a pervasive sense of direction in their lives. In one study involving students at Harvard Medical School, students who were best able to withstand stress were personally committed to a goal of some kind.[62]

Control

As defined by psychologist S. C. Thompson, control is a belief that one has at one's disposal a response that can influence the aversiveness of an event. It is a belief that you can cushion the hurtful impact of a situation by the way you

> *The control that keeps you healthy is a belief that you can control yourself and your reactions to what life hands you.*

look at it and react to it. The kind of control that keeps a person healthy is the opposite of helplessness. It is the firm belief that you can influence how you will react and the willingness to act on that basis. It is the refusal to be victimized.

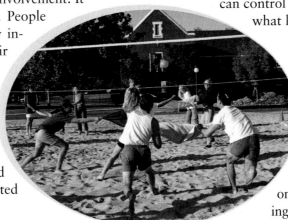

Hardy people are characterized by the "three C's": commitment, control, and challenge.

Control does not mean controlling your environment, your circumstances, or other people. That kind of an attitude leads to illness, not health. The control that keeps you healthy is a belief that you can control yourself and your reactions to what life hands you.

In the Harvard Medical School study, the healthiest students were the ones who approached problem-solving with a sense of control; the least healthy were the ones who were passive.[63] The healthiest and hardiest people are those who focus on what they can control, ignoring the rest. They believe every problem has a solution through skill, planning, and diligent attention to detail.

Challenge

Challenge means the ability to see change as an opportunity for growth and excitement. Excitement is critical, because boredom puts people at a high risk for disease.[64] People who are challenged constructively are healthier. A German philosopher mused that one of the biggest foes of human happiness is boredom.

A person who is not healthy and hardy views change with helplessness and alienation. A healthy, hardy person, in contrast, faces change with confidence, self-determination, eagerness, and excitement. Change becomes an eagerly sought-after challenge, not a threat. Joan C. Post-Gorden, psychologist at

> *One of the biggest foes of human happiness is boredom.*

the University of Southern Colorado, says healthy people don't even *see* the negatives, because they thoroughly *expect* a positive outcome.

In a comprehensive, year-long study of college students, researchers at Boston University School of Medicine concluded that illness is preceded by a

Hardiness   A set of personality traits marked by commitment, control, and challenge.

True Commitment

A perfect example of commitment is Mohandas K. Ghandi, a man who by all standards was a driven workaholic. He went on countless fasts, depriving himself of nourishment, and spent months in prison — one of the most stressful scenarios possible. Yet he was strong and healthy until his assassination at age 77. Many believe this was because of his unwavering commitment to become one of the world's great leaders and to win political freedom for his homeland.

Tips For Action

How to Improve Hardiness

- Figure out what is causing you stress. Make a list. Then divide your list into two columns: things you can control, and things you can't control. Map out a strategy to help you change the things you can control. Then map out a strategy to help you overcome — ignore, move away from — the things you can't control. Don't waste a lot of time and energy pounding against something you can never change.

- Look back on ways you've handled your stress in the last month. Again, it helps to write it down. Summarize the situation, then write down the way you handled it. Now evaluate. Did you respond appropriately? How could you have done it better? Finally, describe how you could have better dealt with the stress. Use that alternative as your blueprint for the future.

- Do a little self-examination a couple of times a day. Are you uptight? Is your stomach tied up in knots? Are you clenching your fists or grinding your teeth? Take a minute and ask yourself why. Then relax. Learn some meditation or relaxation techniques, and use them to take control.

- Learn to change your attitude. When you're confronted with a problem, intentionally tell yourself that it's a challenge instead. Try to see some excitement in it. Try to find some pleasure.

- Do whatever you can to create some situations in your life when you are in control: paint your room, direct a play, take charge of a simple class project. Keeping control over some things in your life reassures you that you can be in control and hones your skills for the times you're not so sure of yourself.

definite series of events.[65] First, a person perceives a distressing life situation. For whatever reason, he or she is not able to resolve the distressing situation effectively. As a result, the person feels helpless and anxious. Those feelings of helplessness weaken the immune system and resistance to disease, and the person becomes more vulnerable to disease-causing agents that are always in the environment.

The traits of a disease-resistant personality interrupt this cycle and, therefore, help prevent illness. Healthy people and ill people look at things in entirely different ways. For example, healthy people tend to maintain reasonable personal control in their lives. If a problem crops up, they look for resources and try out solutions. If one doesn't work, they try another one. People who are frequently ill, on the other hand, leave decisions up to others and try to get other people to solve their problems. Their approach tends to be passive.

According to Yale surgeon Bernie Siegel,

One reason people can undergo tremendous stress and not get sick has a lot to do with meeting your own needs, expressing your own feelings, learning to say "no" without guilt. Now, I'm not suggesting that people blame themselves for an illness. Rather, they should see the illness as a message to redirect their life accordingly — to resolve conflicts with other people, express anger and resentment and other negative emotions they've been bottling up inside, to begin looking out for their own needs. And, in so doing, the immune system becomes stimulated and healing takes place.[66]

NOTES

1. *Love, Medicine, and Miracles,* by Bernie S. Siegel (New York: Harper and Row, 1986).
2. "Feeling Well: A Clinician's Casebook," *Advances,* 6:2, 43–49.
3. "Behaviorally Conditioned Immunosuppression," by R. Ader and N. Cohen, *Psychosomatic Medicine,* 37 (1975).
4. "Research Documents the Mind-Body Connection," *Canyon Ranch Roundup,* 17:3 (June/July 1997), p. 2.
5. "Emotions: How They Affect Your Body," by Gina Maranto, *Discover,* November 1984, p. 35.
6. "Research Documents the Mind-Body Connection," *Canyon Ranch Roundup,* 17:3 (June/July 1997), p. 1.
7. "Accounting for Emotion," by Erica E. Goode, *U.S. News and World Report,* June 27, 1988, p. 53.
8. "Psychoneuroimmunology," by Maureen Groër, *American Journal of Nursing,* August 1991, p. 33.
9. *The Self-Healing Personality* (New York: Henry Holt and Company, 1991), p. 1.
10. "Health's Character," *Psychology Today,* December 1988, p. 28; and "Personality, Stress, and Cancer: Prediction and Prophylaxis," by Hans J. Eysenck, *British Journal of Medical Psychology* (Part 1), 61 (March 1988), pp. 57–75.
11. Grossarth-Maticek's studies are described in "Health's Character," by Eysenck, pp. 30–31.
12. "How Your Personality Affects Your Health," *Good Housekeeping,* June 1983.
13. In "Longevity Predictors: The Personality Link," by Joann Rodgers, *Omni,* February 1989, p. 25.
14. "Is Personality Related to Illness? Cluster Profiles of Aggregated Data," *Advances,* 3:2 (Spring 1986), pp. 4-15.
15. "Heart and Soul," by T. George Harris, *Psychology Today,* p. 50.

16. "Do You Have Type 'A' Behavior?" *Health and Fitness '87* (supplement), pp. S12–S13.
17. *None of These Diseases,* S. I. McMillen, revised edition (Old Tappan, NJ: Fleming H. Revell, 1984).
18. *The Trusting Heart: Great News About Type A Behavior* (New York: Times Books, Division of Random House, 1989), p. 120.
19. "The Cardiac Stress Management Program for Type A Patients," by R. M. Sunin, *Cardiac Rehabilitation,* 5 (1975), pp. 13–15.
20. "Disease as a Reflection of the Psyche," by Marcia Angell, *New England Journal of Medicine,* 312:24 (1985), pp. 1570–1572.
21. "Suppressed Anger and Blood Pressure: The Effects of Race, Sex, Social Class, Obesity, and Age," by Joel E. Dimsdale, Chester Pierce, David Schoenfeld, Anne Brown, Randall Zusman, and Robert Graham, *Psychosomatic Medicine,* 48:6 (July/August 1986), pp. 430–435.
22. *The Trusting Heart.*
23. In *The Healer Within: The New Medicine of Mind and Body* by Steven Locke and Douglas Colligan (New York: E. P. Dutton, 1986), p. 40.
24. *The Healer Within.*
25. *The Healer Within.*
26. *The Healer Within,* p. 134.
27. *The Healer Within.*
28. *The Healer Within;* and *Good Relationships Are Good Medicine* by Barbara Powell (Emmaus, PA: Rodale Press).
29. *Good Relationships Are Good Medicine.*
30. Redford Williams, "The Trusting Heart."

31. "Is There an Ulcer Personality?" *The Wellness Newsletter,* July 1987, p. 2; and *Take Control of Your Life: A Complete Guide to Stress Relief* by Sharon Faelten, David Diamond, and the Editors of Prevention Magazine (Emmaus, PA: Rodale Press, 1988), pp. 206–207.
32. "On the Wisdom of Counting to Ten," by Carol Tavris, in *Review of Personality and Social Psychology,* 5, edited by P. Shaver (Sage, 1984), pp. 170–191.
33. *Anger: The Misunderstood Emotion* by Carol Tavris (New York: Touchstone, 1982).
34. "Mad? How to Work Out Your Anger," by Hendrie Weisinger, *Shape,* January 1988, pp. 86–93.
35. Howard Friedman, in *Good Relationships Are Good Medicine,* by Barbara Powell (Emmaus, PA: Rodale Press, 1987), pp. 158–159.
36. "Mad? How to Work Out Your Anger."
37. *The Complete Guide to Your Health and Your Emotions* by Emrika Padus (Emmaus, PA: Rodale Press, 1986).
38. Padus.
39. "The Physiological and Psychological Effects of Compassion and Anger," by Glen Rein, Mike Atkinson, and Rollin McCraty, *Journal of Advancement in Medicine,* 8:2 (1995), pp. 87–105.
40. *The Healing Brain* by Robert Ornstein and David Sobel (New York: Simon and Schuster, 1987), p. 181.
41. "On the Wisdom of Counting to Ten."
42. *The Complete Guide to Your Emotions and Your Health.*
43. "Is Yours a Hostile Heart?" *Men's Health,* 5:7/8 (August/September 1989), p. 1.
44. Carl E. Thoresen, "The Hostility Habit: A Serious Health Problem?" *Healthline,* April 1984, p. 5.

45. "Hostility, Anger, and Heart Disease," *Drug Therapy,* August 1986, p. 43.
46. "The Hostility Habit."
47. "The Hostility Habit."
48. "The Hostility Habit."
49. "Are You a Chronic Worrier?" by Amy H. Berger, *Complete Woman,* October 1987, p. 58.
50. From a 1997 presentation, "Psychoneuroimmunology: From Biochemistry to Sacred Resonance."
51. *The Complete Guide to Your Emotions and Your Health.*
52. In "The Dark Affliction of Mind and Body," by Winifred Gallagher, *Discover,* May 1986, pp. 66–76.
53. "Depression at an Early Age," by Joseph Alper, *Science,* May 1986, pp. 45–50.
54. "The Dark Affliction."
55. In "The Depression-Stress Link," by Christopher Vaughan, *Science News,* 134 (September 3, 1988), p. 155.
56. "Mortality in Patients with Primary Unipolar Depression, Secondary Unipolar Depression, and Bipolar Affective Disorder: A Comparison with General Population Mortality," by D. W. Black, G. Winokur, and A. Nasrallah, *International Journal of Psychiatric Medicine,* 17 (1987), 351–360.
57. "Heart Disease: The Mind-Body Connection," *Johns Hopkins Medical Letter,* July 1997, p. 4.
58. "Heart Disease: The Mind-Body Connection," *Johns Hopkins Medical Letter,* July 1997, p. 5.
59. "Recovery After Hip Fractures: The Importance of Psychosocial Factors," by Jana M. Mossey, Elizabeth Mutran, Kathryn Knott, and Rebecca Craik, *Advances,* 6:4 (1989), pp. 23–25.
60. *The Self-Healing Personality* (New York: Henry Holt and Company, 1991), p. 99.
61. "Stress: Can We Cope?" by Claudia Wallis, *Time,* June 6, 1983, pp. 48–54.
62. "The Stress-Resistant Person," by Raymond B. Flannery, *Harvard Medical School Health Letter,* February 1989, pp. 1–3.
63. "The Stress-Resistant Person."
64. *The Self-Healing Personality,* p. 111.
65. "Relationship of Life Change, Maladaptive Aggression, and Upper Respiratory Infection in Male College Students," by M. A. Jacobs, A. Spilken, and M. Norman, *Psychosomatic Medicine,* 31:1 (1969), pp. 31–44.
66. "Mind Over Cancer," *Prevention,* March 1988, pp. 61–62.

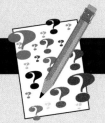

ASSESSMENT 2-1

Hostility Could Harm Your Heart

Name _____ Date _____ Grade _____

Instructor _____ Course _____ Section _____

Experts now conclude that feelings of hostility increase your risk of heart disease. Dr. Redford Williams, Duke University Medical Center, has designed a questionnaire to help you determine whether you have a hostile personality. Circle the answer that most closely fits how you would respond to the given situation:

1. **A teen-ager drives by my yard blasting the car stereo:**

   A. I begin to understand why teen-agers can't hear.
   B. I can feel my blood pressure starting to rise.

2. **A boyfriend/girlfriend calls at the last minute "too tired to go out tonight." I'm stuck with two $15 tickets:**

   A. I find someone else to go with.
   B. I tell my friend how inconsiderate he/she is.

3. **Waiting in the express checkout line at the supermarket where a sign says "No More Than 10 Items Please":**

   A. I pick up a magazine and pass the time.
   B. I glance to see if anyone has more than 10 items.

4. **Most homeless people in large cities:**

   A. Are down and out because they lack ambition.
   B. Are victims of illness or some other misfortune.

5. **At times when I've been very angry with someone:**

   A. I was able to stop short of hitting him/her.
   B. I have, on occasion, hit or shoved him/her.

6. **When I am stuck in a traffic jam:**

   A. I am usually not particularly upset.
   B. I quickly start to feel irritated and annoyed.

7. **When there's a really important job to be done:**

   A. I prefer to do it myself.
   B. I am apt to call on my friends to help.

8. **The cars ahead of me start to slow and stop as they approach a curve:**

   A. I assume there is a construction site ahead.
   B. I assume someone ahead had a fender-bender.

9. **An elevator stops too long above where I'm waiting:**

   A. I soon start to feel irritated and annoyed.
   B. I start planning the rest of my day.

10. **When a friend or co-worker disagrees with me:**

    A. I try to explain my position more clearly.
    B. I am apt to get into an argument with him or her.

11. **At times when I was really angry in the past:**

    A. I have never thrown things or slammed a door.
    B. I've sometimes thrown things or slammed a door.

12. **Someone bumps into me in a store:**

    A. I pass it off as an accident.
    B. I feel irritated at their clumsiness.

13. **When my spouse (significant other) is fixing a meal:**

    A. I keep an eye out to make sure nothing burns.
    B. I talk about my day or read the paper.

14. **Someone is hogging the conversation at a party:**

    A. I look for an opportunity to put him/her down.
    B. I soon move to another group.

15. **In most arguments:**

    A. I am the angrier one.
    B. The other person is angrier than I am.

Score one point for each of these answers: 1. B, 2. B, 3. B, 4. A, 5. B, 6. B, 7. A, 8. B, 9. A, 10. B, 11. B, 12. B, 13. A, 14. A, 15. A. If you scored 4 or more points you may be hostile. Questions 1, 6, 9, 12 and 15 reflect anger. Questions 2, 5, 10, 11, 14, reflect aggression. Questions 3, 4, 7, 8, 13 reflect cynicism. If you scored 2 points in any category, you should work on that area of your personality.

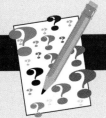

ASSESSMENT 2-2

Temper Test

Name _____ Date _____ Grade _____

Instructor _____ Course _____ Section _____

DIRECTIONS: A number of statements that people have used to describe themselves are given below. Read each statement and then circle the appropriate number to indicate how you generally feel. There are no right or wrong answers. Do not spend too much time on any one statement, but give the answer that seems to describe how you generally feel.

	Almost Never	Some-times	Often	Almost Always
1. I am quick-tempered.	1	2	3	4
2. I feel annoyed when I am not given recognition for doing good work.	1	2	3	4
3. I have a fiery temper.	1	2	3	4
4. I feel infuriated when I do a good job and get a poor evaluation.	1	2	3	4
5. I am a hotheaded person.	1	2	3	4
6. It makes me furious when I am criticized in front of others.	1	2	3	4
7. I get angry when I'm slowed down by others' mistakes.	1	2	3	4
8. I fly off the handle.	1	2	3	4
9. When I get mad, I say nasty things.	1	2	3	4
10. When I get frustrated, I feel like hitting someone.	1	2	3	4

Total Points: _____

Scoring

Add the points from each item (1-4) together to get your total score, somewhere between 10 and 40. A man who scores 17 or a woman who scores 18 is just about average. If you score below 13, you're well down into the safe zone. A score above 20 means you may be a hothead — scoring higher than three-quarters of those tested.

American Health © 1985 by Perry Landon, Ph.D., and Charles D. Spielberger. *American Health*, "Back to Depression."

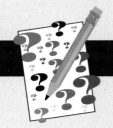

Are You Depressed?

Name _____Date _____Grade _____

Instructor _____Course _____Section _____

Use the chart to check off any symptoms you have had for 2 weeks or more.

- ☐ Loss of interest in things you used to enjoy.
- ☐ Feeling sad, blue, or down in the dumps.
- ☐ Feeling slowed down or restless and unable to sit still.
- ☐ Feeling worthless or guilty.
- ☐ Changes in appetite or weight loss or gain.
- ☐ Thoughts of death or suicide; suicide attempts.
- ☐ Trouble concentrating, thinking, remembering or making decisions.
- ☐ Trouble sleeping or sleeping too much.
- ☐ Loss of energy or feeling tired all of the time.

Other symptoms include:

- ☐ Headaches.
- ☐ Digestive problems.
- ☐ Other aches and pains.
- ☐ Sexual problems.
- ☐ Feeling pessimistic or hopeless.
- ☐ Being anxious or worried.

If you have had five or more of these symptoms for at least 2 weeks, you may have major depressive disorder. See your health care provider for diagnosis.

Even if you have only a few depressive symptoms, you should also tell your health care provider. Sometimes a few symptoms can go on to become major depressive disorder. Some forms of depression are mild, but if symptoms are persistent or chronic, you may need treatment.

Source: National Depressive and Manic-Depressive Association, 730 North Franklin St., Suite 501, Chicago, IL 60610, 312/642-0049 or 800/642-7243 (800-82-NDMDA) has adapted this checklist from the U.S. Department of Health and Human Services booklet, *Depression is a Treatable Illness, A Patient's Guide.*

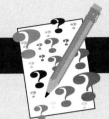

ASSESSMENT 2-4

How Hardy Are You?

Name _____Date _____Grade _____

Instructor _____Course _____Section _____

Evaluating hardiness requires more than this quick test, but this simple exercise should give you some idea of how hardy you are.

DIRECTIONS: Write down how much you agree or disagree with the following statements, using this scale:

0 = Strongly Disagree   2 = Mildly Disagree   3 = Mildly Agree   4 = Strongly Agree

- [ ] **A.** Trying my best at work [or school] makes a difference.
- [ ] **B.** Trusting to fate is sometimes all I can do in a relationship.
- [ ] **C.** I often wake up eager to start on the day's projects.
- [ ] **D.** Thinking of myself as a free person leads to great frustration and difficulty.
- [ ] **E.** I would be willing to sacrifice financial security in my work if something really challenging comes along.
- [ ] **F.** It bothers me when I have to deviate from the routine or schedule I've set for myself.
- [ ] **G.** An average citizen can have an impact on politics.
- [ ] **H.** Without the right breaks, it is hard to be successful in my field.
- [ ] **I.** I know why I'm doing what I'm doing at work [school].
- [ ] **J.** Getting close to people puts me at risk of being obligated to them.
- [ ] **K.** Encountering new situations is an important priority in my life.
- [ ] **L.** I really don't mind when I have nothing to do.

These questions measure control, commitment, and challenge. For half the questions, a high score (such as 4, "strongly agree") indicates hardiness; for the other half, a low score (disagreement) does.

To get your scores on control, commitment, and challenge, first write the number of your answer — 0, 1, 2, or 3 — above the letter of each question on the score sheet below. Then add and subtract as shown. (To get your score on "control," for example, add your answers to questions A and G; add your answers to B and H; and then subtract the second number from the first.)

Add your scores on commitment, control, and challenge together to get a score for total hardiness.

Total Scores: **10-18:** a hardy person; **0-9:** moderate hardiness; **Below 0:** low hardiness

Control Scores.................... □ + □ = □ *MINUS* □ + □ = □ *EQUALS* □
                                        A   G   B   H   +

Commitment Scores □ + □ = □ *MINUS* □ + □ = □ *EQUALS* □
                        C   I   D   J   +

Challenge Scores □ + □ = □ *MINUS* □ + □ = □ *EQUALS* □
                      E   K   F   L

                                                                    EQUALS

TOTAL HARDINESS SCORE: □

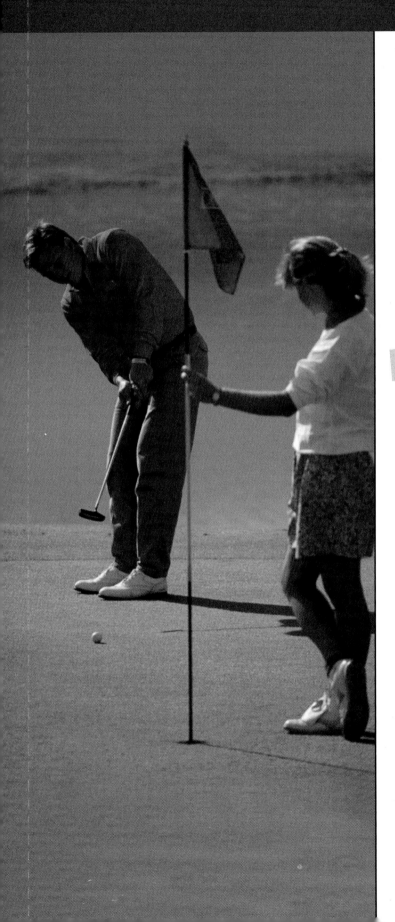

3

Stress and Health

- Learn the definition and characteristics of stress.
- Identify common sources of stress.
- Understand the relationship between stress and illness.
- Recognize the signs and symptoms of stress.
- Identify the body systems affected by stress.
- Recognize the importance of diet, exercise, and sleep in relation to stress.
- Learn some effective time management strategies.
- Define burnout and learn how to help prevent it.
- Become acquainted with stress reduction techniques including meditation, progressive relaxation, autogenics, biofeedback, and the philosophy of yoga.

Our understanding of stress has come a long way in the last four or five decades. Today, we understand that **stress** is the combination of a **stressor** (anything that makes us adapt) and our response to the stressor. Stress can arise from situations that are happy (such as the birth of a baby) or sad (such as the death of a loved one). Stress isn't the same as frustration, anxiety, or conflict, though it can lead to all of those emotions.

Stress is no respecter of persons or situations. It can happen at home, in the classroom, on the job, in families, between friends, and even between us and our surroundings, in the form of extreme heat or cold, noise, pollution, or overcrowding. Stress means different things to different people, and what causes stress for one person may not stress someone else. Stressors can be physical (such as fatigue or a bacterial infection), emotional (such as pent-up anger or hostility), social (such as rejection or embarrassment), intellectual (such as confusion), and spiritual (such as guilt).

Our reaction to stress isn't just mental, either. Stress is an "automatic biological response to demands made upon an individual."[1] Scientifically speaking, stress is "any challenge to homeostasis,"[2] or the body's internal sense of balance. Stress is a biological and biochemical process that begins in the brain and spreads through the autonomic nervous system, causing the release of hormones and influencing the immune system.

The 1949 Conference on Life and Stress and Heart Disease provided the first formal recognition that stress could precipitate chronic disease. Practitioners who gathered at that conference also were among the first to formally define stress by stating that it is "a force which induces distress or strain upon both the emotional and physical makeup."[3]

Stress can be altered by perceptions and outlook. For example, when confronted by the stress of an upcoming final exam in a particularly difficult class, you may react either by becoming extremely anxious and unable to study (distressed) or by taking on the challenge of studying twice as long and enlisting the

Signs and Symptoms of Stress

Cardiovascular
- Pounding of the heart
- Racing of the heart
- High blood pressure
- Irregular heartbeat
- Chest pain
- Cold, sweaty hands

Mental
- Inability to concentrate
- Lack of creativity
- Loss of memory
- Low self-esteem

Respiratory
- Shortness of breath
- Rapid breathing
- Asthma attacks

Sleep Disorders
- Insomnia
- Fatigue
- Nightmares

Emotional
- Nervousness
- Unexplained fearfulness
- Anxiety
- Emotional instability
- Impulsive behavior
- Depression
- Irritability
- Forgetfulness
- Severe mood swings
- Tearfulness
- Urge to hide
- Difficulty in completing tasks
- Changes in eating/smoking/drinking
- Increased dependence on drugs

Skin
- Acne
- Excessive dryness of skin
- Rashes
- Excessive perspiration

Gastrointestinal
- Dryness of the mouth and throat
- Difficulty swallowing
- Grinding of the teeth
- Indigestion
- Nausea or queasiness
- Vomiting
- Loss of appetite
- Excessive appetite
- Diarrhea or constipation
- Abdominal pain
- Increased cravings
- Frequent urination

Musculoskeletal
- Twitching or shakiness
- Neck or back pain
- Headache, including migraine
- Stiffness of the muscles

You want a <u>little</u> stress . . . not too much

Distress	Stress	Distress

1 — 2 — 3 — 4 — 5 — 6 — 7 — 8 — 9

With too little stress we are:	With the right amount of stress we are:	With too much stress we are:
bored	**productive**	burned out
tired	**energetic**	exhausted
unhappy	**happy**	overweight
restless	**creative**	irritable
prone to illness	**healthy**	prone to illness

Reprinted with permission, Hope Publications, Kalamazoo, Michigan (616) 343-0770.

help of study companions (eustressed). These differences in outlook are illustrated beautifully by the Chinese symbol for stress which combines two characters, one representing "danger" and one representing "opportunity."

Austrian-born Dr. Hans Selye, an endocrinologist considered the father of stress research,[4] was the first to explore the notion of "desirable" stress, the stress that keeps life interesting and provides opportunity for growth (such as marriage, birth, new job, new friends, an exciting vacation). This kind of stress, which he termed **eustress**, also is the physiological stress that is essential for maintaining life (such as the churning of the digestive tract and the rhythmic contractions of the heart). **Distress**, on the other hand, is negative. It is an overload of stress — too much stress in a brief time, chronic stress over a long time, or a combination of stressors (even good ones) that eventually throw a person out of balance. How much stress is too much varies from one person to another, and even from one time to another for the same person, depending on how the person perceives the stress.

Stress does not depend as much on what happens *to* us as how we *react* to the things that happen to us. The way you perceive stress has a lot to do with how it affects you. The president of the American Institute of Stress, Paul Rosch, likens stress to a ride on a roller coaster:[5] "There are those at the front of the car, hands over head, clapping, who can't wait to get

on again," he points out, "and those at the back cringing, wondering how they got into this and how soon it's going to be over." Or, to put it another way, one roller coaster passenger "has his back stiffened, his knuckles are white, his eyes shut, jaws clenched, just waiting for it to be over. The wide-eyed thrill-seeker relishes every plunge, can't wait to do it again."

Some stress promotes curiosity and exploration. Stress can be challenging, stimulating, and rewarding. Competitive sport is an excellent example. To gear up for a football game, worry about winning, and then pound across the field for 3 hours is extremely stressful, both physically and emotionally. Many believe the rewards and the thrill are well worth the stress — and millions of fans couldn't agree more.

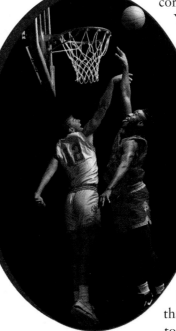

No one is free of stress. According to figures from New York's American Institute of Stress, published in *Time* magazine,[6] 90% of all American adults have high stress levels once or twice a week and a fourth of all American adults are subject to crushing levels of stress nearly every day. The only way to be completely free of stress is to be dead.

Stress is costly. Researchers at the American Institute of Stress estimate that 75% to 90% of all visits to health-care providers result from stress-related disorders. Just among the nation's executives, an estimated $10 to $20 billion are lost each year through absence, hospitalization, and early

Some stress is positive.

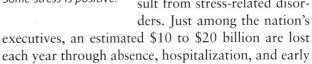

Stress An automatic biological response to demands made on an individual; the result of any event or condition that causes us to adapt.

Stressor Any situation or event that makes us adapt or adjust.

Eustress Positive, desirable stress.

Distress Negative stress, usually consisting of too much stress in a short time, chronic stress over a prolonged time, or a combination of stressors.

death, much of this as a result of stress.[7] The National Council on Compensation Insurance states that stress-related claims account for almost one-fifth of all occupational disease.[8] Fully one-fourth of all workers compensation claims are for stress-related injuries, and researchers estimate that 60% to 80% of all industrial accidents are related to stress.[9] Stress-related symptoms and illnesses are costing industry a conservatively estimated $150 billion a year in absenteeism, company medical expenses, and lost productivity.

SOURCES OF STRESS

Stress has many sources. Some originate within; others are environmental. Some are manmade, others natural. Some of the most difficult stress is self-imposed. For example, low self-esteem, hostility, helpless anger, perfectionism, anxiety, impatience, and suspicion all create stress and at the same time impair the ability to cope with stress.

Organisms that challenge the body are other sources of stress. Infection by bacteria, viruses, parasites, fungi, and protozoa can cause stress. So can fever, pain, trauma, injury, and deformity. Drugs — including tobacco, alcohol, and caffeine — pack a double punch. They are sources of stress and they interfere with the body's ability to recover from stress.

The environment itself can be the source of stress. Temperature, humidity, and weather extremes cause stress. So do pollutants in the air and water. Noise itself can be a significant source of environmental stress; the stress response is triggered by noise over 85 decibels (a loud television, garbage disposal, motorcycle, lawn mower, vacuum cleaner). Something as simple as being in a room that is too hot or too cold can cause stress. More dramatic examples of environmental stress include catastrophic events like severe storms, long-term drought, famine, fires, earthquakes, tornadoes, hurricanes, floods, or war.

One of the most common sources of stress is **conflict**, which occurs when we are faced with incompatible needs, demands, motives, opportunities, or goals.[10] Some of the most pervasive stressors are what researchers call **hassles** — the seemingly minor, irritating annoyances that happen every day, such as losing the car keys, getting stuck behind a dim-witted shopper in a grocery-store line, waking up to a miserable snowstorm, being kept waiting for an appointment, having unexpected company drop in, or getting stuck in a traffic jam. In his now-famous book *Future Shock*, Alvin Toffler listed as among the top 10 reported hassles rising consumer prices, yard work, losing things, and having too many things to do. These seemingly trivial problems actually may be more damaging to health and wellness than major stressors, partly because they eat away at us constantly, piling up until no end is in sight.

Other sources of stress include

— economic factors such as inflation, unemployment, poverty, and debt

— harm or threat of harm

— the pressure of having to intensify or shift behavior to meet increased demands

— the need to perform in the classroom, on the job, or in an interpersonal relationship

— conflict between goals and behavior

— frustration at not attaining goals.

Some factors make any stressor less likely to result in stress. Being able to control the stressor even a little and believing the outcome will be positive reduces the impact of a stressor. Being able to predict an event with certainty also makes it less stressful. In contrast, knowing a stressor could occur but not knowing when causes a state of constant alert much like chronic stress.

Some have extreme reactions; their blood pressure is normal at rest but shoots up to dangerously high levels during stress.[11] As many as one in five people is what cardiologist Robert Eliot calls a *hot reactor*. "They burn a dollar's worth of energy for a dime's worth of trouble," says Eliot, describing them as "pressure cookers without safety valves, literally stewing in their own juices." Worst, says Eliot, they "do not suspect that their bodies are paying a high price for overreacting to stress."[12]

What Makes People the Most Nervous?

1. Making a speech
2. Getting married
3. Getting divorced
4. Going to the dentist

Source: Are You Normal? by Bernice Kanner.

During the last decade, factors on the job have been recognized as significant sources of stress. Stressors in the workplace can include

- — physical demands, such as uncomfortable seating, extremes in temperature, inadequate lighting
- — role demands, such as conflict or ambiguity in an employee's role
- — interpersonal demands, such as an abrasive boss, passive leaders, or abusive co-workers
- — task demands, such as repetition, too few or too many changes, job insecurity, or overload.[13]

> ❝ *Regardless of its source, the stressor itself is not what causes stress. Your reaction to the stressor determines whether stress exists and how intense it is.* ❞

Work overload is such a problem in Japan that the Japanese Labor Ministry recognizes it as a cause of death and allows survivors to sue employers for damages.[14]

STRESS AND DISEASE

Stress has been shown to affect almost all body systems. It can result in cardiovascular disease, neuromuscular disorders, respiratory and allergic ailments, immunologic disorders, gastrointestinal disturbances, skin conditions, dental problems, and a host of other disorders. Because most diseases are caused by a combination of factors instead of only one, stress probably does not in itself *cause* illness. Various studies, however, point to a strong link between stress and the onset of disease.

Stress has been shown to be a major factor in a number of disease conditions, including the following:

- **Cardiovascular diseases.** While recognizing that other factors — such as cigarette smoking and blood cholesterol levels — are certainly important contributors, stress seems to play a significant role in heart disease because of the specific effects it has on the cardiovascular system (discussed later in this chapter). In fact, stress causes an increase in blood cholesterol levels. Friedman and Rosenman, who pioneered the concept of the

Type A coronary-prone personality (discussed in Chapter 2), believe that stress is the major cause of heart disease.[15] High blood pressure, which afflicts approximately a third of all American adults, also has been linked to stress, as has stroke, which often is caused directly by high blood pressure. Other researchers believe that coronary artery disease and congestive heart failure both are partly caused by or aggravated by stress.

- **Gastrointestinal diseases.** Though many ulcers (especially in the stomach) are caused by *Helicobacter pylori* bacteria, some ulcers in the stomach and the small intestine can be caused by stress. Stress also has been shown to have tremendous effect on the colon, producing diarrhea, constipation, and ulcerative colitis (deterioration of the membranes lining the colon). Stress even can affect our eating patterns, causing severe loss of appetite in some people and eating disorders or obesity in others.

- **Musculoskeletal disorders.** One of the most common results of stress is the tension headache, caused by chronic tension in the muscles of the scalp and neck. Another type of headache — the migraine, in which the blood vessels of the scalp become dilated and exert extreme pressure — also is caused by stress. Interestingly, migraines often occur once the stress is relieved instead of during the stressful incident or period.

  Other musculoskeletal disorders associated with stress include rheumatoid arthritis, chronic muscle tension, low back pain, and tempromandibular joint (TMJ) syndrome, which interferes with smooth operation of the joint that connects the upper and lower jaw.

- **Respiratory distress.** Stress may induce shortness of breath and rapid breathing. Also, asthma and hayfever, both allergic reactions, are linked strongly to stress. Significant emotional stress can precipitate an attack even in the absence of the allergen.

Stress also is a factor in a number of skin conditions (such as hives, eczema, and psoriasis), metabolic disorders (such as thyroid malfunctions and diabetes),

Conflict   The stress that results from two opposing and incompatible goals, demands, or needs.

Hassles   Seemingly minor, irritating, everyday annoyances that increase the level of stress.

menstrual irregularity, and gout. Some researchers are finding convincing evidence that stress plays a significant role in the development of some cancers.

HOW THE BODY REACTS TO STRESS

In an ideal state, the body enjoys **homeostasis**, a state of balance in which all systems are functioning smoothly. When the body becomes stressed and homeostasis is disrupted, the body goes through an adaptive response in an effort to reestablish homeostasis. Regardless of the source of stress, the body undergoes the same "**fight-or-flight**" **response** primitive people used when facing threats in their environment, identified first in the early 20th century by physiologist Walter Cannon. It consists of a series of physiological changes that occurred in rapid-fire succession when a cave-dweller was confronted by a saber-toothed tiger. The body systems sped up, and hormones started surging through the bloodstream. The senses sharpened, and levels of energy were high. Everything combined to enable cave-dwellers to face their enemies or run for their life.

While society has become more civilized, our bodies have not. A student with communication anxiety giving an oral presentation in front of a class has the same physiological response as the cave-dweller who faced the saber-toothed tiger. Unfortunately, that kind of response usually isn't appropriate in today's world. As Boston University psychiatrist Peter Knapp pointed out, "When you get a Wall Street broker using the responses a cave man used to fight the elements, you've got a problem."[16]

With stress as an enemy, the body has powerful and intricate weapons to summon in response. "The

How Stress Hormones Affect the Body

- Speed up the heart
- Increase the amount of blood the heart pumps
- Increase fats in the blood
- Increase blood cholesterol levels
- Reduce the white blood cell count
- Decrease production of lymphocytes
- Deplete protein stored in the body
- Raise body core temperature

problem is that many of our battleship's weapons are beautifully designed," one writer commented, "but for the wrong war. The enemy has greatly changed. Our stress responses were programmed for life in the primitive state, thousands of years before we became 'civilized.' No longer are our stresses a simple matter of life and death threats; they now involve much more intricate and complex challenges."[17]

The stress response has been termed the **general adaptation syndrome**. This reaction occurs in three general stages: alarm, resistance, and exhaustion (see Figure 3.1).

Alarm

The first stage of the stress response, **alarm**, begins the second the brain perceives any kind of stress or threat. Following an initial emotional reaction, physical reactions follow rapidly in the classic fight-or-flight syndrome. The brain triggers an immediate response from the autonomic nervous system (the

FIGURE 3.1

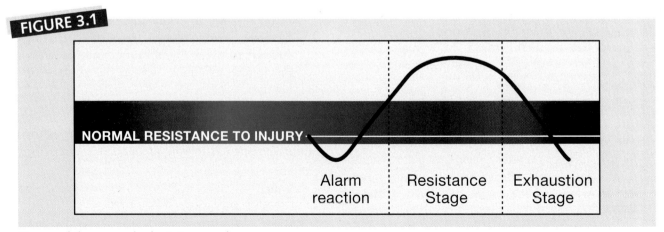

NORMAL RESISTANCE TO INJURY

Alarm reaction | Resistance Stage | Exhaustion Stage

Stages of the general adaptation syndrome.

branch of the nervous system that regulates body functions we can't consciously control). All body systems mobilize and prepare for defense. Manifestations of the alarm reaction are depicted in Figure 3.2.

The mouth gets dry, and the palms get sweaty. Air sacs in the lungs dilate and breathing gets faster, infusing the blood with oxygen. Adrenaline and other hormones are pumped throughout the body, speeding the heart to deliver oxygen-rich blood to the muscles. Digestion shuts down so the much-needed blood is not diverted to the stomach. The liver releases glucose, which the muscles use as fuel. The muscles get tense, prepared for a workout. The senses — sight, hearing, smell, and taste — become

acute, ready to identify any "danger." The brain releases endorphins to relieve pain.

If stress is prolonged, further changes occur during the alarm stage. A hormone released by the pituitary gland causes the adrenal glands to release

Homeostasis   The internal sense of balance.

Fight-or-flight response   A series of rapid-fire physical reactions to stress used originally by primitive people when facing threats in the environment.

General adaptation syndrome   A three-stage attempt of the body to react and adapt to stressors that disrupt its normal balance.

Alarm   The first stage of the general adaptation syndrome, characterized by the release of stress hormones.

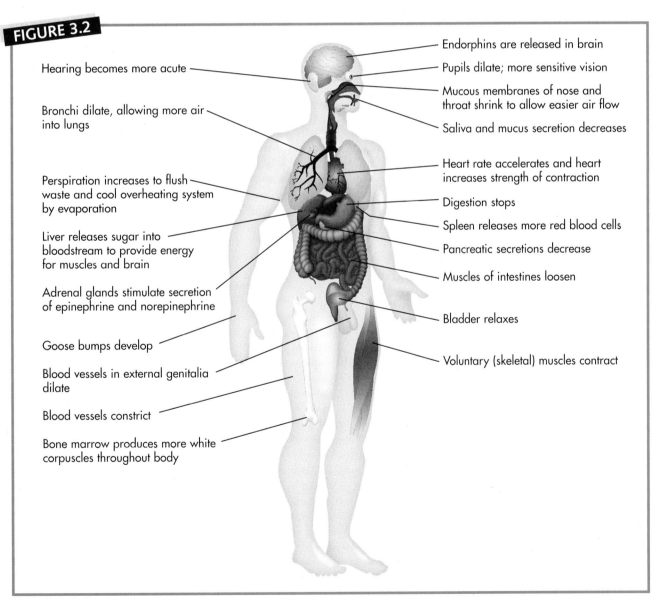

FIGURE 3.2

Hearing becomes more acute

Bronchi dilate, allowing more air into lungs

Perspiration increases to flush waste and cool overheating system by evaporation

Liver releases sugar into bloodstream to provide energy for muscles and brain

Adrenal glands stimulate secretion of epinephrine and norepinephrine

Goose bumps develop

Blood vessels in external genitalia dilate

Blood vessels constrict

Bone marrow produces more white corpuscles throughout body

Endorphins are released in brain

Pupils dilate; more sensitive vision

Mucous membranes of nose and throat shrink to allow easier air flow

Saliva and mucus secretion decreases

Heart rate accelerates and heart increases strength of contraction

Digestion stops

Spleen releases more red blood cells

Pancreatic secretions decrease

Muscles of intestines loosen

Bladder relaxes

Voluntary (skeletal) muscles contract

The alarm reaction.

cortisol. As a result, stored nutrients are made available to the body for energy.

During the alarm stage a person can exhibit "super-human" strength. The physiological reactions of the alarm stage are what enable a small woman to lift a car weighing several tons off the chest of a toddler.

Resistance

The **resistance stage** of the stress response begins almost immediately after the alarm stage begins. During resistance, the body intensifies the physical changes of the alarm stage so you can meet the perceived challenge. The adrenal glands continue to release adrenaline, the thyroid pumps out thyroid hormones, the hypothalamus continues to release endorphins, and the adrenal releases fewer sex hormones (again, to prevent the possibility of any diversion). More glucose and cholesterol are released into the bloodstream, providing instant energy and endurance. Heart and breathing rates increase to boost the supply of oxygen to the body. The blood thickens. The skin "crawls," pales, and sweats. More than 1,400 known physicochemical reactions occur during the alarm and resistance stages of the stress response.

The resistance stage of the stress response is ideally suited to meeting the challenges of short-term stress. Simply stated, the body tries to *adapt* so it can once again achieve the balance (homeostasis) that existed before the stress occurred. The body is on guard, trying to resist the ill effects of the stress.

The goal of the resistance stage is to achieve homeostasis. If the stress is short-term, that's usually what happens. The body is able to adapt and return to a state of balance. If the stress becomes chronic, however, the body eventually loses the ability to adapt.

Exhaustion

Although most people experience the alarm and resistance stages of the stress response frequently, only those with chronic stress experience the **exhaustion stage**, in which the body's resources are depleted and its adaptive abilities are lost. Many of the events of the alarm stage occur again as the body attempts to adjust to higher levels of stress, but the resulting wear and tear knock out the immune system, injure body systems and organs, and lead to illness and disease. The exhaustion stage is when long-term effects of stress set in.

HOW STRESS AFFECTS THE BODY SYSTEMS

The brain usually is the first body system to recognize a stressor. The brain then reacts with split-second timing, instructing the rest of the body how to adjust to the stressor. The brain continues to stimulate the stress reaction as long as 72 hours after the traumatic incident.

The brain is not a discriminator of stressors. It reacts the same whether the stress is physical (you are almost hit by a car) or emotional (your boss calls you in for another one of his "talks"). The result is a virtual cascade of hormones and brain chemicals that take their toll. Elevated levels of stress hormones may kill off significant numbers of vitally important brain cells. When researchers at the University of Kentucky exposed rats to prolonged stress, the rats showed reduced electrical activity in the hippocampus of the brain after only 3 weeks. When examined in autopsies at the end of 6 months, the rats that had been exposed to stress lost twice as many brain cells — 50% of the total brain cells — as same-aged rats who had been spared the stress.[18]

Under chronic stress the endocrine system works overtime, pumping out excess of hormones that increase blood pressure, damage the lining of the heart and blood vessels, inhibit vitamin D activity, cause a loss of calcium, increase the risk of diabetes, and suppress the immune system.

The skin becomes cold, clammy, and pale during stress because the blood vessels nearest the skin constrict (get smaller). The surface temperature of the skin drops, perspiration increases, and the skin is better able to conduct electricity. (The skin's response to electrical current is a main measurement in lie detector tests.)

Stress causes the muscles to contract. Occasional muscle contraction isn't a problem, but during stress the muscles stay contracted so long that they get fatigued. Stress also causes contraction of the involuntary, or smooth, muscles of the body — those lining the stomach, intestines, blood vessels, and other organs. Function is disrupted, and pain results.

Stress and the Digestive System

Stress impacts every aspect of the gastrointestinal system. The mouth stops producing saliva. The regular rhythmic contractions of the esophagus are disrupted, making swallowing difficult. The stomach slows down. Stress causes the stomach to pump out hydrochloric acid and thins the gastric mucus that normally protects the stomach lining, which can cause ulcers. The liver overproduces glucose, and the pancreas becomes chronically inflamed. Increased hydrochloric acid and disruption of normal peristaltic (rhythmic) action in the intestinal tract lead to duodenal ulcers and chronic diarrhea or constipation.

Stress and the Cardiovascular System

The cardiovascular system reacts with increased heart rate, damaged blood vessels, high blood pressure, and a boost in serum cholesterol levels, all of which lead to an increased risk of cardiovascular disease. The heart itself beats more forcefully and pumps a greater volume of blood during stress; severe shock can cause the heart to stop. Research efforts have shown a strong link between stress and all kinds of cardiovascular disease, including deaths attributed to cardiovascular disease. Maryland psychologist David Krantz[19] summarizes heart disease as "some interaction of mind, body, and behavior.

Your coronary risk probably depends on how your body reacts, and how often your behavior leads you into stressful situations."

Stress can cause blood pressure to go up, resulting in permanent hypertension if stress persists over time. In women, blood pressure soars with much less negative stress. The effects of stressors on high blood pressure for both men and women are intensified by caffeine (though the dose does not seem especially important) and by a family history of high blood pressure.

For people with existing heart disease, mental stress may be just as hard on the heart as intense physical exertion is. Physical stress tests and mental stress tests both caused the heart to slow down — with a resulting significant decrease in blood flow to the heart — in more than half the heart disease patients in a UCLA School of Medicine study.[20] The reason is that stress causes blood vessels to constrict instead of expand, reducing the amount of blood that can be circulated. One question asking the heart disease patients to list their own shortcomings caused almost as much stress on the heart as did an intense workout on a stationary bicycle.

Stress may be a strong contributing factor to heart disease. A number of studies have shown that stress causes the body to release cholesterol into the bloodstream. Well-documented evidence shows that high blood cholesterol level is a leading risk factor for the development of coronary artery disease. When the bloodstream carries too much cholesterol or other fats, fatty deposits build up on the walls of the coronary arteries, narrowing them and restricting blood flow to the heart. If the arteries eventually become too clogged, blood flow to a certain part of the heart stops, that part of the heart muscle dies, and the victim has a heart attack.

The effects of stress don't stop there. As part of the fight-or-flight reaction (the alarm stage of the stress response), the blood thickens. As a result, it coagulates more easily. Blood platelets build up along fatty deposits in the coronary arteries, worsening existing arteriosclerosis.

Stress and Heart Attacks

Five times more people than usual had fatal heart attacks the day Los Angeles had its last big earthquake. On the day of the quake — January 17, 1994 — 24 people ages 45 to 92 died of cardiac arrest. Only three of these people were doing something strenuous (such as running from a shaking building) when they died.

Researchers estimate that some sort of outside trigger, such as emotional stress, touches off about 40% of all heart attack deaths. In the case of the L.A. quake, the whole population was simultaneously exposed to enormous stress.

Sudden stress can stop blood circulation in three ways:

1. It can send the heart into unorganized quivering.

2. It can break open a piece of fatty plaque so a clot forms in an artery.

3. It can cause an artery to go into spasms.

People who maintain healthy weight, avoid cigarettes, exercise regularly, and maintain healthy blood pressure and blood cholesterol levels are less at the mercy of stress.

Source: New England Journal of Medicine, 334:7.

Resistance stage   The second stage of the general adaptation syndrome, characterized by meeting the perceived challenge.

Exhaustion stage   The final stage of the general adaptation syndrome, characterized by depletion of the body's resources and loss of adaptive abilities.

STRESS AND THE IMMUNE SYSTEM

Perhaps the greatest effect of stress is on the immune system. During the 40-some years that scientists have been taking a hard look at the immune system, other researchers have become sophisticated at studying the effects of stress on immunity and disease. In one series of studies, reported by Dr. Sheldon Cohen, British volunteers from all walks of life agreed to expose themselves to the common cold virus to see who would get sick. The subjects judged to have been under stress before the study were found to be more than twice as likely to come down with colds than those who were not.[21]

Herpes viruses such as Epstein-Barr offer a helpful model for studying the effects of stress on immunity. These viruses are common, and, unlike some other viruses, herpes viruses never are wiped out completely by the immune system but simply are held in check by the immune response. Diseases caused by herpes viruses often come and go as the virus advances and retreats. Specific herpes viruses are responsible for recurring oral cold sores and genital ulcers, as well as for chicken pox and its recurring form, shingles.

Having more herpes antibodies, or lower immunity, has been associated with many kinds of stress. For example, studies have indicated that students show more herpes antibodies while undergoing exams than they do after summer vacation.

Microorganisms alone do not cause infectious disease. The condition of the person exposed to the microorganism also has a bearing. Scientists are studying more exactly how stress might affect the immune system of people at different stages of life and, in turn, how these immune changes might affect health and disease. Physicians caution that few of these diseases are caused or triggered solely by stress, that other factors also must be considered. Continuing research, however, is clear: Stress plays a moderate to major role in a whole Pandora's box of disease conditions.

Stress is a leading factor in disease because it compromises the immune system, making the body less capable of fighting disease and infection. Stress can literally shut down the immune response. Simply stated, stress suppresses the immune system's ability to produce and maintain lymphocytes (the white blood cells necessary for killing infection) and natural killer cells (the specialized cells that seek out

and destroy foreign invaders), both vital in the fight against infection and disease. Stress affects all the key players in immunity, from the levels of interferon to the organs vital to immune system functioning (such as the thymus).

Also, stress increases the risk of suffering allergic reactions, contracting infectious diseases, and developing autoimmune diseases such as rheumatoid arthritis. One reason is the tendency of stress to suppress the body's production of T lymphocytes, the

---

Stress, the Immune System, and Disease

Conditions caused or aggravated by stress include the following, among others:

- heart disease
- arteriosclerosis
- atherosclerosis
- high blood pressure
- coronary thrombosis
- stroke
- angina
- respiratory ailments
- ulcers
- irritable bowel syndrome
- ulcerative colitis
- gastritis
- pancreatitis
- diabetes
- migraine headache
- myasthenia gravis
- epileptic attacks
- chronic backache
- kidney disease
- chronic tuberculosis
- allergies
- rheumatoid arthritis
- systemic lupus erythematosus
- psoriasis
- eczema
- cold sores
- shingles
- hives
- asthma
- Raynaud's disease
- multiple sclerosis
- cancer
- endocrine and autoimmune problems

immune cells that fight bacterial and viral infections, fungi, and cancer cells.

City University of New York researcher Suzanne Kobasa studied a group of AT&T executives during an 8-year period of extreme stress — the largest corporate reorganization in history. She found that even through debilitating stress, some of the executives didn't get sick. In fact, they suffered less than half the number of illnesses as their co-workers who were under the same amount of job stress. Kobasa and her colleagues determined that the healthy executives had the ability to withstand the negative effects of stress. She coined the term *hardiness* to denote this quality.

Kobasa boiled down the hardiness concept to what she called the three Cs: *commitment, control, and challenge*. The executives who withstood the stress had a strong commitment in their lives. That commitment (to family, work, religious faith, friendships) gave them something to strive toward and work for. They also believed they had some amount of control over their lives, that even when negative things were happening, they were not completely out of control. They trusted that they could get enough information to make intelligent decisions, and that those decisions could help them maintain command. They also saw stressful events as exciting challenges that tested their creativity and resources instead of a debilitating threat that could wipe them out.

Stress doesn't have to result in illness. University of Pennsylvania psychologist Martin E. P. Seligman and his colleague Madelon Visitainer injected laboratory mice with a solution known to lead to the growth of tumors. The next day the mice were randomly divided into three groups. One group was subjected to repeated electric shock that it could not escape — a classic way of creating stress in the laboratory. A second group of mice was subjected to repeated electric shock but was given the opportunity to escape the shocks. The third group of mice was not given any electric shock at all.

When the researchers examined the mice, almost three-fourths of the mice who couldn't escape the shock had developed at least some tumors. Only about one-third of the mice who could escape the shock developed tumors. Seligman blamed the high rate of tumor growth in the stressed animals on *helplessness*, a feeling that they had no control over what happened in their environment.[22]

Ohio State University psychologist Janice Kiecolt-Glaser, known for her work in immune studies, said:

> Just because your immune function goes down during a stressful period doesn't mean you are going to get sick. Where stress seems to have the greatest impact on health is on individuals who already have poor immune function because of age or diseases that impair the immune system, or on individuals who have already been chronically stressed for reasons other than health.[23]

Yale oncologist and surgeon Bernie Siegel, one of the nation's foremost researchers of the link between behavior and disease, pointed out:

> Stresses that we *choose* evoke a response totally different from those we'd like to avoid but cannot. Helplessness is worse than the stress itself. That is probably why the rate of cancer is higher for blacks in America than for whites, and why cancer is associated with grief and depression.[24]

Epidemiologist Leonard Sagan reported that:

> Whether altered conditions are viewed as threatening or challenging, and whether the consequences contribute to personal growth or apathy and despair is the result of the interaction of two factors: the magnitude and quality of the external stressor and the capacity of the individual to cope.[25]

COPING WITH STRESS

Each individual has **adaptation energy stores**, the physical, mental, and emotional reserves that enable us to cope with stress. Researchers think these stores

Adaptation energy stores Reserves of physical, mental, and emotional energy that give us the ability to cope with stress.

The Holmes-Rahe Scale

Thomas Holmes and Richard Rahe listed approximately four dozen social changes that are considered "major" contributors to stress and illness. The top 10 are:

1. Death of a spouse
2. Divorce
3. Marital separation
4. Jail term
5. Death of a close family member
6. Personal injury or illness
7. Marriage
8. Fired at work
9. Marital reconciliation
10. Retirement

occur in two layers: a deep-seated layer surrounded by a superficial layer. The energy stores in the superficial layer are used first and are easy for the body to access. These reserves can be replaced through the coping strategies outlined below. The deep-seated energy stores seem to be determined in part by heredity. They cannot be replaced, and when they are spent, the body dies.

Tips For Action — Some Coping Strategies

The following strategies are designed to reduce the amount and extent of stress in your life, not to cause you more stress. To reach that goal:

- Don't try to incorporate too many strategies at once. Changing old habits and developing new ways of dealing with things require time. If you take on too much at once, you'll end up feeling frustrated and stressed. Another name for stress is *change*, and too much change, even if it's positive, can translate into stress.

- Before you decide on the strategies you want to use, consider your own strengths and skills. Think about what you would *enjoy*. Assess what kind of social support you'll have. Those kinds of considerations can help you choose the most workable and pleasant strategies for you.

- Keep in mind that what works for you won't necessarily work for someone else — and won't even work for you in all situations. Be flexible, be willing to change your coping strategies, and never stop assessing.

- Do not expect a single coping strategy to provide you with enough coping power. Several coping strategies will be required to do the trick.

- Realize that you will not be able to change or control some things. The death of a family member, the diagnosis of a serious illness, the loss of property in a crime — these are examples of things you can't change. The best strategy here is to accept what has happened and determine to move on in a positive way.

- Recognize that even negative stress can have a positive outcome if you meet it head-on and use it as an opportunity for learning and growth. Even a stressful situation can give you insight or help you become more prudent.

Coping with stress successfully allows you to replenish adaptation energy stores. It prepares you to deal with stress. It isn't something that just happens. It's something you have to plan for and work at. Sometimes it involves changing attitudes, ideologies, values, or goals. It may even require making gradual but significant lifestyle changes to eliminate debilitating sources of stress when you can't find any other solutions. Often it requires strategies you develop ahead of time, strategies that help you manage stressful situations. These include eating right, getting plenty of exercise, getting enough rest, changing the way you think about stress, managing time well, preventing burnout, and using relaxation techniques.

> *Another name for stress is change, and too much change, even if it's positive, can translate into stress.*

Balanced Diet

One of the most effective stress-busters is diet. A poor diet not only increases your susceptibility to disease in general but also increases your susceptibility to the negative effects of stress. Some foods (especially those that contain caffeine) cause a stresslike response. Certain things in your diet can exaggerate stress by making you more uptight. Overeating, undereating, or eating the wrong foods can upset your body's balance, making all your systems more apt to suffer the ill effects of stress.

Stress may change your nutritional requirements, too. Chronic stress may influence your body's stores of important vitamins and minerals. It also can increase the amount of fats in your bloodstream, requiring you to eat a diet lower in fats and may boost your protein requirements. If you're under chronic stress, you may need more than the normal amount of protein. You also may need more calories, as stress makes your body cells less capable of metabolizing the energy released from the food you eat and causes you to burn up your food more quickly.

You should eat three sensible meals a day containing foods low in fat and high in fiber. A balanced diet follows the guidelines in the U.S. Department of Agriculture's food pyramid. Most of your calories should come from complex carbohydrates: grains, pastas, vegetables, and fruits. If you are under

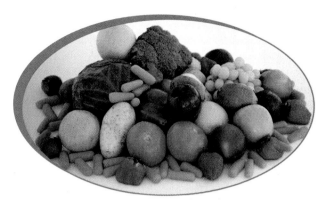

*Proper nutrition is a key element
to overall stress management.*

chronic stress, you should boost your protein intake with the leanest possible protein sources: fish, poultry, lean cuts of beef, and low-fat or skim dairy products.

Follow these specific dietary guidelines:

■ Cut back on sugar and foods containing sugar. The stress response changes metabolism, which leads to higher levels of sugar in the bloodstream. Corn syrup, corn sweeteners, sucrose, and honey are examples of sugars in processed foods. Even though sugar provides calories for energy, it may be followed by a "crash" as the rapid effects of the sugar wear off.

■ Avoid all products containing nicotine: cigarettes, cigars, pipes, chewing tobacco, snuff. Nicotine is a stimulant that can make you high-strung and irritable.

■ Cut back on or eliminate caffeine, a stimulant that increases your sensitivity to stress. Caffeine is found not only in coffee and tea but also in cola drinks, chocolate, and a number of both prescription and over-the-counter medications.

■ Reduce the amount of salt in your diet. Major culprits are processed foods, including some that don't even taste salty, such as canned soup and powdered gelatin.

Regular Physical Activity and Exercise

Physical activity and exercise decrease the intensity of stress, lessen its effects, cut down the time to recover from stress, and even minimize the physiological reactions of the stress response. An active lifestyle reduces the risk of getting sick, even for those under severe or chronic stress. Exercise reduces hostility, improves mental acuity, increases energy, eases muscle tension, and floods the system with endorphins.

Various tests have proven just how much exercise can reduce the effects of stress. In one, University of Washington psychologist Jonathon Brown studied stress levels among students there. He found that those with the most stress also were those most likely to develop a wide range of medical problems. Also, those who exercised regularly reported far fewer visits to the university student health center, even when under extreme stress.[26]

To get the maximum stress-reducing benefit from a regular physical activity routine:

■ Increase your overall amount of daily physical activity. While a regular structured exercise routine (jogging, swimming, cycling, aerobics, strength training) is important, you should attempt to accumulate at least 30 minutes of moderate-intensity physical activity on most days of the week. Examples of moderate-intensity activity include: walking, gardening, mowing the lawn, washing the car by hand, fast dancing, golfing, tennis, and doing household chores.

■ Choose a form of exercise you *like*. Not only will you be more prone to stick with it, but you'll enjoy yourself, too — an essential factor in alleviating stress.

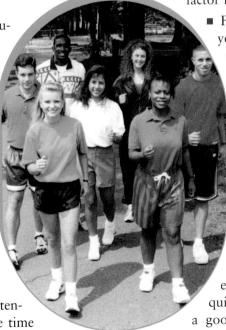

*An active lifestyle
buffers the effects of stress.*

■ Find an activity suited to your personality. Consider whether you'd like an exercise that requires keen concentration or one that allows you to daydream; whether you want some time alone or want to exercise with a partner or as part of a team; and whether you'd rather engage in a competitive or a noncompetitive exercise.

■ Consider how much equipment the exercise requires. Walking requires only a good pair of shoes, whereas golf requires a set of clubs, a handful of tees, and plenty of fresh balls. Consider, too, where you'll have to go to exercise. Walking and bicycling can be done almost anywhere. If you want to swim, though, you'll have to go to a pool. Consider options for different weather conditions. You can walk in almost any weather, but you'll need certain seasons and conditions for skiing, golfing, or swimming outdoors. For greatest versatility, choose several activities so you won't be limited by locale, weather, and equipment needs.

- Don't feel limited to what you can do already. If you think fencing sounds like fun, take a class. If you think golf sounds challenging and enjoyable, sign up for lessons.

- Don't overlook team sports as a good form of exercise. Not only do you get to vent your stress, frustrations, and aggression, but you'll also enjoy some good social support — another proven stress-buster. Team sports don't have to involve competition; you might join a group of classmates in an informal football contest every Saturday or play some "parking-lot basketball" just for fun.

- If you haven't been exercising, start slowly. If you try too much at first, you're more likely to get injured, or, at the least, stiff and sore. The resulting discouragement might keep you from exercising at all. If you're just starting out, take it easy. Try 10 to 15 minutes at a time, then work up as you get more conditioned. Challenge yourself, but don't overdo it.

- Consider aerobic exercises that help condition your heart and lungs — walking, jogging, running, bicycling, swimming, racquetball.

- Exercise regularly. In addition to daily physical activity, experts think 3 to 5 times a week of structured exercise is ideal.

- Consider exercising more often for shorter periods. Dr. Irving Dardik, a founding chairman of the U.S. Olympic Sports Medicine Council, has found that exercising in 5-minute chunks followed by relaxation techniques (what he calls "recovery") can be more beneficial in relieving stress than a continuous 30-minute workout.

- Don't overdo it. People who get addicted to exercise are vulnerable to injury, fatigue, and over-exertion, all of which can lead to depression and anxiety instead of stress relief. If you start to feel anxious about your exercise, cut back and ease off until you find you're enjoying yourself again.

Additional information on developing and implementing an active lifestyle and a regular exercise program is provided in Chapter 7.

Plenty of Rest

Sleep is essential to coping with stress. If you've had your rest, it's easier to face almost anything. Sleep offers other, not-so-obvious benefits, too, including the relaxation so important to minimizing the effects of the stress response.

If you're feeling fatigued:

- Try to establish a sleep pattern. Go to bed at about the same time every night and wake up at the same time every morning instead of skimping on sleep during the week and sleeping until noon on weekends.

- If you really need to, take a *short* nap during the day; 20 minutes is optimal. Shorter than that doesn't give you enough sleep, and longer than that can make you drowsy.

- If you're having trouble falling asleep at night, don't nap during the afternoon, eat a light dinner, and avoid caffeine after 6 p.m.

- Use your bedroom only for sleeping. Don't watch television, study, or do work in bed. You need to associate your bed and your bedroom with sleep.

Sleep Stealers

- Stress
- Depression
- Alcohol
- Nicotine
- Caffeine
- Exercising too close to bedtime
- Going to bed/getting up at differing times
- Shift work
- Jet lag
- Bed partner with sleep problems
- Bedroom that's too hot/too cold/too noisy/too bright
- Arthritis, hormonal shifts (e.g., menopause), asthma, sleep apnea, pain
- Medications (side effect)

Source: National Sleep Foundation.

- Most people need 6 to 8 hours of sleep a night to function well and feel refreshed, but that requirement can vary from one person to another. To discover how much sleep you *really* need, go to sleep at the same time every night, then sleep until you wake up. It will take a couple of weeks to determine what you need. Once you've figured it out, discipline yourself and set a goal to get the rest you need.

> **One in three Americans say they have "sleep problems."**

Reframing Thoughts

Reframing entails changing the way you look at things, learning to be an optimist instead of a pessimist. The way you think often determines what really happens, and under stress it can help change the way stress impacts your body.

To help reframe your own thinking:

- Listen carefully to the words you use to describe yourself and your situation. Are they positive or negative? Listen for a few weeks. Then, if you need to, use different phrases and descriptions.

- Role play, either by yourself or with a friend. Start by relating a stressful situation you have experienced lately; tell how you reacted. Then come up with some different ways in which you could have reacted to the situation. If you're role playing with a friend, ask for feedback or suggestions. Next, imagine some plausible stressful situations and outline how you'd handle them. Concentrate on positive responses.

Planning and prioritizing your daily activities simplifies your days.

- For one week, look for the good in every person and every situation you encounter. This can be tough, but you always can find something! This kind of exercise is like conditioning your attitudes. Before long, it can become a habit.

- Avoid words that signal defeat: *always, never, should have, ought to.* Replace them with more benign choices. Instead of saying, "I *always* fail quizzes in class," say, "I'm *sometimes* unprepared when the teacher springs a quiz on us."

Effective Time Management

One of the leading sources of stress is simply too much to do in too little time. We are living in the fastest-paced society of this century, and the mere speed at which we move can be a significant stressor. Learning to manage the time you have can alleviate stress and reduce anxiety.

To better manage your time:

- Figure out how you're spending your time: Keep a diary for 2 weeks. You might be stunned to find out how much time you're spending on the phone or watching television programs. You can't outline realistic goals until you know what you're really doing.

- Try to figure out your peak time. Are you a "morning person," or do you get your second wind when most people are quitting for the day? Plan your most demanding tasks — studying, working — for the time you're at your peak. If you have to take a particularly challenging class and you're generally sluggish in the morning, see if you can schedule it for the afternoon, or find out if it's offered at night.

- Before you schedule anything else on your daily calendar, schedule time for a break. Plan on several periods for doing what you *want* to do — soaking in a hot tub, reading a good book, watching a football game on TV, or talking to a friend. Knowing you can look forward to a few breaks can help you more easily face the more stressful periods of your day.

- Learn to prioritize. Not every demand is a top priority. You usually can split up tasks into those that are essential, important, and unimportant or trivial. Spend your time and attention on the ones that are essential and important. If you have time left over, you can go for the trivial ones.

- Attack things one at a time. If you are faced with a number of things to do, don't try to accomplish everything at once. Instead, decide on a course of action that lets you move through the list calmly. Limit the number of interruptions you have, but

Reframing Changing the way you look at things.

don't schedule yourself so tightly that a few interruptions throw you off completely.

- Learn to realistically judge how long a task will take. Most people underestimate by about 50%, so get into the habit of adding 50% to the time you think it will take. Once you learn how to estimate realistically the time different tasks take, you can stop overcrowding your day with too much to handle.

- If some things don't require your personal attention, delegate them to someone else.

- Before you go to bed each night, write down your schedule for the next day. Think through what *has* to be done — classes you need to attend, your part-time job, a commitment at the community crisis center. Prioritize. Figure out which are most important, and make the time for those. Include times for leisure.

- Set realistic goals. Write them down, and break them up into chunks you can accomplish more readily. Keep track of your progress, and reward yourself for a job well done.

- Protect against boredom by setting a satisfying, realistic goal and doing something toward it every day.

- Don't feel guilty if you have to say "no" to a request. You can do only so much in a single day. If you start to get overwhelmed, back off. Going to the movies with a few friends might be fun, but not if you have to stay up half the night to study for an exam in exchange.

- The ability to say "no" relates in another way to stress management: Stress diminishes when you can feel good about expressing yourself and satisfying your own needs (assertive behavior). Stress increases when you deny your own needs or wishes to satisfy someone else (nonassertive behavior) or try to get your own way at the expense of someone else (aggressive behavior).

Burnout Prevention

Stress — especially chronic stress — can lead to **burnout**, a state of physical and mental exhaustion with few remaining resources. Accompanying physical symptoms may include headache, indigestion, fatigue, and muscle soreness. Mental symptoms might be depression, apathy, or loss of enjoyment in life.

To prevent burnout:

- Surround yourself with a strong network of social support. Have at least one friend in whom you can confide.

- Distract yourself from your routine by developing a new interest, trying a new hobby, or volunteering for something new. Two hours a week telling animated stories to a group of captivated preschoolers at the local library might be just what you need to get a fresh perspective on things.

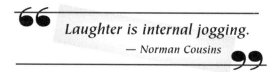

Laughter is internal jogging.
— Norman Cousins

- Take the time to have fun. With all the demands of everyday life, a person can get bogged down in things that aren't always enjoyable. Go fly a kite, wade in a ditch, or have a picnic in the middle of a downtown park. Aim for fun, silly things you can laugh over at least once a day. Laughter has been shown to actually strengthen the immune system.

Laughter as Medicine

The benefits of laughter are many. It lowers blood pressure, increases muscle flexibility, and triggers a flood of beta endorphins, the brain's natural compounds that induce euphoria.

Laughter's most profound effects are on the immune system. Gamma-interferon, a disease-fighting protein, rises with laughter — as do B-cells, which produce disease-destroying antibodies, and T-cells, which orchestrate the immune response.

Laughter also shuts off the flow of stress hormones, the fight-or-flight compounds that come into play during times of stress, hostility, and rage.

Stress hormones suppress the immune system, raise blood pressure, and increase the number of platelets, which can cause fatal blockages in the arteries.

The average child laughs hundreds of times a day. The average adult laughs a dozen times. We need to find these lost laughs — and use them to our advantage.

Sources: American Association for Therapeutic Humor; Lee Berk, M.D. and Stanley Tan, M.D., Loma Linda University.

■ If you've got a strenuous class load, take a class just for fun. Go for something you've always wanted to do — maybe a water color class, or bowling.

Relaxation Techniques

One of the best and most *immediate* ways of breaking the stress response is to use a relaxation technique. This may be any one of a host of techniques that bring on what researcher Herbert Benson calls "the relaxation response, an inborn bodily reaction that counteracts the harmful effects of stress."[27]

Invoking the relaxation response not only breaks up stress, but it also gives you a more positive mental outlook, eases anxiety, and brings on a sense of control (essential to overcoming the negative aspects of stress). Regular relaxation exercises can reduce stress, increase resistance to stress-induced illness, minimize the symptoms of illness (such as headache), lower your blood pressure, and alleviate pain.

Of the number of relaxation exercises, some are based on deep relaxation with a myriad of benefits, and others (such as deep breathing and a quick massage) reduce stress and are a good way of leading into more extensive relaxation exercises. As with physical exercise, learning about various relaxation exercises takes some time. Before you decide which ones to try, you should consider your likes and dislikes, your personality, and your situation. You can learn some techniques on your own and you will need some training for others. The techniques include, among others, meditation, progressive relaxation, deep breathing, autogenics, biofeedback training, and yoga.

As a note of caution, if you are taking medication for high blood pressure, heart conditions, diabetes, epilepsy, or psychological conditions, consult with your health care practitioner *before* you begin practicing relaxation techniques. These exercises can cause physiological changes.

Meditation

Simply stated, **meditation** is an exercise in which you control your thoughts and thus affect certain body processes. Meditation originated in India and Tibet

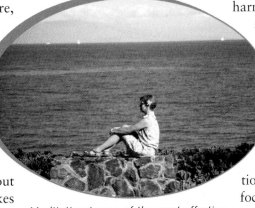

Meditation is one of the most effective stress-coping techniques.

and first became popular in the United States during the 1960s, when the Maharishi Mahesh Yogi introduced it as *transcendental meditation* (TM). The exercise got its name because of the practitioner's ability to effortlessly "transcend" (go beyond) everyday thought. Among the various types of meditation are:

— Zen, which focuses on counting breaths

— Soto Zen, which focuses on an external object (like a flower)

— Rinzai Zen, which focuses on unanswerable riddles

— Tibetan Buddhism, which focuses on a geometric figure that has spiritual significance.

Today, meditation is recognized as one of the most effective ways to reduce stress. More than 700 scientific studies have verified that meditation induces the relaxation response and alleviates the harmful physiological effects of stress. Whereas basic meditation requires little training, TM is a little more specialized. TM classes usually require several sessions. "Mindfulness meditation" is another type of meditation. It requires total concentration and prevents mental distraction, drifting attention, and unfocused thoughts. It is being used to promote safety and prevent accidents.

The meditator focuses exclusively on a specific thought or object. Heartbeat and breathing slow down, blood pressure drops (often for 12 to 24 hours after the meditative period), and the body's metabolism slows, decreasing its need for oxygen and other nutrients. As the person becomes relaxed, blood flow to the arms and legs increases, which helps to ease muscle tension. Laboratory studies have shown that people who meditate have fewer blood lactates, the enzymes associated with stress and anxiety.

Burnout   A state of physical and mental exhaustion in which few resources remain.

Meditation   A mental exercise that helps the meditator gain control over thoughts.

Meditation has psychological benefits, too. It lessens anxiety, produces better sleep, and promotes less fear, fewer phobias, greater internal locus of control, and more positive mental health. Meditation also has helped people stop drug abuse and cigarette smoking. And people who meditate have been found to have a more positive outlook immediately after a stressful experience.[28]

The most essential element of meditation is something to focus on: a word or phrase repeated silently (a *mantra*) or an unchanging object on which to focus. To be effective, meditation has to be done in a comfortable position in a quiet place, free of distractions. No specific posture is required for meditation, but because the physiological processes of meditation are different from those of sleep, meditators sit so they won't fall asleep during meditation.

The goal of meditation is relaxation, which involves diverting blood to the arms and legs. After a meal, blood pools in the abdomen, where it is used to help digestion. Therefore, it's best to meditate *before* you eat. Also, avoid using any stimulants, including tobacco and caffeine, before you meditate, as they can interfere with relaxation.

For maximum effects, experts recommend meditating 20 minutes at a time, twice during the day. The procedure is as follows.

1. Find a quiet room as free from distraction as possible. Lighting and temperature are a matter of individual preference. Just make sure you're comfortable. Turn off the phone. Alert others that you don't want to be disturbed. (At first, it's important to have quiet surroundings; later, after you've practiced for a while, you will be able to meditate in almost any situation.)

2. Loosen your clothing if it is tight, especially at the wrists, neck, and waist. Get in the most comfortable position you can, in a chair or on a couch. Some recommend a straight-backed chair to prevent you from falling asleep. Place your feet flat on the floor, and rest your hands in your lap.

3. Inhale slowly and deeply through your nose, hold your breath briefly, then exhale slowly. As you begin to breathe deeply, let the tension flow out of your body. Don't force it or concentrate on it. Just let it happen.

4. If you are concentrating on an unchanging object, close your eyes partially so the object appears blurred. Softly focus on it without bringing in any of the sharp details. If you are focusing on

a mantra, begin repeating it silently and rhythmically as you breathe in and out. Repeat the word *slowly* with the rhythm of your breathing. Gradually focus all your attention on that object or mantra. Do not let any other thoughts invade your meditation.

5. Continue meditating for approximately 20 minutes. Don't worry about the exact time. You'll probably have to work up to it at first. Learning to sit still for 20 minutes at a time takes a lot of practice, especially when you are focusing so intensely on a single object or phrase.

6. When you are finished meditating, give yourself time to readjust. Open your eyes, focus on various objects around the room, and return gradually to your normal rate and pattern of breathing. While still seated, stretch your arms, legs, back, shoulders, and neck. Finally, stand up slowly.

It's important to let your body readjust after meditating. If you stand up too soon or too quickly, you may get dizzy, because your heart rate and blood pressure drop during meditation.

Progressive Relaxation

Progressive relaxation is a technique for relaxing the nerves and muscles pioneered by Edmund Jacobson, a physician who wanted to help patients with stress-induced muscle tension. He showed patients how to recognize muscle tension and how to differentiate it from muscle relaxation. His three-step technique is simple: Patients first contract (tense) a small muscle group, then relax the muscle group, and finally concentrate on determining how different the two sensations feel.

Progressive relaxation helps relieve tension headache, migraine headache, back pain, and other conditions related to muscle tension. It even has been shown to relax the smooth, or involuntary, muscles (like those in blood vessels and the digestive tract). It also has been shown to reduce anxiety, relieve depression, and improve sleep patterns.

Progressive relaxation is simple. In essence, you contract, then relax the muscles of the body, progressing from one group of muscles to another. You can design your own routine — working from your head to your toes, for example, or from your feet to your head — as long as all major groups in the body are involved eventually. When you start doing progressive relaxation, you should first tense the muscles as hard as you can, then relax them. Once you become practiced, you can relax the muscles easily and effortlessly without having to first contract them.

Unlike meditation, in which you should *not* think about what's happening to your body, progressive relaxation requires you to *concentrate on what's happening to your muscles*. For the best results, you have to be acutely aware of the relaxed condition of your body.

Regardless of your individual routine, the following steps apply:

1. Take off your shoes, and loosen any restrictive clothing. Stretch out on the floor on your back in the most comfortable position possible. Support your neck with a small pillow. If you need it, put a pillow under your knees. Close your eyes and rotate your ankles outward. Depending on which helps you relax best, either put your arms at your sides or rest your hands on your abdomen. You need to be completely relaxed before you start.

2. First tense, then relax each muscle group. (Make sure you move to all major muscle groups in the body.) Don't forget your face — including your forehead, eyes, nose, mouth, cheeks, and tongue.

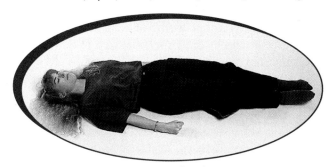

Progressive muscle relaxation is an effective stress management technique.

3. As you move to each muscle group, contract the muscles as tightly as you can and hold the contraction for 20 or 30 seconds. If you experience pain or cramping, release the contraction immediately.

4. Concentrate on the dramatic difference in feeling between a tensed muscle and a relaxed one. With practice, you'll be able to achieve relaxation without first tensing the muscle.

Breathing Techniques

Breathing exercises also can be an antidote to stress. These exercises have been used for centuries in the Orient and India as a means to develop better mental, physical, and emotional stamina. Breathing exercises can be learned in only a few minutes and require considerably less time than other forms of stress management.

In breathing exercises, the person concentrates on "breathing away" the tension and inhaling fresh oxygen to the entire body. To be effective, the breathing must be so deep that the belly is expanded with each breath — a sign that the diaphragm is being expanded.

As an example of a breathing exercise:

1. Lie in a comfortable position on your back, with your hands placed lightly over your lower stomach.

2. Keeping your eyes open, imagine a balloon lying beneath your hands.

3. Begin to slowly inhale through your nose, concentrating on the warm air entering your nose and slowly filling the balloon. You should be able to feel your lower abdomen rise as you breathe in. When the "balloon" is full (this should take 3 to 4 seconds initially), pause for a second, then slowly exhale to empty the balloon, feeling your chest and abdomen relaxing.

4. Repeat the entire process two or three times.

5. When finished, sit quietly for a few minutes before rising. If you feel dizzy at any point, stop the procedure.[29]

Autogenics

Similar to progressive relaxation, **autogenics** is self-induced relaxation that causes all major muscle groups in the body to feel relaxed, heavy, and warm. It begins with a routine that relaxes all the major muscles (much like that of progressive relaxation), followed by imagery (vivid mental visualization) that extends the relaxed state. It is actually a form of self-hypnosis that was developed by German psychiatrist Johannes Shultz in 1932, who used it to treat patients with psychosomatic illness. Today, it is recognized as an effective relaxation technique for managing stress.

Progressive relaxation   A method of reducing stress that consists of tensing, then relaxing small muscle groups.

Autogenics   A relaxation technique in which the person is trained, with the aid of specialized equipment, to relax all major muscle groups through a form of self-hypnosis, followed by imagery.

Autogenics and meditation both result in relaxation, but they do it in different ways. In meditation, you first relax the mind, which causes the body to relax. In autogenics, you first relax the body, which causes the mind to relax.

The benefits of autogenics exceed those of progressive relaxation because it goes a step farther to invoke the relaxation response. The general sensations resulting from autogenics are feelings of warmth and heaviness, especially in the arms and legs, caused by dilation of blood vessels and relaxation of muscles. Autogenics and the associated imagery reduce heartbeat and breathing rates, ease muscle tension, and increase the brainwaves associated with deep relaxation. Autogenics can help relieve migraine headache, tension headache, low back pain, and asthma, and can improve high blood pressure. Autogenics also can relieve anxiety, reduce depression, increase resistance to stress, and increase pain tolerance.

Autogenics requires time, motivation, commitment, and practice. Commercial tapes are available to guide you through the relaxation exercises. You also can make your own tape, or simply repeat the phrases aloud as you move through the exercises. As with progressive relaxation, you can design your own routine.

1. In a quiet room with mild temperature, free of distractions, sit in the most comfortable position you can. Experts recommend sitting in a straight-backed but comfortable chair with your feet flat on the floor, your head hanging loosely forward, your eyes closed, and your hands in your lap with your palms turned upward. Loosen any restrictive clothing.

2. Imagine you have just had a strenuous workout. You might begin with your legs. As you inhale and exhale deeply and slowly, repeat, "My legs are so tired. My legs are so heavy. My legs are very heavy and warm." As you repeat these phrases, feel the heaviness and warmth in your legs. With practice, your legs should become so heavy and relaxed that you can lift them only with considerable struggle.

3. Move to other muscle groups — buttocks, abdomen, chest, arms, shoulders, and so on. You even might imagine your internal organs, such as your stomach and your heart, relaxed and warm.

4. Concentrate on how cool your forehead feels. For you to feel refreshed and alert, your forehead must feel cool.

5. Once your entire body is relaxed, visualize an image that you find relaxing. It might be waves lapping against a sandy beach, a cloud drifting lazily across the afternoon sky, an eagle soaring silently across a ravine. The image is different for everyone, but it should lead you to total relaxation.

For the greatest benefit, experts recommend that you practice autogenics twice a day for 10 minutes at a time. As with other kinds of relaxation exercises, autogenics requires practice, starting out slowly, then working up to a 10-minute period of visualization and relaxation.

Biofeedback Training

Essentially, **biofeedback** training is a method of measuring physiological functions you're not normally aware of (such as skin temperature and blood pressure) and then training you to control those functions. It has three basic stages:

1. Measuring the physiological function
2. Converting the measurement into something meaningful
3. Feeding back the information

Unlike some other forms of relaxation exercises, you can't learn biofeedback training on your own. It requires that you be monitored by extremely sensitive equipment, then taught to regulate your own physiological responses. Biofeedback training is valuable as a stress management technique, as it allows you to control your body's responses to stress. Most people can learn effective biofeedback techniques in a few sessions from a trained therapist using sensitive biofeedback equipment.

Within a few sessions most people are able to competently control physiological effects of stress such as higher blood pressure, increasing heart rate, and muscle contraction. An obvious disadvantage is the necessity of using expensive machinery and trained therapists. Most people, however, quickly gain the ability to control their own physiological responses without the biofeedback machinery.

Yoga

Yoga, an ancient exercise technique known to induce calm and invigorate the mind, has been shown in scientific studies to reduce the biological effects of stress. Some use it to increase intelligence or activate the nervous system. In addition, yoga is an excellent exercise for improving muscular strength, flexibility, and endurance.

There are many different styles of yoga, which comes from a Sanskrit word meaning "union." The most common type of yoga used in the western world is **Hatha Yoga,** which involves stretching exercises to induce relaxation.

Unlike other relaxation exercises, you can't design your own technique or routine in yoga. It consists of precise postures done in a specific sequence combined with an exact breathing rhythm designed to reduce tension and inflexibility.

The yoga postures are difficult and complex and require training and practice. Few people can assume the postures at first, and you may not be able to complete the sequence properly for as long as 3 months. The goal of yoga is relaxation, so you should not force positions that make you tense or could cause injury.

A number of good yoga instruction books are on the market, and yoga classes are taught throughout the United States. Most experts recommend practicing yoga for 15 to 45 minutes a day in a place free of distraction. Many people sign up for classes, where they actually perform yoga daily.

CHECKMATE FOR STRESS

Like improving your game of chess, you can develop strategies to put stress in check. You don't want to *eliminate* stress completely. Too little stress, say researchers at Seattle's Hope Heart Institute, leaves you feeling restless, bored, unhappy, and tired. Conversely, with too much stress, you feel exhausted, irritable, and burned out. Just the right amount of stress can help you feel energetic, creative, happy, and productive. The key is to achieve the middle ground.

Based on years of researching why some people stay cool while others buckle, Salvatore Maddi, professor of psychology at the University of California, Irvine, founded the Hardiness Institute in Irvine, which offers training courses throughout the United States. It utilizes three key techniques for "hardy coping":

1. *Situational reconstruction:* When a stressful event occurs, replay it in your mind to gain understanding and pinpoint where the anxiety is coming from. If you've had an argument, what contribution did you make? What did the other person do? Next, get some perspective by imagining both how the situation could get worse and how it could get better. Finally, ask yourself what you could do to increase the likelihood of it getting better, and put your answer into action.

2. *Focusing:* If you can't get your imagination going in the first exercise, the situation may be evoking emotions you're not acknowledging. For example, you assume you are angry when, in fact, you're frightened. In this case, let your body cue you in. Focus on your center, the chest-abdomen area, and ask yourself, "What is it about this situation that stands in the way of my feeling good?" If you come up with an answer that seems familiar, put it aside, refocus, and ask the question again. When an unexpected thought or feeling pops into your mind, that's probably the information you've been burying. Acknowledge it, and try the first step again.

3. *Compensatory self-improvement:* When you can't think of anything you could do to make the situation better, you may be confronting something you can't change. That's rarely the case, but if it is, accept the reality gracefully without falling into bitterness and self-pity. One way to do this is by choosing another problem related to the first one and work on that instead. Rather than feeling victimized or overwhelmed, say to yourself, "I may not be able to fix everything, but I can improve some things."

In short, start with yourself. There are few situations that can't be improved by working on your own personal changes. For example, try seeking greater understanding by identifying with the people who are causing you the stress. In this way they become human again, no longer monsters. They'll also be more likely to listen to you and to help find a solution that will ease your stress.

Biofeedback   A relaxation technique that involves measuring and controlling physiological functions.

Hatha Yoga   An ancient exercise technique involving stretching, used today to relieve stress and induce calm.

NOTES

1. Ari Kiev, "Managing Stress to Achieve Success," *Executive Health*, 24:1 (October 1987), 1–4.
2. Kiev.
3. Marc K. Lewen and Harold L. Kennedy, "The Role of Stress in Heart Disease," *Hospital Medicine*, August 1986, pp. 125–138.
4. Randall R. Ross and Elizabeth M. Altmaier, *Intervention in Occupational Stress* (London: Sage Publications, 1994), p. 4.
5. Paul Rosch, "Good Stress: Why You Need It to Stay Young," *Prevention*, April 1986, p. 29.
6. *Time* Magazine.
7. Ari Kiev, "Managing Stress to Achieve Success," *Executive Health*, 24:1, 1987, pp. 1–4.
8. Ruthan Brodsky, "Identifying Stressors is Necessary to Combat Potential Health Problems," *Occupational Health & Safety*, pp. 30–32.
9. Michael T. Matteson and John M. Ivancevich, *Controlling Work Stress: Effective Human Resource and Management Strategies* (San Francisco: Jossey-Bass Publishers, 1987), p. 6.
10. R.C. Kessler, K.S. Kendler, A.C. Heath, M.C. Neale, and L.J. Eaves, "Social Support, Depressed Mood, and Adjustment to Stress: A Genetic Epidemiological Investigation," *Journal of Personality and Social Psychology* 62 (1992), pp. 257–272.
11. Susan Jenks: "Further Clues to CAD-Stress Link," *Medical World News*, June 13, 1988, p. 108.
12. Robert S. Eliot and Dennis L. Breo, "Are You a Hot Reactor? Is It Worth Dying For?" *Executive Health*, 20:10, 1984, pp. 1–4.
13. Susan Kripke Byers, "Organizational Stress: Implications for Health Promotion Managers," *American Journal of Health Promotion*, Summer 1987, pp. 19–32.
14. *New York Times*, March 12, 1994.
15. Friedman/Rosenman.
16. Claudia Wallis, "Stress: Can We Cope?" *Time*, June 6, 1983, pp. 48–54.
17. Peter G. Hanson, *The Joy of Stress* (Kansas City: Andrews, McMeel, and Parker, 1986).
18. Workplace Warning: Stress May Speed Brain Aging." *New Sense Bulletin*, 16:11, Aug. 1991, p. 1.
19. David Krantz, cited in John Tierney, "Stress Success and Samoa," *Hippocrates*, May/June 1987, p. 84.
20. Editors of *Prevention* Magazine, *Positive Living and Health: The Complete Guide to Brain/Body Healing and Mental Empowerment* (Emmaus, PA: Rodale Press, 1990).
21. Brendan O'Regan, Caryle Hirshberg, Nola Lewis, Barbara McNeill, and Winston Franklin, *The Heart of Healing* (Atlanta: Turner Publishing, 1993).
22. Seligman.
23. In "The Stress-Free Personality," by Betty Weider, *Shape*, July 1990, p. 18.
24. *Love, Medicine, and Miracles* (New York: Basic Books, 1987).
25. In *The Health of Nations* (New York: Basic Books, 1987).
26. Jonathon Brown, University of Washington.
27. Herbert Benson.
28. D.H. Shapiro and D. Giber, "Meditation and Psychotherapeutic Effects," *Archives of General Psychiatry*, 35 (1978), pp. 294–302.
29. Adapted from Daniel A. Girdano, George S. Everly, and Dorothy Dusek, *Controlling Stress and Tension*, 3d edition (Englewood Cliffs, NJ: Prentice Hall, 1990), p. 219.

ASSESSMENT 3-1

How Stressed Are You?

Name _____ Date _____ Grade _____

Instructor _____ Course _____ Section _____

To find out your stress level take the "stress scale" — a test developed by University of Washington researchers Thomas Holmes and Richard Rahe. The test rates life events known to produce stress. Check off the events that have happened to you in the past year. Add them up. If you score 300 or more, you are at highest risk of developing stress-induced disease.

Stress	Points	Stress	Points
1. Death of spouse	100	23. Son or daughter leaving home	29
2. Divorce	73	24. Trouble with in-laws	29
3. Marital separation	65	25. Outstanding personal achievement	28
4. Jail term	63	26. Spouse beginning or stopping work	26
5. Death of close family member	63	27. Beginning or ending school	26
6. Personal injury or illness	53	28. Change in living conditions	25
7. Marriage	50	29. Revision of personal habits	24
8. Fired from job	47	30. Trouble with boss	23
9. Marital reconciliation	45	31. Change in work hours or conditions	20
10. Retirement	45	32. Change in residence	20
11. Change in health of family member	44	33. Change in schools	20
12. Pregnancy	40	34. Change in recreation	19
13. Sexual difficulties	39	35. Change in worship activities at church or temple	19
14. Gain of new family member	39	36. Change in social activities	18
15. Business readjustment	39	37. Mortgage or loan less than $10,000	17
16. Change in financial state	38	38. Change in sleeping habits	16
17. Death of close friend	37	39. Change in number of family get-togethers	15
18. Change to different line of work	36	40. Change in eating habits	15
19. Change in number of arguments with spouse	35	41. Vacation	13
20. Mortgage over $10,000	31	42. Christmas	12
21. Foreclosure of mortgage or loan	30	43. Minor violation of the law	11
22. Change in responsibilities at work	29		

Total Points [ ]

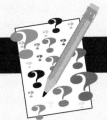

How Does Stress Affect Your Susceptibility?

Name _____ Date _____ Grade _____

Instructor _____ Course _____ Section _____

Ever wonder why tense times are often accompanied or followed by a cold, sore throat, or flu? Stress lowers resistance to infection by temporarily inhibiting some facets of the immune response. Keeping stress under control likewise may have positive results in a person's resistance against enemies such as cancer, heart disease, and accidents.

Listen to Your Body!

Some people become so accustomed to chronic stress that they fail to recognize the symptoms as abnormal. Consider stopping and listening. Your body is "talking" to you all the time about how you manifest stress. It is important to understand your own responses to pressure so you can take advantage of the positive ones and minimize the ones that work against you.

Recognizing your body symptoms and signs is a good first step to knowing your stress strengths and susceptibilities. It will also cue you to select skills and strategies that best address your needs. Complete the Symptoms of Stress activity below before reading on.

THE ART OF LISTENING TO YOUR BODY: THE SYMPTOMS OF STRESS

Circle the number that most accurately describes how often you experience each of the following symptoms or behaviors in response to stress.

1 = Rarely		2 = Sometimes		3 = Frequently	
Listen To Your Body		**Observe Your Actions**		**Listen To Your Emotions**	
Change in breathing	1 2 3	Yelling	1 2 3	Worrying	1 2 3
Rapid or abnormal pulse	1 2 3	Crying	1 2 3	Depression	1 2 3
Muscle tension	1 2 3	Hostility	1 2 3	Impatience	1 2 3
Headaches	1 2 3	Decreased productivity	1 2 3	Loneliness	1 2 3
Upset or queasy stomach	1 2 3	Use of alcohol	1 2 3	Powerlessness	1 2 3
Fatigue	1 2 3	Use of drugs	1 2 3	Boredom	1 2 3
Dry throat or sweaty palms	1 2 3	Increased smoking	1 2 3	Poor self-esteem	1 2 3
Difficulty sleeping	1 2 3	Eat more/eat less	1 2 3	Frustration	1 2 3
Frequent colds or flu	1 2 3	Forgetfulness	1 2 3	Overwhelmed	1 2 3
Total [ ]		**Total** [ ]		**Total** [ ]	

If your total in any category is greater than 10, or your total for all categories is greater than 20, there's a good chance that your symptoms and actions are controlling you. Most of us are somewhere along a spectrum: our symptoms neither totally control us, nor do we totally control our symptoms. Because it tells us where we stand, symptom recognition is one of the most important steps in gaining control over stress.

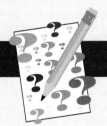

ASSESSMENT 3-3

Take Your Stress Temperature

Name _____ Date _____ Grade _____

Instructor _____ Course _____ Section _____

How Stressed Are You?

Let's play 20 questions. Check "yes" or "no" for the following:

		YES	NO
1.	Do you prefer to do everything yourself rather than let people help you?	☐	☐
2.	For you, is there only one right way to do things?	☐	☐
3.	Do you find it hard to make decisions?	☐	☐
4.	Do you forget to laugh?	☐	☐
5.	Do you never have time to daydream?	☐	☐
6.	Is it important to you that everyone likes you?	☐	☐
7.	When little things go wrong, does it ruin your whole day?	☐	☐
8.	Do you constantly feel exhausted?	☐	☐
9.	Have you had problems with insomnia?	☐	☐
10.	Do you grind your teeth?	☐	☐
11.	In the last year have you had three or more illnesses that could have been triggered by stress — headaches, diarrhea, colds, flus?	☐	☐
12.	Do you hate it when the plan changes?	☐	☐
13.	Do you get upset when you have to wait in line?	☐	☐
14.	Are you easily bored?	☐	☐
15.	Do you find it hard to say no?	☐	☐
16.	Do you hate the shape your body is in but can't seem to do anything about changing it?	☐	☐
17.	Does your life feel out of control?	☐	☐
18.	Are you resentful that so many people make demands on your time?	☐	☐
19.	Have you moved, broken up with a boyfriend/girlfriend, lost a parent, or gone through any other big changes in the last year?	☐	☐
20.	Was the last time you had a vacation over a year ago?	☐	☐

Count one point for each "yes." The closer your total is to 20, the higher your stress level. If you rate 10 or above, be sure you do *something* because, with this level of stress in your life, you have a high risk of getting sick unless you learn to manage it.

Reprinted with permission from *Shape*, 1992, April issue.

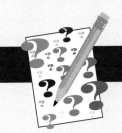

ASSESSMENT 3-4

Stress Management Skills: What Do You Do?

Name _____ Date _____ Grade _____

Instructor _____ Course _____ Section _____

For each skill, circle the number that corresponds to your typical skill use.

I use the following skills . . .	Never	Rarely	Occasionally	Regularly
Personal Management Skills: Organizing Yourself				
Valuing: Investing self appropriately				
Planning: Moving toward goals	1	2	3	4
Commitment: Saying yes and sticking to it	1	2	3	4
Time Use: Setting priorities	1	2	3	4
Pacing: Controlling the tempo	1	2	3	4
Relationship Skills: Changing The Scene				
Contact: Reaching out	1	2	3	4
Listening: Tuning in to others	1	2	3	4
Assertiveness: Saying no	1	2	3	4
Fight: Standing your ground	1	2	3	4
Flight: Leaving the scene	1	2	3	4
Nest-Building: Creating a home	1	2	3	4
Outlook Skills: Changing Your Mind				
Relabeling: Turning a spade into a diamond	1	2	3	4
Surrendering: Saying goodbye	1	2	3	4
Faith: Accepting your limits	1	2	3	4
Imagination: Laughing, creativity	1	2	3	4
Whispering: Talking nicely to oneself	1	2	3	4
Physical Stamina: Building Your Strength				
Exercise: Fine-tuning your body	1	2	3	4
Nourishment: Feeding your body	1	2	3	4
Gentleness: Wearing kid gloves	1	2	3	4
Relaxation: Cruising in neutral	1	2	3	4

Look down the column of 1's. These are your underdeveloped skills. Underline the ones you would like to use more often. **Look at the column of 4's.** These are probably your skills of habit. Mark those you tend to overuse. Which three individual coping skills do you use most often? For what kinds of stressors? As you identify your pattern of skill use, what insights and observations strike you?

Reprinted with permission from *Kicking Your Stress Habits*, copyright 1981, 1989. Donald A. Tubesing. Published by Whole Person Associates Inc., 210 West Michigan, Duluth, MN 55802, (218) 727-0500. Used by permission.

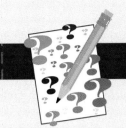

ASSESSMENT 3-5

Burnout Quiz

Name _____ Date _____ Grade _____

Instructor _____ Course _____ Section _____

Take a look at all three aspects of your life: career (school), personal, and relationships, and ask yourself the following questions. If the answer is an emphatic *yes*, score 5 points. If it's definitely no, give yourself 0 points. If you're in between, score 1 to 4 points, depending on your level of discomfort.

Score

1. I feel more negative than positive lately. ☐

2. I feel more fatigued than energetic. ☐

3. I work harder and harder and accomplish less and less. ☐

4. Joy is elusive, and I'm often invaded by a sadness I can't explain. ☐

5. I'm increasingly irritable and choosing not to be with people. ☐

6. I suffer from physical complaints (legs feel heavy, backache, headache, lingering colds). ☐

7. I'm unable to laugh at a joke about myself. ☐

8. I feel a loss of self-esteem, confidence and can-do attitude. ☐

9. Sex seems like more trouble than it's worth. ☐

10. I'm increasingly judgmental, short-tempered, and disappointed in the people around me. ☐

Total Points ☐

SCORING

    0–15: You're doing fine.

  16–25: Oops! There are things you should be watching.

  26–35: You're a candidate for burnout.

  36–45: You're burning out.

46 and over: Take special note. There are distinct threats to your health and well-being.

Reprinted with permission from *Shape*, May 1991 issue.

ASSESSMENT 3-6

Scoring Your Stress:
A Test to Pinpoint What's Eating You

Name _____Date _____Grade _____

Instructor _____Course _____Section _____

How stressed are you?

The answer depends in part on what's going on in your life. But it also depends on some other factors — like what your *attitudes* are about those events and how much control you feel over what happens.

The first step in managing stress, of course, is to *identify* it — and the test below will help you do just that. It's simple: read each question, then circle the number that most closely describes your situation or attitude. If you're completely neutral, circle **5**; if a question doesn't apply to you at all, skip it.

Ready?

Sharpen your pencil, and go to work:

1 How often do you suffer stress-related physical symptoms, such as headaches, jaw pain, neck pain, back pain, indigestion, abdominal pain, diarrhea, loss of appetite, excessive perspiration, fatigue, or a pounding in your chest?

Rarely or never   Every day

1   2   3   4   5   6   7   8   9   10

2 Do you wash your hands before you eat?

Always   Rarely or never

1   2   3   4   5   6   7   8   9   10

3 Do you take measures to keep your food safe, such as cooking it adequately, storing it properly, and avoiding obvious contaminants?

Almost always   Rarely or never

1   2   3   4   5   6   7   8   9   10

4 How often do you eat fresh fruits, fresh vegetables, whole grains, and foods high in fiber?

Every day   Rarely or never

1   2   3   4   5   6   7   8   9   10

5 How often do you eat high fat or high-sugar foods — including candy, pastry, soft drinks, and food from fast-food restaurants?

Occasionally   Every day

1   2   3   4   5   6   7   8   9   10

6 How often do you exercise?

Every day   Rarely or never

1   2   3   4   5   6   7   8   9   10

7 How many hours of sleep do you get each day?

Eight or more   Less than four

1   2   3   4   5   6   7   8   9   10

8 How many cups of coffee or caffeinated soft drinks do you drink each day?

None   Five or more

| 1 | 2 | 3 | 4 | 5 | 6 | 7 | 8 | 9 | 10 |

9 How often do you use alcohol, tobacco, over-the-counter drugs, or prescription drugs to relieve stress?

Never   Every day

| 1 | 2 | 3 | 4 | 5 | 6 | 7 | 8 | 9 | 10 |

10 If you have a relationship with a significant other, how would you describe that relationship?

Mutually satisfying in many ways   Marked by jealousy or insecurity

| 1 | 2 | 3 | 4 | 5 | 6 | 7 | 8 | 9 | 10 |

11 How do you feel when you have to say "no" to a request for your time, energy, talents, or money?

Confident and at ease   Anxious and guilt-ridden

| 1 | 2 | 3 | 4 | 5 | 6 | 7 | 8 | 9 | 10 |

12 How would you characterize your support system?

Broad-based, many sources   Limited or no sources

| 1 | 2 | 3 | 4 | 5 | 6 | 7 | 8 | 9 | 10 |

13 What kinds of friendships do you have?

At least several close friends/confidants   No close friends

| 1 | 2 | 3 | 4 | 5 | 6 | 7 | 8 | 9 | 10 |

14 What do you do if you have a problem you can't solve on your own?

Seek help immediately   Suffer on my own

| 1 | 2 | 3 | 4 | 5 | 6 | 7 | 8 | 9 | 10 |

15 How many major changes (such as entering or ending an intimate relationship, the death of a family member, a change in your financial status, moving, starting a new job, a change in sleeping habits, a change in living conditions, or a change in the number of arguments you have with roommates) have occurred in your life during the last year.

None   Many

| 1 | 2 | 3 | 4 | 5 | 6 | 7 | 8 | 9 | 10 |

16 How do you react when confronted with a problem or stressful situation?

Put it aside to gain perspective,   Feel overwhelmed
then focus on solutions   or panic-stricken

| 1 | 2 | 3 | 4 | 5 | 6 | 7 | 8 | 9 | 10 |

17 How often do you "retreat" temporarily when you start to feel overwhelmed by stress?

Most of the time   Never

| 1 | 2 | 3 | 4 | 5 | 6 | 7 | 8 | 9 | 10 |

18 How do you normally feel at the end of the day?

I got the important things done   I didn't accomplish anything

| 1 | 2 | 3 | 4 | 5 | 6 | 7 | 8 | 9 | 10 |

19 How many "hassles" do you have in a typical day?

A few   A lot

1   2   3   4   5   6   7   8   9   10

20 How much noise are you exposed to every day?

Not very much   Most of the day is noisy

1   2   3   4   5   6   7   8   9   10

21 How comfortable is your environment? (Consider temperature extremes, humidity, crowding, and environmental pollutants.)

Very comfortable   Very uncomfortable

1   2   3   4   5   6   7   8   9   10

22 Overall, how satisfying is your life?

Very satisfying   Very disappointing

1   2   3   4   5   6   7   8   9   10

Scoring

Time to take a look at your stress level. This exercise will tell you *two* things: first, it will indicate your general stress level. Then it will help pinpoint the specific things that are causing you stress.

First, total up your score by adding every number you circled. Now divide it by the number of questions you answered. This is one test on which you don't want a high score: The closer your average creeps toward 10, the higher your stress level is likely to be. (By the way, it's important to "average" your stress score this way; a high level of stress in a few areas won't cause your *general* stress level to skyrocket.

Next, go back and isolate what's causing you problems. Look back through your responses. Find those in which you circled a number higher than 5. Simple — you've found your problem areas.

Finally, determine some stress-busting strategies. Check out your problematic question number, then find the corresponding number among the tips below. The rest is up to you!

Stress-Savvy Tips

1 Obviously, stress-related physical symptoms are just that: related to stress. The best way to get rid of them is to get rid of the stress that causes them? In the meantime, there are a few things you *can* do to manage your most troublesome symptoms. **For headaches:** keep a "headache diary"; it will help you identify what triggers your headaches, a first step in prevention. Until you can do that, try deep breathing, relaxation, stretching muscles to relieve tension in your neck and jaw, or a warm bath. **For back pain:** try deep breathing combined with gentle stretching exercises, soaking in a warm bath, or meditation. **For irritable bowel syndrome:** stay away from high-fat foods, avoid caffeine (including chocolate), add fiber to your diet (eat plenty of whole grains), and try relaxation exercises. **For indigestion:** eat smaller meals more often during the day; stick to foods that are mild and easy to digest. Watching what you eat can also ease **fatigue** — eat foods rich in vitamins, potassium, calcium, iron, and zinc.

2 Washing your hands before you eat dramatically reduces your chance of picking up an infection — an obvious stressor. Other simple things you can do: Keep your hands out of your mouth, don't share eating utensils or drinking glasses, avoid contact with people you know are ill, limit sexual contact and use safe sexual practices, and make sure your immunizations are up to date.

3 You can avoid the physical stress of food-borne illness by scrubbing fruits and vegetables thoroughly; preparing raw meat on surfaces that can be easily cleaned; preparing raw meats separate from other foods; avoiding raw or rare meats or fish; cooking hamburger until it's no longer pink; boiling canned foods before you eat them; refrigerating leftovers immediately; avoiding foods that contain raw eggs; avoiding foods that are obviously spoiled; and avoiding wild nuts, berries, mushrooms, and plants unless you are certain they are edible.

4 Stress robs your body of certain nutrients — if you're under stress from *any* source, you need an extra shot of certain vitamins and minerals. Especially important are the B vitamins (found in nuts, seeds, beans, peas, meat, and whole grains), vitamin C (found in citrus fruits, green peppers, dark-green vegetables, strawberries, and tomatoes), calcium (found in milk and dairy products, citrus fruits, dark-green leafy vegetables, and dried beans), and protein (found in meat, fish, poultry, dairy products, and eggs). Don't forget that you can get a "complete" protein by combining certain plant foods — rice with legumes, wheat with soybeans, or legumes with corn, rice, wheat, or oats, for example.

5 Stress robs your body of some vital nutrients, and sugars and fats speed up the process! Sugars, in fact, tend to strip out certain B vitamins and actually make you more *susceptible* to stress. Concentrate on eating a balanced diet of foods low in fats and sugars; check labels, and steer clear of foods that list sugar in any form as the first or second ingredient. Avoid skipping meals; eat a hearty breakfast and light supper; drink plenty of water; and check with your physician about nutritional supplements if you're under a lot of stress.

6 Research proves that regular exercise diminishes the effects of stress — even stress you can't avoid. The best kind of stress-busting exercise is continuous, rhythmic, aerobic exercise — walking, running, bicycling, swimming, or cross-country skiing are good choices. To avoid injury, make sure you allow for warm-up and cool-down time. And if your joints are a little creaky from inactivity, start slowly and build up gradually. Wear light-colored clothing in the summer, and several light layers of dark-colored clothing in the winter. Drink plenty of fluid before and after you exercise. You should feel energized, not tired, when you finish exercising; you're pushing too hard if you feel a heaviness in your arms or legs, soreness in your muscles or joints, or extreme fatigue.

7 Sleep relieves stress. How? While you're asleep, you breathe more deeply, your heart slows down, your blood pressure drops, and your muscles relax. To get better sleep, review the suggestions earlier in this section; in a nutshell, try to relax for an hour or so before you go to bed, do your best to stick to a regular sleep schedule, avoid eating a big meal right before you go to sleep, and do what you can to make your sleep environment comfortable.

8 Caffeine actually *increases* your sensitivity to stress by stimulating the central nervous system, charging up the autonomic nervous system, and lowering your ability to tolerate stress. Avoid caffeine or use it only in moderation. Remember, too, that caffeine is found in more than just coffee and cola drinks — cut back on chocolate, cocoa, and over-the-counter medications that contain caffeine, too. Try drinking decaffeinated coffee or switching to a soothing herbal tea.

9 Alcohol might relax you at first — but research shows that, over the long term, alcohol actually *increases* stress by causing your body to churn out stress-related hormones. Keep a diary of your alcohol intake for a few weeks; if you're drinking too much (more than an occasionally drink, or more than 12 ounces of beer or 4 ounces of wine at a time), take measures to stop. Find some other ways to relieve stress, and try substituting another kind of drink for alcohol — exotic fruit juices or sparkling mineral water can be fun.

And don't forget tobacco: we know that smoking causes a long list of health problems. What you may not know is that smoking *combined with stress* escalates the situation. Take measures to stop; ask your doctor or the college health center about local problems that can help you quit.

10 The least stressful relationship is one in which your combination is also your *friend* — someone with whom you share your feelings, triumphs, disappointments, goals, and dreams. If appropriate, healthy sexual expression should be part of that relationship; aside from being a way to communicate within a committed relationship, the physiological processes involved in sex work to relieve stress and tension. Finally, remember that no matter how well matched you are, no two people can fill *every* need for each other; maintain separate friends and interests to avoid becoming too dependent on each other.

11 The ability to assert yourself means you usually meet your own needs without destroying interpersonal relationships. Assertive behavior allows you to protect your own rights — essential to avoiding stress. If you're not very assertive now, start by respecting yourself. You're responsible for yourself, and others need to live with your decisions. If you need to say "no," just say it; don't feel obligated to offer excuses. And remember the nonverbals that go along with it: speak in a firm, steady voice without hesitation, stand straight, and look at the other person directly in the eye.

12 The larger your network of support the better you will be able to manage stress. Ideally, your network of support should be broad, stemming from your family, church, neighborhood, school, social and political organizations, and friends. Try organizing or joining a study group (students in a class or within a major area of study), service group, sports team, hobby group, campaign team, social group, or simply a group of friends who share a favorite activity — bicycling, kite-flying, or watercolors, for example. Remember — the most valuable type of social support from groups like these often happens from the informal contacts, such as riding to a meeting with someone or getting together for dinner after the meeting.

13 Research shows that one of the best ways to prevent stress-related illness is to have good friends — people you can really talk to, people with whom you can share your joys, concerns, apprehensions, and love. If you need to expand your circle of friends, start by expanding your contacts: in other words, go where the people are. Draw people into conversation, invite people to informal get-togethers, show people you care, and get involved with others.

14 An important part of social support — and stress reduction — is your willingness to seek help when you need it *and* the assurance that there are people who can help you. Close friends can act as confidants, but you should also know that there are others in your support network to whom you can turn — a clergyman, school counselor, or therapist.

15 Research has shown that your chance of developing a stress-induced illness increase with the number of "life crises" you have during any given time. (Check the list of specific crises earlier in this section for an idea of what we're talking about.) Whenever you can, avoid too many changes at once: If you've just ended an important relationship, for example, don't move to a new apartment and start a part-time job, too. For the best coping strategy, try to anticipate likely changes — then slow down your pace, be gentle on yourself, avoid as many new commitments as you can, and stay flexible. Still another strategy is called *stress-inoculation*: in essence, you imagine —vividly — the worst thing that could happen, then map out how you'd handle it. Then, no matter what happens, you know you can do *something* to cope.

16 Your ability to *adapt* to situations and problems directly affects your ability to manage stress. Boost your odds by trying the following: Put the problem aside long enough to get perspective — what long-range effects will it have? Who does it involve? Then focus in on what you can do to solve the problem, and try to come up with several different alternatives. (Having several different plans for confronting the situation gives you flexibility and removes the anxious possibility of your *only* plan failing.) Above all, relax and keep a sense of humor; and, when you've successfully met the challenge, reward yourself for succeeding!

17 There's nothing wrong with retreat — it's a coping skill that can help you buffer the effects of stress. Don't run away from problems or avoid responsibility — that's not what we're talking about. But when you're feeling overwhelmed, buy yourself some breathing space by going for a long walk, taking in a new movie, putting together a challenging puzzle, going to lunch with a friend, reading a favorite book, or taking a nap. The key is to get a mini-escape or time-out: something that will divert your thoughts and recharge your batteries. You'll go back to the problem renewed and strong enough to handle the challenge!

18 If you want to manage stress, learn to manage your time. There are some excellent pointers earlier in this section. One of the most important tactics is prioritizing: figure out which tasks are most important, then *do those things first*. It helps to make a list of everything you need to do — then assign each a "priority" (for example, **1** for things you *must* get done today if you want to avoid problems, **2** for things that *must* be done but that could wait, and **3** for things you'd like to do but that are not essential). Start out with the things that are the highest priority; get them done first. Then move to the second category;. If you have time left over, start on the last category — but, if not, no big deal. For maximum effectiveness, schedule your time, delegate things that someone else could do for you, limit the number of interruptions you have, and plan for some breaks.

19 *Hassles* are defined as the irritants and annoyances — most of them fairly minor — that all of us encounter on a daily basis. Simply stated, they're part of living. Hassles can include things like having to wait for someone, getting caught in traffic, not being able to find a parking space, having to stand in lines, being bothered by a fly, not being able to find the book you need at the library, conflicts with a roommate, having to endure a boring professor, sleeping in and missing breakfast, or not having enough change to do laundry. One or two aren't bad. But when your day gets filled with hassles, your stress skyrockets.

There's not a lot you can do to prevent hassles — but you *can* work smart to defuse them. Think ahead; anticipate what you can. If you think you might get stuck in traffic, leave fifteen minutes early. If you know the parking on campus is a nightmare, ride the bus, ride your bike, walk, or join a carpool. If it's laundry day, stop at the bank on the way home and buy a couple of rolls of quarters. If you've had trouble finding resource materials for a paper, start early. For the rest — those things you can't circumvent — try to change your expectations. Don't expect to avoid traffic problems; don't expect to get your groceries without standing in line. If you learn to look at things differently, you'll be able to wait patiently, sit calmly, and think of something pleasant instead of getting uptight.

20   Everyone knows that noise is irritating. But did you know that *noise actually increases stress*? How? It boosts the heart rate, increases blood pressure, tenses the muscles, and causes the body to secrete stress-related hormones. At certain decibels (a jet plane engine, a pneumatic riveter, a guitar amplifier), noise can permanently damage hearing; if you're trying to concentrate on a difficult task, even a little noise can be stressful. The most stressful is noise that constantly changes in intensity, frequency, or pitch.

There's a lot you can do to reduce your stress from noise. If you can, choose an apartment away from a busy street, a convenience store, a fast-food restaurant, or an industrial area. Look for a carpeted apartment — you at least want carpet in the rooms that are directly adjacent to other units. Choose upholstered instead of hard-surfaced furniture, heavy drapes instead of aluminum blinds. Put a small foam pad under noisy appliances, such as blenders. Turn down the TV and the stereo. And, if you're exposed to chronic noise, use cotton or ear plugs to protect your ears and filter out some of the sound.

21   The environment you live in can either soothe you or add to your stress. You can't control some things — like air pollution — but you *can* clean up clutter, keep your room at the most comfortable temperature, and use adequate lighting, for example. Do whatever you can to limit your exposure to pollutants, insecticides, pesticides, food additives, gasoline exhaust, industrial wastes, and glazes or paints that contain lead.

22   You'll do best at coping with stress if you are generally satisfied: you feel some control over your life, you are able to set and meet goals, you have aspirations you believe you'll fulfill, the people closest to you are affectionate and caring, you feel valued, and you are able to make a meaningful contribution. Generally, satisfaction leads to optimism — and optimists suffer fewer symptoms of stress. If you're not optimistic and satisfied, try to figure out why. Change the things you can. Work to accept the things you can't change. Most importantly, learn to concentrate on your successes and use what you learned from them to meet your challenges head-on.

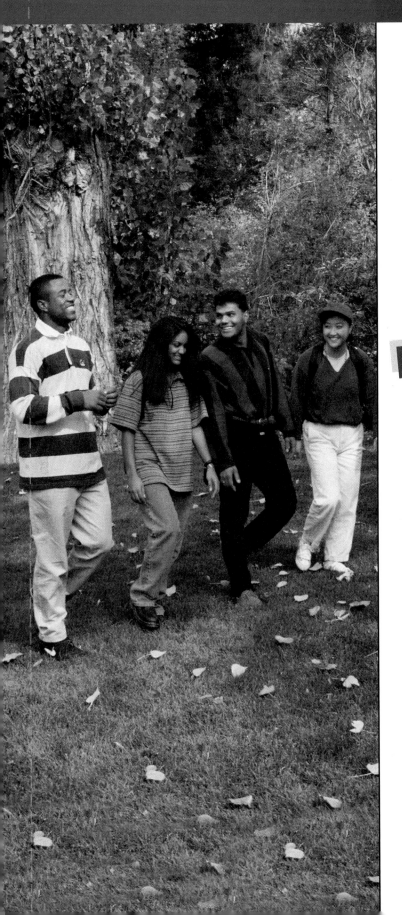

4

Social Support and Health

OBJECTIVES

■ Illustrate how social support systems contribute to health and well-being.

■ Point out the benefits of friends, confidants, and mates.

■ Understand the differences between loneliness and aloneness.

■ Know the connection between loneliness and health.

■ Become familiar with the health hazards of divorce.

■ Compare the health of divorced people with those who are unhappily married.

■ Learn the health benefits of marriage.

■ Learn how family life can contribute to the health of its members, including children.

The claim that social support is important to health is not new. What is new is the collection of hard evidence that proves the case — proof positive that social support indeed can protect people in crises from a wide variety of diseases.

A group of researchers went to Alameda County, California, and gathered data on more than 7,000 people over a 9-year period. At the end of the study, they found the common denominator that most often led to good health and long life: social support.[1] The researchers who conducted the study concluded that people with social ties — regardless of their source — lived longer than people who were isolated. And people who have a close-knit network of intimate personal ties with other people seem to be able to avoid disease, maintain higher levels of health, and in general deal more successfully with life's difficulties.

The people in the study with many social contacts — a mate, a close-knit family, a network of friends, church or other group affiliations — lived longer and had better health. People who were socially isolated had poorer health and died earlier. In fact, those who had few ties with other people died at rates two to five times higher than those with good social ties.[2] The link between social ties and death rate held up regardless of gender, race, ethnic background, or socioeconomic status.[3]

Some well-loved people fall ill and die prematurely, and some isolates live long and healthy lives. For the most part, though, people tied closely to others are better able to stay well.[4]

SOCIAL SUPPORT DEFINED

Social support consists of the resources that other people provide. It's a person's perception that he or she can count on other people for help with a problem or in time of crisis.[5]

According to University of Michigan researchers James House and Robert Kahn, the following factors are necessary to fulfill our social needs:[6]

1. *Social network:* the size, density, durability, intensity, and frequency of social contacts.

A network of social support can enhance and protect health.

2. *Social relationships:* the presence of relationships, number of relationships, and type of relationships.

3. *Social support:* the type, source, number, and quality of resources.

The resources a social network provides may come in the form of tangible, instrumental aid — lending you money, running an errand for you, studying with you. Another kind of resource that is equally important is the emotional, intangible kind of help — affection, understanding, acceptance, respect.

No one knows for certain how social support works to protect health, but two conclusions seem to be standing up to close scrutiny.

1. *Social support enhances health and well-being no matter how much stress a person is under.* The enhancement may result from an overall positive feeling and a sense of self-esteem, stability, and control over one's environment.

2. *Social support acts as a buffer against stress* by protecting a person from the diseases that often result from stress.

Strong social ties might give people still another edge in good health. The range of problems people bring to friends and neighbors is much broader than those brought to doctors, says Dr. Eva Salber, professor emeritus of Duke University's School of Medicine. Fewer than 5% of all visits to a physician are for psychological problems, she says, because we learn that if we want a doctor's attention, we must

> **Happy relationships depend not on finding the right person but on being the right person.** — Eric Butterworth

focus on a physical symptom. A woman might tell her doctor, for example, that she has a bladder infection, but she'll tell a friend that she's gotten a low grade, had a fight with her boyfriend, and has a bladder infection. What it boils down to, says Dr.

Relationships Fend Off Colds

Loners are four times more likely to come down with a cold than people rich in relationships. This is the conclusion of a study probing the mind-body connection. The study strengthens the notion that an active network of family, friends, neighbors, and even co-workers can bolster resistance to disease, perhaps by activating the immune system.

"This is the first time that anyone has directly linked personal relationships with an immunologically relevant disease outcome," said Janice Kiecolt-Glaser, clinical psychologist at the Ohio State University Medical Center.

The researchers who conducted the study, led by psychologist Sheldon Cohen of Carnegie Mellon University in Pittsburgh, cannot explain precisely why socially deprived people were comparatively worse at warding off a cold virus.

Source: "Relationships Fend Off Colds, Study Finds," Los Angeles Times, June 25, 1997.

Salber, is that most human ills are never seen by a doctor. The real primary care is provided by one's family, close friends, and neighbors.[7] These natural helpers may prove to be our most important health resource.

Early researchers who struggled to determine what sort of patient has disease found striking similarities in the circumstances of people with conditions as diverse as depression, tuberculosis, high blood pressure, multiple accidents, and even complications in pregnancy. The people who were ill usually lacked a strong supportive network or had experienced a recent disruption in their traditional social support network. The number of people in that category seems to be increasing, not decreasing. In comparing people in the United States today with those of earlier generations, a disturbing trend is evident. People today are more likely to live alone, less likely to be married, and less likely to belong to a social organization. The result is a generation of people with weaker social ties — and poorer health.

The Tenderloin Senior Outreach Project was a 10-year study delving into San Francisco's seedy Tenderloin District — a cluster of low-priced, single-room-occupancy hotels crammed with poverty-stricken elderly people.[8] The district was characterized by skyrocketing crime rates, deteriorating housing conditions, poor access to food, and remarkably bad physical and mental health among its occupants. For the study, researchers from the University of California at Berkeley School of Public Health organized weekly support groups for the elderly residents of the district. They formed Safehouse Project, in which more than 80 stores and agencies in the neighborhood became places of refuge to which residents could flee in emergencies. Buoyed by each others' strength, the residents themselves soon began working on their problems.

The results were dramatic. Several resident groups formed "mini-markets" in the lobbies of their hotels so residents had access to fresh fruit and vegetables. Other groups successfully blocked landlords' attempts to increase rents. Others were able to get the hotel food service restored. Still others succeeded in getting the City to enhance public transportation access to the district.

In the 18 months following start-up of the project, crime dropped by a startling 26%. Nutritional status of hotel residents improved dramatically. So did their physical and mental health.

The sense of control and the social networking that came out of the project have been studied and acclaimed for their health-enhancing benefits. One elderly resident checked himself into a mental institution every month or so for "reality orientation." After 2 years of involvement with the program, the habitual check-ins stopped altogether. When researchers asked him about it, he quipped, "I'm a co-leader of my hotel support group, a found of the anti-crime project, and a member of the Mayor's Task Force on Aging. I don't have time for reality!"

RESEARCH INTO SOCIAL SUPPORT

A scientific panel convened by the U.S. government found that social support not only reduced mortality but was a key to protecting health as well. According to the panel, the number and strength of an individual's close relationships are related closely to an individual's health and longevity.[9]

Individuals who lack the comfort of another human being may very well lack one of nature's most

Social support   The human resources that people provide to each other.

Finding a Support Group

You can locate a support group through your physician, psychologist, or health-care worker; through local chapters of national organizations; or through newspaper ads. To determine if a group is right for you:

- Attend one of its meetings; check out who is there and whether you feel welcome and free to participate.
- Decide whether you feel free to express your own ideas and thoughts. A good group should provide for open discussion without judgment or criticism.
- You should leave the group feeling uplifted and helped. If you are not, the group probably is not for you.

powerful antidotes to stress.[10] In summing up the results of his research, Dr. James Lynch remarked:

> The mandate to love your neighbor as you love yourself is not just a moral mandate. It's a physiological mandate. Caring is biological. One thing you get from caring for others is you're not lonely; and the more connected you are to life, the healthier you are.[11]

Nearly 3,000 adults in Tecumseh, Michigan, were the subjects of one long-term study.[12] At the beginning of the study, each adult was given a thorough physical examination to rule out any existing illness that would force a person to become isolated. Researchers then watched these people closely for the next 10 years, making special note of their social relationships and group activities. Those who were socially involved were found to have the best health. When social ties were interrupted or broken, the incidence of disease increased significantly. The researchers noticed particularly that certain conditions seemed to be related to marginal social ties. Among them were coronary heart disease, cancer, arthritis, strokes, upper respiratory infections, and mental illness. The researchers concluded that interrupted social ties seemed to actually suppress the body's immune system. Those who conducted the study called close personal relationships a safety net and said that people without this safety net are more vulnerable to a wide variety of diseases.

If we want to live longer, we need to surround ourselves with at least a few good people as friends and confidants.

Studies involving the elderly underscore the importance of social support not only to physical health but also to morale. A study of 60 women living alone in the central Appalachian area showed that the stronger the social support, the better their morale. And those with the best morale also had the best physical health.[13] In a separate study involving more than 4,700 adults aged 65 and older, even a perceived lack of social support was strongly related to depression, poorer health, and a lower quality of life.[14]

If we want to live longer, we need to surround ourselves with at least a few good people as friends and confidants. This is true across the board.[15] People who are socially isolated — unmarried, divorced, widowed, people with few friends, and people who have few church or social contacts — are three times as likely to die of a wide variety of diseases than those who have happy, fulfilling social lives. Social support is such a powerful factor in mortality that it even lowers mortality among those who are unhealthy (such as survivors of heart attacks). One reason may be its effect on the immune system. Stress generally decreases the number and function of natural killer cells and reduces the percentage of T-lymphocytes. Strong interpersonal relationships protect the functioning of the immune system, even in the face of stress.

SOCIAL CONNECTIONS AND THE HEART

Even the simplest social support seems to have a particular effect on the heart. This was shown in a landmark study in the close-knit Italian-American community of Roseto, Pennsylvania. Its residents had average incidence of exercise, cigarette smoking, obesity, high blood pressure, and stress. Their diets were higher in fat, cholesterol, and red meat than the average American diet. The men in Roseto, however, had only about one-sixth the incidence of heart disease and deaths from heart disease as random population groups in the United States. The rates for Roseto's women were even better.

The researchers concluded that the protective factor was the residents' strong sense of community and their strong social ties. Stewart Wolf, a professor of medicine at Temple University School of Medicine in Philadelphia and one of the study's researchers, reported:

> More than any other town we studied, Roseto's social structure reflected old-world values and traditions. There was a remarkable cohesiveness and sense of unconditional support within the community. Family ties were very strong. And what impressed us the most was the attitude toward the elderly. In Roseto, the older residents weren't put on a shelf; they were promoted to "supreme court." No one was ever abandoned.[16]

Sadly, when the younger generations started changing — moving away, marrying "outsiders," severing the close emotional ties to the "old neighborhood" — their physical health began to deteriorate. By the mid-1970s, the mortality and heart disease rates of the Rosetans were comparable to those in surrounding Pennsylvania communities. Tremendously strong social ties had protected the hearts of community members. When those social ties started to vanish, so did the protection.

> The experience clearly demonstrates that the most important factors in health are the intangibles — things like trust, honesty, loyalty, team spirit. In terms of preventing heart disease, it's just possible that morale is more important than jogging or not eating butter.[17]

Social support may help reduce or modify risk factors for heart disease. In one study, researchers used coronary angiography to determine the health of the coronary arteries. They found that Type A men who had strong social support were on an even par with the Type B men when it came to coronary health.[18]

Social ties play an important role in good health.

TOUCH: A CRUCIAL ASPECT OF SOCIAL SUPPORT

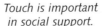

Touch is important in social support.

As important as social support is to health, perhaps one of its most powerful components is also one of its simplest: People who touch others and are touched themselves enjoy the best health. People who enjoy regular, satisfying touch — a pat on the back, a hug — enjoy health benefits as a result. The good health that emanates from touch is both psychological and physical. Those who are touched have stronger hearts, lower blood pressure, lower stress levels, and less overall tension.

LONELINESS AND HEALTH

Loneliness has been characterized as an unpleasant experience that occurs when a person's network of social relationships is significantly deficient in either quality or quantity.[19] Loneliness is not necessarily a consequence of living alone. Of the more than 22,000 American adults responding to a survey in five major newspapers, almost a fourth of those who lived alone fell into the "least lonely" category.[20] On the other hand, loneliness can exist even when we're surrounded by people. Loneliness is associated less with the number of people in our lives than the satisfaction with those relationships. Loneliness sets in when our current relationships fall short of our ideal.[21]

Feelings of loneliness are worse when the lonely person is surrounded by people who don't seem to be lonely — people who seem to have interpersonal attachments — or when the lonely person has low self-esteem. And, though loneliness can stem from lack of attachment to someone else, it can be just as intense as if the person has a sense of not belonging within an accepting community. Factors that help determine when someone is alone is also lonely are general attitude, boredom, and attitude toward self.

Even though being alone doesn't necessarily mean people are lonely, many people who are alone *are* lonely. And more people than ever are living

Loneliness A condition that occurs when a person's network of social relationships is significantly deficient in either quality or quantity.

Landmark Spiegel Study

Dr. David Spiegel is a well-known figure in researching the mind-body connection. He conducted a landmark study with women whose breast cancer had metastasized. One group was given counseling and social support in addition to the proper medical care. The comparison group of women received only the appropriate medical care without the counseling or peer support. The latter group reported more pain and did not live as long as the group that had received social support from friends and family.

Source: *Healing and the Mind*, by Bill Moyers (New York: Doubleday, 1993), p. 157.

their living arrangements affected their health. They found that patients who lived by themselves were nearly twice as likely to have another attack, or die of one, within 6 months.[26] None of the known risk factors for second heart attacks — advanced age, low socioeconomic status, and severe heart damage — accounted for the ill health of those who lived alone. Nearly 16% of that group had another heart attack within 6 months. Only 9% of the patients who shared living quarters were stricken. Led by Dr. Robert Case of Manhattan's St. Luke's-Roosevelt Hospital, the study suggests that human contact may subtly affect heart function, or simply may improve one's chances of getting quick medical attention in an emergency. In any case, these people didn't live alone.

alone — more than 20 million in the United States alone. Between 1950 and 1980 the figure rose by 385%. The most radical change has been in the number of men living alone: today, slightly more than 25% of adult men live alone. More than 23% of the households in the United States now are headed by singles; 85% of the single-parent households are headed by women.[22]

Loneliness carries with it a big risk for health problems. James Lynch says loneliness is "the greatest unrecognized contributor to premature death in the United States."[23] Loneliness, and the stress that accompanies it, has been connected not only to premature death but to a host of physical and mental disorders as well. People who are not lonely have a better chance of staying healthy or recovering from disease than people who are lonely.

Loneliness is a more prevalent and serious problem among adolescents than any other age group.[24] As loneliness increases, so do psychological and physical problems. One study of 325 adolescents aged 12 to 21 showed that loneliness correlated strongly with introspection, a poor perception of health, and a number of physical symptoms including headaches, nausea, sleep disorders, and eating disorders. Adolescent girls had more health problems related to loneliness than did adolescent boys.[25]

Researchers at three hospitals in New York state followed 1,200 heart-attack survivors to see whether

> *I find there is a quality to being alone that is incredibly precious. Life rushes back into the void, richer, more vivid, fuller than before. It is as if in parting one did actually lose an arm. And then, like starfish, one grows it anew; one is whole again, complete and round — more whole, even, than before, when the other people had pieces of one.*
>
> — Anne Morrow Lindbergh

The Importance of Good Friends

Close friendships clearly buffer stress and help overcome the health effects of loneliness. Friendship involves certain attitudes that may in themselves help boost health.[27] Friends enjoy trust, respect, and acceptance. A friend accepts you as you are, without trying to make you into a different person. Friends support and help each other, act in the other's best interests, and have a deep sense of what is important to the other. Friends share feelings and experiences with each other that they don't share with other people. And, despite occasional

Loneliness and the Immune System

Bill Moyers interviewed David Felten, Professor of Neurobiology and Anatomy at the University of Rochester, about loneliness and health. Loneliness consistently emerges as a predictor of diminished immune response in patients, leaving them vulnerable to a number of diseases. For example, in one study involving medical students, those who said they were lonely and had poor social support also had chronically diminished immune responses.

Source: *Healing and the Mind*, by Bill Moyers (New York: Doubleday, 1993), pp. 220–221.

annoyance or anger, friends enjoy each other most of the time.

Friends contribute to health by providing all the functions of the family. In some cases, friends may be closer confidants than family members are. And people who are able to build close relationships with friends have greater health protection against stress.

James Pennebaker, a professor of psychology at Southern Methodist University in Dallas, believes that confiding — having a confidant — forges a powerful and lasting bond and can provide many health benefits. He warns, however, of some risks involved in confiding and urges that you consider the following before you begin to confide in someone:[28]

- Realize your friendship may be at risk. In most cases, confiding in someone helps the two of you grow closer. Your friend, however, might feel threatened or hurt by what you say, changing the nature of the relationship.

- Recognize that your own traumas may traumatize the listener, too. If the information you

Loneliness is a factor that may increase the risk of disease and health problems.

divulge is upsetting enough, the listener may be so burdened by what you say that he or she, in turn, may need to tell someone else.

- Understand that what you say and how you say it depends on how your confidant reacts to you. In the best possible situation, your friend will allow you to express all your feelings and frustrations freely without judging or criticizing you.

- Realize that you might have a twisted motive for confiding in a certain person. A surprising number of people confide out of revenge (You hurt me, so I'm going to hurt you). You know why you should choose someone as a confidant. Revenge, anger, and hurt are *not* good reasons.

- Recognize that there might be a better way to solve a problem than disclosing or confiding. You might be able to take direct action, for example. If so, do it. Don't spend your time and energies discussing your grievances instead.

The Importance of Pets

Comfort does not always have to come only from people. Pets fulfill a variety of needs for their human owners. They provide a chance for interaction with another living thing and fulfill the natural craving for emotional relationships. They meet our need to care and our desire to be loved. As anyone who owns a pet knows, pets also give affection in return.

The University of Pennsylvania's Center for Interaction of Animals and Society showed that coronary disease patients with pets had one-third the death rate of people who did not have pets. The patients actually had lower heart rates when they were with their pets. The researchers concluded that "even small reductions in the heart rate repeated thousands of times per week could provide direct health benefits by decreasing the frequency of arterial damage, and thus slowing the arteriosclerotic process."[29]

Even though the health benefits of pets are obvious, that doesn't mean you should rush into pet ownership without weighing the pros and cons. Owning a pet requires a tremendous commitment, and you have to be in a position to handle it before you take on the care of a pet.

Developing a Lasting Relationship

Here are some things you can do to develop a lasting friendship with someone you care about:

- Start with someone you feel close to or *want* to feel close to.

- Learn trust. It's tough to face possible rejection when you let someone in on your deepest secrets, but a true friend will love and accept you regardless of your flaws.

- Be willing to share your most personal thoughts and feelings, as well as your time, your possessions, and other things that are important to you.

- Spend plenty of time together; it's what helps you develop a closeness. If you have to, make adjustments in your schedule.

- Be a good listener. Your friend needs a confidant, too.

What is the downside to owning a pet? Consider some of the following:

- Pets cost money. There's the initial expense of purchasing the pet, plus bills for food and for veterinarian expenses (inoculations, neutering or spaying, and inevitable illnesses). Added to those are the expenses of licensing your pet and purchasing any related paraphernalia, such as food bowls, collars, and leashes.

- Pets also can ruin carpets and furniture, dig up flowers or shrubs, and damage other personal items.

Tips For Action   Choosing the Right Pet

Pets provide rewards, but they also require attention! Carefully consider your schedule and the demands on your time before you choose a pet. You can expect the following from these pets:

- **Birds, fish, hamsters, guinea pigs.** These and other similar pets require much less time and direct care than dogs and cats. You have to make sure they have food and you have to clean their cages or bowls. Although these kinds of pets require less care, they also provide less intense interaction.

- **Cats.** Cats require more care than the pets listed above, but less care than dogs. You can leave a large amount of water and dry food if you need to be gone for extended periods, and a cat will do just fine. You also can train cats to use an indoor litter box, so cats can adapt to staying indoors. Cats preen themselves, so they do not need grooming and do not require you to provide exercise. Cats can adjust to even a small apartment. Even though they provide interaction, they also can be independent.

- **Dogs.** Dogs offer the most intense interaction and also require the most care. They must be fed at the same time each day, must be exercised twice a day, and must be groomed several times a month. Larger dogs need plenty of space for exercise, and you must clean up after dogs.

- Some pets are difficult to housebreak. You can overcome this by purchasing a pet that is housebroken already, but you should expect some minor accidents as the pet adjusts to its new surroundings.

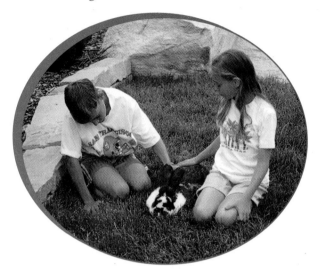

Pets can help meet our need and desire to be loved.

- A pet can interfere with *your* independence. If you have a dog, for example, and want to travel for a week, you have to take the dog with you or pay to board the dog at a kennel or pay someone to come to your home and care for the dog every day.

- Pets can generate anxiety and concern. Many pet owners fear their pets will be injured or get sick. Pets also die eventually, which means a period of bereavement as you grieve the loss of your pet.

Irrespective of the downsides, owning a pet has great advantages in addition to the health benefits already discussed, including the following:

- Pets bring cheerfulness, play, and laughter to your life. There's nothing like watching a cat get intoxicated on a catnip mouse!

- Pets help boost your self-esteem. After a hard day away from home, when all the world seems to be against you, a bounding greeting from your dog is quite a treat.

- If you choose a pet that needs exercise, your own exercise will increase, too. You're the one who has to walk the dog twice a day.

- Some pets, such as watchdogs, can contribute to your safety.

MARRIAGE AND HEALTH

For the first time since 1990 and only the second in a decade, the U.S. marriage rate rose slightly in 1994 (see Figure 4.1). A good marriage can help protect people from illness and disease, help them bounce back more quickly if they do get sick, and even help people live longer. Divorced people and those who are unhappily married don't fare nearly as well in terms of health and long life.

What does "happily married" mean?[30]

1. The partners find their prime source of joy in each other, but they maintain separate identities. They are independent; they have outside interests and hobbies that don't depend on their partner.

2. They are generous and giving out of love, not because they expect repayment or are keeping score.

3. The partners enjoy a healthy and vigorous sexual relationship.

4. The partners fight — that's right! — in a constructive way. For people in a healthy marriage, verbal fighting offers a chance to air feelings and frustrations without implying that the other person is wrong or at fault.

5. The partners communicate with each other openly and honestly. There's a risk in it, but experts claim it's worth the risk.

6. The two partners in the marriage trust each other. Even after a lapse in the relationship, trust can be reestablished if both work at it.

7. Both partners talk about their future together, a future they will share because they want to. They

> *Marriage is our last, best chance to grow up.*
> — Joseph Barth

may dream about a house on the beach, a vacation to Europe, or a child they want to have late in their 30s. This kind of planning and talking indicates that both people intend to be together later on — again, because they want it more than anything else.

Health Hazards of Divorce

As a country, the United States has the highest divorce rate in the world, between 50% and 55%. The divorce rate in the United States almost doubled between 1965 and 1995.[31] The parents of more than 1 million children divorce in the United States each year. About 23% of America's children and 40% of America's Black children spend at least part of their formative years in post-divorce, single-parent families.[32] Increasingly, too, children are being subjected to a second divorce during their childhood.

A number of factors lead to divorce in today's society. Consider the following:

- Divorces are easier to get today than ever before. Many states have no-fault divorces, in which one partner does not have to prove the other is to blame. In some states, "do-it-yourself divorce kits" enable couples to split property and even custody without the assistance of an attorney.

- The strong social stigma against divorce three or four decades ago no longer exists.

- Many people go into marriage without the proper preparation. The resulting unrealistic expectations can make adjustment to marriage extremely difficult. An amazing number of couples think they should never argue, for example, when in reality constructive fighting is a characteristic of a healthy relationship. As a result, they abandon the marriage when they begin fighting.

- A large percentage of married women work outside the home, making them less financially dependent on their husbands and thus making divorce a less devastating option.

Perhaps because of the emotional repercussions, divorce seems to pose particular health hazards. Men and women who are separated or divorced have poorer physical health than do comparable widowed, married, or single adults. Of all these

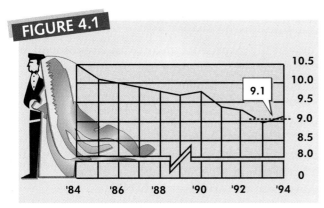

FIGURE 4.1

10.5
10.0
9.5
9.0
8.5
8.0
0

9.1

'84   '86   '88   '90   '92   '94

Marriages per 1,000 population.

groups, the divorced have the most medical complaints, chronic medical conditions, and overall disability, even when taking age, race, and income into account.

People who are divorced — and others who are separated from their mates — experience more mental and physical illness than those who are married. Psychologically, divorce is related significantly to depression, alcoholism, increased incidence of traffic accidents and accidental death, higher rates of admission to psychiatric facilities, and more suicides and homicides. Physically, divorced people have higher rates of cancer, heart disease, diabetes, pneumonia, and high blood pressure than do married, single, or widowed persons.

Negotiating an Argument

If you find yourself in an argument with someone important to you, try the following negotiation tactics to avoid a "knock-down, drag-out":

■ State your needs or wants clearly. If you've already given up something, say so.

■ Ask your partner to do the same; communication has to be open and honest.

■ Listen carefully and honestly until your partner is ready to listen to you.

■ Figure out whether your needs or wants are compatible. If they are, the argument is over! If not, you have four choices:

1. Both of you can maintain your position. That's okay, as long as it doesn't happen all the time.

or

2. You can compromise. Both of you get a little of what you want.

or

3. Both of you get *all* of what you want, but you take turns. You might get everything you wanted tonight, and your partner might get everything he or she wanted tomorrow night.

or

4. You can *freely* give up on your position in deference to the other person. That's okay, too, as long as you're doing it freely and as long as it doesn't happen all the time either.

Factors Leading to a Happy Marriage

Your attitudes about marriage and the person you choose to marry determine how happy you'll be. Your marriage is more likely to be happy if you *both* want the marriage to succeed and you share the following attitudes about marriage with your partner:

■ Marriage is a long-term commitment (we're in this for good).

■ Marriage is a spiritual, sanctified institution between two people.

Your chances for marital happiness are highest if you marry:

■ Your best friend.

■ Someone you genuinely *like* as a person.

■ Someone who grows more interesting to you as time goes on.

■ Someone who shares your basic dreams, goals, and aspirations.

Divorce actually can compromise the immune system, which helps explain why illness and death rates are higher among divorced people. This is especially apparent the first year following divorce. A study of divorced or separated women during the first year following divorce or separation showed that they had poor cellular immune function, a lower number of natural killer cells, and a deficit in the ability to fight disease with responsive lymphocytes.[33]

Children of divorce are often the ones who suffer the most profoundly. Divorce is one of the most disruptive of all life events for children, and it leads to changes in their biological health. Children almost universally experience divorce as a profound personal, familial, and social loss. In addition to health problems, most children involved in divorce suffer emotional and behavioral changes that also can impact health.

Children of divorce visit health clinics and physicians more often. Some childhood cancers and other alterations in physical health as a result of injury have been associated strongly with divorce. Divorce is particularly damaging to a child's emotional and physical health if it involves a move.

Divorce Versus Unhappy Marriage Versus Happy Marriage

Unhappily married people may be the worst off in terms of good health and long life. Research results from a number of cross-sectional studies are all saying the same thing: Unhappily married people have poorer health then their single counterparts, even the ones who are divorced.[34]

Preliminary evidence shows that actual physical damage occurs during marital conflict. Marital conflict apparently causes a sharp increase in blood pressure, a much higher risk for all kinds of illness, and reduced functioning of the immune system. Interactions characterized by hostility, sarcasm, and blame (refusing to take responsibility and demeaning the other partner) seem to be the most damaging. Not surprising, marital dissatisfaction has a real bearing not only on physical health, but on mental health as well.

> ❝ *The great secret of a successful marriage is to treat all disasters as incidents and none of the incidents as disasters.* — Harold Nicholson ❞

The greatest benefits regarding health and long life come to those who are happily married. They seem healthier, overall, than any other group. The health benefits of marriage result from a number of factors: good integration into the community, social support, the tendency to eat more regular and nutritionally balanced meals, and higher economic status.

One study looked at a group of students enrolled in a theological seminary in Australia. Those who had the strongest, happiest marriages when they entered the seminary had the lowest levels of accumulated stress by the end of their first year of study. Even though the students all had the same perceived quality of health, time, finances, housing, and neighborhood, a happy marriage contributed significantly to health, whereas friendships outside the marriage did not have the same effect.[35]

FAMILIES AND HEALTH

A **family** is a group that shares common goals and values and works together to achieve those goals. A family may be a dual-career family, a single-parent family, or a "bi-nuclear family" (in which the father and mother no longer live together but both provide a place for the children). What goes on in a family — the relationships between its members — can have a profound effect on the health and longevity of each member.

How children are perceived in the family can have great impact, even on their physical growth. According to researcher Leonard Sagan, "Children raised in an affectionate environment grow more rapidly and reach greater size as adults. On the other hand, there is ample evidence that emotional deprivation can have a deleterious effect on growth."[36]

Health Problems in Weak or Stressed Families

Health problems can be traced to weak or stressed families, and many of those families have characteristics that help us identify them. Physical symptoms of stress in the family include:

— stuttering
— bed-wetting
— nail-biting
— burnout, in which the family becomes a burden instead of a joy
— lack of communication between family members
— "controlled" arguments in which true disagreements are buried in silence
— too-tight or too-loose construction of the family
— lack of affection
— sexual infidelity

The top 10 stressors for families are said to be:[37]

1. Economics
2. Children's behavior, discipline, and sibling fighting
3. Insufficient couple time
4. Lack of shared responsibility within the family
5. Communicating with children
6. Insufficient "me" time for individual members
7. Guilt for not accomplishing more
8. Poor spatial relationships

Family A unique cluster of people who enjoy a special relationship by reason of love, marriage, procreation, and mutual dependence.

9. Insufficient family play time

10. An overscheduled family calendar.

Marital stress and tension, troubled family life, and other problems in the family unit can be a direct cause of illness and stress in individual family members. A study conducted at Duke University Medical Center indicated that, in general, people from weak families tend to have weak health. Families that were weak in structure and support produced people with more symptoms, impaired physical health, and weakened emotional health.[38]

The Health Benefits of Strong Families

Just as weak or stressed families can contribute to illness, strong families can contribute to good health and long lives. And just as weak families show signs of distress, healthy families have characteristic signs. Strong families show:

— positive listening and communication
— strong feelings of affirmation and support
— respect for all family members
— high levels of trust
— great enjoyment of each other
— positive and equal interaction
— plenty of leisure times together

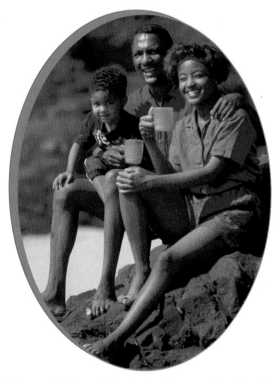

A strong family contributes to a long and healthy life.

Tips For Action

Twelve Ways to Build Strong Family Values

1 Eat together as a family as often as possible, certainly several full family dinners a week. Involve everyone (for example, younger children can set the table and older ones can clear up).

2 Hold weekly gatherings to plan family activities, trips, and vacations, and discuss immediate and persistent problems.

3 Schedule daily stress-reduction periods when the entire household is quiet — no TV or CDs. According to your family values, read, meditate, pray, exercise, or whatever works for your family.

4 Volunteer time and talent to worthy causes in the church or community.

5 Participate in school. Become involved with teachers and administrators. Help with after-school and summer programs.

6 Do recreational activities as a family. Take walks, bike rides together.

7 Make or build things together. Share creative activities, and let children take the lead in some of these. Go for accomplishment, not perfection.

8 Take organized trips to sporting events, concerts, local fairs. Include everyone.

9 Bring children to work on occasion to let them see their parents' life away from home.

10 At least once a year travel away from home. Discuss vacation ideas with children.

11 Limit TV watching. Watch TV with children, monitor what they watch, and discuss what they see.

12 Stay involved. Keep informed about community and national issues that concern you and your children. Let children know your concerns and opinions, and listen to theirs.

Copyright by Dr. Benjamin Spock, in *A Better World for Children* (New York: National Press Books, 1994); excerpted from the *Denver Post*.

— shared responsibility among family members

— a strong sense of right and wrong

— traditions and rituals

— a strong religious core

— respect for the privacy of all family members

— service to others, both within and outside the family circle

— the ability to solve problems.

Individuals in a healthy family have lower stress levels, significantly less illness, and the ability to recover from illness and disease much more rapidly than those in unhealthy families. A strong family helps an individual cope with stress, reducing the risk of illness and disease. Evidence of the buffering effect of healthy families abounds. Because children experience less stress from hospital visits when parents are there, many hospitals now allow parents to stay in the room with sick infants and children. People in strong families recover more quickly from surgery, tend to follow medical instructions, maintain treatment recommendations, take prescribed medications, and get better more quickly with fewer complications. People in strong families also tend to manage chronic illness better. They tend to live longer than people in weak families or people without children.

To Have or Not to Have Children?

Should your family include children? That's a difficult question that depends on you, your partner, your lifestyle, and your goals. Before you decide whether to have children:

■ Talk openly and honestly with your partner. Is your relationship healthy? Do you both want a child? If one partner wants a child and the other doesn't, but caves in from pressure or a desire to make the other person happy, problems could result.

■ Discuss your philosophies about children. You should share pretty much the same views about discipline and techniques for rearing

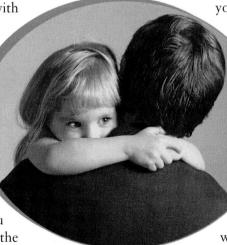

The decision to have a child should be given thought and care.

How to Develop Parenting Skills

If you're thinking about becoming a parent, parent education is available — and well worth the effort. You'll find out ahead of time what to expect, how to react, and how you can best build a healthy relationship between you and your child. To find a parent education course, check the following:

■ Local public schools

■ Local churches or synagogues

■ Local community centers

■ Local institutions offering adult education courses, including school districts and local colleges

■ YMCA

■ Your physician or health-care provider

---

children. What about religion? Do you share the same religious views? If not, in which church will the child be reared?

■ Consider *why* you want to have a child. If you want to share your life with someone and want to share your love, that's fine. It's not so fine to help to realize a goal or dream through a child that you couldn't realize on your own, or to have a child because you're being pressured. Worst of all is to have a child because you hope the child will make you happy or take care of you.

■ Consider your lifestyle carefully. If you're both working, do you both want to keep working after you have a child? How will that impact you? If one of you decides to quit, can you get along on just one income? If you both decide to keep working, can you afford day care, and how will you work it out? If you're going to school, will having a child interfere with your education? Are you ready to give up some of your freedom and independence in making a commitment to a child?

■ Assess your personal characteristics. How do you express yourself when you're angry? Would you take it out on a child? Are you a person who gives love easily? Can you share? Do you enjoy teaching other people? Do you get along pretty well with your parents and your brothers and sisters? Most important, do you like children? If you've been miserable around children, you might need to take a hard look at your own decision to become a parent.

LOSS, GRIEF, AND HEALTH

For more than 2,000 years people have recognized that **grief** can make people sick. Even longer ago, philosophers and physicians knew that grief alone could kill. Today, loss and the grief that follows it still are recognized as a precursor to distress, depression, and disease. Loss even has been implicated in premature death.

In one study, Dr. Arthur Schmale studied 42 consecutive patients admitted to the Rochester Memorial Hospital with conditions as diverse as cardiovascular disease and skin problems. He interviewed each regarding the events that led up to the illness and found a common thread: loss. Approximately three-fourths of the patients had developed their disease within a week after the loss of a loved one. The loss led to feelings of helplessness and hopelessness, and illness followed.[39]

Loss seems to have a particularly strong influence in the development of cancer. A vast number of long-range studies point to loss and the grief that follows it as a contributing factor in cancer. Renowned general and pediatric surgeon Bernie Siegel, well-known for his work with cancer patients, said:

> One of the most common precursors of cancer is a traumatic loss or a feeling of emptiness in one's life. When a salamander loses a limb, it grows a new one. In an analogous way, when a human being suffers an emotional loss that is not properly dealt with, the body often responds by developing a new growth. It appears that if we can react to loss with personal growth, we can prevent growth gone wrong within us.[40]

Some kinds of loss are especially devastating. For the elderly, loss of possessions

Grieving increases our vulnerability to illness but social support can lessen the chances of a negative physical response to loss.

What's "Normal" Grief?

When you experience a loss significant enough to cause grief, you can expect the following:

■ *For the first few days*, you'll be in a state of shock and denial. It probably will be difficult to accept the loss, and you're likely to feel numb. You'll probably cry a lot during this time, too, which usually lasts about 3 days.

■ *For the next 2 or 3 months*, you'll go through a series of emotions — including anger. You may "bargain" with God, offering all kinds of things in exchange for what was lost. You'll feel sad, tearful, and preoccupied. You may have vivid memories of the lost person and may even sense his or her presence. You may lose your appetite, as well as interest in things you used to enjoy. These feelings generally peak about a month after the loss and usually last for 3 or 4 months but can last as long as a year.

■ *Within a year after the loss*, you'll be able to resume your ordinary activities and will be able to generate happy memories about the lost person. You'll feel sad less often and finally will be able to resolve the loss within yourself.

poses high risk for illness. Parents who lose children are at risk, as are children who lose parents. The loss of a parent through death, separation, or divorce can lead to later health problems. From what researchers can determine, *early* loss of a parent is associated with both physical and psychological illness. One study of cardiac patients in Philadelphia revealed that a significant number of the coronary disease patients had lost their fathers, most of them between the time they were 5 and 17 years old.[41]

Stages in Grieving

Grief is necessary to healing. For grief to progress "normally," a person needs to pass systematically through six stages:

1. Denial
2. Anger
3. Bargaining

4. Depression

5. Acceptance

6. Hope for the future

> *The human spirit has an innate ability to bounce back from loss and despair.*

Those stages don't occur in rapid-fire succession. The average recovery time from a major loss ranges from 18 to 24 months.

Grieving is hard work, but it's essential when suffering a significant loss. People who don't go through the stages of grieving can get stuck in a stage and experience what professionals call "abnormal grief." The result can be serious illness and premature death.

In the denial stage of grief, the person literally can't believe the loss happened. That kind of denial should last only a few days. After that, it's necessary to face up to the loss and admit that it happened. In the case of death, attending a funeral service, viewing the body, and hearing tributes to the person's life help mourners accept the reality of the death.

Even though memories of the lost person will remain, the bonds with the person have to be severed. This is why grieving individuals box up or give away shoes, clothing, and personal possessions.

Grieving saps a tremendous amount of emotional and physical strength. As soon as feasible, grieving individuals should get active in something they really enjoy. They might develop a new interest or hobby.

Tips For Action Coping With Loss

- Try to keep things in your life as *status quo* as possible. Avoid other things that could cause stress right now, such as a new job, a vacation, or moving to a new house or apartment.

- Postpone decisions that can wait until later. You'll be thinking more clearly, and won't be reacting under duress.

- Keep in touch with other people. Social support is especially important now. Let other people express their concern and help you out.

- Avoid the temptation to use drugs or alcohol to ease your feelings of grief; they only make things worse.

- Believe in yourself and your ability to recover. You have the right to go through the stages of grief, so don't be too hard on yourself.

This helps them move on and gives them something pleasant to look forward to.

Bereavement is a special kind of grief. The intense and pivotal grief involved in bereavement has been shown to pose significant health risks, ranging all the way from immune system disorders to sudden deaths and increased death rates from all causes.

Immune Disorders

Immune system disorders associated with bereavement include a lower activity level of lymphocytes, diminished natural killer cell activity, and feeble T-cell strength, among others. One source of immune system dysfunction during bereavement may be a simple hormone. During periods of active mourning, **corticosteroid** levels increase vastly. In the bloodstream, corticosteroids put a damper on the immune

Protecting Your Immune System While You Grieve

To keep your immune system in shape:

- Get plenty of rest. Take naps if you need them, and try to maintain your normal sleep pattern at night.

- Eat a balanced diet: three solid meals a day with choices from all four food groups. When you feel hungry in between meals, eat low-fat snacks high in complex carbohydrates.

- Get plenty of fluids, but avoid those that contain alcohol or caffeine. Both alcohol and caffeine increase dehydration.

- Exercise regularly. Choose an activity you enjoy, and do it for at least half an hour at least three times a week. Bicycling, walking, and swimming are good choices.

Above all, *stay connected to other people!* Social support is especially important during grief to keep your immune system healthy.

Grief   The overwhelming sorrow that follows a loss.

Bereavement   The process of "disbonding" from someone who played an important role in one's life and is now gone.

Corticosteroid   A hormone released during stress that affects immunity.

system's antibody response, preventing the immune system from completely kicking into gear. This lowers the immune response and increases susceptibility to all kinds of illnesses.

Sudden Deaths

Those who are mourning a loss have a higher than expected rate of sudden death. In one study, researchers investigated sudden deaths among Eastman Kodak employees in Rochester, New York. In at least half of the sudden deaths studied, the deaths were preceded by the departure of the last or only child in the family for college or marriage.[42]

In another study, Dr. George Engle studied newspaper reports of sudden deaths in the Rochester area over 6 years. In more than half of the sudden deaths he investigated, he was able to document that the death was immediately preceded by some kind of interpersonal loss. In men and women alike, most of the deaths occurred after the collapse or death of a loved one, during acute grief (within 16 days of the loss), or during the threat of loss of a loved one. Many of the deaths were of young, apparently healthy people.[43] Several interesting studies involving twins have shown that when one twin dies, the other twin, though healthy, dies within minutes or hours.

General Mortality Rates

When considering all causes of death, bereaved people have a much higher death rate than people of the same age whose mates are living. Although the exact statistics vary according to the specific study, the results are the same: People who are widowed are more likely to die early.

In addition to findings that death rates are higher overall for bereaved people, studies reveal unusually high death rates for certain conditions. Bereaved women tend to die more often than expected from cancer, heart disease, tuberculosis, cirrhosis, and alcoholism. Bereaved women over age 60 have a higher death rate from accidents, suicide, and diabetes. Bereaved men have a higher risk of dying from heart disease, tuberculosis, influenza, pneumonia, cirrhosis, alcoholism, accidents, and suicide.

The best protection for the bereaved is good social support, strong religious beliefs, rituals, and a conviction that one can control the bereavement. These factors all increase the odds of good health and long life.

NOTES

1. *The Complete Guide to Your Emotions and Your Health,* Emrika Padus (Emmaus, PA: Rodale Press, 1986).

2. "The Social Component of Health," Meredith Minkler, *American Journal of Health Promotion,* Fall 1986, pp. 33–38.

3. "The Social Component of Health."

4. *The Healing Web,* Marc Pilisuk and Susan Hillier Parks (Hanover, NH: University Press of New England, 1986).

5. "Social Support and Physical Illness," Sheldon Cohen, *Advances,* 7:1 (1990); original source, *Healthy Psychology,* 7:3 (1988).

6. "Social Support and Physical Illness."

7. In "The Invisible Health Care System," by Tom Ferguson, January/February 1988.

8. *The Healing Brain: A Scientific Reader,* Robert Ornstein and Charles Swencionis, editors (New York: Guilford Press, 1990).

9. *The Health of Nations,* Leonard A. Sagan (New York: Basic Books, 1987).

10. *The Broken Heart: The Medical Consequences of Loneliness* (New York, Basic Books, 1977).

11. In *People Who Need People Are the Healthiest People: The Importance of Relationships,* by Brent Q. Hafen and Kathryn J. Frandsen (Provo, UT: Behavioral Health Associates).

12. *People Who Need People.*

13. "Functional Health, Social Support, and Morale of Older Women Living Alone in Appalachia," Janet M. Collins and Penelope B. Paul, *Journal of Women & Aging,* 6:3 (1994), pp. 39–51.

14. "Social Support as a Mediator in the Relation Between Functional Status and Quality of Life in Older Adults," Jason T. Newsom and Richard Schulz, *Psychology and Aging,* 11:1 (1996), pp. 34–44.

15. "Social Support and Physical Illness."

16. *People Who Need People.*

17. *People Who Need People.*

18. "Friendship: Heart Saver for Type A's," *Men's Health,* November 1987, p. 4.

19. "Loneliness: A Healthy Approach," *Longevity,* April 1990, p. 22.

20. Boris Blai, "Health Consequences of Loneliness: A Review of the Literature," *JACH,* January 1989, p. 162.

21. *The Complete Guide to Your Emotions and Your Health.*

22. U.S. Bureau of the Census, *Statistical Abstract of the U.S.: 1993* (Washington, DC: U.S. Government Printing Office, 1993).

23. *People Who Need People.*

24. "Health Consequences of Loneliness in Adolescents," Noreen E. Mahon, Adela Yarcheski, and Thomas J. Yarcheski, *Research in Nursing and Health,* 16 (1993), pp. 23–31.

25. *"Health Consequences of Loneliness in Adolescents."*

26. "Living Alone Could Shorten Your Life," *Newsweek,* February 3, 1992.

27. *Contemporary Human Sexuality,* J. Turner and L. Rubinson, (Englewood Cliffs, NJ: Prentice Hall, 1993), p. 457.

28. J. W. Pennebaker et al., *Psychosomatic Medicine,* 51 (September-October 1989), p. 577.

29. Shelley Levitt, "Take Two Poodles and Call Me in the Morning," *50 Plus,* July 1988, pp. 56–61.

30. *Positive Living and Health: The Complete Guide to Brain/Body Healing and Mental Empowerment,* Editors of *Prevention* magazine (Emmaus, PA: Rodale Press, 1990), p. 154.

31. National Center for Health Statistics, 1995.

32. U.S. Bureau of the Census, 1993.

33. *Social Support: An Interactional View,* by Barbara R. Sarason, Irwin G. Sarason, and Gregory R. Pierce (New York: John Wiley and Sons, 1990), p. 257.

34. *Social Support,* p. 258.

35. "Relational Resources as Buffers Against the Impact of Stress: A Longitudinal Study of Seminary Students and Their Partners," Alan E. Craddock, *Journal of Psychology and Theology,* 24:1 (1996), pp. 38–46.

36. *The Health of Nations* (New York: Basic Books, Inc., Publishers, 1987).

37. Dolores Curran, *Stress and the Healthy Family* (Minneapolis: Winston Press, 1985).

38. "Associations Among Family Support, Family Stress, and Personal Functional Health Status," G. R. Parkerson, Jr., J. L. Michener, and L. R. Wu et al., *Journal of Clinical Epidemiology,* 42:3 (1989), pp. 217–229.

39. *The Broken Heart.*

40. *Love, Medicine, and Miracles* (New York: Harper and Row, 1986).

41. *The Broken Heart.*

42. *Who Gets Sick: Thinking and Health,* Blair Justice, (Houston: Peak Press, 1987), p. 189.

43. *Who Gets Sick,* pp. 192–193.

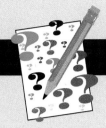

ASSESSMENT 4-1

Do You Have the Qualities of Friendship?

Name _____ Date _____ Grade _____

Instructor _____ Course _____ Section _____

Friendship is a two-way business. To make friends, you have to be a friend. The better friend you are, the more friends you are likely to have. This questionnaire lists some of the qualities of friendship.

Check "yes" or "no" to the questions. Then look at the scoring key at the end.

YES **NO**

☐ ☐ 1. Are people able to depend on you to keep your word?

☐ ☐ 2. Can they rely on you to respect their confidences?

☐ ☐ 3. Do you keep the friends you make?

☐ ☐ 4. Do you often put yourself to trouble and inconvenience to oblige other people?

☐ ☐ 5. Suppose they want to do something you are not particularly keen on. Would you go along with them and do what they want to do?

☐ ☐ 6. Are you quick to pay your share of the expenses?

☐ ☐ 7. Are you generous with your praise and appreciation?

☐ ☐ 8. Do you show affection when you feel it?

☐ ☐ 9. Is it easy for you to forgive and forget?

☐ ☐ 10. Do you readily give people the benefit of the doubt and make allowances?

☐ ☐ 11. In a sharp difference of opinion, would you speak first?

☐ ☐ 12. Do you own up when you are wrong and say you are sorry?

☐ ☐ 13. You may like somebody very much, but would you feel the same if he or she were to become unpopular?

☐ ☐ 14. Are you quick off the mark to give sympathy and practical help when people need it?

☐ ☐ 15. Do you like to see others praised and fussed over?

☐ ☐ 16. Can you agree to differ and stay on the best of terms?

☐ ☐ 17. Are you an attentive and sympathetic listener?

☐ ☐ 18. Are you always the same, not full of welcome today and too busy to bother tomorrow?

☐ ☐ 19. Do you mind people having other friends and interests that you do not share?

☐ ☐ 20. Can you say you are much more interested in other people than in yourself?

SCORING

Count 5 points for every "yes." A score of 70 or over is good, and 60-70 is satisfactory. Under 60 is not satisfactory. You are not likely to be a good friend. Usually, when we are like this, we're wrapped up in ourselves. We like only the individuals who notice us and make a fuss over us and dislike anybody who is not interested in us or who will not do what we want. If you desire to be a good friend, you will have to be more interested in other people than in yourself and put them first.

Adapted from Singer Communications, Inc., Anaheim, California. Used by permission.

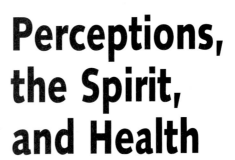

Perceptions,
the Spirit,
and Health

OBJECTIVES

- Define *explanatory style* and explain the differences between a pessimistic style and an optimistic style, as well as their effects on health.

- Explain the differences between an internal locus of control and an external locus of control, together with their health effects.

- Understand the connection between self-esteem and health.

- Learn how to protect health with a fighting spirit.

- Understand the connection between spirituality and health, including the power of prayer, forgiveness, and faith.

- Describe the altruistic personality and health benefits of volunteerism.

- Contrast the health effects of hope and hopelessness.

The habitual manner in which people explain the things that happen to them is their **explanatory style**. It is a way of thinking when all other factors are equal and when there are no clear-cut right and wrong answers. The contrasting explanatory styles are pessimism and optimism.

People with a pessimistic explanatory style interpret events negatively. People with an optimistic explanatory style interpret them in a positive light — every cloud has a silver lining.

The pessimistic explanatory style can be identified by three thought patterns that give clues during conversation.

1. Assuming a problem is never-ending, convinced it will never go away.

2. Believing a problem is global, that it applies across the board instead of being an isolated incident.

3. Internalizing everything ("It's my fault"), often placing the wrong blame at the wrong time.

Whether explanatory style is endemic and unchangeable is a matter of considerable controversy in the professions. Many believe that we have the same explanatory style throughout our life. Some evidence supports that notion. University of Pennsylvania psychologist Martin Seligman believes, however, that explanatory style can be changed, and he supports this position using the results of his own work.[1]

A growing body of evidence suggests that explanatory style can be a potent predictor of physical health. It affects both emotional and physical well-being. In the emotional arena, a negative explanatory style can lead to anxiety, eating disorders, and dysphoria, in the form of depression, guilt, anger, or hostility. In the physical realm a negative explanatory style can halt the healing process.

A pessimistic explanatory style can influence healing time and the course of the illness in several major diseases. For example, it can impact the circulatory system and outlook for people with coronary heart disease. Sophisticated instruments and testing procedures have enabled researchers to watch the brain in action. Blood flow to the brain actually changes as thoughts, feelings, and attitudes change. Findings from a variety of studies show that people with a pessimistic explanatory style have higher risk for atherosclerosis, blockage of coronary arteries, and heart attack.

Studies of explanatory style conducted at Yale University and the University of Pennsylvania verify that a negative explanatory style compromises immunity. Blood samples taken from people with a negative explanatory style revealed suppressed immune function, a low ratio of helper/suppressor T-cells, and fewer lymphocytes (the cells responsible for waging war against disease or infection).[2]

In contrast, an optimistic style tends to increase the strength of the immune system. Robert Good, former president and director of the Memorial Sloan-Kettering Cancer Hospital in New York, maintains that an optimistic explanatory style and the positive attitude it fosters can alter our ability to resist infections, allergies, autoimmunities, and even cancer. Bernie Siegel, who works with patients to help them change their explanatory style and to resolve stress and conflict in their lives, says a change in explanatory style has been accompanied by remarkable changes in the course of disease.[3] He maintains that an optimistic explanatory style and the positive emotions it embraces — such as love, acceptance, and forgiveness — stimulate the body's own healing systems.

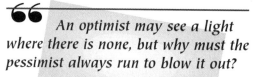

An optimist may see a light where there is none, but why must the pessimist always run to blow it out?
— *Michel de Saint-Pierre*

Michael A. Lerner, founder of Commonweal and winner of a MacArthur Foundation Genius Award, says that attitudes linked to an optimistic explanatory style can boost the immune system enough to help fight cancer, that attitudes themselves have a potent effect on the immune system. You become the person who developed the cancer, he says. Becoming a different personality may change the environment the cancer grew in; it may become so inhospitable that the cancer shrinks.[4]

To boost your own optimism:

- Before you start to change your attitudes, surround yourself with people who care about you and can help you. Ideally, they are optimistic people. When you surround yourself with optimists, you begin to "catch" their attitude. Tell others you want to change, and solicit their help and suggestions.

- Learn to genuinely like other people. Look for their good qualities, and respect their differences.

- Realize that changing your explanatory style is a big commitment. In essence, it's a change in lifestyle. You didn't develop an explanatory style overnight, and you won't be able to change it overnight, either. Be patient with yourself and expect some hard work. Get past the inevitable setbacks and disappointments. Look at these as challenges and don't let them debilitate you.

- Look for evidence to support the way you want to feel. You'll be surprised to find it! Too often, we adopt pessimistic or negative attitudes based on faulty beliefs when the evidence really suggests otherwise.

> *If the theme song of the external is "Cast Your Fate to the Winds," the theme song of the internal is "I Did It My Way."*
> — *Phillip Rice*

- Set small, attainable goals, then reward yourself richly when you meet those goals. Celebrate your accomplishments.

- Look beyond yourself. The world does not revolve around you. Get involved in volunteerism to expand your horizons.

- Guard against overexaggeration. An argument with a friend doesn't mean the friendship is collapsing. One poor exam score doesn't mean your college career is doomed. Don't blow things out of proportion.

- Gather all the facts before you form a conclusion. Take the time to research things. You'll probably develop a whole new set of ideas!

- Avoid overgeneralization. Just because you couldn't get a professor you wanted doesn't mean that nothing ever turns out right. Recount all the successes, all the good things that have happened to you.

- Face your problems head-on. Develop strategies for solving them instead of trying to escape them.

- Above all, have fun. Learn to laugh at yourself, to relax, to enjoy and respect yourself.

LOCUS OF CONTROL

The concept of **locus of control** originated several years ago with the work of Julian Rotter. It relates to the extent we believe we can master or control the environment surrounding us. Control does not mean that we need to control *everything* around us — other people, our circumstances, good or bad. Control *does* entail the perception of how much we can impact a situation. We can choose how to react and respond. If we regard a loss with gloom and doom, for example, we allow it to hurt us. If we view it as a chance for growth and opportunity, we minimize its ability to hurt us.

Each person lies somewhere along a continuum. At one end of the continuum shown in Figure 5.1 is the **external locus of control**. At the opposite end is the **internal locus of control**. Where a person is along the continuum relates to his or her health. People with an external locus of control believe the things that happen to them are unrelated to their own behavior and, therefore, are beyond their control. People with an internal locus of control, in contrast, believe that negative events are a consequence of their personal actions, and, thus, potentially can be controlled.

Explanatory style The way people perceive the events in their lives, from an optimistic or a pessimistic perspective.

Locus of control The extent to which a person believes he or she can control the external environment.

External locus of control One's prevailing belief that the things that happen are unrelated to one's own behavior.

Internal locus of control One's prevailing belief that negative events are a consequence of one's own actions and, thus, potentially can be controlled.

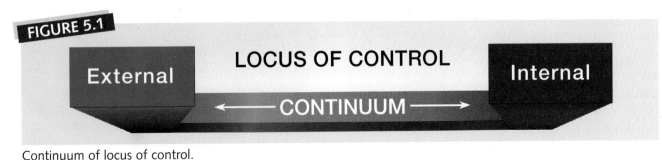

FIGURE 5.1

LOCUS OF CONTROL

External   ← CONTINUUM →   Internal

Continuum of locus of control.

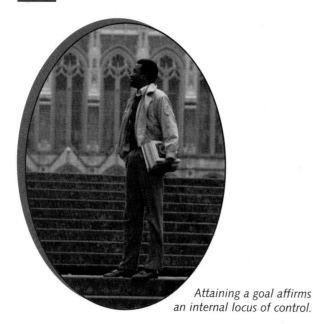

Attaining a goal affirms an internal locus of control.

As a whole, people with a greater sense of control are at less risk of illness. Scientists are realizing that an internal locus of control has an even more profound role in protecting health than we once thought. Former *Saturday Review* editor Norman Cousins, renowned for his work linking attitudes and health, maintained that, in general:

> Anything that restores a sense of control to a patient can be a profound aid to a physician in treating serious illness. That sense of control is more than a mere mood or attitude, and may well be a vital pathway between the brain, the endocrine system, and the immune system. The assumed possibility is that it may serve as the basis for what may well be a profound advancement in the knowledge of how to confront serious illness.[5]

An internal locus of control has a significant influence over the body's release of hormones, which has been found to be a powerful determinant of health. Three of the hormones influenced by a lack of control are:

1. *Serotonin*, which regulates moods, relieves pain, and helps control the release of the pain-killing endorphins;

2. *Dopamine*, largely responsible for a sense of reward and pleasure;

3. *Norepinephrine*, which, when depleted, causes depression.

When a person has little sense of control, the level of corticosteroids in the bloodstream soars. The corticosteroids, released by the body during stress, have a variety of negative physical effects. They lower the body's resistance to disease and suppress the body's manufacture of the three hormones above, making lack of control a two-edged sword. A sense of lack of control may have an even stronger influence over health than does a high level of stress.

A person in a stressful situation who believes he or she has some control over the situation has far less of the physiological damage normally associated with stress. And control acts as a buffer against stress when we *believe* we have control, even if we really don't.

SELF-ESTEEM

Self-esteem is a way of viewing oneself as a good person who is well in all aspects. It is a sense of feeling good about one's capabilities, physical limitations, goals, place in the world, and relationship to others. Self-esteem is a powerful determinant, as perceptions about self set the boundaries for what we can and cannot do. Self-esteem might be called the blueprint for behavior.

> *We can secure other people's approval if we do right and try hard; but our own is worth a hundred of it.*
> — *Mark Twain*

American humorist and author Samuel Clemens — the legendary Mark Twain — believed that approving of ourselves is a hundred times more valuable than having the approval of others. A century after he penned that advice, it is proving to be true.

Healthy self-esteem is one of the best things a person can do for overall health, both mental and

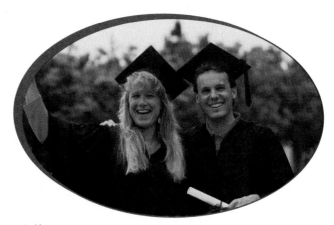

Self-esteem can contribute to mental and physical health.

physical. A good, strong sense of self can boost the immune system, protect against disease, and aid in healing.

Whether people do or do not get sick — and how long they stay that way — may depend in part on the strength of their self-esteem. A growing body of evidence indicates, for example, that low self-esteem often is a factor in chronic pain. Several studies show that recovery from infectious mononucleosis is related to "ego strength." The higher the self-esteem, the more rapid the recovery. If we have strong self-esteem, the outlook is good. The more positive the life events, the better our health. If our self-esteem is poor, however, our health can decline in direct proportion as our life becomes peppered with more negative life events.

> **"**
> *What wise people and grandmothers have always known is that the way you feel about yourself, your attitudes, beliefs, values, have a great deal to do with your health and well-being.*
> — *Madeline Gershwin*
> **"**

The way people regard themselves and their own health can serve as sort of a self-fulfilling prophecy. When Canadian researchers asked more than 3,500 elderly people to rate their own health and then followed the volunteers for 7 years, they found that actual health 7 years later correlated to the self-ratings. Actually, the ratings the elderly people gave themselves were more accurate and predictive than the health measures provided by physicians who examined the patients.[6]

Belief in oneself is one of the most powerful weapons people have in protecting health and living longer. It has a startling impact on wellness, and we are able to harness it to our advantage.

To boost your self-esteem:

- Use **affirmations**. Boost your sense of esteem by saying positive things about you to yourself, such as, "I'm honest and open in expressing my feelings." Write some affirmations of your own and use them every day.

- List the things you would like to have or experience. Construct the statements as if you already were enjoying those situations, beginning each sentence with "I am. . . ." For example: "I am feeling great about doing well in my classes" or "I am enjoying the opportunity to meet new people." Visualize each situation, and get in the habit of repeating this process several times a day.

- When your "internal critic" — the negative inner voice we all have — starts putting you down, tune it out. Force yourself to think of a situation that you handled well or something about yourself that you're especially proud of.[7]

A FIGHTING SPIRIT

A **fighting spirit** requires the open expression of emotions, whether they are negative or positive. At the other extreme is hopelessness, a surrender to despair. In between these are attitudes of denial and stoic acceptance, as shown in Figure 5.2.

Fighting spirit can play a major role in recovery from disease. People with a fighting spirit accept the diagnosis fully, adopt an optimistic attitude filled with faith, seek information about how to help themselves, and are determined to fight the disease.

Self-esteem   A sense of positive self-regard.

Affirmations   Positive statements that help reinforce the most positive aspects of personality and experience.

Fighting spirit   Determination; the open expression of emotions, whether negative or positive.

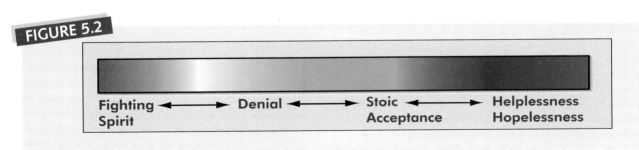

FIGURE 5.2

Fighting Spirit ⟷ Denial ⟷ Stoic Acceptance ⟷ Helplessness Hopelessness

Continuum showing attitudes toward serious illness.

Case Study of a Fighting Spirit

In discussing the power of a fighting spirit, psychoneuroimmunology pioneer Dr. George Solomon told the story of a Harvard professor who had been stricken with cancer; he had lesions in his head, lungs, and liver. Nonetheless, the professor continued teaching his classes, reassuring his friends and students.

Solomon says of the professor, "It was thrilling to see how powerful the fighting spirit can be. For most of a year, he battled that cancer. And he won. The most important thing he had to teach us came not out of his medical lectures but out of his own experience and example. He won against all the odds — against the predictions of the specialists and against the reports based on sophisticated technology."

What the professor taught all around him was, in essence, that if we are willing to fight, we *can* win.

A fighting spirit may be the underlying factor in what is called **spontaneous remission** from incurable illness. More and more physicians believe that the phenomenon is real, and that the patient is the key in spontaneous remission. They believe the patient's attitude, especially the presence of a fighting spirit, is responsible for victory over disease. "The forces exist in the body to arouse its natural disease-fighting abilities," says Dr. Lloyd Old of Memorial Sloan-Kettering Cancer Center in New York City. "The task ahead is to find ways to unleash them."

Fighters aren't stronger or better or more capable than the rest of the people. They simply don't give up easily. In study after study, they have been shown to enjoy better health and live longer, even when physicians and laboratory tests say they shouldn't.

Specific factors bolster a fighting spirit and promote survival.[8] A fighting spirit makes a person take charge. When illness or disease is present, that makes a big difference. As heart surgeon Dr. Wayne Eisom of New York Hospital-Cornell Medical Center points out, "A fighter gets out of bed earlier and walks, even with painful incisions. A non-fighter doesn't, and gets an infection in his lungs."[9] Fighters are intrinsically different from people who give up, and their health reflects those differences.

Probably the most remarkable studies involving the effect of a fighting spirit have dealt with cancer, a disease that, by its very name, evokes terror in many people. The spirit with which a patient accepts the diagnosis apparently is a major determinant in how the disease will progress. According to some researchers, an overall fighting spirit may help stave off cancer.

A style of giving up, as contrasted with an active, fighting style, has been shown repeatedly to affect the prognosis in cancer cases significantly. Siegel used the example of a patient who invested people's life savings according to statistics. "His oncologist told him what statistics said about his chances, and from then on he refused to fight for his life. He said, 'I've spent my life making predictions based on statistics. Statistics tell me I'm supposed to die. If I don't die, my whole life doesn't make sense.' And he went home and died."[10]

The immune system may bear some of the greatest impact of a fighting spirit, and it may be the reason why fighters do better in all kinds of disease situations. Convincing evidence from a host of studies indicates that a fighting spirit boosts immune function, mobilizing the body and empowering it to fight off disease and infection.

SPIRITUALITY

You always have a choice about how you feel. Listen to Jesse Jackson say that you may not have chosen to be down, but you have a choice as to whether you want to try to get up. . . . Listen to Mahatma Gandhi, who said, "Let us not kill our enemies but kill their desire to kill." And so you have a choice about how you behave, whether you are in prison, whether you are in a concentration camp, or whether you are sick. You have a choice.[11]

A 1995 conference in Leesburg, Virginia, organized by the National Institute for Healthcare Research, was devoted to exploring how much is known about spirituality and health. One of the speakers — Dale Matthews, associate professor of medicine at Georgetown University School of Medicine — called spirituality and medicine "the twin guardians of healing through the ages."[12] And National Institute for Healthcare Research President David Larson called for more detailed studies of spirituality and health, saying that the question today is not whether spirituality has health benefits but how these benefits can be obtained.[13]

Spiritual health is the ability to discover and articulate our own basic purpose in life and to learn how to experience love, joy, peace, and fulfillment.

It's the experience of helping ourselves and others achieve full potential.[14] Through the spiritual dimension we emphasize our connectedness to other members of the human family.

Influences on Health

The cultivation of spiritual health — which is a process or journey, not an endpoint — can have a significant influence on physical, mental, and emotional health, sometimes in dramatic ways. Among the scientists pioneering research into the effect of spirituality on health is Kenneth Pelletier. He began his research by studying men and women he deemed to be "successful." He found, first, that most of the professionally successful men and women had strong spiritual values and beliefs. Further, virtually all of them had suffered a major psychological or physical trauma early in life but, perhaps because of their spirituality, had been able to weather the crisis and develop a more effective style of coping with life crises.[15] Preliminary findings from the study found the correlation between good spiritual health and good physical health "striking."

> 66 *Psychiatrists no longer dismiss out of hand the importance of religious faith in recovery from emotional illness and the healing power of forgiveness; there is a recognition of the connection between prayer and healing. A strong faith can have a profound effect on our lifestyles and outlook in terms of health.* — Pollster George Gallup, Jr. 99

Spirituality seems to buffer stress. People with a deep sense of spirituality are not defeated by crises. Spirituality helps people interpret crises in a growth-producing way. As a result, they are able to use illness as a means of spiritual growth. Even when disease claims a life, spirituality can make the experience one of positive growth.

Spirituality entails a belief in a power higher than oneself.

Not everyone will attain a cure from disease, Siegel points out. At some time or another, everyone will die. Nevertheless, people who are busy living, who are trying to make changes in their lives, experience great growth even in the face of serious illness. People who face disease with that attitude define their disease as a gift, a challenge, a wake-up call, a new beginning, and a beauty mark. And they are not necessarily saying, "I am cured." The exceptional people accept their mortality. They have heard they're going to die, but they don't take it as a sentence. So they don't go home and die. They take it as an opportunity to live until they die.[16]

Prayer

Prayer signals a commitment to a set of moral and ethical values. It is a signpost of our spirituality, at the core of most spiritual experiences. Prayer also has powerful physiological effects on the body. In a

> 66 *Large majorities of Americans say that prayer is an important part of their lives, that they believe that miracles are performed by the power of God, and that they are sometimes conscious of the presence of God.* — Pollster George Gallup, Jr. 99

nationwide poll asking doctors whether they believe patients benefit from prayer, half the doctors questioned said they believe prayer helps patients, and two-thirds of the doctors responding said they pray for their patients.

Dr. Herbert Benson, associate professor of medicine at the Harvard Medical School and chief of the

Spontaneous remission　Inexplicable recovery from incurable illness.

Spiritual health　The ability to develop our spiritual nature to its fullest potential.

Section on Behavioral Medicine at the New England Deaconess Hospital, has described the **relaxation response**.[17] According to Benson, the relaxation response, with all its physiological benefits, has been elicited most often and most effectively through forms of prayer.

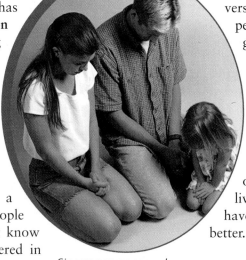

Sincere prayer can enhance health and buffer stress.

Prayer can have a powerful impact on people even when they don't know prayers are being offered in their behalf. One San Francisco cardiologist arranged for a group of people around the country to pray daily for 192 coronary care unit patients at San Francisco General Hospital, without telling the patients that anyone was praying for them. A second group of 201 control patients had no one praying for them. The praying continued for 10 months. Cardiologist Randy Byrd, who engineered the study, reported that the patients who were prayed for had significantly fewer complications while they were in the coronary care unit.[18]

Forgiveness

Essential to a spiritual nature is **forgiveness**. It means accepting the core of every human being the same as yourself and giving them the gift of not judging them.[19] To understand the health benefits of forgiveness, we must understand what happens when we *don't* forgive: The body releases masses of "high-voltage" hormones that cause the heart to pound, blood pressure to skyrocket, muscles to contract, and abdominal pains to develop. If the situation continues unchecked, gastric ulcers, gastritis, or irritable bowel syndrome can result. With forgiveness, the anger and resentment dissolve. The body stops pouring high-voltage chemicals into the bloodstream, and the healing begins.

Church Affiliation

Religion is "the personal beliefs, values, and activities pertinent to that which is supernatural, mysterious, and awesome, which transcends immediate situations, and which pertains to questions of final causes and ultimate ends of man and the universe."[20] People with active religious faith and people who are strongly affiliated with a church generally enjoy better health.

Those who participate actively in a church or synagogue boost their immune system and health and may even live longer. People who attend a church or synagogue regularly have a much lower rate for a number of diseases than those who attend less frequently or not at all. Churchgoers have especially low rates of heart disease, lung disease, cirrhosis of the liver, and some kinds of cancer. Religious people have been shown consistently to heal faster and better.

Learning to Forgive

For day-to-day mishaps — a roommate offended you, you were served cold food in a restaurant — you can learn to forgive, and it may be easier than you think.

- Start practicing forgiveness of minor infractions, things that are easy to forgive. Once you've learned the technique, it's easier to transfer to more difficult problems.

- Set aside a "forgiveness hour." For that hour, forgive *everything* that happens, even the things *you* do. Expand it to a "forgiveness day." Realize how great you feel to forgive someone instead of lugging around a burden of grudges and hard feelings.

- Take a hard look at the way you judge others. Your own judgment, not the actions of someone else, often is what makes forgiveness difficult. Make it a policy to reserve judgment until you have all the facts. Better yet, make a hard-and-fast rule to postpone all judgments for one year. (Chances are good that you will have forgotten the whole thing by then.)

- Don't say you've "forgiven" someone, then tell your roommates what happened. Forgiving entails forgetting.

- Learn to forgive yourself. If you have to, say it aloud ("I forgive myself for cutting class and not being up front with the professor"). Learn from your mistakes, and turn them into positives instead of using them as ammunition against yourself forever.

Researcher Jeffrey Levin, associate professor of family and community medicine at Eastern Virginia Medical School, conducted in-depth studies of the influence of religion on health. All but one of the studies that included a religious variable — such as church affiliation or regular religious involvement — reported a positive effect of religion on health. Based on the studies, Levin suggests that lack of religious involvement seems to be a risk factor for poorer health.[21]

Religion — *if* it requires a lifestyle commitment — offers a life that is better physically, emotionally, and mentally. Various studies show that religious people, regardless of denomination, generally have stronger marriages, stronger families, a stronger inclination to help other people, a greater sense of happiness, and better physical health. One of the keys may be the tendency of religious people to find hope and meaning, rather than hopelessness and emptiness, in life and its challenges.

Even though no one knows for certain how religious participation protects health, probable reasons have been advanced:

1. Many churches prescribe behavior that prevents illness or assists in the treatment of illness and discourage behavior that is harmful to health.

2. Organized churches provide social support, reduce loneliness, and offer support groups for people in times of need.

3. Most religions place strong emphasis on marriage and the family, both of which have health benefits.

4. Religious people more often have a strong sense of self-esteem and control, as well as a deep sense of spiritual well-being. One study that concentrated on Blacks found a strong association between religion and well-being that is consistent throughout life.[22]

5. Churches promote more positive approaches toward illness, pain, or disability, which can influence the outcome of disease. A study of older adults showed that those with chronic disabling conditions, such as heart disease and diabetes, are less likely to become depressed if they use religion (such as prayer, faith in God, and Bible reading) to adapt to stress.[23]

6. Religious faith and activity improve coping skills and generally give people a value system that helps them prioritize in times of indecision.

Faith and religious devotion together are indicators of happiness and a worthwhile life. A Gallup poll showed that religious faith and practice is a primary source of happiness. Of those who characterized themselves as "deeply religious," more than 90% also characterized themselves as "very happy." Many religious people even find hope in suffering, which inspires a fighting spirit and optimism.

Regardless of *why* religion works to boost health, regular attendance or participation seems to be a key. Regular participation has been shown to increase lifespan and decrease mortality, even after controlling for age and various other risk factors. More than 200 studies on religion and health show that religion has a strong positive influence on mortality, even from cancer.[24] The higher the level of religious commitment, as measured by church attendance and prayer, the better the health.

Regular church attendance apparently has an impact on a number of specific diseases, too, especially cardiovascular disease. The more active in a religion a person is, the less chance that person has of incurring a heart attack. Regular church attenders also are at lower risk for myocardial degeneration, chronic endocarditis, arteriosclerotic heart disease, and degenerative heart disease. People with high conformity to religious belief have lower blood pressure, a slower, steadier heartbeat, and a healthier cardiovascular system overall.

Altruism

One aspect of spirituality is **altruism**, giving oneself to other people out of genuine concern. During a selfless career, physician and philosopher Albert Schweitzer proclaimed that true happiness is to be found only by serving others.

The ability to put another's needs above one's own also seems to contribute to a longer and healthier life. Doing good for others is good for a person, especially for the nervous system and the immune system. Whereas stress can undermine the immune system, the positive emotions related to altruism

Relaxation response   The body's ability to enter a scientifically defined state of relaxation.

Forgiveness   The ability to release from the mind all past hurts and failures, all sense of guilt and loss.

Religion   The science of how to know God.

Altruism   The act of giving of oneself out of a genuine concern for other people.

help stabilize the immune system against the normal immunosuppressing effects of stress.

What makes a person altruistic? Some believe it's instinct, stemming from the time when people lived in small groups of hunters and gatherers. Growing numbers believe that altruism is a capacity everyone shares to some extent. Some believe in an altruistic "personality" that enables them to reach out to others.

Based on a study of rescuers who provided help to the Jews during Hitler's reign of terror, Samuel P. Oliner and Pearl M. Oliner developed a summary of the traits they believe are common to all altruistic people.[25] They:

— never regard others as inferiors;

— value human relationships more than money;

— believe that ethical values should be applied universally;

— believe in the right of innocent people to be free from persecution;

— have a healthy perspective about themselves;

— are "connected" to others;

— have a profound commitment to caring;

— believe they can control events and shape their own destiny but are willing to risk failure.

University of Massachusetts psychologist Ervin Staub believes that altruistic people share three general traits:

1. They have a positive view of people in general.

2. They are concerned about others' welfare.

3. They take personal responsibility for how other people are doing.

In studying outstanding altruists, Christie Kiefer found that background and family values help determine the altruistic personality. The altruists she studied came from families that were warm and nurturing. The emotional self-acceptance they developed in that environment liberated them to be generative, creative, playful, and relaxed.[26]

Elderly people who engage in volunteer work have better health, visit the doctor less often, and have fewer complaints.[27] This is because volunteerism causes a release of endorphins resulting in a "helper's high," similar in nature to the "runner's high" that runners experience.[28] Harvard cardiologist Herbert Benson says the sensation comes from the ability to forget oneself.

The "healthy-helper syndrome," as Allan Luks and Howard Andrews dubbed it, starts with a physical high, (reported by 95% of the volunteers surveyed). This physical sensation has been likened to the sense of fitness and well-being people experience during and immediately after exercise. This is followed by a longer-lasting sense of calm and heightened emotional well-being. Together the two stages are a powerful antidote to stress, a key to happiness and optimism, and a way to combat feelings of helplessness and depression. Further, the helper's high isn't restricted to the time a volunteer is helping. Luks found that 82% of the volunteers had a less intense helper's high just by remembering the helping.[29]

The volunteers who experienced the healthy-helper syndrome noticed an improvement in their own ills, including arthritis, lupus symptoms, asthma attacks, migraine headaches, colds, and bouts of flu. Based on their study, the researchers also believe that volunteerism alleviates the stress and other physiological conditions that lead to heart attack.[30]

Characteristics of Volunteers

A true volunteer has the following characteristics:

■ The helper actually *connects with people* (one-on-one contact). Writing out a check to a charity doesn't provide the same health benefits as working for a few hours at the local food bank.

■ The helper has a *desire* to help (the word "volunteer" is a key).

■ The helper *likes* what he or she is doing.

■ The helper is *consistent* (the greatest health benefits have been reaped by those who do regular volunteer work at least once a week).

■ The helper *gives freely*, not out of a sense of obligation. A person who swings a hammer on low-income housing because of her desire to see better housing for the poor will have better health benefits than a person who cleans up litter along the interstate as part of court-enforced community service requirements.

■ The volunteer work is part of a *balance* in the helper's life. If volunteer work begins to interfere with school, work, or family obligations, the helper may have more, not fewer, health problems.

Guidelines for Volunteers

To guard against burnout, volunteers should adhere to the following guidelines:

- Don't try to do too much. A good goal is roughly 2 hours of volunteer work a week. With a tight schedule, just an hour a week may be advisable.

- Do something you enjoy and something you'd feel comfortable doing. A suicide hotline may be begging for volunteers, but if that kind of work makes you extremely uncomfortable, another volunteer option would be better.

- Realize that any line of work, volunteer or paid, has occasional setbacks or bad experiences, but that plenty of good happens in the meantime.

- Realize that you are not responsible for anyone else. You can't keep a person from committing suicide or an addict from returning to cocaine. You can provide help and support, but the responsibility is up to the person being helped.

- Get out of any situation that isn't right for you; look for something else. Just because the other volunteers seem to be doing well and enjoying themselves, it doesn't mean this specific situation is the best one for everybody.

Motive is important. People do not fare as well if they expect something in return. Some expect monetary reward; others expect payment in terms of increased status.

Places that use volunteers include schools, churches/synagogues, homeless shelters, food pantries, thrift shops, libraries, zoos/animal shelters, museums, hospitals, and nursing homes. The best volunteer opportunities:

— provide a regular schedule and a specific description of what the volunteers are expected to do.

— provide personal contact with the people the volunteers are going to help.

— utilize skills the volunteers have already or train them for something they'd like to be able to do.

— fall within volunteers' area of interest. It's easier to stick with the volunteer work if it's something they really enjoy doing.

— expect a reasonable commitment; 2 hours a week is a good goal to shoot for.

Before making a commitment, the volunteer should check out what's available in the area, visit the facilities, watch what goes on, then narrow the choices. Before signing up for volunteer work, the volunteer should get as much information as possible and not be afraid to ask questions. This will enable the prospective volunteer to find the most satisfying outlet for altruism.

Volunteering to help others can bring tremendous health benefits. If people overextend themselves or get involved in the wrong kind of activity for them, however, they will get burned out and run the risk of getting sick instead of protecting their health.

A Secret of Longevity

In the early 1960s Bruce Randolph was almost 60 years old and nearly broke when he headed to Denver to be near his son. He began his little barbecue restaurant out of a house, using his mother's "secret" sauce recipe. Four years later he started a holiday meal tradition, feeding a few hundred people out of the back of a truck.

By the time he died in 1994, he was a household name in Denver. "Daddy Bruce" was the only name he needed. Each year he organized giant Thanksgiving dinners for 30 years for thousands of needy people who had nowhere else to go for the holiday. His philanthropy didn't end there. He often served free meals on Christmas and 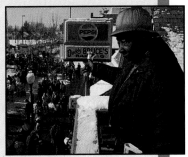 on his birthday. He collected and distributed clothing for the poor, and he organized Easter egg hunts in the park for children.

After his death at age 93, a street was named in his honor. A handpainted sign on the closed restaurant reads, "It is more blessed to give than to receive." No one would argue that one of Daddy Bruce's secrets to a long life was altruism, a giving spirit.

Faith

What exists is not as important as what we believe to exist. Personal belief gives us an unseen power that enables us to do the impossible, to perform miracles, even to heal ourselves. History is replete with examples of people who have been affected by the healing power of **faith**. It has relieved headaches, reduced angina pains, controlled hypertension, overcome insomnia, prevented hyperventilation attacks, alleviated backaches, enhanced cancer treatment, controlled panic attacks, reduced cholesterol levels, lowered overall stress, and alleviated symptoms of anxiety, including nausea, vomiting, diarrhea, and constipation. A good example of faith's power over physiological processes is its influence over blood pressure. Devoutly faithful groups of people tend to have lower blood pressure.[31]

The power of faith is apparent in the healing process. Daniel Goleman maintains that faith is the hidden ingredient in Western medicine and every traditional system of healing. A large number of illnesses can be treated more successfully if the patient believes in a cure.[32]

> *[Faith] is an excitement and an enthusiasm: it is a condition of intellectual magnificence to which we must cling as a treasure, and not squander in the small coin of empty words.* — George Sand, French authoress

One of the best-known healing shrines is Lourdes, a healing spring in the French countryside that attracts more than 2 million pilgrims each year, who travel to the site from all corners of the world in the hope of being healed. For most, the journey is a last resort. They have been told there is no cure for their conditions. Many people are, indeed, healed, probably as a result of the expectant faith of the pilgrim who comes to be healed.

One of the most striking and profound examples of how faith influences even the course of medication is the well-known story of a patient treated by Dr. Bruno Klopfer in the late 1950s. The patient was suffering from a widespread lymphoma — a serious cancer of the immune system — that was in its late stages. At the time, a drug called Krebiozen was being touted as a cure for cancer. The patient demanded that Klopfer administer Krebiozen, and the doctor agreed. Within 2 days of receiving the Krebiozen, the patient had a remarkable turnaround. According to one account, the large tumors that covered his body began "melting like snowballs." After 10 days of treatment with Krebiozen, the patient was released from the hospital, apparently free of disease. Klopfer believed a medical miracle had occurred, but it was the patient's faith in the Krebiozen, not the drug itself.

A few months after the patient was released from the hospital, newspapers around the country announced that Krebiozen was worthless. The patient's tumors promptly reappeared. Klopfer was fascinated by this turn of events. Based on the patient's history, he strongly suspected the patient's *belief* was what had cured him and that the drug had nothing to do with it. Klopfer became convinced that he could once again harness the man's faith if the conditions were right. He called his patient in, reassured him, told him the newspaper accounts were inaccurate, and that an extra-strength, improved, refined form of the drug had just been released to physicians.

Klopfer offered this "refined" form of the drug to his eager patient. Klopfer didn't actually have any improved Krebiozen. What he gave his patient was actually distilled water. With distilled water coursing through his veins, the patient who believed that he had a new super Krebiozen staged another remarkable recovery. Within days, his tumors again disappeared. He was released from the hospital a second time, apparently disease-free.

Unfortunately, that didn't last, either. Three months after his recovery, the patient read a newspaper report citing the American Medical Association as stating that definitive tests had proven beyond a doubt that Krebiozen was worthless. The patient, who had left the hospital 3 months earlier free of tumors, was shattered. His tumors ballooned. Two days after he read the newspaper report, he literally laid down and died.

Hope

Hope — a wealth of optimism, a want of fear — apparently is one of the strongest influences on health and the human body. Medical lore is replete with examples of "terminal" patients who, awash with hope, defied all medical odds. Some lived months or years longer than predicted. Some were able to remain symptom-free and enjoyed comfort for the last period of their lives. Some lived and were healed. More and more, physicians are finding that hope is a powerful tool in their work with patients.

Psychologist Robert Ornstein and physician David Sobel define hope as:

> . . . a special type of positive expectation. Unlike denial, which involves a negation of reality, hope is an active way of coping with threatening situations by focusing on the positive. No matter how dark or grim a situation may appear, certain people seem to be able to extract the positive aspects and concentrate on them. They fill their mind with hopeful scenarios, stories with happy endings, or lucky outcomes.[33]

Hope has a powerful influence on physical health and well-being. It can bring not only enhanced health but a longer life as well. Dr. Elisabeth Kübler-Ross, whose work with dying patients revolutionized the medical profession, stressed the importance of hope. Even though they can't hope for a cure, she says, patients can

> hope for a few more days or hours of life, for contact with loved ones, for freedom from pain, or for peaceful death with dignity. . . Hope is a satisfaction unto itself and need not be fulfilled to be appreciated.[34]

If hope can influence health profoundly for the better, its opposite — hopelessness — can have the opposite effect. **Hopelessness** is marked by negative future expectations and the belief that the future holds nothing good or positive. It also is characterized by the inability to reach a desired goal, futility in planning for goals, and a lack of motivation for using constructive action to gain control of life. People who feel hopeless usually feel despondent, desperate, and despairing; they feel they have lost control and feel helpless about what the future holds.[35]

Los Angeles physician Alexandra M. Levine gives a poignant example of what happens when hope is lost.[36] She remembers a 55-year-old woman who was admitted to the hospital with a lesion in the upper lobe of her lung. Levine describes her as "a real dynamo, vigorous and friendly. She became the extra pair of hands on the ward, helping to pass the meal trays, running minor errands. We all came to love her."

When the woman underwent biopsy, it revealed a deadly cancer that already had invaded the nodes. The surgeons could not remove it, so they closed the incision. The next day a group of residents and interns surrounded her bed. One of them looked down and said, "Well, it's cancer, and we couldn't really resect it, so we just opened and closed."

The patient kept repeating the question, "Opened and closed?" As the intern nodded and repeatedly confirmed the procedure, she finally asked, "You mean you left the cancer in there?" "Yes," he replied. She closed her eyes and told the interns she was tired. They left the room.

The woman died that night. The autopsy revealed no specific cause of death, just the cancer — but it had been there for months. Levine wrote, "I have never been able to get her words out of my mind. . . . I don't really know why she died, but to be honest, I will always believe that she died because all hope had been taken away from her. . . . The resident's words took away her hope, and I honestly believe, as crazy as it may seem, that those words took away some of her potential lifetime."

> *Hope is the essential ingredient. Without it, patients find no reason for struggling to survive; without it, we find it easy to give up and stay in bed.*
> — *Journalist Natalie Davis Springarn*

An attitude such as hope is not just a mental state; it causes specific electrochemical changes in the body that influence not only the strength of the immune system but the workings of individual organs in the body as well. Norman Cousins is perhaps best known for his work with what he calls "the biology of hope." As he explains it, hope is tremendous expectation, and expectation can have powerful influence over the human body. One of his favorite examples of expectation occurred when a man collapsed on the Rancho Golf Course near Cousins's home. Paramedics were there, and from the monitor Cousins could see that the man was experiencing premature contractions of the heart. The paramedics were not talking to the man. Cousins leaned over and assured the man that he was in good hands and would be just fine within a few minutes. Cousins kept his eye on the cardiac monitor. Within 30 seconds, the cardiogram began to change. In just 2 minutes, the man's heartbeat had slowed, and his pulse was under 100 beats per minute.

Hope is so powerful and so real that it can even influence the outcome of supposedly terminal and irreversible diseases, such as cancer.

Faith What we perceive or believe to be real.

Hope Optimism in the absence of fear; positive expectation.

Hopelessness A mental state marked by negative expectations about the future.

If there is one thing I learned from my years of working with cancer patients, it's that there is no such thing as false hope. Hope is real and physiological. It's something I feel perfectly comfortable giving people — no matter what their situation. I know people are alive today because I said to them, "You don't have to die."[37]

Although denial usually is considered to be a negative emotion, it can be positive, especially for health. Denial makes room for hope. As Norman Cousins remarked, "Don't deny the diagnosis. Try to defy the verdict."[38]

There is a difference between total denial — the kind that does not leave room for hope — and "informed" denial, which allows for and actually inspires hope. According to psychologist Richard S. Lazarus of the University of California at Berkeley:

Illusion can sometimes allow hope, which is healthy. The critical determinant is whether you're denying facts or the implications. Let's say I get a biopsy that says I have a malignant tumor. I can face the facts, decide that this is a terrible illness, that I'm in trouble, will die very soon, and so give up hope. Or I can face the fact that this is a serious illness but acknowledge the ambiguity; people sometimes recover; it's curable. I've got to be treated, but I don't have to give up.[39]

In summing up the importance of hope, Cousins leaves us with this thought:

Hope, faith, love, and a strong will to live offer no promise of immortality, only proof of our uniqueness as human beings and the opportunity to experience full growth even under the grimmest circumstances. The clock provides only a technical measurement of how long we live. Far more real than the ticking of time is the way we open up the minutes and invest them with meaning. Death is not the ultimate tragedy in life. The ultimate tragedy is to die without discovering the possibilities of full growth.[40]

NOTES

1. *Learned Optimism* (New York: Alfred A. Knopf, 1991), p. 178.

2. "Explanatory Style and Cell-Mediated Immunity in Elderly Men and Women," Leslie Kaman-Siege, Judith Rodin, Martin E. P. Seligman, and John Dwyer, *Health Psychology*, 10:4 (1991), pp. 229–235.

3. "Mind Over Cancer: An Exclusive Interview with Yale Surgeon Dr. Bernie Siegel," *Prevention*, March 1988, pp. 59–64.

4. In "The Mind Over the Body," by Daniel Goleman, *New Realities*, March/April 1988, pp. 14–19.

5. *Head First: The Biology of Hope* (New York: E. P. Dutton, 1989), p. 120.

6. Cited in *The Healing Brain*, Robert Ornstein and David Sobel, (New York: Simon and Schuster, 1987), pp. 246–248.

7. *Society and the Adolescent Self-Image*, Morris Rosenberg.

8. "Absolutely, Positively, Refusing to Die," Steve Fishman, *Longevity*, September 1990, p. 69.

9. In "Mind Over Disease: Your Attitude Can Make You Well," by Donald Robinson, *Reader's Digest*, April 1987, pp. 73–78.

10. *The Complete Book of Cancer Prevention*, by Editors of Prevention Magazine Health Books (Emmaus, PA: Rodale Press).

11. "The High Priest of Healing," by Florence Graves, *New Age Journal*, May/June 1989, p. 34.

12. "Should Physicians Prescribe Prayer for Health? Spiritual Aspects of Well-Being Considered," Charles Marwick, *Journal of the American Medical Association*, 273:20 (May 24/31, 1995), p. 1561.

13. "Should Physicians Prescribe Prayer?" p. 1562.

14. "Developing a Useful Perspective on Spiritual Health: Love, Joy, Peace, and Fulfillment," Larry S. Chapman, *American Journal of Health Promotion*, Fall 1987, p. 12.

15. From "The Spirit of Health," *Advances: Journal of the Institute for the Advancement of Health*, 5:4 (1988), p. 4.

16. "The High Priest of Healing."

17. *Your Maximum Mind* (New York: Times Books/Random House, 1987), p. 6.

18. "Does Prayer Help Patients?" MD, December 1986, p. 35; and *Who Gets Sick: Thinking and Health*, Blair Justice (Houston: Peak Press, 1987), p. 284.

19. *Minding the Body, Mending the Mind*, Joan Borysenko, (Reading, MA: Addison-Wesley, 1987), p. 176.

20. "Religion and Well-Being in Later Life," Harold G. Koenig, James N. Kvale, and Carolyn Ferrel, *Gerontologist*, 28:1 (1988), pp. 18–27.

21. In "Should Physicians Prescribe Prayer for Health? Spiritual Aspects of Well-Being Considered," Charles Marwick, *Journal of the American Medical Association*, 273:20 (May 24/31, 1995), p. 1562.

22. "Religious Effects on Health Status and Life Satisfaction Among Black Americans," Jeffrey S. Levin, Linda M. Chatters, and Robert Joseph Taylor, *Journal of Gerontology*, 50B:3 (1995), pp. S154–163.

23. "Should Physicians Prescribe Prayer for Health?"

24. "Religious Effects on Health Status and Life Satisfaction Among Black Americans."

25. *The Altruistic Personality: Rescuers of Jews in Nazi Europe* (New York: Macmillan/Free Press, 1988).

26. "Research: Altruism and Transformation," *Noetic Sciences Review*, Autumn 1990, p. 33.

27. "Helper's High," by Allan Luks with Peggy Payne, *The Healing Power of Doing Good: The Health and Spiritual Benefits of Helping Others* (New York: Ballantine Books, 1991).

28. "Helper's High."

29. "Helper's High."

30. "Helper's High."

31. "Extend Your Hand, Extend Your Life," Sarah Long, *Longevity*, March 1989, p. 18.

32. In "Another Look at Altruism: Notes on an International Conference," by Tom Hurley, *Noetic Sciences Bulletin*, August/September 1989, p. 3.

33. "Another Look at Altruism."

34. "Hope: That Sustainer of Man," *Executive Health*, Section II, 20:3 (December 1983), pp. 1–4.

35. *Journal of Psychosocial Nursing*, 25:2 (1987), p. 21.

36. "The Importance of Hope," *Western Journal of Medicine*, 150 (May 1989), p. 609.

37. "Mind Over Cancer."

38. *Head First*.

39. In *The Healing Brain*, by Ornstein and Sobel.

40. *Head First*, pp. 65–66.

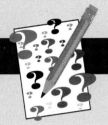

The Life Orientation Test: Are You an Optimist?

Name _____ Date _____ Grade _____

Instructor _____ Course _____ Section _____

In the following spaces, write how much you agree with each of the items, using the following scale:

4 = strongly agree   **3 = agree**   **2 = neutral**   **1 = disagree**   **0 = strongly disagree**

1. In uncertain times, I usually expect the best.   _____

2. If something can go wrong for me, it will.   _____

3. I always look on the bright side of things.   _____

4. I'm always optimistic about my future.   _____

5. I hardly ever expect things to go my way.   _____

6. Things never work out the way I want them to.   _____

7. I'm a believer in the idea that "every cloud has a silver lining."   _____

8. I rarely count on good things happening to me.   _____

How to Score

For items 2, 5, 6, and 8, you will need to reverse the numbers. For example, if you strongly agree with statement 8, "I rarely count on good things happening to me," change your score from 0 to 4. Now total up your score.

Interpreting Your Results

This test seems to demonstrate a relationship between an optimistic or a pessimistic outlook and physical well-being. When college students completed this test 4 weeks before final exams, the higher-scoring optimists (with 20 points and over) reported far fewer health problems. The pessimists complained of more dizziness, fatigue, sore muscles, and coughs.

Adapted from R. Ornstein and D. Sobel, *Healthy Pleasures* (Reading, MA: Addison-Wesley, 1989), pp. 162–163. © 1990 Robert Ornstein/David Sobel. Reprinted by permission of Addison-Wesley Publishing Co.

How Do You Feel About Yourself?

Name _____ Date _____ Grade _____

Instructor _____ Course _____ Section _____

This scale is designed to assist you in understanding your self-image. Positive attitudes toward oneself are important components of maturation and emotional well-being.

Self-image aspect	Strongly agree	Agree	Disagree	Strongly disagree
1. I feel that I'm a person of worth, at least on an equal plane with others.	A	B	C	D
2. I feel that I have a number of good qualities.	A	B	C	D
3. All in all, I am inclined to feel that I am a failure.	A	B	C	D
4. I am able to do things as well as most other people.	A	B	C	D
5. I feel I do not have as much to be proud of as others.	A	B	C	D
6. I take a positive attitude toward myself.	A	B	C	D
7. On the whole, I am satisfied with myself.	A	B	C	D
8. I wish I could have more respect for myself.	A	B	C	D
9. I certainly feel useless at times.	A	B	C	D
10. At times I think I am no good at all.	A	B	C	D

How to Score

Use the following table to determine the number of points to assign to each of your answers. To determine your total score, add up all the numbers that match the letter (A, B, C, or D) you circled for each statement.

Statement	A	B	C	D
1.	4	3	2	1
2.	4	3	2	1
3.	1	2	3	4
4.	4	3	2	1
5.	1	2	3	4
6.	4	3	2	1
7.	4	3	2	1
8.	1	2	3	4
9.	1	2	3	4
10.	1	2	3	4

Total: _____ **This is your self-esteem score.**

Interpreting Your Score

Classify your score in the appropriate score range.

Score range	Current self-esteem level
Less than 20	Low self-esteem
20-29	Below-average self-esteem
30-34	Above-average self-esteem
35-39	High self-esteem
40	Highest self-esteem

The higher your score, the more positive your self-esteem.

High self-esteem means that individuals respect themselves, consider themselves worthy, but do not necessarily consider themselves better than others. They do not feel themselves to be the ultimate in perfection; on the contrary, they recognize their limitations and expect to grow and improve.

Self-esteem is the most important variable in regard to human development and maturation. It is the master key that can open the door to the actualization of an individual's human potential.

M. Rosenberg, *Society and the Adolescent Self-Image* (Hanover, NH: Wesleyan University Press, 1986). Used by permission.

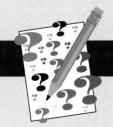

ASSESSMENT 5-3

Are Your Thoughts Helping or Hurting Your Longevity?

Name _____ Date _____ Grade _____

Instructor _____ Course _____ Section _____

Does an extraordinary challenge make you freeze up with fear? Do you let yourself dwell on minor slights? If so, you're prone to destructive thinking patterns that can prevent you from doing your best, fostering successful relationships and, in general, coping well and living long. Pessimists are less likely to survive major surgery, for example. And anyone who's easily offended will have trouble enjoying the camaraderie that is a key to living a long life.

The antidote for destructive thoughts is cultivating constructive ones. To help you do that, Seymour Epstein, Ph.D., professor of psychology at the University of Massachusetts and author of *You're Smarter Than You Think*, adapted the following quiz from a psychological test he uses to help patients strengthen their coping skills. This exercise will tell how constructive a thinker you are overall and identify the areas that could stand some pumping up.

Rate each statement from 1 to 5 according to this scale:

1 = completely false　　**2 = mainly false**　　**3 = undecided**　　**4 = mainly true**　　**5 = completely true**

Be honest. Don't answer according to how you think you should be but how you naturally are.

1. I don't worry about things I can do nothing about. _____

2. I am the kind of person who takes action, not just complains about things. _____

3. I don't let little things bother me. _____

4. If I have an unpleasant chore to do, I try to make the best of it by thinking in positive terms. _____

5. I don't feel I have to perform exceptionally well in order to consider myself a worthwhile person. _____

6. I look at challenges not as something to fear, but as opportunities to test myself and learn. _____

7. I tend to dwell more on pleasant than unpleasant incidents from the past. _____

8. When I have a difficult task, I think encouraging thoughts that help me do my best. _____

9. I tend not to take things personally. _____

10. When faced with upcoming unpleasant events, I usually think carefully how I will deal with them. _____

Total A _____

11. I feel that if people treat you badly, you should treat them in kind. _____

12. Talking about something I want to succeed at all but ensures failure. _____

13. I believe in astrology. _____

14. There are two kinds of people: good and bad. _____

15. When something good happens to me, I believe it will be balanced by something bad. _____

16. I have at least one good-luck charm. _____

17. There are many wrong ways to do something, but only one right way. _____

18. I believe in good and bad omens. _____

19. I believe in ghosts. _____

20. I tend to classify people as being either for or against me. _____

21. I sometimes think that if I want something to happen too badly, it probably won't. _____

22. I believe some people are able to read other people's thoughts. _____

23. I tend to be very judgmental. _____

24. I've learned not to hope for something too much — that usually means it won't happen. _____

Total B (90 minus total for 11-25) _____

25. I believe there are people who can literally see into the future. _____

Grand Total (A + B) _____

SCORING

Above 99 = VERY HIGH. You are a very constructive thinker. Keep up the good work.

89-99 = HIGH. You are a better-than-average constructive thinker. You usually expect good things to happen and they often do. But there's room for improvement.

74-88 = AVERAGE. Like most people, you're prone to some destructive thoughts. Go back through the exercise and try to identify a pattern. For example, statements 11, 14, 17, 20 and 23 represent categorical thinking — seeing situations and people as either good or bad; statements 12, 15, 18, 21 and 24 are examples of superstitious thinking; and 13, 16, 19, 22 and 25 show a kind of thinking that relies on belief in the paranormal. If you gave more than a 3 to these questions, try to catch yourself before lapsing into your usual assumptions. In addition, shore up your constructive thinking by reviewing the positive statements, 1 through 10, paying particular attention to those to which you gave less than a 3.

63-73 = LOW. Your habitual thinking is somewhat more destructive than most people's, and it interferes with your happiness and efficiency. Follow the advice given for average scorers. You have much to gain from working hard to improve your constructive thinking.

Below 63 = VERY LOW. Your destructive thinking is likely to be the source of serious problems. Work at identifying and correcting it. If you have trouble doing so, consider seeing a therapist. But regardless, don't expect your destructive thoughts to go away overnight.

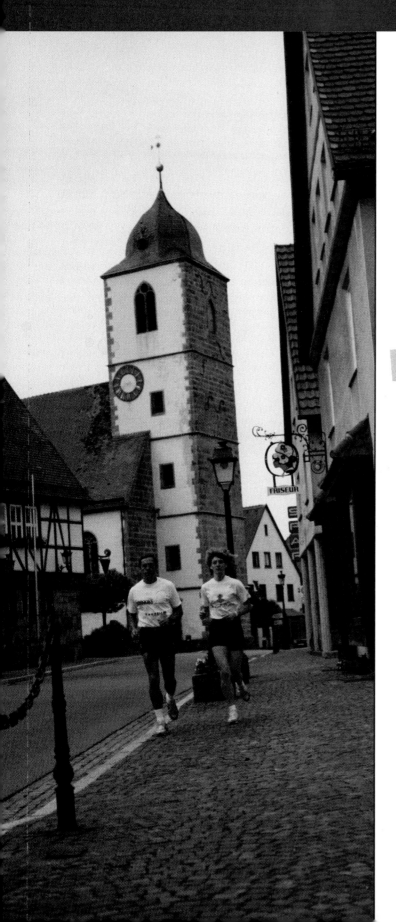

6

Fitness Assessment for Wellness

OBJECTIVES

■ Understand the significance of the U.S. Surgeon General's Report on Physical Activity and Health.

■ Explain the differences between physical activity, exercise, and physical fitness.

■ Understand the benefits and the significance of lifetime physical activity.

■ Identify risk factors that may interfere with safe participation in exercise.

■ Learn the difference between health and physical fitness standards.

■ Identify the components of health-related and skill-related fitness.

■ Learn to assess cardiorespiratory endurance, strength endurance, and flexibility.

■ Be able to interpret health-related fitness test results.

Advances in modern technology have almost completely eliminated the need for physical activity in the daily life of most people. Physical activity no longer is a natural part of our existence. We live in an automated society, in which most of the activities that used to require strenuous physical exertion can be accomplished by machines with the simple pull of a handle or push of a button. Physical inactivity and a sedentary lifestyle pose a serious threat to our health and accelerate the deterioration rate of the human body. Physically active people live longer than their inactive counterparts, even if they become active later in life. More than 250,000 deaths each year are attributed to lack of regular physical activity.[1] A similar trend is found in most industrialized nations throughout the world.

> **More than 250,000 deaths each year are attributed to lack of regular physical activity.**

During the late 1960s and in the 1970s, scientists began to realize that good fitness was important in the fight against chronic diseases, which had replaced infectious diseases as the leading causes of death.

We now recognize that health is largely self-controllable and that the leading causes of premature death and illness in the United States can be prevented by adhering to a healthy lifestyle. Physical activity is a crucial component.

PHYSICAL ACTIVITY VERSUS EXERCISE

Based on the abundance of scientific research on physical activity and exercise over the last three decades, a clear distinction has been established between physical activity and exercise. **Physical activity** is bodily movement produced by skeletal muscles that requires energy expenditure and produces progressive health benefits.[2] Examples of physical activity are walking to and from class, taking stairs instead of elevators and escalators, gardening, dancing, and washing the car by hand. Physical inactivity, on the other hand, implies a level of activity that is lower than that required to maintain good health.

Exercise is a type of physical activity that requires "planned, structured, and repetitive bodily movement done to improve or maintain one or more components of physical fitness."[3] Examples of exercise are regular, ongoing walking, jogging, cycling, aerobics, swimming, strength training, and stretching exercises.

1993 Summary Statement

The importance of regular physical activity in preventing disease and enhancing quality of life started to gain recognition by the nation's leaders in 1993 at a news briefing held at the National Press Club in Washington, DC. At this briefing, the U.S. Centers for Disease Control and Prevention and the American College of Sports Medicine, in conjunction with the President's Council on Physical Fitness and Sports, set forth recommendations on the types and amounts of physical activity that are needed for maintenance and promotion of health.

This summary statement encourages the American people to accumulate at least 30 minutes of moderate-intensity physical activity (walking part or all the way to and from work, walking up stairs, gardening, raking leaves, dancing fast) on an almost daily basis. Such a daily routine is suggested as an effective way to improve health. The 30 minutes of physical activity also can be conducted during a planned exercise program (for example, jogging, cycling, or swimming). The entire content of this statement on the benefits of physical activity is given in Figure 6.1.

Surgeon General's Report on Physical Activity and Health

Subsequently, a landmark report on the influence of regular physical activity on health was released in July of 1996 by the U.S. Surgeon General.[4] The significance of this historic document cannot be underestimated. Until 1996, the Surgeon General had released only two previous reports — one on smoking and health in 1964 and a second one on nutrition and health in 1988. More than 1,000 scientific

Physical activity Bodily movement produced by skeletal muscles that requires energy expenditure and produces progressive health benefits.

Exercise Physical activity that requires planned, structured, and repetitive bodily movement done to improve or maintain one or more components of physical fitness.

FIGURE 6.1

— SUMMARY STATEMENT —
Workshop On
Physical Activity and Public Health

Sponsored By:
U. S. Centers for Disease Control and Prevention
and
American College of Sports Medicine

In Cooperation with the President's Council on Physical Fitness and Sports

Regular physical activity is an important component of a healthy lifestyle — preventing disease and enhancing health and quality of life. A persuasive body of scientific evidence, which has accumulated over the past several decades, indicates that regular, moderate-intensity physical activity confers substantial health benefits. Because of this evidence, the U.S. Public Health Service has identified increased physical activity as a priority in Healthy People 2000, our national health objectives for the year 2000.

A primary benefit of regular physical activity is protection against coronary heart disease. In addition, physical activity appears to provide some protection against several other chronic diseases such as adult-onset diabetes, hypertension, certain cancers, osteoporosis, and depression. Furthermore, on average, physically active people outlive inactive people, even if they start their activity late in life. It is estimated that more than 250,000 deaths per year in the U.S. can be attributed to lack of regular physical activity, a number comparable to the deaths attributed to other chronic disease risk factors such as obesity, high blood pressure, and elevated blood cholesterol.

Despite the recognized value of physical activity, few Americans are regularly active. Only 22% of adults engage in leisure time physical activity at the level recommended for health benefits in Healthy People 2000. Fully 24% of adult Americans are completely sedentary and are badly in need of more physical activity. The remaining 54% are inadequately active and they too would benefit from more physical activity. Participation in regular physical activity appears to have gradually increased during the 1960s, 1970s, and early 1980s, but has plateaued in recent years. Among ethnic minority populations, older persons, and those with lower incomes or levels of education, participation in regular physical activity has remained consistently low.

Why are so few Americans physically active? Perhaps one answer is that previous public health efforts to promote physical activity have overemphasized the importance of high-intensity exercise. The current low rate of participation may be explained, in part, by the perception of many people that they must engage in vigorous, continuous exercise to reap health benefits. Actually the scientific evidence clearly demonstrates that regular, moderate-intensity physical activity provides substantial health benefits. A group of experts brought together by the U.S. Centers for Disease Control and Prevention (CDC) and the American Col-

lege of Sports Medicine (ACSM) reviewed the pertinent scientific evidence and formulated the following recommendation:

Every American adult should accumulate 30 minutes or more of moderate-intensity physical activity over the course of most days of the week. Incorporating more activity into the daily routine is an effective way to improve health. Activities that can contribute to the 30-minute total include walking up stairs (instead of taking the elevator), gardening, raking leaves, dancing, and walking part or all of the way to or from work. The recommended 30 minutes of physical activity may also come from planned exercise or recreation such as jogging, playing tennis, swimming, and cycling. One specific way to meet the standard is to walk two miles briskly.

Because most adult Americans fail to meet this recommended level of moderate-intensity physical activity, almost all should strive to increase their participation in moderate or vigorous physical activity. Persons who currently do not engage in regular physical activity should begin by incorporating a few minutes of increased activity into their day, building up gradually to 30 minutes of additional physical activity. Those who are irregularly active should strive to adopt a more consistent pattern of activity. Regular participation in physical activities that develop and maintain muscular strength and joint flexibility is also recommended.

This recommendation has been developed to emphasize the important health benefits of moderate physical activity. But recognizing the benefits of physical activity is only part of the solution to this important public health problem. Today's high-tech society entices people to be inactive. Cars, television, and labor-saving devices have profoundly changed the way many people perform their jobs, take care of their homes, and use their leisure time. Furthermore, our surroundings often present significant barriers to participation in physical activity. Walking to the corner store proves difficult if there are no sidewalks; riding a bicycle to work is not an option unless safe bike lanes or paths are available.

Many Americans will not change their lifestyles until the environmental and social barriers to physical activity are reduced or eliminated. Individuals can help to overcome these barriers by modifying their own lifestyles and by encouraging family members and friends to become more active. In addition, local, state, and federal public health agencies; recreation boards; school groups; professional organizations; and fitness and sports organizations should work together to disseminate this critical public health message and to promote national, community, worksite, and school programs that help Americans become more physically active.

The American College of Sports Medicine and the U.S. Centers for Disease Control and Prevention, in cooperation with the President's Council on Physical Fitness and Sports, released this statement July 29, 1993, at the National Press Club in Washington, D.C.

Summary Statement: Workshop on Physical Activity and Public Health.

studies from the fields of epidemiology, exercise physiology, medicine, and the behavioral sciences are summarized in the 1996 document on physical activity and health.

The report states that regular moderate physical activity provides substantial benefits in health and well-being for the vast majority of Americans who are not physically active. Among these benefits are a significant reduction in the risk of developing or dying from heart disease, diabetes, colon cancer, and high blood pressure. Regular physical activity also is important for health of muscles, bones, and joints; and it seems to reduce symptoms of depression and anxiety, improve mood, and enhance the ability to perform daily tasks throughout life. For individuals who are moderately active already, greater health benefits can be achieved by increasing the amount of physical activity.

According to the Surgeon General, more than 60% of adults do not achieve the recommended amount of physical activity, and 25% are not physically active at all. Further, almost half of all people between ages 12 and 21 are not vigorously active on a regular basis. This report has become a call to nationwide action. Regular moderate physical activity can prevent premature death, unnecessary illness, and disability. It also can help control health-care costs and help to maintain a high quality of life into old age.

While acknowledging that participation in exercise (higher-intensity activity) provides slightly better health benefits and greater fitness benefits, the main objective of the Surgeon General's report is to get people to participate in at least moderate-intensity activities. In the report, **moderate intensity physical activity** is defined as physical activity that uses 150 calories of energy per day, or 1,000 calories per week. People should strive to achieve at least 30 minutes of physical activity per day most days of the week. Examples of moderate physical activity are walking, cycling, playing basketball or volleyball, swimming, water aerobics, dancing fast, raking leaves, shoveling snow, washing or waxing a car, and washing windows or floors.

FITNESS AND HEALTH

Several significant research studies linking physical activity habits and mortality rates have shown a decrease in premature mortality rates among physically active people. A study conducted by Dr. Ralph Paffenbarger and his colleagues involving 16,936 Harvard alumni showed that as the amount of weekly physical activity increased, the risk of cardiovascular deaths decreased.[5] The greatest decrease in cardiovascular deaths was observed among alumni who used in excess of 2000 calories per week through physical activity (see Figure 6.2).

Another major study, conducted by Dr. Steve Blair and his associates,[6] upheld the findings of the Harvard alumni study. Based on data from 13,344 people who were followed over

The U.S. Surgeon General has determined that moderate-intensity physical activity is beneficial to a person's health and well-being.

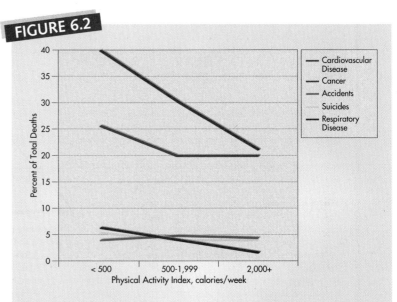

FIGURE 6.2

Based on 10,000 man-years of observation. One person-year indicates one person followed up 1 year later.

From "A Natural History of Athleticism on Cardiovascular Health," by R. S. Paffenbarger, R. T. Hyde, A. L. Wing, and C. H. Steinmetz, *Journal of the American Medical Association*, 252 (1984), pp. 491–495.

Death rates according to physical activity index.

an average of 8 years, the results confirmed that the level of cardiorespiratory fitness is related to mortality from all causes. In essence, the higher the level of cardiorespiratory fitness, the longer the life (see Figure 6.3). Death-rate from all causes for the least fit (group 1) men was 3.4 times higher than it was for the most fit men. For the least fit women, the death rate was 4.6 times higher than it was for the most fit women.

The same study reported a much lower rate of premature deaths even at the moderate fitness levels most adults can achieve. Even greater protection was attained when a higher fitness level was combined with elimination of other risk factors such as hypertension, high cholesterol, cigarette smoking, and excessive body fat.

Additional research that looked at changes in fitness and mortality found a substantial (44%) reduction in mortality risk when people abandoned a sedentary lifestyle and became moderately fit.[7] The lowest death rate was found in people who were fit and remained fit, and the highest rate was found in men who remained unfit (see Figure 6.4).

Subsequent research on the Harvard alumni study published in 1995 substantiated the previous findings and also indicated that primarily vigorous activities are associated with greater longevity.[8]

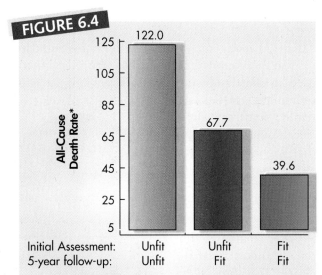

FIGURE 6.4

| Initial Assessment: | Unfit | Unfit | Fit |
| 5-year follow-up: | Unfit | Fit | Fit |

* Death rate per 10,000 man-years observation. Based on data from "Changes in Physical Fitness and All-Cause Mortality: A Prospective Study of Healthy Men," *Journal of the American Medical Association*, 273 (1995), pp. 1193–1198.

Source: "Health Practices and Cancer Mortality Among Active California Mormons,", by J. E. Enstrom, *Journal of the National Cancer Institute*, 81 (1989), pp. 1807–1814.

Five-year follow-up in mortality rates associated with maintenance and improvements in fitness.

Moderate intensity physical activity Physical activity that uses 150 calories of energy per day, or 1,000 calories per week.

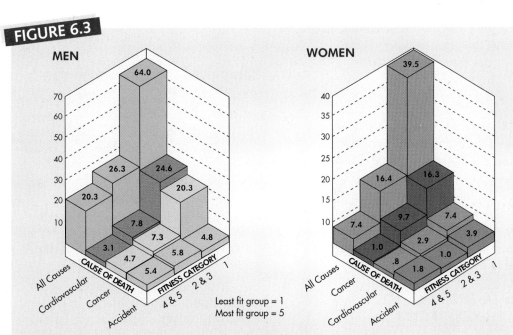

FIGURE 6.3

Least fit group = 1
Most fit group = 5

Based on data from "Physical Fitness and All-Cause Mortality: A Prospective Study of Healthy Men and Women, by S. N. Blair, H. W. Kohl III, R. S. Paffenbarger, Jr., D. G. Clark, K. H. Cooper, and L. W. Gibbons, *Journal of the American Medical Association* 262 (1989), 2395–2401.

Note: Study included 13,344 people, followed for 10,000 person-years 1970°1985. One person-year indicates one person followed up 1 year later.

Death rates by physical fitness groups.

Vigorous activity was defined as any activity that requires a MET* level equal to or greater than 6 METs (21 ml/kg/min — see Health Fitness Standards later in this chapter). Examples of vigorous activities used in that study include brisk walking, jogging, swimming laps, squash, racquetball, tennis, and shoveling snow. The results also indicated that vigorous exercise is as important as not smoking and main- taining recommended weight.

The results of all these studies indicate clearly that fitness im- proves health, wellness, and longevity. If people are able to do vigorous exer- cise, it is preferable because it is most clearly associated with longer life.

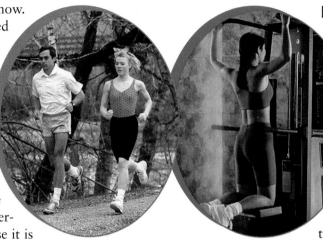

Regular participation in a lifetime exercise program increases quality of life and longevity.

IMPACTS OF PHYSICAL FITNESS

Most people exercise because it improves their per- sonal appearance and makes them feel good about themselves. The greatest benefit of all, however, is that physically fit individuals enjoy a better quality of life. These people live life to its fullest potential, with fewer health problems than inactive individuals who also may indulge in negative lifestyle patterns.

Health-Care Costs

The economic impact of sedentary living has left a strong impression on the nation's economy. As the need for physical exertion decreased steadily during the last century, the nation's health-care expenditures increased dramatically. Health-care costs in the United States rose from $12 billion in 1950 to more than $1 trillion in 1997.

If the rate of escalation continues, health-care expenditures could double every 5 years. The 1993 figure represents about 14% of the gross national product (GNP), and it is projected to reach 17% by the year 2000 and 37% by 2030. The 1989 average

health-care cost per person in the United States ($2,354) was almost twice as high as most other in- dustrialized nations, including Great Britain ($836), (West) Germany ($1,232), France ($1,274), and Switzerland ($1,376).

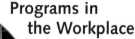

Programs in the Workplace

As a result of the stag- gering rise in medical costs, many organiza- tions are beginning to realize that it costs less to keep employees healthy than to treat them once they are sick. Consequently, con- taining health-care costs through fitness and wellness programs has become a major issue for many organizations around the country.

The Prudential Insurance Company of Houston, Texas, released the findings of a study conducted on its 1,386 employees. Those who participated for at least a year in the company's fitness program aver- aged 3.5 days of disability, compared to 8.6 days for nonparticipants. A further breakdown by level of fit- ness showed no disability days for those in the high

Company Programs in Europe

- Research in Germany (West Germany prior to reunification) reported 68.6% less absentee- ism by workers with cardiovascular symptoms who participated in a fitness program. In Ger- many, the law mandates that corporations em- ploying workers for sedentary jobs must provide an in-house facility for physical exercise.

- The Goodyear Company in Norrkoping, Swe- den, indicated a 50% reduction in absentee- ism following implementation of a fitness program.

- Studies in the former Soviet Union reported increased physical work capacity and motor coordination, lower incidence of disease, shorter duration of illness, and fewer relapses by individuals participating in industrial fitness programs.

---

* MET is the energy expenditure at rest, or approximately 3.5 ml/kg/min.; six or more METs represents exercising at an oxygen uptake (VO_2) equal to or greater than 6 times the resting energy requirement.

fitness group, 1.6 days for the good fitness group, and 4.1 disability days for the fair fitness group.

Data analysis conducted by Tenneco Inc., also of Houston, showed that annual medical-care costs for male and female exercisers were about 44% to 58% lower than for the nonexercising group. Sick leave also was lower for the men and women exercisers. Furthermore, the company reported that individuals with high job performance ratings also rated high in exercise participation — providing evidence that job productivity is related to fitness.

PRE-EXERCISE SCREENING AND GOALS

Even though exercise testing and participation are relatively safe for most apparently healthy individuals under age 40, the reaction of the cardiovascular system to more intense levels of physical activity cannot always be predicted. Consequently, people face a small but real risk of some bodily changes during exercise testing or participation. These changes may include abnormal blood pressure, irregular heart rhythm, fainting, and, rarely, a heart attack or cardiac arrest.

Before you start an exercise program or participate in any exercise testing, you should fill out the Physical Activity Readiness Questionnaire (PAR-Q) in Assessment 6-1. This questionnaire, developed by the British Columbia Ministry of Health in Canada, is used widely in the United States and Canada as a screening instrument prior to fitness testing.

If your answer to any of the PAR-Q questions is positive, you should consult a physician before participating in fitness testing or a fitness program. Exercise testing or participation is not advised under some of the conditions listed in the questionnaire and may require a stress electrocardiogram (ECG) test (see Chapter 7). If you have any questions regarding your current health status, you should consult your doctor before initiating, continuing, or increasing your level of physical activity.

As you work through this chapter and assess the various components of fitness, you will be able to develop a fitness profile. When you obtain the information pertaining to each component of fitness, you can enter your results on the profile found in Assessment 6-2.

Once the results for each component have been established, either with your instructor's help or using your own judgment, you can set the target goals to achieve over the next 10 to 14 weeks. You then may proceed with an exercise program as outlined in Chapter 7. Following 8 to 12 weeks of exercise training, you should retest each component to assess improvements in physical fitness.

PHYSICAL FITNESS

Physical fitness has been defined in several ways and has meant different things to different people. Perhaps the most comprehensive definition has been given by the American Medical Association, which defined **physical fitness** as the general capacity to adapt and respond favorably to physical effort. This implies that individuals are physically fit when they can meet the ordinary and the unusual demands of daily life safely and effectively, without being overly fatigued, and still have energy left for leisure and recreational activities.

As the fitness concept gained ground in the last two decades or so, it became clear that no single test was sufficient to assess overall fitness. Rather, a battery of tests was necessary because several specific components have to be established to determine an individual's overall level of fitness.

Most authorities agree that physical fitness can be classified into health-related and motor skill-related fitness. As illustrated in Figure 6.5, the four fitness components, from a health point of view, are cardiorespiratory (aerobic) endurance, muscular strength and endurance, muscular flexibility, and body composition. The first three components of health-related fitness are discussed in this chapter. Body composition is discussed in Chapter 9.

The motor skill-related components of fitness are identified mostly with athletics. Motor skill-related fitness encompasses agility, balance, coordination, power, reaction time, and speed. Although these components are important in achieving success in athletics, they are not crucial for developing better health.

In terms of health and wellness, the main emphasis of fitness programs should be placed on the health-related components, and that is the focus of the fitness information in this book.

Vigorous activity   Any activity that requires a MET level equal to or greater than 6 METs (21 ml/kg/min).

Physical fitness   The general capacity to adapt and respond favorably to physical effort.

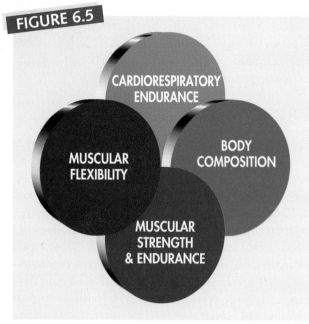

FIGURE 6.5

Health-related components of physical fitness.

FITNESS STANDARDS

A meaningful debate has arisen to determine recommended fitness standards for the nation. The debate focuses on determining sound age- and gender-related fitness standards for the general population. Two standards have started to develop in this regard: a health fitness standard (criterion-referenced) and a physical fitness standard.

Health Fitness Standards

As illustrated in Figure 6.6, although fitness (see VO_{2max} discussion below) improvements with a moderate aerobic activity program are not as notable, significant health benefits are reaped with such a program. Only slightly better health benefits are obtained with a more intense exercise program. Benefits include a reduction in blood lipids, lower blood pressure, decreased risk for diabetes, weight loss, stress release, and lower risk for disease and premature mortality.

The health fitness or criterion-referenced standards proposed here are based on epidemiological data linking minimum fitness values to disease prevention and health. Attaining the health fitness standards requires only moderate amounts of physical activity. For example, a 2-mile walk in less than 30 minutes, five to six times per week, seems to be sufficient to achieve the health-fitness standard for cardiorespiratory endurance.

> *Attaining the health fitness standards requires only moderate amounts of physical activity.*

Cardiorespiratory endurance is measured in terms of the maximal amount of oxygen the body is able to utilize per minute of physical activity, called **maximal oxygen uptake**, or VO_{2max}. VO_{2max} commonly is expressed in milliliters of oxygen per kilogram of

FIGURE 6.6

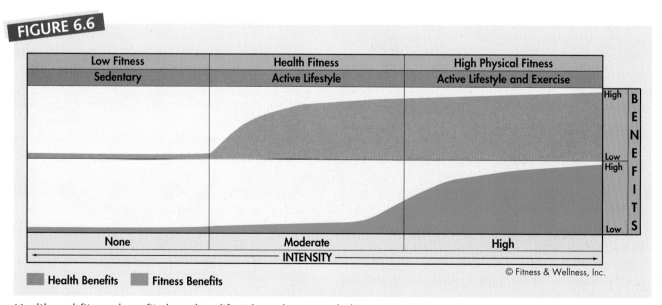

Low Fitness	Health Fitness	High Physical Fitness
Sedentary	Active Lifestyle	Active Lifestyle and Exercise

None	Moderate	High

INTENSITY

Health Benefits Fitness Benefits

© Fitness & Wellness, Inc.

Health and fitness benefits based on lifestyle and exercise habits.

body weight per minute (ml/kg/min). Individual values can range from about 10 ml/kg/min in cardiac patients to approximately 80 to 90 ml/kg/min in world-class runners and cross-country skiers.

Data from the research study presented in Figure 6.3 indicate that VO_{2max} values of 35 and 32.5 ml/kg/min for men and women, respectively, may be sufficient to lower the risk for all causes of mortality significantly. Although greater improvements in fitness yield a slightly lower risk for premature death, the largest drop is seen between the least fit (group 1) and the moderately fit (groups 2 and 3). Therefore, the 35 and 32.5 ml/kg/min values could be selected as the health fitness standards.

Physical Fitness Standards

Physical fitness standards are set higher than the health fitness norms and require a more vigorous exercise program. Many experts believe that people who meet the criteria of "good" physical fitness should be able to do moderate to vigorous physical activity without undue fatigue and to maintain this capability throughout life. In this context, physically fit people of all ages will have the freedom to enjoy most of life's daily and recreational activities to their fullest potential. Current health fitness standards may not be enough to achieve these objectives.

Sound physical fitness gives the individual a degree of independence throughout life that many people in North America no longer enjoy. Most older people should be able to carry out activities similar to those conducted in their youth, though not with the same intensity. Although a person does not have to be an elite athlete, activities such as changing a tire, chopping wood, climbing several flights of stairs, playing a vigorous game of basketball, mountain biking, playing soccer with grandchildren, walking several miles around a lake, and hiking through a national park require more than the current "average fitness" level of the American people.

In this book, fitness standards for cardiorespiratory endurance, strength, flexibility, and body composition provide both a health fitness standard and a

A high level of fitness is needed to enjoy many of life's recreational and leisure physical activities.

physical fitness standard. You will have to decide your own objectives. If the main objective of a fitness program is to lower the risk of disease, attaining the health fitness standards may be enough to ensure better health. If you want to participate in moderate to vigorous fitness activities, achieving a high physical fitness standard is recommended.

ASSESSMENT OF CARDIORESPIRATORY ENDURANCE

Cardiorespiratory endurance has been defined as the ability of the lungs, heart, and blood vessels to deliver adequate amounts of oxygen to the cells to meet the demands of prolonged physical activity. As you breathe, part of the oxygen in the air is taken up in your lungs and transported in the blood to your heart. The heart then pumps the oxygenated blood through your circulatory system to all organs and tissues of your body. At the cellular level, oxygen is used to convert food substrates, primarily carbohydrates and fats, into energy necessary to conduct body functions and maintain a constant internal equilibrium.

During physical exertion, a greater amount of energy is needed to perform the activity. As a result, the heart, lungs, and blood vessels have to deliver more oxygen to the cells to supply the required energy. During prolonged exercise, an individual with a high level of cardiorespiratory endurance is able to deliver the required amount of oxygen to the tissues quite easily. The cardiorespiratory system of a person with a low level of endurance has to work much harder, because the heart has to pump more often to supply the same amount

Maximal oxygen uptake (VO_{2max}) The maximum amount of oxygen the body is able to utilize per minute of physical activity, commonly expressed in ml/kg/min. The best indicator of cardiorespiratory or aerobic fitness.

Cardiorespiratory endurance The ability of the lungs, heart, and blood vessels to deliver adequate amounts of oxygen to the cells to meet the demands of prolonged physical activity.

of oxygen to the tissues and, consequently, fatigues faster. A higher capacity to deliver and utilize oxygen (oxygen uptake), then, indicates a more efficient cardiorespiratory system.

A sound cardiorespiratory endurance program greatly enhances health. With the exception of older adults, cardiorespiratory endurance is the single most important component of health-related physical fitness. Certain levels of muscular strength and flexibility are necessary in daily activities to lead a normal life. Even so, a person can get by without a lot of strength and flexibility but cannot do without a good cardiorespiratory system.

Again, the level of cardiorespiratory endurance, cardiorespiratory fitness, or **aerobic capacity** is determined by the maximal amount of oxygen the human body is able to utilize per minute of physical activity (usually expressed in ml/kg/min). Because all tissues and organs of the body require oxygen to function, higher oxygen consumption indicates a more efficient cardiorespiratory system.

The most precise way to determine VO_{2max} is through **open circuit indirect calorimetry** or **direct gas analysis**. This is done using a metabolic cart through which the amount of oxygen the body consumes can be measured directly. Because this type of equipment is not available in most health/fitness centers, several alternative methods of estimating VO_{2max} have been developed.

Even though most cardiorespiratory endurance tests probably are safe to administer to apparently healthy individuals (those with no major coronary risk factors or symptoms), the American College of Sports Medicine[9] recommends that a physician be present for any **maximal exercise test** on apparently healthy men over age 40 and women over age 50. A maximal test is any test that requires the participant's all-out or nearly all-out effort. For submaximal exercise tests a physician should be present when testing higher risk/symptomatic individuals or diseased people, regardless of the participant's current age.

Two exercise tests frequently used to assess cardiorespiratory fitness are the 1.5-Mile Run test and the 1.0-Mile Walk test. Depending on fitness level and personal preference, you may choose either or both of these. The running test is recommended for individuals who exercise regularly, whereas the walking test is preferred for those who have not yet initiated an exercise program. Because these are field tests to estimate VO_{2max}, each test will not necessarily yield exactly the same results. To make valid comparisons, the same test should be used for pre- and post-assessments.

The 1.5-Mile Run Test

The 1.5-Mile Run test is used most frequently to predict cardiorespiratory fitness according to the time it takes to run (or walk) a 1.5-mile course. VO_{2max} is estimated based on the time required to cover the distance (see Table 6.1).

The only equipment necessary to conduct this test is a stopwatch and a 440-yard track (6 laps to complete the 1.5 miles) or a premeasured 1.5-mile course. A person should be cautious prior to doing the 1.5-mile run. Because the objective of this test is to cover the distance in the shortest time, it is considered a maximal exercise test. Therefore, its use should be limited to conditioned individuals who have been cleared for exercise. The 1.5-Mile Run test is not recommended for unconditioned beginners, men over age 40 and women over age 50 without proper medical clearance, symptomatic individuals, and those with known disease or coronary heart disease risk factors. Unconditioned individuals should participate in at least 6 weeks of aerobic training before taking this test.

Before the actual run, you should warm up properly by doing some stretching exercises, walking, and slow jogging. Equally important, at the end of the 1.5-mile run, you should cool down by walking slowly or jogging another 3 to 5 minutes. You should not sit or lie down after the test. If any unusual symptoms arise during the run, the test should be terminated immediately and you should cool down through slow jogging or walking. You may retake the test following 6 weeks of aerobic training.

Table 6.1 can be consulted to find the estimated VO_{2max}. The corresponding fitness categories, based on VO_{2max} are found in Table 6.2. You can record the results of your 1.5-Mile Run test in the fitness profile in Assessment 6-2.

Aerobic capacity   The maximal amount of oxygen the human body is able to utilize per minute of physical activity (usually expressed in ml/kg/min).

Open circuit indirect calorimetry (direct gas analysis)   The most precise way to determine VO_{2max} using a metabolic cart to measure the amount of oxygen consumed by the body.

Maximal exercise test   Any test that requires the participant's all-out or nearly all-out effort.

TABLE 6.1 Estimated Maximal Oxygen Uptake for the 1.5-Mile Run Test

Time	VO$_{2max}$ (ml/kg/min)	Time	VO$_{2max}$ (ml/kg/min)	Time	VO$_{2max}$ (ml/kg/min)	Time	VO$_{2max}$ (ml/kg/min)
6:10	80.0	9:30	54.7	12:50	39.2	16:10	30.5
6:20	79.0	9:40	53.5	13:00	38.6	16:20	30.2
6:30	77.9	9:50	52.3	13:10	38.1	16:30	29.8
6:40	76.7	10:00	51.1	13:20	37.8	16:40	29.5
6:50	75.5	10:10	50.4	13:30	37.2	16:50	29.1
7:00	74.0	10:20	49.5	13:40	36.8	17:00	28.9
7:10	72.6	10:30	48.6	13:50	36.3	17:10	28.5
7:20	71.3	10:40	48.0	14:00	35.9	17:20	28.3
7:30	69.9	10:50	47.4	14:10	35.5	17:30	28.0
7:40	68.3	11:00	46.6	14:20	35.1	17:40	27.7
7:50	66.8	11:10	45.8	14:30	34.7	17:50	27.4
8:00	65.2	11:20	45.1	14:40	34.3	18:00	27.1
8:10	63.9	11:30	44.4	14:50	34.0	18:10	26.8
8:20	62.5	11:40	43.7	15:00	33.6	18:20	26.6
8:30	61.2	11:50	43.2	15:10	33.1	18:30	26.3
8:40	60.2	12:00	42.3	15:20	32.7	18:40	26.0
8:50	59.1	12:10	41.7	15:30	32.2	18:50	25.7
9:00	58.1	12:20	41.0	15:40	31.8	19:00	25.4
9:10	56.9	12:30	40.4	15:50	31.4		
9:20	55.9	12:40	39.8	16:00	30.9		

Adapted from "A Means of Assessing Maximal Oxygen Intake" by K. H. Cooper, *Journal of the American Medical Association* 203 (1968), pp. 201-204; *Health and Fitness Through Physical Activity,* by M. L. Pollock et al. (New York: John Wiley and Sons, 1978), and *Training for Sport and Activity* by J. H. Wilmore (Boston: Allyn and Bacon, 1982).

TABLE 6.2 Cardiorespiratory Fitness Classification According to Maximal Oxygen Uptake

Gender	Age	Fitness Classification (in ml/kg/min)				
		Poor	Fair	Average	Good	Excellent
Men	<29	<24.9	25–33.9	34–43.9	44–52.9	>53
	30–39	<22.9	23–30.9	31–41.9	42–49.9	>50
	40–49	<19.9	20–26.9	27–38.9	39–44.9	>45
	50–59	<17.9	18–24.9	25–37.9	38–42.9	>43
	60–69	<15.9	16–22.9	23–35.9	36–40.9	>41
Women	<29	<23.9	24–30.9	31–38.9	39–48.9	>49
	30–39	<19.9	20–27.9	28–36.9	37–44.9	>45
	40–49	<16.9	17–24.9	25–34.9	35–41.9	>42
	50–59	<14.9	15–21.9	22–33.9	34–39.9	>40
	60–69	<12.9	13–20.9	21–32.9	33–36.9	>37

■ High physical fitness standard
■ Health fitness standard

The 1.0-Mile Walk Test*

For the walking test, either a 440-yard track (4 laps to a mile) or a premeasured 1.0-mile course can be used. A stopwatch is required to determine total walking time and exercise heart rate. Prior to the walk, you have to know your body weight in pounds.

You should walk the 1.0-mile course at a brisk pace in such a way that the exercise heart rate at the end of the test is above 120 beats per minute. At the end of the 1.0-Mile Walk, walking time is checked and the pulse is counted immediately for 10 seconds.

You can take your pulse on the wrist by placing two fingers over the radial artery (inside of the wrist on the side of the thumb) or over the carotid artery in the neck just below the jaw next to the voice box. Next, the 10-second pulse count is multiplied by 6 to obtain the exercise heart rate in beats per minute (bpm).

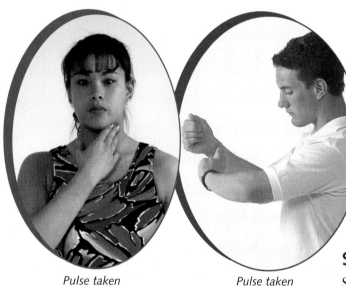

Pulse taken at the carotid artery.   *Pulse taken at the radial artery.*

Now the walking time is converted from minutes and seconds to minute units. Because each minute has 60 seconds, the seconds are divided by 60 to obtain the fraction of a minute. For instance, a walking time of 12 minutes and 15 seconds equals 12 + (15 ÷ 60) or 12.25 minutes.

---

*Source: G. Kline et al., "Estimation of VO_{2max} from a One-Mile Track Walk, Gender, Age, and Body Weight," *Medicine and Science in Sports and Exercise* (19(3):253–259, 1987. © American College of Sports Medicine. Used by permission.

To obtain the estimated VO_{2max} in ml/kg/min for the 1.0-Mile Walk test, plug your values into the following equation:

$$VO_{2max} = 132.853 - (.0769 \times W) - (.3877 \times A) + (6.315 \times G) - (3.2649 \times T) - (.1565 \times HR)$$

Where:

W	= weight in pounds
A	= age in years
G	= gender (use 0 for women and 1 for men)
T	= total time for the mile walk in minutes
HR	= exercise heart rate in beats per minute at the end of the mile walk

For example, a 19-year-old female weighing 140 pounds completed the mile walk in 14 minutes and 39 seconds with an exercise heart rate of 148 beats per minute. The estimated VO_{2max} is:

W	= 140 lbs
A	= 19
G	= 0 (female gender = 0)
T	= 14:39 = 14 + (39 ÷ 60) = 14.65 min
HR	= 148 bpm
VO_{2max}	= 132.853 - (.0769 × 140) - (.3877 × 19) + (6.315 × 0) - (3.2649 × 14.65) - (.1565 × 148)
VO_{2max}	= 43.7 ml/kg/min

As with the 1.5-Mile Run test, the fitness categories, based on VO_{2max} are found in Table 6.2. The cardiorespiratory fitness test results are recorded in Assessment 6-2.

ASSESSMENT OF MUSCULAR STRENGTH AND ENDURANCE

Strength, a basic component of fitness and wellness, is crucial for optimal performance in daily activities such as walking, running, lifting and carrying objects, doing housework, and even enjoying recreational activities. Strength also is of great value in improving posture, personal appearance, and self-image, in developing sports skills, and in meeting certain emergencies in life in which strength is necessary to cope effectively.

From a health standpoint, strength helps to maintain muscle tissue and a higher resting metabolism (see Chapter 10), facilitates weight loss and weight control, decreases the risk for injury, helps to prevent and correct chronic low back pain, and is thought to help with childbearing and delivery. Adequate strength is especially critical in maintaining functional independent living in advanced age. Many older adults lack sufficient strength to move about and be able to perform simple tasks of daily living such as being able to stand up or get out of bed without help, walk up a flight of stairs, or lift and carry small objects. Additional information on strength training and older adults is presented in Chapter 7.

Strength Versus Endurance

When discussing strength, the difference between muscular strength and muscular endurance has to be clarified. Although these components are interrelated, they have a basic difference. **Strength** is the ability to exert maximum force against resistance. **Endurance** is the ability of a muscle to exert submaximal force repeatedly over a period of time.

Muscular endurance (also referred to as localized muscular endurance) depends to a large extent on muscular strength. Weak muscles cannot repeat an action several times or sustain it for a long time. Keeping these two principles in mind, strength tests and training programs have been designed to measure and develop absolute muscular strength, muscular endurance, or a combination of both.

Muscular strength usually is determined by the maximal amount of resistance — **one repetition maximum**, or 1 RM — that an individual is able to lift in a single effort. This assessment gives a good measure of absolute strength, but it does require a considerable amount of time, as the 1 RM is determined through trial and error.

For example, the strength of the chest muscles frequently is measured with the bench press exercise. If the individual has not trained with weights, he or she may try 100 pounds and lift this resistance quite easily. Then 50 pounds are added, but the person fails to lift the resistance. The resistance then is decreased by 10 or 20 pounds, and finally, after several trials, the 1 RM is established. Fatigue also becomes a factor, because by the time the 1 RM is established, several maximal, or near-maximal attempts have been performed already.

Muscular endurance is commonly established by the number of repetitions an individual can perform against a submaximal resistance such as lifting 80 pounds 20 times. It also can be determined by the length of time a given contraction is sustained — for example, how long the chin can be maintained

above a bar while holding onto the bar with the hands and while the body is freely suspended from the ground.

Muscular Endurance Test

We live in a world in which muscular strength and endurance both are required. Because muscular endurance depends to a large extent on muscular strength, a muscular endurance test has been selected to determine strength.

Three exercises that assess the endurance of the upper body, lower body, and abdominal muscle groups have been selected for the muscular endurance test. A stopwatch, a metronome, a bench or gymnasium bleacher 16¼ inches high, and a partner are needed to administer the three test (exercise) items. The exercises conducted for this test are bench-jump, modified-dip (men) or modified push-up (women), and bent-leg curl-up (or abdominal crunch for individuals prone to low-back pain).

Bench-jump

Using a bench or gymnasium bleacher 16¼ inches high, attempt to jump up onto and down off of the bench as many times as possible in a 1-minute period. If you cannot jump the full minute, step up and down. A repetition is counted each time both feet return to the floor.

Modified-dip

This upper-body exercise is performed by men only. Using the same bench or gymnasium bleacher 16¼ inches high, place the hands on the bench with the fingers pointing forward. Have a partner hold your feet in front of you. Your hips should be bent at approximately 90°. Lower your body by flexing your elbows until you reach a 90° angle at

Bench-jump.

Strength The ability to exert maximum force against resistance.

Endurance The ability of a muscle to exert submaximal force repeatedly over a period of time.

One repetition maximum (1 RM) The maximal amount of resistance (weight) that an individual is able to lift in a single effort.

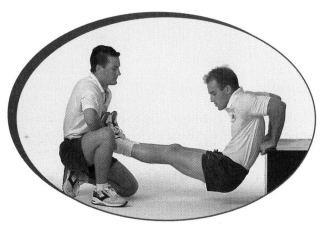

Modified-dip.

this joint, and then return to the starting position. (A repetition does not count if you do not reach 90°.) Perform the repetitions to a two-step cadence (down-up), regulated with a metronome set at 56 beats per minute. Perform as many continuous repetitions as possible. The test is terminated if you fail to follow the metronome cadence.

Modified push-up

Women are to perform the modified push-up exercise instead of the modified-dip exercise. Lie down on the floor (face down), bend your knees (feet up in the air), and place your hands on the floor by the shoulders with your fingers pointing forward. The lower body will be supported at the knees (rather than the feet) throughout the test. The objective is to raise and lower the upper body by fully extending and flexing the elbows. The chest must touch the floor on each repetition.

As with the modified-dip exercise, the repetitions are performed to a two-step cadence (up-down) regulated with a metronome set at 56 beats per minute. Perform as many continuous repetitions as possible. The test is stopped when you can't do any more repetitions or you can no longer follow the metronome cadence.

Bent-leg curl-up

Lie down on the floor (face up) and bend both legs at the knees at approximately 100°. Your feet should be on the floor, and you must hold them in place yourself throughout the test. Cross the arms in front of your chest, each hand on the opposite shoulder. Now raise the head off the floor, placing the chin against your chest. This is the starting and finishing position for each curl-up. The back of the head may not come in contact with the floor, the hands cannot be removed from the shoulders, nor may the feet or hips be raised off the floor at any time during the test. The test is terminated if any of these four conditions occur.

When you curl up, the upper body must come to an upright position before going back down. The

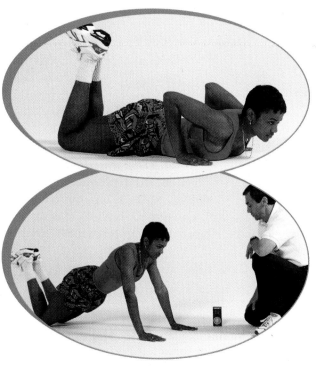

Modified push-up.

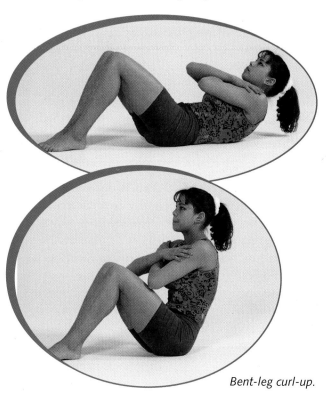

Bent-leg curl-up.

repetitions are performed to a two-step cadence (up-down) regulated with the metronome set at 40 beats per minute. For this exercise, you should allow a brief practice period of 10 to 15 seconds to familiar-ize yourself with the cadence. The up movement is initiated with the first beat, then you must wait for the next beat to initiate the down movement; one repetition is accomplished every two beats of the metronome. Count as many repetitions as you are able to perform following the proper cadence. This test is also terminated if you fail to maintain the ap-propriate cadence or if you accomplish 100 repeti-tions. Have your partner check the angle at the knees throughout the test to make sure the 100° angle is maintained as closely as possible.

Abdominal crunch

This test is very difficult to administer. Individuals often gain an unfair advantage by bending the el-bows, shrugging the shoulders, or sliding the body during the test.[10,11,12] Test results are not valid unless the test procedure and the exercise form are moni-tored carefully.[13,14] Further, a large upper body mass and lack of spinal flexibility make the abdominal crunch impossible or difficult to perform for some individuals.[15,16] This test, therefore, should be used only by individuals who, because of back pain or risk for low back injury, cannot perform the bent-leg curl-up test.

To administer the test, tape a 3½ x 30-inch strip of cardboard onto the floor. Lie down on the floor in a supine position (face up) with the knees bent at ap-proximately 100° and the legs slightly apart. The feet should be on the floor, and you must hold them in place yourself throughout the test. Straighten your arms and place them on the floor alongside the trunk with the palms down and the fingers fully ex-tended. The fingertips of both hands should barely touch the closest edge of the cardboard. Bring the head off the floor until the chin is 1 inch to 2 inches away from your chest. Your head should remain in this position during the entire test (do not move the head by flexing or extending the neck). You are now ready to begin the test.

The repetitions are performed to a two-step ca-dence (up-down) regulated with a metronome set at 60 beats per minute. As you curl up, slide the fingers over the cardboard until the fingertips reach the far end (3½ inches) of the board, then return to the starting position.

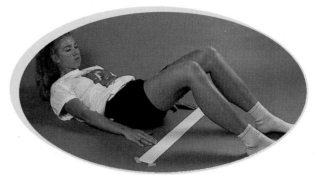

The fingertips of both hands should barely touch the closest edge of the cardboard.

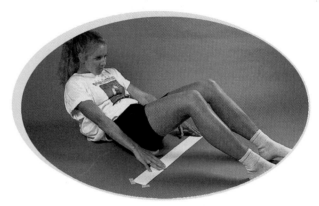

As you curl up, slide the fingers over the cardboard until the fingertips reach the far end of the board.

Allow a brief practice period of 5 to 10 seconds to familiarize yourself with the cadence. The up movement is initiated with the first beat, and the down movement with the next beat. One repetition is accomplished every two beats of the metronome. Count as many repetitions as you are able to per-form following the proper cadence. You may not count a repetition if the fingertips fail to reach the distant end of the cardboard.

The test is terminated if: (a) you fail to maintain the appropriate cadence, (b) your heels come off the floor, (c) your chin is not kept close to the chest, (d) you accomplish 100 repetitions, or (e) you can no longer perform the test. Have your partner check the angle at the knees throughout the test to make sure that the 100° angle is maintained as closely as possible.

For this test you may also use a Crunch-Ster Curl-Up Tester, available from Novel Products.*

According to your results, look up the percentile rank based on the number of repetitions performed on each test and the respective strength fitness

---

* Novel Products Figure Finder Collection, P.O. Box 408, Rockton, IL 61072-0408, (800) 624-4888.

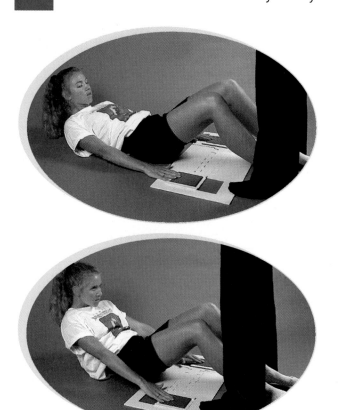

Abdominal crunches using a Crunch-Ster Curl-Up Tester.

categories in Table 6.3. Record this information in Assessment 6-2.

ASSESSMENT OF MUSCULAR FLEXIBILITY

Flexibility is defined as the ability of a joint to move freely through its full range of motion. Sports medicine specialists believe that many muscular/skeletal problems and injuries, especially in adults, may be related to a lack of flexibility. Improving and maintaining good range of motion in the joints throughout life enhances the quality of life.

> *Improving and maintaining good range of motion in the joints throughout life enhances functional independence.*

Because flexibility is joint-specific — good flexibility in one joint does not necessarily indicate the same is true in other joints — two tests are used to obtain an indication of current flexibility levels: the Modified Sit-and-Reach and the Total Body

TABLE 6.3 — **Percentile Ranks and Fitness Standards for the Muscular Endurance Test**

Percentile Rank	MEN Bench Jump	MEN Modified Dip	MEN Bent-leg Curl-up	MEN Abdominal Crunch*	WOMEN Bench Jump	WOMEN Modified Push-up	WOMEN Bent-leg Curl-up	WOMEN Abdominal Crunch*	Fitness Classification
99	66	54	100	100	58	95	100	100	
95	63	50	81	100	54	70	100	100	Excellent
90	62	38	65	100	52	50	97	69	
80	58	32	51	66	48	41	77	49	Good
70	57	30	44	45	44	38	57	37	
60	56	27	31	38	42	33	45	34	Average
50	54	26	28	33	39	30	37	31	
40	51	23	25	29	38	28	28	27	Fair
30	48	20	22	26	36	25	22	24	
20	47	17	17	22	32	21	17	21	
10	40	11	10	18	28	18	9	15	Poor
5	34	7	3	16	26	15	4	0	

◼ High physical fitness standard

◼ Health fitness standard

* Use this exercise only if you are unable to perform a bent-leg curl-up due to back pain or risk of lower back injury.

Rotation tests. Before doing any flexibility testing, participants should warm up properly with a few stretching exercises. Assistance from another person is necessary to administer both tests.

Modified Sit-and-Reach Test

To administer the Modified Sit-and-Reach test, an Acuflex I flexibility tester is needed, or you may design your own equipment by placing a yardstick on top of a box 12 inches high. To perform the test, remove your shoes and sit on the floor with your hips, back, and head against a wall. Fully extend your legs with the bottom of your feet placed against the box.

Position one hand on top of the other, and reach forward as far as possible without letting your head or back come off the wall. The person assisting with the test then should slide the reach indicator (or yardstick) until the zero (end) point of the scale touches your fingers. He or she then must hold the indicator firmly in place throughout the rest of the test.

Your head and back now can come off the wall, and you should gradually reach forward as far as possible on the indicator, holding the final position at least 2 seconds. Be sure that, during the test, you keep the back of your knees flat against the floor.

Flexibility The ability of a joint to move freely through its full range of motion.

Two trials are necessary and the average of the two scores, each recorded to the nearest half inch, is used as the final test score. Flexibility fitness categories for this test are provided in Table 6.4.

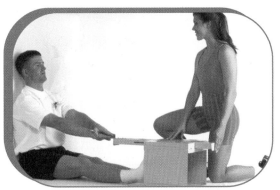

Determining the starting position for the Modified Sit-and-Reach test.

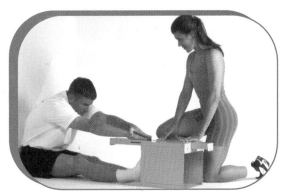

Modified Sit-and-Reach test.

TABLE 6.4 Percentile Ranks and Fitness Standards for the Modified Sit-and-Reach Test

MEN						WOMEN					
Percentile Rank	Age Category				Fitness Category	Percentile Rank	Age Category				Fitness Category
	<18	19–35	36–49	>50			<18	19–35	36–49	>50	
99	20.8	20.1	18.9	16.2		99	22.6	21.0	19.8	17.2	
95	19.6	18.9	18.2	15.8	Excellent	95	19.5	19.3	19.2	15.7	Excellent
90	18.2	17.2	16.1	15.0		90	18.7	17.9	17.4	15.0	
80	17.8	17.0	14.6	13.3	Good	80	17.8	16.7	16.2	14.2	Good
70	16.0	15.8	13.9	12.3		70	16.5	16.2	15.2	13.6	
60	15.2	15.0	13.4	11.5	Average	60	16.0	15.8	14.5	12.3	Average
50	14.5	14.4	12.6	10.2		50	15.2	14.8	13.5	11.1	
40	14.0	13.5	11.6	9.7	Fair	40	14.5	14.5	12.8	10.1	Fair
30	13.4	13.0	10.8	9.3		30	13.7	13.7	12.2	9.2	
20	11.8	11.6	9.9	8.8		20	12.6	12.6	11.0	8.3	
10	9.5	9.2	8.3	7.8	Poor	10	11.4	10.1	9.7	7.5	Poor
05	8.4	7.9	7.0	7.2		05	9.4	8.1	8.5	3.7	
01	7.2	7.0	5.1	4.0		01	6.5	2.6	2.0	1.5	

■ High physical fitness standard   ■ Health fitness standard

Total Body Rotation Test

An Acuflex II* flexibility tester or a measuring scale with a sliding panel is needed to administer this test. The Acuflex II or scale is placed on the wall at shoulder height and should be adjustable to accommodate individual differences in height.

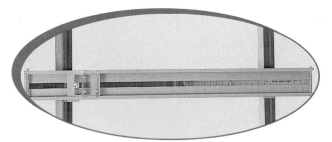

Acuflex II measuring device for the Total Body Rotation test.

If you need to build your own scale, use two measuring tapes, each at least 30 inches long, and glue them above and below the sliding panel, centered at the 15-inch mark. If no sliding panel is available, simply tape the measuring tapes onto a wall. Also, draw a line centered with the 15-inch mark on the floor.

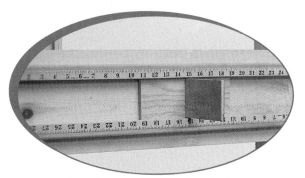

*Homemade measuring device
for the Total Body Rotation test.*

Stand sideways, an arm's length away from the wall, your feet straight ahead, slightly separated, and your toes right up to the corresponding line drawn on the floor. Hold out the arm opposite to the wall horizontally from your body, making a fist with your hand. The Acuflex II, measuring scale, or tapes should be shoulder height at this time. Rotate your trunk, the extended arm going backward (always maintaining a horizontal plane) and making contact with the panel, gradually sliding it forward as far as

Acuflex I and II flexibility equipment can be obtained from Novel Products Figure Finder Collection, P.O. Box 408, Rockton, IL 61072-0408, (800) 624-4888.

possible. If no panel is available, slide your fist alongside the tapes as far as possible. Hold the final position for at least 2 seconds.

Your hand should be positioned with the little finger side forward during the entire sliding movement. It is crucial to have the proper hand position. Many people attempt to open the hand or push with extended fingers or slide the panel with the knuckles, none of which is an acceptable test procedure. During the test, the knees can be slightly bent, but the

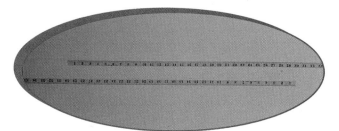

Measuring tapes for the Total Body Rotation test.

feet cannot be moved; they always must point straight forward. The body must be kept as straight (vertical) as possible.

Conduct the test on either the right or the left side of the body. You are allowed two trials on the selected side. The farthest point reached, measured to the nearest half inch and held for at least 2 seconds, is recorded. The average of the two trials becomes the final test score. Flexibility fitness categories for the test are provided in Table 6.5.

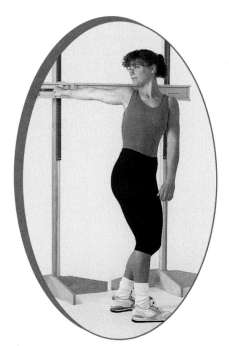

Total Body Rotation test.

After obtaining your flexibility scores, record your percentile ranks and flexibility fitness categories in the fitness profile provided in Assessment 6-2.

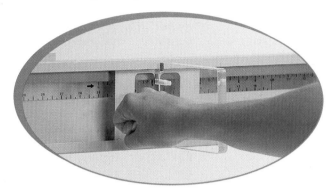

Proper hand position for the Total Body Rotation test.

EXERCISE PRESCRIPTION

Upon completing the health-related fitness assessment, Chapter 7 will help you learn how to develop and implement your own exercise programs for cardiorespiratory endurance, muscular strength, and muscular flexibility. In Chapter 9 you also will learn how to assess your body composition (the fourth component of health-related fitness) and compute your recommended body weight based on your current percent body fat. Guidelines for a weight management program are provided in Chapter 10.

TABLE 6.5 Percentile Ranks and Fitness Standards for the Total Body Rotation Test

	Percentile Rank	Left Rotation				Right Rotation				Fitness Category
		<18	19–35	36–49	>50	<18	19–35	36–49	>50	
Men	99	29.1	28.0	26.6	21.0	28.2	27.8	25.2	22.2	
	95	26.6	24.8	24.5	20.0	25.5	25.6	23.8	20.7	Excellent
	90	25.0	23.6	23.0	17.7	24.3	24.1	22.5	19.3	
	80	22.0	22.0	21.2	15.5	22.7	22.3	21.0	16.3	Good
	70	20.9	20.3	20.4	14.7	21.3	20.7	18.7	15.7	
	60	19.9	19.3	18.7	13.9	19.8	19.0	17.3	14.7	Average
	50	18.6	18.0	16.7	12.7	19.0	17.2	16.3	12.3	
	40	17.0	16.8	15.3	11.7	17.3	16.3	14.7	11.5	Fair
	30	14.9	15.0	14.8	10.3	15.1	15.0	13.3	10.7	
	20	13.8	13.3	13.7	9.5	12.9	13.3	11.2	8.7	
	10	10.8	10.5	10.8	4.3	10.8	11.3	8.0	2.7	Poor
	05	8.5	8.9	8.8	0.3	8.1	8.3	5.5	0.3	
	01	3.4	1.7	5.1	0.0	6.6	2.9	2.0	0.0	
Women	99	29.3	28.6	27.1	23.0	29.6	29.4	27.1	21.7	
	95	26.8	24.8	25.3	21.4	27.6	25.3	25.9	19.7	Excellent
	90	25.5	23.0	23.4	20.5	25.8	23.0	21.3	19.0	
	80	23.8	21.5	20.2	19.1	23.7	20.8	19.6	17.9	Good
	70	21.8	20.5	18.6	17.3	22.0	19.3	17.3	16.8	
	60	20.5	19.3	17.7	16.0	20.8	18.0	16.5	15.6	Average
	50	19.5	18.0	16.4	14.8	19.5	17.3	14.6	14.0	
	40	18.5	17.2	14.8	13.7	18.3	16.0	13.1	12.8	Fair
	30	17.1	15.7	13.6	10.0	16.3	15.2	11.7	8.5	
	20	16.0	15.2	11.6	6.3	14.5	14.0	9.8	3.9	
	10	12.8	13.6	8.5	3.0	12.4	11.1	6.1	2.2	Poor
	05	11.1	7.3	6.8	0.7	10.2	8.8	4.0	1.1	
	01	8.9	5.3	4.3	0.0	8.9	3.2	2.8	0.0	

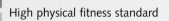 High physical fitness standard   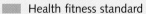 Health fitness standard

NOTES

1. U.S. Centers for Disease Control and Prevention and American College of Sports Medicine, "Summary Statement: Workshop on Physical Activity and Public Health," *Sports Medicine Bulletin*, 28:4, p. 7.

2. National Institutes of Health, *Consensus Development Conference Statement: Physical Activity and Cardiovascular Health*, Washington, DC, December 18–20, 1995.

3. National Institutes of Health.

4. U.S. Department of Health and Human Services, "Physical Activity and Health: A Report of the Surgeon General," Atlanta; U.S. Department of Health and Human Services, Centers for Disease Control and Prevention, National Center for Chronic Disease Prevention and Health Promotion, 1996.

5. R. S. Paffenbarger, Jr., R. T. Hyde, A. L. Wing, and C. H. Steinmetz. "A Natural History of Athleticism and Cardiovascular Health," *Journal of the American Medical Association* 252 (1984), pp. 491–495.

6. S. N. Blair, H. W. Kohl III, R. S. Paffenbarger, Jr, D. G. Clark, K. H. Cooper, and L. W. Gibbons. "Physical Fitness and All-Cause Mortality: A Prospective Study of Healthy Men and Women," *Journal of the American Medical Association* 262 (1989), 2395–2401.

7. S. N. Blair, H. W. Kohl III, C. E. Barlow, R. S. Paffenbarger, Jr., L. W. Gibbons, and C. A. Macera, "Changes in Physical Fitness and All-Cause Mortality: A Prospective Study of Healthy and Unhealthy Men," *Journal of the American Medical Association*, 273 (1995), pp. 1193–1198.

8. I. Lee, C. Hsieh, and R. S. Paffenbarger, Jr., "Exercise Intensity and Longevity in Men: The Harvard Alumni Health Study," *Journal of the American Medical Association*, 273 (1995), pp. 1179–1184.

9. *Guidelines for Exercise Testing and Prescription* (Philadelphia: Lea & Febiger, 1995).

10. R. A. Faulkner, E. J. Sprigings, A. McQuarrie, and R. D. Bell, "A Partial Curl-Up Protocol for Adults Based on Analysis of Two Procedures," *Canadian Journal of Sports Science*, 14 (1989), 135–141.

11. P. A. Macfarlane, "Out with the Sit-Up, in with the Curl-Up!" *Journal of Physical Education, Recreation, and Dance*, 64 (1993), 62–66.

12. D. Knudson and D. Johnston, "Validity and Reliability of a Bench Trunk-Curl-Up Test of Abdominal Endurance," *Journal of Strength and Conditioning Research*, 9 (1995), 165–169.

13. R. Kjorstad. "Validity of Two Field Tests of Abdominal Strength and Muscular Endurance," unpublished master's thesis, Boise State University, 1997.

14. G. L. Hall, R. K. Hetzler, D. Perrin, and A. Weltman, "Relationship of Timed Sit-Up Tests to Isokinetic Abdominal Strength," *Research Quarterly for Exercise and Sport*, 63 (1992), 80–84.

15. L. D. Robertson and H. Magnusdottir, "Evaluation of Criteria Associated with Abdominal Fitness Testing," *Research Quarterly for Exercise and Sport*, 58 (1987), 355–359.

16. Macfarlane.

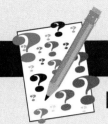

ASSESSMENT 6-1

Physical Activity Readiness Questionnaire (PAR-Q)

Name _____ Date _____ Grade _____

Instructor _____ Course _____ Section _____

NECESSARY LAB EQUIPMENT: None required.

OBJECTIVE: To determine safety of exercise participation.

INSTRUCTIONS: It is important that you answer all questions honestly. The PAR-Q is a scientifically and medically researched preexercise selection device. It complements exercise programs, exercise testing procedures, and the liability considerations attendant with such programs and testing procedures. PAR-Q, like any other preexercise screening device, will misclassify a small percentage of prospective participants, but no preexercise screening method can entirely avoid the problem.

Par-Q is designed to help you help yourself. Many health benefits are associated with regular exercise, and the completion of PAR-Q is a sensible first step to take if you are planning to increase the amount of physical activity in your life.

For most people physical activity should not pose any problem or hazard. PAR-Q has been designed to identify the small number of adults for whom physical activity might be inappropriate or those who should have medical advice concerning the type of activity most suitable for them.

Common sense is your best guide in answering these few questions. Please read them carefully and check the ☑ yes or no opposite the question if it applies to you.

YES NO

☐ ☐ 1. Has a doctor ever said that you have a heart condition and recommended only medically supervised activity?

☐ ☐ 2. Do you have chest pain brought on by physical activity?

☐ ☐ 3. Have you developed chest pain in the last month?

☐ ☐ 4. Do you tend to lose consciousness or fall over as a result of dizziness?

☐ ☐ 5. Do you have a bone or joint problem that could be aggravated by the proposed physical activity?

☐ ☐ 6. Has a doctor ever recommended medication for your blood pressure or a heart condition?

☐ ☐ 7. Are you aware through your own experience, or a doctor's advice, of any other physical reason against your exercising without medical supervision?

Note: If you have a temporary illness, such as a common cold, or are not feeling well at this time — **Postpone**

If you answered YES to one or more questions:

If you have not recently done so, consult with your personal physician BEFORE increasing your physical activity and/or taking a fitness test. Tell him what questions you answered YES on PAR-Q, or show him your copy.

After medical evaluation, seek advice from your physician as to your suitability for:

- unrestricted physical activity, probably on a gradually increasing basis.
- restricted or supervised activity to meet your specific needs, at least on an initial basis. Check in your community for special programs or services.

If you answered NO to all questions:

If you answered PAR-Q accurately, you have reasonable assurance of your present suitability for:

- **A graduated exercise program** — A gradual increase in proper exercise promotes good fitness development while minimizing or eliminating discomfort.
- **An exercise test** — Simple tests of fitness or more complex types may be undertaken if you so desire.

Postpone

If you have a temporary minor illness, such as a common cold.

---

*Developed by the British Columbia Ministry of Health, Revised, 1991.
Reference: PAR-Q Validation Report, British Columbia Ministry of Health,. May, 1978.
Produced by the British Columbia Ministry of Health and the Department of National Health and Welfare.

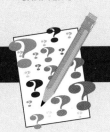

ASSESSMENT 6-2

Physical Fitness Profile

Name _____ Date _____ Grade _____

Instructor _____ Course _____ Section _____

Age _____ Male or Female   M / F   Body Weight _____

NECESSARY LAB EQUIPMENT: Pre-measured 1.5-mile or 1.0 mile course, stopwatch, metronome, and modified sit-and-reach box (Acuflex I), and total body rotation scale (Acuflex II).

OBJECTIVE: To assess your current level of cardiorespiratory endurance, muscular strength endurance, and muscular flexibility fitness.

LAB PREPARATION: Wear appropriate exercise clothing including a good pair of athletic (jogging/walking) shoes. Avoid strenuous physical activity for 36 hours prior to this lab.

PRETEST

Fitness Component	Test Data	Test Results	Fitness Classification
Cardiorespiratory Endurance	Time	$VO_{2\ max.}$	
1.5-Mile Run	____ : ____	____ . ____	_____
	Time		
1.0-Mile Walk	____ : ____		
	Heart Rate	$VO_{2\ max.}$	
	_____	____ . ____	_____
Muscular Strength / Endurance	Reps	Percentile	
Bench Jumps	_____	_____	_____
Chair Dips / Mod. Push-Ups	_____	_____	_____
Bent-Leg Curl-Ups or Abdominal Crunches	_____	_____	_____
Average Percentile		_____	_____
Muscular Flexibility	Inches	Percentile	
Modified Sit-and-Reach	_____	_____	_____
Body Rotation (R/L)	_____	_____	_____
Average Percentile		_____	_____

POST-TEST

Fitness Component	Test Data	Test Results	Fitness Classification
Cardiovascular Endurance	Time	VO2 max.	
1.5-Mile Run	_____ : _____	_____ . _____	_____
	Time		
1.0-Mile Walk	_____ : _____		
	Heart Rate	$VO_{2\ max.}$	
	_____	_____ . _____	_____
Muscular Strength / Endurance	Reps	Percentile	
Bench Jumps	_____	_____	_____
Chair Dips / Mod. Push-Ups	_____	_____	_____
Bent-Leg Curl-Ups or Abdominal Crunches	_____	_____	_____
Average Percentile		_____	_____
Muscular Flexibility	Inches	Percentile	
Modified Sit-and-Reach	_____	_____	_____
Body Rotation (R/L)	_____	_____	_____
Average Percentile		_____	_____

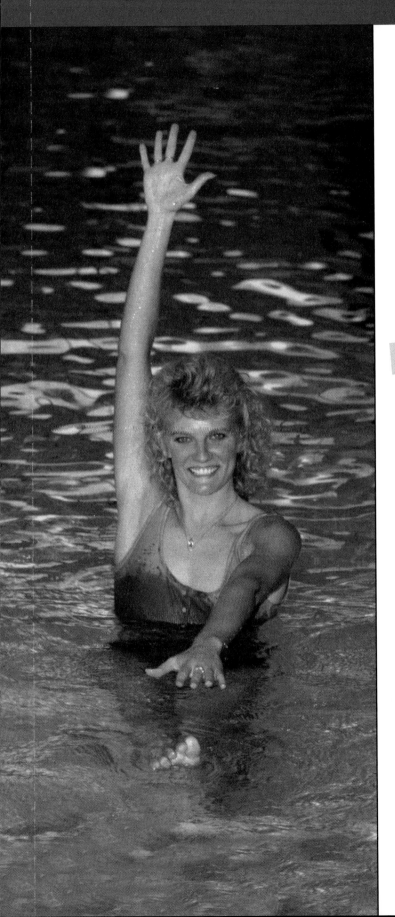

7

Exercise Prescription for Wellness

- Understand the benefits of an active lifestyle.
- Define aerobic and anaerobic exercise.
- Learn the guidelines for cardiorespiratory, strength, and flexibility exercise prescription.
- Recognize the different types of muscle fibers.
- Understand the overload principle for strength development.
- Clarify misconceptions related to exercise training programs.
- Become familiar with concepts for preventing and treating injuries.
- Learn basic skills to enhance motivation and exercise adherence.

No drug in current or prospective use holds as much promise for sustained health as a lifetime program of physical exercise.[1] A physically active lifestyle and participation in a lifetime exercise program contribute greatly to good health (see Chapter 6). When they take a battery of fitness tests, though, many individuals who are active and exercise regularly find that they may not be as conditioned as they thought they were. Although these individuals may be exercising regularly, they most likely are not following the basic principles for exercise prescription and, therefore, are not reaping the full benefits of their activity and exercise programs.

> **All programs must be individualized to obtain optimal results.**

A key principle in exercise prescription is that all programs must be individualized to obtain optimal results. Our bodies are not all alike, and fitness levels and needs vary from individual to individual. The information presented in this chapter provides the necessary guidelines to write a personalized cardiorespiratory endurance, muscular strength, and muscular flexibility exercise program that promotes and maintains physical fitness. Information on weight control to achieve and maintain recommended body weight and body composition — a key component of good physical fitness — is given in Chapter 10.

At age 45, George Snell of Sandy, Utah, weighed approximately 400 pounds, his blood pressure was 220/180, he was blind because of diabetes he didn't know he had, and his blood glucose level was 487. Snell had determined to do something about his physical and medical condition, so he started a walking/jogging program.

After about 8 months of conditioning, Snell had lost almost 200 pounds, his eyesight had returned, his glucose level was down to 67, and he was taken off medication. Two months later, less than 10 months after initiating his personal exercise program, he completed his first marathon, a running course of 26.2 miles.

CARDIORESPIRATORY ENDURANCE

Cardiorespiratory endurance refers to the ability of the lungs, heart, and blood vessels to deliver adequate amounts of oxygen to the cells to meet the demands of prolonged physical activity. Because the body uses oxygen to convert food (carbohydrates and fats) into energy, a greater capacity to deliver and utilize oxygen (oxygen uptake or VO_2) indicates a more efficient cardiorespiratory system.

Cardiorespiratory endurance activities also are called **aerobic exercise**. The word *aerobic* means "with oxygen." Whenever an activity requires oxygen to produce energy, it is considered an aerobic exercise. Examples of cardiorespiratory or aerobic exercise are walking, jogging, swimming, cycling, cross-country skiing, water aerobics, and rope skipping.

Anaerobic activities, on the other hand, are carried out without oxygen. The intensity of anaerobic exercise is so high that oxygen is not utilized to produce energy. Because energy production is limited without oxygen, these activities can be carried out for only a short time of 2 to 3 minutes. The higher the intensity of the activity, the shorter the duration.

Activities such as the 100, 200, and 400 meters in track and field, the 100 meters in swimming, gymnastics routines, and weight training are good examples of anaerobic activities. Anaerobic activities will not contribute much to development of the cardiorespiratory system. Only aerobic activities will enhance cardiorespiratory endurance.

Physical activity is no longer a natural part of our existence. If we need to go to a store only a couple of blocks away, most people drive their cars and then spend a couple of minutes driving around the parking lot to find a spot 10 yards closer to the store's entrance. We do not even have to carry out the groceries any more. A youngster working at the store usually takes them out in a cart and places them in your vehicle. During a normal visit to a multilevel shopping mall, almost everyone chooses to ride the escalators instead of taking the stairs. Automobiles, elevators, escalators, telephones, intercoms, remote controls, and electric garage door openers — all are modern-day commodities that minimize body movement and effort.

One of the most detrimental effects of modern-day technology has been an increase in chronic conditions related to a lack of physical activity. Some examples are hypertension, heart disease, chronic low-back pain, and obesity. These conditions also

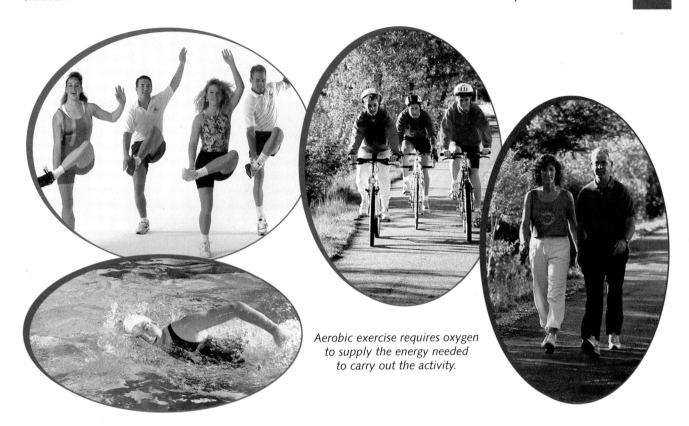

Aerobic exercise requires oxygen to supply the energy needed to carry out the activity.

are called **hypokinetic diseases.** "Hypo" means low or little, and "kinetic" denotes motion.

To compensate for the lack of adequate physical activity and expect to live life to its fullest, a personalized lifetime exercise program must become part of daily living. Based on current estimates, more than 60% of adults do not achieve the recommended amount of physical activity, and 25% are not physically active at all.[2]

Aerobic exercise is especially important in preventing coronary heart disease. A poorly conditioned heart that has to pump more often just to keep a person alive is subject to more wear-and-tear than a well-conditioned heart. In situations that place strenuous demands on the heart, such as doing yard work, lifting heavy objects or weights, or running to catch a train, the unconditioned heart may not be able to sustain the strain.

In addition, regular participation in cardiorespiratory endurance activities helps achieve and maintain recommended body weight, the fourth component of health-related physical fitness. (Weight management is the topic of Chapter 10.)

Physiological Adaptations

Everyone who initiates a cardiorespiratory or aerobic exercise program can expect a number of physiological adaptations from training. Among the most significant adaptations are:

1. *A higher maximal oxygen uptake* (VO_{2max}). The amount of oxygen the body is able to use during physical activity increases significantly. This allows the individual to exercise longer and at a higher rate before becoming fatigued.

   Small increases in VO_{2max} can be observed in as few as 2 to 3 weeks of aerobic training. Depending on the initial fitness level, VO_{2max} may rise as much as 30%, although higher increases have been reported in people with very low initial levels of fitness.

2. *A decrease in resting heart rate and an increase in cardiac muscle strength.* During resting conditions, the heart ejects between 5 and 6 liters of blood per minute (a liter is slightly larger than a quart). This amount of blood, also referred to as

Aerobic exercise Exercise that requires oxygen to produce the necessary energy (ATP) to carry out the activity.

Anaerobic activity Activity that does not require oxygen to produce the necessary energy (ATP) to carry out the activity.

Hypokinetic disease Condition associated with a lack of physical activity (for example, hypertension, coronary heart disease, obesity, and diabetes).

cardiac output, meets the energy demands in the resting state.

Like any other muscle, the heart responds to training by gaining strength and size. As the heart gets stronger, the muscle can produce a more forceful contraction. A stronger contraction causes more blood to be ejected with each beat (stroke volume), yielding a lower heart rate. This reduction in heart rate also allows the heart to rest longer between beats.

Physical work capacity, measured through an oxygen uptake test, increases with aerobic training.

The **resting heart rate** frequently decreases 10 to 20 beats per minute (bpm) after only 6 to 8 weeks of training. A reduction of 20 bpm saves the heart about 10,483,200 beats per year. The average heart beats between 70 and 80 bpm. Resting heart rates in highly trained athletes frequently are around 45 bpm.

3. *A lower heart rate at given workloads.* When compared with untrained individuals, a trained person has a lower heart rate response to a given task, because of higher efficiency of the cardiorespiratory system. Following several weeks of training, a given workload (let's say a 10-minute mile) elicits a much lower heart rate response as compared to the response when training first started.

4. *An increase in the number and size of the mitochondria.* All energy necessary for cell function is produced in the mitochondria. As the size and number increase, so does the potential to produce energy for muscular work.

5. *An increase in the number of functional capillaries.* These smaller blood vessels allow for the exchange of oxygen and carbon dioxide between the blood and the cells. As more vessels open up, more gas exchange can take place, thereby decreasing the onset of fatigue during prolonged exercise. This increase in capillaries also speeds up the rate at which waste products of cell metabolism can be removed. Increased capillarization also is seen in the heart, which enhances the oxygen delivery capacity to the heart muscle itself.

6. *Faster recovery time.* Trained individuals have a faster recovery time following exercise. A fit system is able to more rapidly restore any internal equilibrium disrupted during exercise.

7. *A decrease in blood pressure and blood lipids.* A regular aerobic exercise program will result in lower blood pressure and fats such as cholesterol and triglycerides, linked to the formation of the atherosclerotic plaque, which obstructs the arteries. This reduction lowers the risk for coronary heart disease (see Chapter 11). High blood pressure also is a leading risk factor for strokes.

8. *An increase in fat-burning enzymes.* Fat is lost primarily by burning it in muscle. As the concentration of the enzymes increases, so does the ability to burn fat.

Guidelines for Cardiorespiratory Exercise Prescription

To develop the cardiorespiratory system, the heart muscle has to be overloaded (see discussion under Muscular Strength) like any other muscle in the human body. Just as the biceps muscle in the upper arm is developed through strength-training exercises, the heart muscle has to be exercised to increase in size, strength, and efficiency. To better understand how the cardiorespiratory system can be developed, we have to be familiar with four basic principles: intensity, mode, duration, and frequency of exercise. These principles are discussed separately in this section, and Figure 7.1 summarizes the cardiorespiratory exercise prescription guidelines of the American College of Sports Medicine (ACSM), the leading sports medicine organization in the world.[3]

The ACSM recommends that a medical exam and a diagnostic exercise stress test or stress ECG be administered prior to vigorous exercise by apparently healthy men over age 40 and women over age 50. The American College of Sports Medicine has defined vigorous exercise as an exercise intensity above 60% of VO_{2max}.[4] This intensity is the equivalent of exercise that provides a "substantial challenge" to the participant or one that cannot be maintained for 20 continuous minutes.

FIGURE 7.1

Activity:	Aerobic (examples: walking, jogging, cycling, swimming, aerobics, racquetball, soccer, stair climbing)
Intensity:	60–90% of maximal heart rate
Duration:	20–60 minutes of continuous aerobic activity
Frequency:	3 to 5 days per week

"The Recommended Quantity and Quality of Exercise for Developing and Maintaining Cardiorespiratory and Muscular Fitness in Healthy Adults," by the American College of Sports Medicine, *Medical Science in Sports and Exercise,* 22(1990); 265–274.

Cardiorespiratory exercise prescription guidelines.

Intensity of Exercise

When trying to develop the cardiorespiratory system, the **intensity of exercise** perhaps is the most commonly ignored factor. It refers to how high the heart rate has to be during exercise to improve cardiorespiratory endurance.

Muscles have to be overloaded to a given point for them to develop. The stimulus for the cardiorespiratory system comes from making the heart pump at a higher rate for a certain period of time. Research has shown that cardiorespiratory development occurs when the person is working between 60% and 90% of maximal heart rate. Faster development can be obtained by working closer to the higher end of the range. For this reason, many experts prescribe exercise between 70% and 90% for young people.

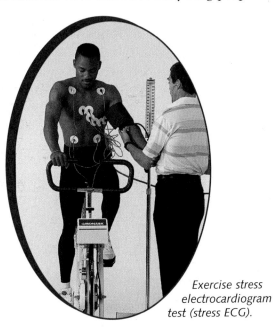

Exercise stress electrocardiogram test (stress ECG).

Exercise intensity can be calculated easily and training can be monitored by checking your pulse. To determine the intensity of exercise or cardiorespiratory training zone:

1. Estimate your **maximal heart rate** (MHR). The maximal heart rate depends on the person's age and can be estimated according to the following formula: MHR = 220 minus age (220 − age)

2. Calculate the training intensities (TI) at 60%, 70%, and 90%. Multiply MHR by the respective 60%, 70%, and 90%. For example, the 60%, 70%, and 90% training intensities for a 20-year-old person are:

MHR: 220 − 20 = 200 beats per minute (bpm)
    60% TI = (200 × .60) = 120 bpm
    70% TI = (200 × .70) = 140 bpm
    90% TI = (200 × .90) = 180 bpm
Cardiorespiratory training zone: 120 to 180 bpm

According to your present age, you also may look up your cardiorespiratory training zone in Table 7.1. The training zone indicates that whenever you exercise to improve the cardiorespiratory system, you should maintain the heart rate between the 60% and 90% training intensities to obtain adequate development.

Monitor your exercise heart rate regularly during exercise to make sure you are training in the respective zone. Wait until you are about 5 minutes into the exercise session before taking your first rate. When checking exercise heart rate, count your pulse for 10 seconds. Next, multiply the 10-second count by 6 to obtain the rate in beats per minute. Exercise heart rate will remain at the same level for about 15 seconds following exercise. After 15 seconds, heart rate will drop rapidly. Do not hesitate to stop during your exercise bout to check your pulse. If the rate is too low, increase the intensity of exercise. If the rate is too high, slow down.

Cardiac output Amount of blood ejected by the heart in 1 minute.

Resting heart rate Rate after a person has been sitting quietly for 15–20 minutes.

Intensity of exercise In cardiorespiratory exercise, how hard a person has to exercise to improve or maintain fitness.

Maximal heart rate (MHR) Highest heart rate for a person, primarily related to age.

TABLE 7.1

Recommended Cardiorespiratory Exercise Intensities

Age	Estimated Max HR*	60% HR* Intensity	70% HR* Intensity	90% HR* Intensity
15	205	123	144	185
20	200	120	140	180
25	195	117	137	176
30	190	114	133	171
35	185	111	130	167
40	180	108	126	162
45	175	105	123	158
50	170	102	119	153
55	165	99	116	149
60	160	96	112	144
65	155	93	109	140
70	150	90	105	135
75	145	87	102	131

*HR = Heart Rate

To develop the cardiorespiratory system, you do not have to exercise above the 90% rate. From a *fitness* standpoint, training above this percentage will not yield extra benefits and actually may be unsafe for some people.

For unconditioned people and older adults, cardiorespiratory training should be conducted at about the 60% rate. This lower rate is recommended to reduce potential problems associated with high-intensity exercise.

Training benefits obtained by exercising at the 60% training intensity may place a person only in an average or "moderately fit" category (see Table 6.2, Chapter 6). Even though it is not an excellent cardiorespiratory fitness rating, exercising at this lower intensity does significantly decrease the risk for cardiovascular mortality and other chronic diseases. An excellent fitness rating is obtained by exercising closer to the 90% threshold.

If you have been physically inactive and the objective is to attain a high physical fitness standard (see Chapter 6), you should train around 60% intensity during the first 4 to 6 weeks of the exercise program. After the first few weeks, you can exercise between 70% and 90% training intensity.

Rate of Perceived Exertion. Many people do not check their heart rate during exercise, so an alternative method of prescribing intensity of exercise has become more popular recently. This method uses a **rate of perceived exertion (RPE)** scale developed by

Gunnar Borg.[5] Using the scale in Figure 7.2, a person subjectively rates the perceived exertion or difficulty of exercise when training in the appropriate target zone. The exercise heart rate then is associated with the corresponding RPE value.

If the training intensity requires a heart rate zone between 150 and 170 bpm, for example, this is associated with training between "hard" and "very hard" (15 and 17, respectively, on the scale). Some individuals perceive less exertion than others when training in the correct zone. Therefore, you should associate your own inner perception of the task with the phrases on the scale. You then may proceed to exercise at that rate of perceived exertion.

Whether you monitor the intensity of exercise by checking your pulse or through rate of perceived exertion, changes in normal exercise conditions affect the training zone. For example, exercising on a hot or humid day or at high altitude increases the heart rate response to a given task. Therefore, you may have to adjust the intensity of your exercise.

Mode of Exercise

The **mode of exercise** that develops the cardiorespiratory system has to be aerobic in nature. Once you have established your cardiorespiratory training zone, any activity or combination of activities that will get your heart rate up to that training zone and keep it

FIGURE 7.2

6	
7	Very, very light
8	
9	Very light
10	
11	Fairly light
12	
13	Somewhat hard
14	
15	Hard
16	
17	Very Hard
18	
19	Very, very hard
20	

From "Perceived Exertion: A Note on History and Methods," by Gunnar Borg, *Medicine and Science in Sports and Exercise* (1993), pp. 90–93.

Rate of perceived exertion scale.

there for as long as you exercise will produce adequate development. Examples are walking, jogging, aerobics, swimming, water aerobics, cross-country skiing, rope skipping, cycling, racquetball, stair climbing, and stationary running or cycling. Most of these activities can be used for either moderate- or high-intensity programs. Additional moderate-intensity activities include raking leaves, washing a car, golfing, tennis, and volleyball.

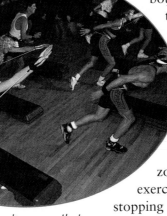

The more muscle groups that are involved during aerobic exercise, the greater are the benefits.

The activity you choose should be based on your personal preferences, what you enjoy doing most, and your physical limitations. Different activities may affect the amount of strength or flexibility developed, but as far as the cardiorespiratory system is concerned, the heart doesn't know whether you are walking, swimming, or cycling. All the heart knows is that it has to pump at a certain rate, and as long as that rate is in the desired range, cardiorespiratory development will take place.

Duration of Exercise

The general recommendation is that a person should train between 20 and 60 minutes per session. **Duration of exercise** is based on how intensely a person trains. If the training is done around 90%, 20 minutes are sufficient. At 60% intensity, a person should train at least 30 minutes. As mentioned, unconditioned people and older adults should train at lower percentages; therefore, the activity should be carried out over a longer time.

Although most experts recommend 20 to 60 minutes of aerobic exercise per session, 1990 research[6] indicates that three 10-minute exercise sessions per day (separated by at least 4 hours), at approximately 70% of maximal heart rate, also produce training benefits. Increases in VO_{2max} with this program were not as large (only 57%) as those in a group performing a continuous 30-minute bout of exercise per day, but the researchers concluded that moderate-intensity exercise training, conducted for 10 minutes three times per day, does benefit the cardiorespiratory

system. The results of this study are meaningful because people often mention lack of time as the reason for not taking part in an exercise program. Many think they must exercise at least 20 minutes to get any benefits at all. Even though 20 to 60 minutes are ideal, short, intermittent bouts of exercise also are beneficial to the cardiorespiratory system.

The training session always should include a 5-minute warm-up and a 5-minute cool-down period (see Figure 7.3). The warm-up should consist of general **calisthenics**, stretching exercises, or exercising at a lower intensity than the actual target zone. To cool down, the intensity of exercise is decreased gradually. Abruptly stopping causes blood to pool in the exercised body parts, diminishing the return of blood to the heart. Less blood return can cause dizziness and faintness or even bring on cardiac abnormalities.

Frequency of Exercise

As to **frequency of exercise**, a person should engage in aerobic exercise three to five times per week.[7] When starting an exercise program, a program consisting of three to five 20- to 60-minute training sessions per week improves VO_{2max}. When training is conducted more than 5 days per week, further improvements are minimal.

For people on a weight-loss program, a regimen of 45- to 60-minute exercise sessions of low to moderate intensity, conducted 5 or 6 days a week, is recommended. Longer exercise sessions increase caloric expenditure for faster weight reduction (see Chapter 10).

Ideally, a person should engage in physical activity six to seven times a week. To reap both the high-fitness and health-fitness benefits of physical activity,

---

Rate of perceived exertion (RPE)   A perception scale to monitor or interpret the intensity of aerobic exercise.

Mode of exercise   Form of exercise.

Duration of exercise   How long a person exercises.

Calisthenics   The exercise of muscles for the purpose of gaining health, strength, and grace of form and movement.

Frequency of exercise   How often a person engages in an exercise session.

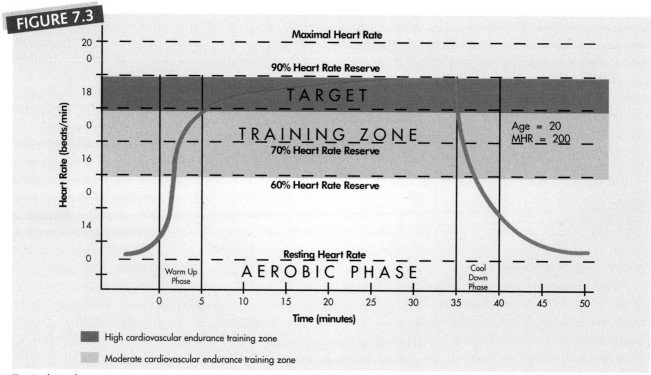

FIGURE 7.3

Typical cardiorespiratory training pattern.

a person needs to exercise a minimum of three times per week in the appropriate target zone to maintain high fitness and three to four additional times per week in moderate-intensity activities to enjoy the full benefits of health fitness. As indicated in the Surgeon General's Report on Physical Activity and Health,[8] you should strive to attain at least 30 minutes of physical activity per day most days of the week.

Maintaining Cardiorespiratory Fitness

A decrease in cardiorespiratory fitness has been observed in as little as 2 weeks without training. Depending on how long you have participated in the aerobic program, complete loss of training benefits is seen between 3 and 8 months after discontinuing the program. Following an aerobic conditioning program, a person must continue a regular training program to maintain cardiorespiratory fitness.

The key to maintaining fitness seems to be the intensity of training.[9] While the duration and frequency of training can be reduced, VO_{2max} does not decline as long as the proper intensity is maintained.

> *The key to maintaining fitness seems to be the intensity of training.*

Three 20-minute training sessions per week, on nonconsecutive days, maintains cardiorespiratory fitness as long as the heart rate is in the appropriate target zone.

Personal Cardiorespiratory Exercise Prescription

Having learned the basic principles of cardiorespiratory exercise prescription, you can proceed to Assessment 7-1 at the end of this chapter and fill out your own prescription. This exercise prescription calls for a gradual increase in intensity, duration, and frequency.

If you have not been exercising regularly, you could go ahead and attempt to train five or six times a week for 20 to 60 minutes at a time. You may find this discouraging, however, and may drop out before getting too far because you probably will develop some muscle soreness and stiffness and possibly incur minor injuries. Muscle soreness and stiffness and the risk for injuries can be lessened or eliminated by increasing the intensity, duration, and frequency of exercise progressively as outlined in Assessment 7-1.

Once you have determined your exercise prescription, the difficult part begins: starting and sticking to a lifetime exercise program. Although you may be motivated after reading the benefits to be gained from physical activity, lifelong dedication and perseverance are necessary to reap and maintain good fitness.

The first few weeks are probably the most difficult, but where there's a will, there's a way. Once you begin to see positive changes, it won't be as hard. Soon you will develop a habit for exercise that will be deeply satisfying and will bring about a sense of self-accomplishment.

MUSCULAR STRENGTH

An adequate level of strength is an important component of good physical fitness. The two forms of strength, as defined in Chapter 6, are muscular strength and muscular endurance. Muscular strength is the ability to exert maximum force against resistance; muscular endurance is the ability of a muscle to exert submaximal force repeatedly over a period of time. For example, a person may have the muscular strength to lift 100 pounds once but may not have the muscular endurance to lift 80 pounds 12 times.

The capacity of muscle cells to exert force increases and decreases according to the demands placed upon the muscular system. If muscle cells are overloaded beyond their normal use, such as in strength-training programs, the cells increase in size, called **hypertrophy**, and strength. If the demands placed on the muscle cells decrease, such as in sedentary living or required rest because of illness or injury, the cells decrease in size and lose strength, termed **atrophy**.

Benefits of Strength Training

Strength is important for optimal performance in daily tasks and recreational activities, to improve personal appearance and self-image, to lessen the risk of injury, and to cope with emergency situations in life. Adequate strength levels also contribute to weight control and enhanced overall health and well-being.

Perhaps one of the most significant benefits of maintaining a good strength level is its relationship to human **metabolism**, all energy and material transformations that occur within living cells.

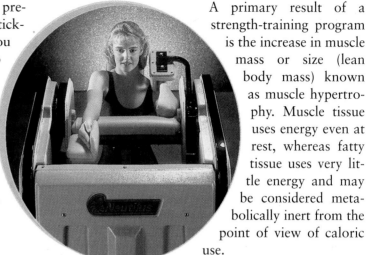

A regular strength-training program helps to increase and maintain a higher resting metabolic rate.

A primary result of a strength-training program is the increase in muscle mass or size (lean body mass) known as muscle hypertrophy. Muscle tissue uses energy even at rest, whereas fatty tissue uses very little energy and may be considered metabolically inert from the point of view of caloric use.

As muscle size increases, so does the **resting metabolism**, the amount of energy (expressed in calories) an individual requires during resting conditions to sustain proper cell function. Even small increases in muscle mass may affect resting metabolism.

Each additional pound of muscle tissue is estimated to increase resting metabolism by approximately 35 calories per day.[10] All other factors being equal, if two individuals at 150 pounds have different amounts of muscle mass — let's say 5 pounds — the one with the greater muscle mass will have a higher resting metabolic rate. A higher metabolic rate indicates that this person can afford to eat more calories to maintain the additional muscle tissue.

Loss of lean tissue is thought to be the main reason for the decrease in metabolism as people grow older. Contrary to some beliefs, metabolism does not slow down that much with aging. We slow down!

Lean body mass declines with sedentary living, which, in turn, slows down the resting metabolic rate. If people continue eating at the same rate, body fat increases. The average decrease in resting metabolism for a 60-year-old individual is about 300 to 400

Hypertrophy An increase in the size of the cell (for example, muscle hypertrophy).

Atrophy Decrease in size of a cell.

Metabolism All energy and material transformations that occur within living cells necessary to sustain life.

Resting metabolism The amount of energy (expressed in milliliters of oxygen per minute or total calories per day) an individual requires during resting conditions to sustain proper body function.

calories per day, as compared to a 25-year-old person. Hence, participating in a strength-training program is a means of preventing and reducing obesity.

Another benefit of strength training, accentuated even more when combined with aerobic exercise, is a decrease in adipose (fatty) tissue. The decrease in fatty tissue often is greater than the amount of muscle hypertrophy gained through strength training. Therefore, losing inches but not body weight is a typical outcome.

Because muscle tissue is denser than fatty tissue, and despite the fact that inches are being lost, people, especially women, often become discouraged because they cannot see the results on the scale. This discouragement can be offset by determining body composition to monitor changes in percent body fat rather than simply measuring total body weight changes.

Adequate strength levels are especially critical in older age. Functional independence, the physical capacity to meet ordinary and unexpected demands of daily life safely and effectively, is related to a large extent to a person's level of strength. Older adults with good strength enjoy greater freedom of movement and functionality than their inactive counterparts. Simple daily tasks such as getting out of bed, getting in and out of a tub, doing household chores, climbing a flight of stairs, and crossing a street safely and effectively are enhanced through a strength-training program.

Older adults can increase their strength levels. The amount of muscle hypertrophy achieved decreases with age. Strength gains as high as 200% have been found in previously inactive adults over age 90.[11] Suddenly, many of these individuals, previously dependent on others, can perform most of life's daily tasks without restrictions or functional dependence.

Overload

Strength gains are achieved in two ways: (a) through greater ability of individual muscle fibers to get a stronger contraction, and (b) by recruiting a greater proportion of the total available fibers for each contraction. These two factors combine in the concept of **overload**, in which, for strength to improve, the demands placed on the muscle must be increased systematically and progressively over a period of time, and the resistance must be of a magnitude significant enough to cause physiologic adaptation. In simpler terms, just like all other organs and systems of the human body, muscles have to be taxed beyond their accustomed loads to increase in physical capacity.

Specificity of Training

According to the concept of **specificity of training**, for a muscle to increase in strength or endurance, the training program must be specific to obtain the desired effects. In like manner, to increase static (isometric) versus dynamic strength (discussed next), an individual must use static against dynamic training procedures to achieve the desired results.

Guidelines for Strength Development

The principles necessary to develop a strength-training program have to be followed, as in the prescription of cardiorespiratory exercise. These principles are built around mode, resistance, sets, and frequency of training.

Mode of Training

Two basic **modes of training** are used to improve strength: isometric and dynamic. **Isometric** training refers to a muscle contraction producing little or no movement, such as pushing or pulling against immovable objects. **Dynamic** training refers to a muscle contraction with movement, such as lifting an object over your head.

Isometric training does not require much equipment. Used commonly several years ago, its popularity has waned. As strength gains with isometric training are specific to the angle of muscle contraction, this type of training is beneficial in a sport such as gymnastics, which requires regular static contractions during routines.

Dynamic training programs can be conducted without weights or with free weights (barbells and dumbbells), fixed resistance machines, variable resistance machines, and isokinetic equipment.

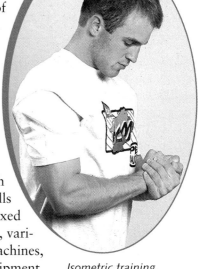

Isometric training.

When performing dynamic exercises without weights (for example, pull-ups or push-ups), with free weights, or with fixed resistance machines, a constant resistance (weight) is moved through a joint's full range of motion.

A limitation of dynamic training is that the greatest resistance that can be lifted equals the maximum weight that can be moved at the weakest angle of the joint. This is because of changes in muscle length and angle of pull as the joint moves through its range of motion.

As strength training became more popular, new strength-training machines were developed. This technology brought about isokinetic and variable resistance training. These training programs require special machines equipped with mechanical devices that provide varying amounts of resistance, with the intent of overloading the muscle group maximally through the entire range of motion.

Isokinetic training.

should be better because maximum resistance is applied at all angles, research has not shown this type of training to be more effective than other modes of dynamic training.

A possible advantage of isokinetic training is that specific speeds used in various sport skills can be duplicated more closely with this type of training, which may enhance performance through specificity of training. A disadvantage is that the equipment is not readily available to many people.

Resistance

Resistance in strength training is the equivalent of intensity in cardiorespiratory exercise prescription. The amount of resistance, or weight lifted, depends on whether the individual is trying to develop muscular strength or muscular endurance.

To stimulate strength development, a resistance of approximately 80% of the maximum capacity (1 RM) is recommended.[12] For example, a person who

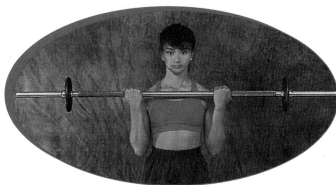

Dynamic training.

A distinction of **isokinetic** training is that the speed of the muscle contraction is kept constant because the machine provides resistance to match the user's force through the range of motion. The mode of training an individual uses depends mainly on the type of equipment available and the specific objective the training program is attempting to accomplish.

Dynamic training is the most popular mode for strength training. The main advantage is that strength is gained through the full range of motion. Most daily activities are dynamic in nature, involving lifting, pushing, and pulling. Strength is needed through a complete range of motion. Another advantage is that improvements are measured easily by the amount lifted.

The benefits of isokinetic and variable resistance training are similar to the other dynamic training methods. Although, theoretically, strength gains

Overload   Training concept stating that the demands placed on a system (cardiorespiratory, muscular) must be increased systematically and progressively over time to cause physiologic adaptation (development or improvement).

Specificity of training   Targeting the specific area the person is attempting to improve (aerobic, anaerobic, strength, flexibility).

Modes of training   Form of training used to improve strength.

Isometric   Strength-training method that refers to a muscle contraction producing little or no movement, such as pushing or pulling against immovable objects.

Dynamic   Strength training method referring to a muscle contraction with movement.

Isokinetic   Strength-training method in which the speed of the muscle contraction is kept constant because the equipment (machine) provides an accommodating resistance to match the user's force (maximal) through the range of motion.

Resistance   Amount of weight lifted in strength training.

can press 150 pounds should work with at least 120 pounds (150 x .80). Using less than 80% will increase muscular endurance rather than strength. Because of the time factor involved in constantly determining the 1 RM on each lift to ensure that you indeed are working above 80%, a rule of thumb that many authors and coaches accept is that individuals should perform between 3 and 12 repetitions maximum (3 to 12 RM) for adequate strength gains.

> *We live in a dynamic world in which muscular strength and endurance both are required to lead an enjoyable life.*

For example, if a person is training with a resistance of 120 pounds and cannot lift it more than 12 times, the training stimulus is adequate for strength development. Once the person can lift the weight more than 12 times, the resistance should be increased by 5 to 10 pounds and the person again should build up to 12 repetitions. If training is conducted with more than 12 repetitions, primarily muscular endurance will be developed.

The closer a person trains to the 1 RM, the greater are the strength gains. A disadvantage of constantly working at or near the 1 RM is that it increases the risk for injury.

Highly trained athletes seeking maximum strength development often use 3 to 6 repetitions maximum. Working around 10 repetitions maximum seems to produce the best results in terms of muscular hypertrophy. From a health-fitness point of view, 8 to 12 repetitions maximum are ideal for adequate development. We live in a dynamic world in which muscular strength and endurance both are required to lead an enjoyable life. Therefore, working near a 10-repetition threshold seems best to improve overall performance.

Sets

In strength training, a **set** is the number of repetitions performed for a given exercise. For example, a person lifting 120 pounds 8 times has performed 1 set of 8 repetitions (1 × 8 × 120). The number of sets recommended for optimum development is 3 sets per exercise.

Because of the characteristics of muscle fiber, the number of sets that can be done is limited. As the number of sets increases, so does muscle fatigue and subsequent recovery time. Therefore, if too many sets are performed, strength gains may be lessened. A recommended program for beginners in their first year of training is 3 heavy sets, up to the maximum number of repetitions, preceded by 1 or 2 light warm-up sets using about 50% of the 1 RM.

To make the exercise program more time-effective, two or three exercises that require different muscle groups may be alternated. In this way, you will not have to wait too long before proceeding to a new set on a different exercise. For example, you may combine bench press, leg extensions, and abdominal crunches so you can go almost directly from one set to the next.

To avoid muscle soreness and stiffness, new participants ought to build up gradually to the 3 sets of maximal repetitions. This can be done by doing only 1 set of each exercise with a lighter resistance on the first day. During the second session, 2 sets of each exercise can be performed, one light and the second with the regular resistance. On the third session, 3 sets could be performed, one light and two heavy. After that, you should be able to do all 3 heavy sets.

Women and Strength Training

One of the most common misconceptions about physical fitness relates to women and strength training. Because of the increase in muscle mass commonly seen in men, some women think that if they participate in strength-training, they, too, will develop large muscles. Even though the *quality* of muscle in men and women is the same, endocrinological differences will not allow women to achieve the same amount of muscle hypertrophy (increase in size) as men. Men also have more muscle fibers, and because of the male sex-specific hormones, each fiber has a greater potential for hypertrophy.

As the number of women who participate in sports has increased steadily in the last few years, the myth that strength training for women leads to larger muscle size has waned. In recent years, better body appearance has become the rule rather than the exception for women who participate in strength-training programs. Some of the most attractive women movie stars and many beauty pageant participants train with weights to further improve their personal image.

Frequency of Training

Strength training should be done either with a total body workout three times per week, or more frequently if using a split-body routine (upper body one day, lower body the next). After a maximum strength workout, the muscles should be rested for about 48 hours to allow adequate recovery.

People who are not completely recovered in 2 or 3 days most likely are overtraining and, therefore, not reaping the full benefits of their program. In that case, decreasing the total number of sets or exercises performed during the previous workout is recommended.

To achieve significant strength gains, a minimum of 8 weeks of consecutive training is needed. Once an ideal level of strength is achieved, one training session per week will be sufficient to maintain the new strength level.

Designing a Strength-Training Program

Two strength-training programs are illustrated in this chapter. Only a minimum of equipment is required for the first program, "Strength-Training Exercises Without Weights" (Exercises 1 through 11). This program can be done within the walls of your own home. Your body weight is used as the primary resistance for most exercises. A few exercises call for a friend's help or some basic implements from around the house to provide more resistance.

The program "Strength-Training Exercises With Weights" (Exercises 12 through 20) requires machines such as those shown in the photographs. Some of these machines use fixed resistance; others use variable resistance. Many of these exercises also can be done with free weights.

Depending on the facilities available to you, you should be able to choose one of the two training programs outlined in this chapter. The resistance and the number of repetitions you use should be based on whether you want to increase your muscular strength or your muscular endurance. Do up to 10–12 repetitions maximum for strength gains and muscle hypertrophy, and more than 12 for muscular endurance.

As pointed out, a regimen of three training sessions per week on nonconsecutive days is an ideal arrangement for proper development. Because both strength and endurance are required in daily activities, 3 sets of about 8 to 12 repetitions maximum for each exercise are enough. In doing this, you will

obtain good strength gains and yet be close to the endurance threshold.

Perhaps the only exercises that call for more repetitions are abdominal exercises. The abdominal muscles are considered primarily antigravity or postural muscles. Hence, a little more endurance may be required. When doing abdominal work, most people do about 20 repetitions.

If time is a concern in completing a strength-training exercise program, the American College of Sports Medicine recommends as a minimum: (a) 1 set of 8 to 12 repetitions performed to near fatigue, and (b) 8 to 10 exercises involving the major muscle groups of the body, conducted twice a week[13] (see Figure 7.4). This recommendation is based on research showing that this training generates 70% to 80% of the improvements reported in other programs using 3 sets of about 10 RM. You may now proceed to write your own strength-training prescription using Assessment 7-2 at the end of this chapter.

MUSCULAR FLEXIBILITY

Flexibility is the ability of a joint to move freely through its full range of motion. Health-care professionals and practitioners generally have underestimated and overlooked the contribution of good muscular flexibility to overall fitness and preventive

FIGURE 7.4

Mode:	8 to 10 dynamic strength-training exercises involving the body's major muscle groups.
Resistance:	Enough resistance to perform 8 to 12 repetitions to near fatigue.
Sets:	A minimum of one set.
Frequency:	At least two times per week.

Source: "The Recommended Quantity and Quality of Exercise for Developing and Maintaining Cardiorespiratory and Muscular Fitness in Healthy Adults," by the American College of Sports Medicine, *Medicine Science in Sports and Exercise*, 22 (1990), pp. 265–274.

Minimum guidelines for strength-training.

Set Number of repetitions in strength training (e.g., 1 set of 12 repetitions).

Flexibility Ability of a joint to move freely through its full range of motion.

health care. In daily life we often have to make rapid or strenuous movements we are not accustomed to making, which may cause injury. Improper body mechanics often are the result of poor flexibility.

Approximately 80% of all low-back problems in the United States are attributable to improper alignment of the vertebral column and pelvic girdle, a direct result of inflexible and weak muscles. This backache syndrome costs American industry billions of dollars each year in lost productivity, health services, and workers compensation.[14]

Participating in a regular flexibility program helps a person maintain good joint mobility, increases resistance to muscle injury and soreness, prevents low-back and other spinal column problems, improves and maintains good postural alignment, promotes proper and graceful body movement, improves personal appearance and self-image, and helps to develop and maintain motor skills throughout life. In addition, flexibility exercises have been prescribed successfully to treat dysmenorrhea (painful menstruation) and general neuromuscular tension (stress).[15]

Furthermore, stretching exercises in conjunction with calisthenics are helpful in warm-up routines to prepare the human body for more vigorous aerobic or strength-training exercises, as well as cool-down routines following exercise to help the person return to a normal resting state. Fatigued muscles tend to contract to a shorter than average resting length, and stretching exercises help fatigued muscles reestablish their normal resting length.

Adequate flexibility helps to develop and maintain sports skill throughout life.

Total range of motion around a joint is highly specific and varies from one joint to the other (hip, trunk, shoulder), as well as from one individual to the next. The amount of muscular flexibility relates primarily to genetic factors and the index of physical activity. Other factors that influence range of motion about a joint include joint structure, ligaments, tendons, muscles, skin, tissue injury, adipose tissue (fat), body temperature, age, and gender. Because of the specificity of flexibility, to indicate what constitutes an ideal level of flexibility is difficult. Nevertheless, flexibility is important to everyone's health, and even more so during the aging process.

Guidelines for Flexibility Development

Although the role of genetics in body flexibility is considerable, range of joint mobility can be increased and maintained through a regular flexibility exercise program. Because range of motion is highly specific to each body part (ankle, trunk, shoulder), a comprehensive stretching program that includes all body parts and adheres to the basic guidelines for flexibility development should be followed to obtain optimal results.

Overload and specificity of training, discussed in conjunction with strength development, also apply to the development of muscular flexibility. To increase the total range of motion around a joint, the specific muscles surrounding that joint have to be stretched progressively beyond their accustomed length. The principles of mode, intensity, repetitions, and frequency of exercise also can be applied to flexibility programs.

Mode of Exercise

Three modes of exercise can be used to increase flexibility: (a) ballistic stretching, (b) slow-sustained stretching, and (c) proprioceptive neuromuscular facilitation (PNF) stretching. Although all three types of stretching are effective in developing better flexibility, each technique has certain advantages.

Ballistic (or dynamic) **stretching** exercises are performed using jerky, rapid, and bouncy movements that provide the necessary force to lengthen the muscles. This type of stretching helps to develop flexibility; however, the ballistic actions may cause muscle soreness and injury because of small tears to the soft tissue.

Precautions must be taken not to overstretch ligaments, as they will undergo plastic (permanent) elongation. If the stretching force cannot be controlled, as in fast, jerky movements, ligaments can be easily overstretched. This, in turn, leads to excessively loose joints, heightening the risk for injuries, including joint dislocation and subluxation (partial dislocation). Most authorities, therefore, do not recommend ballistic exercises for development of flexibility.

With **slow-sustained stretching** technique, muscles are lengthened gradually through a joint's complete

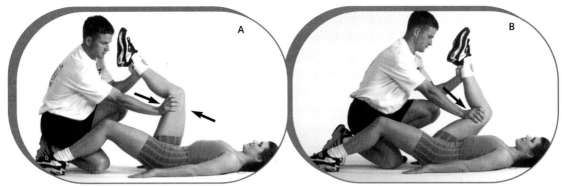

Proprioceptive neuromuscular facilitation (PNF) stretching technique (a) isometric phase and (b) stretching phase.

range of motion, and the final position is held for a few seconds. Using a slow-sustained stretch causes the muscles to relax and thereby lengthen. This type of stretch causes little pain and has a low risk for injury. Slow-sustained stretching exercises are recommended for flexibility development programs.

Proprioceptive neuromuscular facilitation (PNF) stretching has become more popular in the last few years. This technique, based on a contract and relax method, requires the assistance of another person. The procedure is as follows:

1. The person assisting with the exercise provides an initial force by slowly pushing in the direction of the desired stretch. The initial stretch does not cover the entire range of motion.

2. The person being stretched then applies force in the opposite direction of the stretch, against the assistant, who tries to hold the initial degree of stretch as closely as possible. An isometric contraction is being performed at that angle.

3. After 4 or 5 seconds of isometric contraction, the muscle(s) being stretched are relaxed completely. The assistant then slowly increases the degree of stretch to a greater angle.

4. The isometric contraction then is repeated for another 4 or 5 seconds, after which the muscle is relaxed again. The assistant then can increase the degree of stretch slowly one more time.

This procedure is repeated two to five times, until the exerciser feels mild discomfort. On the last trial, the final stretched position should be held for several seconds.

Theoretically, with the PNF technique, the isometric contraction helps relax the muscle(s) being stretched, which results in greater muscle length. Some fitness leaders believe that PNF is more effective than slow-sustained stretching. Another benefit

of PNF is an increase in strength of the muscle(s) being stretched. Recent research showed an approximate 17% and 35% increase in absolute strength and muscular endurance, respectively, in the hamstring muscle group through 12 weeks of PNF stretching.[16] The results were consistent in men and women. These increases are attributed to the isometric contractions performed during PNF. The disadvantages are more pain with PNF, a second person (preferably) has to assist, and more time is necessary to conduct each session.

Intensity of Exercise

Before starting any flexibility exercises, the muscles should be warmed up using some calisthenic exercises. A good time to do flexibility exercises is after aerobic workouts when the higher body temperature can increase joint range of motion significantly. Failing to do a proper **warm-up** increases the risk for muscle pulls and tears.

When doing flexibility exercises, the intensity or degree of stretch should be only to a point of mild discomfort. The stretching routine should not be to the point of pain. Pain is an indication that the load is too high and may lead to injury. As you reach the point of pain, you should try to relax the muscle or muscles being stretched as much as possible. After

Ballistic stretching Exercises performed using jerky, rapid, and bouncy movements.

Slow-sustained stretching Technique whereby the muscles are lengthened gradually through a joint's complete range of motion and the final position is held a few seconds.

Proprioceptive neuromuscular facilitation (PNF) Stretching technique in which muscles are stretched out progressively with intermittent isometric contractions.

Warm-up Starting a workout slowly.

completing the stretch, bring back the body part to the starting point.

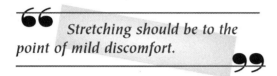

Stretching should be to the point of mild discomfort.

Repetitions

In an exercise session, the time required for flexibility development is based on the number of repetitions performed and the length of time each repetition (final stretched position) is held. The general recommendation is that each exercise be done four or five times, holding the final position each time for about 10 to 30 seconds.

As flexibility increases, you gradually can increase the time each repetition is held, to a maximum of one minute. Individuals who are susceptible to flexibility injuries should limit each stretch to 20 seconds.

Frequency of Training

Flexibility exercises should be conducted five to six times a week in the initial stages of the program. After a minimum of 6 to 8 weeks of almost daily stretching, flexibility levels can be maintained with only two sessions per week, using about 3 repetitions of 10 to 15 seconds each. Figure 7.5 provides a summary of flexibility development guidelines.

FIGURE 7.5

- **Mode**

  Static stretching or proprioceptive neuromuscular facilitation (PNF) to include every major joint of the body

- **Intensity**

  Stretch to the point of mild discomfort

- **Repetitions**

  Repeat each exercise three to five times and hold the final stretched position for 10 to 30 seconds

- **Frequency**

  At least three days per week

Source: *ACSM's Guidelines for Exercise Testing and Prescription* (Baltimore: Williams & Wilkins, 1995).

Guidelines for developing flexibility.

DESIGNING A FLEXIBILITY PROGRAM

To improve body flexibility, each major muscle group should be subjected to at least one stretching exercise. A complete set of exercises for developing muscular flexibility is presented at the end of this chapter. With some of the exercises, you may not be able to hold a final stretched position (examples are lateral head tilts and arm circles), but you still should perform the exercise through the joint's full range of motion. Depending on the number and the length of the repetitions, a complete workout will last between 15 and 30 minutes. You can use Assessment 7-3 at the end of this chapter to design your own stretching program.

PREVENTING AND REHABILITATING LOW-BACK PAIN

Few people make it through life without having low back pain at some point. An estimated 75 million Americans currently have chronic low-back pain each year. About 80% of the time, backache syndrome is preventable and is caused by any or some combination of: (a) physical inactivity, (b) poor postural habits and body mechanics, or (c) excessive body weight.

Lack of physical activity is the most common contributor to chronic low-back pain. Deterioration or weakening of the abdominal and gluteal muscles, along with tightening of the lower back (erector spine) muscles, brings about an unnatural forward tilt of the pelvis. This tilt puts extra pressure on the spinal vertebrae, causing pain in the lower back. Accumulation of fat around the midsection of the body contributes to the forward tilt of the pelvis, which further aggravates the condition.

Low-back pain frequently is associated with faulty posture and improper body mechanics (body positions in all of life's daily activities, including sleeping, sitting, standing, walking, driving, working, and exercising). Incorrect posture and poor mechanics, as explained in Figure 7.6, increase strain not only on the lower back but on many other bones, joints, muscles, and ligaments as well.

The incidence and frequency of low-back pain episodes can be reduced greatly by including some specific stretching and strengthening exercises in the regular fitness program. In most cases, back pain is present only with movement and physical activity.

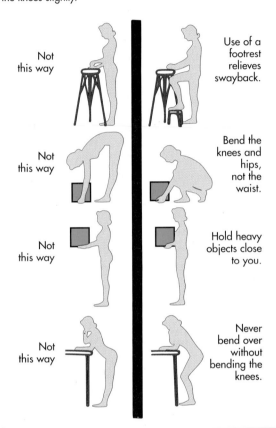

FIGURE 7.6

Your Back and How to Care For It

HOW TO STAY ON YOUR FEET WITHOUT TIRING YOUR BACK

To prevent strain and pain in everyday activities, it is restful to change from one task to another before fatigue sets in. Housewives can lie down between chores; others should check body position frequently, drawing in the abdomen, flattening the back, bending the knees slightly.

Not this way

Use of a footrest relieves swayback.

Not this way

Bend the knees and hips, not the waist.

Not this way

Hold heavy objects close to you.

Not this way

Never bend over without bending the knees.

HOW TO PUT YOUR BACK TO BED

For proper bed posture, a firm mattress is essential. Bedboards, sold commercially, or devised at home, may be used with soft mattresses. Bedboards, preferably, should be made of 3/4 inch plywood. Faulty sleeping positions intensify swayback and result not only in backache but in numbness, tingling, and pain in arms and legs.

Incorrect:
Lying flat on back makes swayback worse.

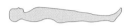

Use of high pillow strains neck, arms, shoulders.

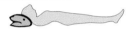

Sleeping face down exaggerates swayback, strains neck and shoulders.

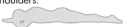

Bending one hip and knee does not relieve swayback.

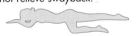

Correct:
Lying on side with knees bent effectively flattens the back. Flat pillow may be used to support neck, especially when shoulders are broad.

Sleeping on back is restful and correct when knees are properly supported.

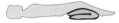

Raise the foot of the mattress eight inches to discourage sleeping on the abdomen.

Proper arrangement of pillows for resting or reading in bed.

HOW TO SIT CORRECTLY

A back's best friend is a straight, hard chair. If you can't get the chair you prefer, learn to sit properly on whatever chair you get. To correct sitting position from forward slump: Throw head well back, then bend it forward to pull in the chin. This will straighten the back. Now tighten abdominal muscles to raise the chest. Check position frequently.

Relieve strain by sitting well forward, flatten back by tightening abdominal muscles, and cross knees.

Use of footrest relieves swayback. Aim is to have knees higher than hips.

Correct way to sit while driving, close to pedals. Use seat belt or hard backrest, available commercially.

TV slump leads to "dowager's hump," strains neck and shoulders.

If chair is too high, swayback is increased.

Keep neck and back in as straight a line as possible with the spine. Bend forward from hips.

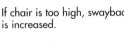

Driver's seat too far from pedals emphasizes curve in lower back.

Strained reading position. Forward thrusting strains muscles of neck and head.

**Reproduced with permission of Schering Corporation.
Copyright Schering Corporation, Kenilworth, NJ**

If the pain is severe and persists even at rest, the first step is to consult a physician, who can rule out any disc damage and most likely will prescribe proper bed rest using several pillows under the knees for leg support. This position helps release muscle spasms by stretching the muscles involved.

The physician also may prescribe a muscle relaxant or anti-inflammatory medication (or both) and some type of physical therapy. Once the individual is pain-free in the resting state, he or she needs to start correcting the muscular imbalance by stretching the tight muscles and strengthening the weak ones. Stretching exercises always are performed first.

Several exercises for preventing back pain and rehabilitating the back are given at the end of this chapter. These exercises can be done twice or more daily when a person has back pain. Under normal circumstances, three to four times a week is sufficient to prevent the syndrome.

MANAGING EXERCISE-RELATED INJURIES

To enjoy and maintain physical fitness, you must do what you can to prevent injury during a conditioning program. Exercise-related injuries are common in exercise programs. Surveys show that more than half of all new participants will incur injuries during the first 6 months of the conditioning program.

The four most common causes of injuries are: (a) high-impact activities, (b) rapid conditioning programs (doing too much too quickly), (c) improper shoes or training surfaces, and (d) anatomical predisposition (body propensity). Of these, high-impact activities and a substantial increase in quantity, intensity, and duration of activities comprise the most common causes of injuries, by far. The body requires time to adapt to more intense activities. Most of these injuries could be prevented through a more gradual and proper conditioning program.

The best treatment always has been prevention itself. If an activity is causing unusual discomfort or chronic irritation, you need to treat the cause by decreasing the intensity, switching activities, or using better equipment such as proper-fitting shoes.

In cases of acute injury, the standard treatment is cold application, compression or splinting (or both), and elevation of the affected body part. This commonly is referred to as ICE (I = Ice application, C = Compression, and E = Elevation). Cold should

be applied three to five times a day for 15 to 20 minutes at a time during the first 24 to 36 hours, by submerging the injured area in cold water, using an icebag, or applying ice massage to the affected part. An elastic bandage or wrap can be used for compression. Elevating the body part decreases blood flow to it.

The purpose of these three types of treatment is to minimize swelling in the area, which hastens recovery time. After the first 36 to 48 hours, heat can be used if swelling or inflammation has abated. If you have doubts regarding the nature or seriousness of the injury (such as suspected fracture), seek a medical evaluation.

Obvious deformities (such as in fractures, dislocations, or partial dislocations) call for splinting, cold application with an icebag, and medical attention. Never try to reset any of these conditions by yourself, as that could further damage muscles, ligaments, and nerves. Treatment of these injuries always should be in the hands of specialized medical personnel. A quick reference guide for the signs or symptoms and treatment of exercise-related problems is provided in Table 7.2.

EXERCISE INTOLERANCE

As you start your exercise program, be sure to stay within the safe limits for exercise participation. The best way to determine whether you are exercising too strenuously is to check your heart rate and make sure it does not exceed the limits of your target zone. Exercising above this target zone may not be safe for unconditioned or high-risk individuals. You do not need to exercise beyond your target zone to gain the desired benefits for the cardiorespiratory system.

> ❝ *One of the basic things you will need to learn with exercise is to listen to your body.* ❞

In addition, several physical signs will tell you when you are exceeding functional limitations. These include a rapid or irregular heart rate, difficult breathing, nausea, vomiting, lightheadedness, headaches, dizziness, pale skin, flushness, extreme weakness, lack of energy, shakiness, sore muscles, cramps, and tightness in the chest. If you notice any of these symptoms, you should seek medical attention before continuing your exercise program. One of the basic things you will need to learn with exercise is to listen to your body.

Your recovery heart rate also can be an indicator of overexertion. To a certain extent, recovery heart rate is related to fitness level. The higher your cardiorespiratory fitness level, the faster your heart rate will decrease following exercise. As a rule of thumb, heart rate should be below 120 beats per minute 5 minutes into recovery. If your heart rate is above 120, you likely have overexerted yourself or possibly could have some other cardiac abnormality. If you decrease the intensity or duration of exercise and still have a fast heart rate 5 minutes into recovery, consult your physician.

LEISURE-TIME PHYSICAL ACTIVITY

Although notable differences are found across the population, the average person in developed countries has about 3.5 hours of "free" or leisure time daily. In the current automated society, most of this time is spent in sedentary living. Leisure-time physical activity usually is viewed as any activity undertaken during an individual's discretionary time that helps to increase resting energy or caloric expenditure. Which activities are selected are personal choices. Among the motivations for participation are health, aesthetics, weight control, competition and challenge, fun, social interaction, mental arousal, relaxation, and stress management.

TABLE 7.2 **Reference Guide For Exercise-Related Problems**

Injury	Signs/Symptoms	Treatment*
Bruise (contusion)	Pain, swelling, discoloration	Cold application, compression, rest
Dislocations Fractures	Pain, swelling, deformity	Splinting, cold application, seek medical attention
Heat cramps	Cramps, spasms and muscle twitching in the legs, arms, and abdomen	Stop activity, get out of the heat, stretch, massage the painful area, drink plenty of fluids
Heat exhaustion	Fainting, profuse sweating, cold/clammy skin, weak/rapid pulse, weakness, headache	Stop activity, rest in a cool place, loosen clothing, rub body with cool/wet towel, drink plenty of fluids, stay out of heat for 2–3 days
Heat stroke	Hot/dry skin, no sweating, serious disorientation, rapid/full pulse, vomiting, diarrhea, unconsciousness, high body temperature	*Seek immediate medical attention*, request help and get out of the sun, bathe in cold water / spray with cold water / rub body with cold towels, drink plenty of cold fluids
Joint sprains	Pain, tenderness, swelling, loss of use, discoloration	Cold application, compression, elevation, rest, heat after 36 to 48 hours (if no further swelling)
Muscle cramps	Pain, spasm	Stretch muscle(s), use mild exercises for involved area
Muscle soreness and stiffness	Tenderness, pain	Mild stretching, low-intensity exercise, warm bath
Muscle strains	Pain, tenderness, swelling, loss of use	Cold application, compression, elevation, rest, heat after 36 to 48 hours (if no further swelling)
Shin splints	Pain, tenderness	Cold application prior to and following any physical activity, rest, heat (if no activity is carried out)
Side stitch	Pain on the side of the abdomen below the rib cage	Decrease level of physical activity or stop altogether, gradually increase level of fitness
Tendonitis	Pain, tenderness, loss of use	Rest, cold application, heat after 48 hours

* Cold should be applied 3 to 4 times a day for 15 minutes
Heat can be applied 3 times a day for 15 to 20 minutes

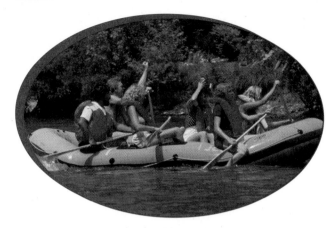

Leisure-time activities should promote energy expenditure and enhance overall health and fitness.

Frequently, leisure-time physical activity is not the same as exercise performed during a regular exercise program. During leisure time, people may walk, hike, garden, and participate in sports such as tennis, table tennis, badminton, golf, and croquet.

Every small increase in daily physical activity contributes to the development of health and wellness. Small increases in physical activity have a large impact in decreasing the risk for disease and premature death. Therefore, a new, concerted effort must be made to spend leisure time in activities that promote energy expenditure, provide a break from daily tasks, and contribute to health-related fitness.

BEHAVIOR MODIFICATION

Over the course of many years, we all develop habits that at some point in time we would like to change. Old habits die hard. **Behavior modification** requires considerable effort. The following principles can be adopted to help change behavior.

1. *Self-analysis.* The first step in behavior modification is a decisive desire to do so. If you have no interest in changing a behavior, you won't do it. A person who has no intention of quitting smoking will not quit, regardless of what anyone may say or how strong the evidence is against it. In your self-analysis, prepare a list of reasons for continuing or discontinuing a certain behavior. When the reasons for change outweigh the reasons for not changing, you are ready for the next step.

2. *Behavior analysis.* Determine the frequency, circumstances, and consequences of the behavior to be altered or implemented. If the desired outcome is to decrease your consumption of fat, you first must find out what foods in your diet are high in fat, when you eat them, and when you don't eat them. Knowing when you don't eat them points to circumstances under which you can exert control over your diet and will help you set goals.

3. *Goal setting.* Goals motivate change in behavior. The stronger the goal (desire), the more motivated you'll be to either change unwanted behaviors or implement new, healthy behaviors. The discussion on goal setting that follows will help you write goals and prepare an action plan to achieve those goals and will aid behavior modification.

4. *Social support.* Surround yourself by people who either will work toward a common goal with you or will encourage you along the way. When attempting to quit smoking, it may help to do so with others who are trying to quit. You also may get help from friends who already have quit. Peer support is a strong incentive for behavioral change. Avoid people who will not support you. Friends who have no desire to quit smoking actually may tempt you to smoke and encourage a relapse. People who are beyond the goal you are trying to reach may not be supportive either. For instance, someone may say: "I can do six consecutive miles." Your response should be: "I'm proud that I can jog three consecutive miles."

5. *Monitoring.* Continuous behavior monitoring increases awareness of the desired outcome. Sometimes this in itself is sufficient to generate change. For example, keeping track of your daily food intake will reveal sources of fat in the diet. It can help you cut down gradually or completely eliminate high-fat foods before consuming them. If the goal is to increase daily fruit and vegetable intake, keeping track of the number of servings you eat each day will raise your awareness and may help increase your intake of fruits and vegetables.

6. *Positive outlook.* Take a positive approach from the beginning and believe in yourself. Look at the outcomes — how much healthier you will be, how much better you will look, or how you will be able to jog a certain distance, for instance.

7. *Reinforcement.* People tend to repeat behaviors that are rewarded and disregard those that are not rewarded or are punished. If you have been successful in cutting down your fat intake during the week, reward yourself by going to a show or

buying a new pair of shoes. Do not reinforce yourself with destructive behaviors such as eating a high-fat dinner. If you fail to change a desired behavior (or to implement a new one), put off buying the new shoes as you had planned for that week. When a positive behavior becomes habitual, give yourself an even better reward. Treat yourself to a vacation weekend or go on a short trip.

SETTING GOALS

Goals are critical in initiating change. They motivate behavioral change and entail a plan of action. Goals are most effective when they are:

- *Well-planned.* Only a well-conceived action plan will help you attain your goal. In doing this, you also must set both general and specific objectives. The general objective is the ultimate goal you intend to achieve. The specific objectives are the smaller steps required to reach this general objective. For example, a general objective might be to achieve recommended body weight. Several specific objectives could be to:

  (a) lose an average of one pound (or one fat percentage point) per week

  (b) monitor body weight before breakfast every morning

  (c) assess body composition every 2 weeks

  (d) limit fat intake to less than 25% of total calories

  (e) eliminate all pastries from the diet during this time

  (f) exercise in the proper target zone for 45 minutes, five times per week.

- *Personalized.* Goals that you set for yourself are more motivational than goals someone else sets for you.

- *Written.* An unwritten goal is simply a wish. A written goal, in essence, becomes a contract with yourself. Show this goal to a friend or an instructor and have him or her witness, by way of a signature, the contract you made with yourself.

- *Realistic.* Goals should be within reach. If you have not exercised regularly, it would be unrealistic to start a daily exercise program consisting of 45 minutes of step aerobics at a vigorous intensity level. Unattainable goals lead to discouragement and loss of interest. Setting smaller, attainable goals works better.

At times, even with realistic goals, problems arise. Try to anticipate potential difficulties as much as possible, and plan for ways to deal with them. If your goal is to jog 30 minutes on 6 consecutive days, what are the alternatives if the weather turns bad? Possible solutions are to jog in the rain, find an indoor track, jog at a different time of day when the weather improves, or participate in a different aerobic activity, such as stationary cycling, swimming, or step aerobics.

- *Measurable.* Write your goals so they are clear and state specifically the objective to accomplish. "I will lose weight" is not clear enough and is not measurable. A better example is: "I will decrease my body fat to 17%."

- *Time-specific.* A goal always should have a specific date set for completion. This date should be realistic but not too distant in the future.

- *Monitored.* Monitoring your progress as you move toward a goal reinforces behavior. Keeping a physical activity log or doing a body composition assessment periodically determines where you are at at any given time.

- *Evaluated.* Periodic reevaluations are vital for success. You may find that a given goal is unreachable. If so, reassess the goal. On the other hand, if a goal is too easy, you will lose interest and may stop working toward it. Once you achieve a goal, set a new one to improve or maintain what you have achieved. Goals keep you motivated.

ENHANCING ADHERENCE TO EXERCISE

Different things motivate different people to join and remain in a fitness program. Regardless of the initial reason for beginning a physical activity or an exercise program, you now need to plan for ways to make your workout fun. The psychology behind it is simple. If you enjoy an activity, you will continue to do it. If you don't, you will quit. Some of the following suggestions may help:

1. *Start your exercise program slowly.* Adhering to new behaviors takes time. Don't be discouraged

Behavior modification A process to permanently change destructive or negative behaviors and replace them with positive behaviors that will lead to better health and well-being.

if you can exercise only a few minutes or if you miss one or more exercise sessions. The key to success is perseverance.

2. *Select aerobic activities you enjoy doing.* Picking an activity you don't enjoy makes you less likely to keep exercising. At the same time, don't be afraid to try out a new activity, even if that means learning new skills.

3. *Combine different activities.* You can train by doing two or three activities the same week. Some people find that this counteracts the monotony of repeating the same activity every day. Many endurance sports, such as racquetball, basketball, soccer, badminton, in-line skating, cross-country skiing, and surfing (paddling the board), provide a nice break from regular workouts.

4. *Set aside a regular time for exercise.* If you don't plan ahead, it's a lot easier to skip exercise. Holding your exercise hour "sacred" helps you adhere to the program.

5. *Obtain the proper equipment for exercise.* A poor pair of shoes, for example, can increase the risk for injury, discouraging you right from the beginning.

6. *Find a friend or a group of friends to exercise with.* Social interaction makes exercise more fulfilling. Besides, it's harder to skip exercise if someone else is waiting for you.

7. *Set goals and share them with others.* Quitting is tougher when someone else knows what you are trying to accomplish. When you reach a specific goal, reward yourself with a new pair of shoes or a jogging suit.

8. *Don't become an exercise addict.* Learn to listen to your body. Overexercising can lead to chronic fatigue and injuries. Exercise should be enjoyable, and in the process you will need to stop and smell the roses.

9. *Exercise in different places and facilities.* This adds variety to your workouts.

10. *Keep a regular record of your activities.* Keeping a record allows you to monitor your progress and compare it with previous months and years.

11. *Conduct periodic assessments.* Improving to a higher fitness category is a reward in itself.

12. *If health problems arise, see a physician.* When in doubt, it's better to be safe than sorry.

13. *Exercise for a lifetime.* To stay fit, you need to maintain a regular exercise program, even during vacations. If you have to interrupt your program for reasons beyond your control, do not attempt to resume your training at the same level you left off. Instead, build up gradually again.

The real challenge will come now: a lifetime commitment to physical activity and exercise. To make the commitment easier, enjoy yourself and have fun along the way. Implement your program based on your interests and what you enjoy doing most. Then adhering to your new active lifestyle will not be difficult.

Your activities over the next few weeks or months should help you develop positive behaviors that will carry on throughout life. If you truly commit to an active lifestyle and experience the feeling of being physically fit, there will be no looking back. If you don't get there, you won't know what it's like.

You need to put forth a constant and deliberate effort to achieve and maintain a higher quality of life. Improving the quality of your life, and most likely your longevity, is in your hands. Only you can take control of your lifestyle and thereby reap the benefits of wellness.

NOTES

1. W. M. Bortz II, "Disuse and Aging," *Journal of the American Medical Association*, 248 (1982), 1203–1208.

2. U.S. Department of Health and Human Services, *Physical Activity and Health: A Report of the Surgeon General* (Atlanta: U.S. Department of Health and Human Services, Centers for Disease Control and Prevention, National Center for Chronic Disease Prevention and Health Promotion, 1996).

3. *Guidelines for Exercise Testing and Prescription* (Baltimore: Williams & Wilkins, 1995).

4. *Guidelines for Exercise Testing and Prescription.*

5. "Perceived Exertion: A Note on History and Methods," *Medicine and Science in Sports and Exercise*, 5 (1983), pp. 90–93.

6. R. F. DeBusk, U. Stenestrand, M. Sheehan, and W. L. Haskell, "Training Effects of Long Versus Short Bouts of Exercise in Healthy Subjects," *American Journal of Cardiology*, 65 (1990), pp. 1010–1013.

7. American College of Sports Medicine, "The Recommended Quantity and Quality of Exercise for Developing and Maintaining Cardiorespiratory and Muscular Fitness in Healthy Adults," *Medicine and Science in Sports and Exercise*, 22 (1990), pp. 265–274.

8. U. S. Department of Health and Human Services.

9. American College of Sports Medicine (1990).

10. W. W. Campbell, M. C. Crim, V. R. Young, and W. J. Evans, "Increased Energy Requirements and Changes in Body Composition with Resistance Training in Older Adults," *American Journal of Clinical Nutrition*, 60 (1994), pp. 167–175.

11. W. S. Evans, "Exercise, Nutrition and Aging," *Journal of Nutrition*, 122 (1992), pp. 796–801.

12. W. W. K. Hoeger, D. R. Hopkins, S. L. Barette, & D. F. Hale, "Relationship Between Repetitions and Selected Percentages of One Repetition Maximum: A Comparison Between Untrained and Trained Males and Females" *Journal of Applied Sport Science Research*, 4:2 (1990), pp. 47–51.

13. *Guidelines for Exercise Testing and Prescription.*

14. S.A. Plowman, "Physical Fitness and Healthy Low Back Function," *President's Council on Physical Fitness and Sports: Physical Activity and Fitness Research Digest*, Series 1:3 (1993), p. 3.

15. University of California at Berkeley, *The Wellness Guide to Lifelong Fitness* (New York: Random House, 1993), p. 198.

16. J. Kokkonen and S. Lauritzen, "Isotonic Strength and Endurance Gains Through PNF Stretching," *Medicine and Science in Sports and Exercise*, 27 (1995), S22, 127.

Strength-Training Exercise Without Weights

Step-Up

Action Step up and down using a box or chair approximately 12 to 15 inches high (a). Conduct one set using the same leg each time you go up, and then conduct a second set using the other leg. You also could alternate legs on each step-up cycle. You may increase the resistance by holding an object in your arms (b). Hold the object close to the body to avoid increased strain in the lower back.

Muscles Developed Gluteal muscles, quadriceps, gastrocnemius, and soleus

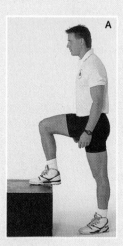
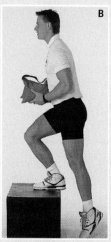

High-Jumper

Action Start with the knees bent at approximately 150° (a) and jump as high as you can, raising both arms simultaneously (b).

Muscles Developed Gluteal muscles, quadriceps, gastrocnemius, and soleus

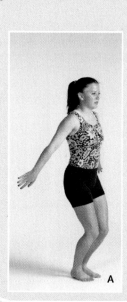
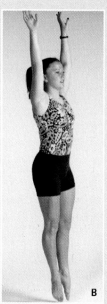

Push-Up

Action Maintaining your body as straight as possible (a), flex the elbows, lowering the body until you almost touch the floor (b), then raise yourself back up to the starting position. If you are unable to perform the push-up as indicated, decrease the resistance by supporting the lower body with the knees rather than the feet (c) or using an incline plane and supporting your hands at a higher point than the floor (d). If you wish to increase the resistance, have someone else add resistance to your shoulders as you are coming back up (e).

Muscles Developed Triceps, deltoid, pectoralis major, erector spinae, and abdominals

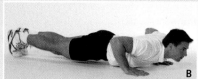
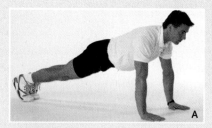
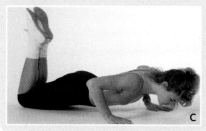
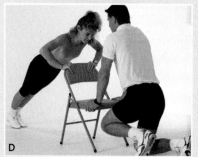
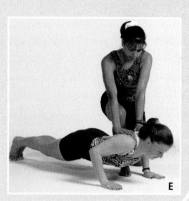

4   Abdominal Crunch and Bent-Leg Curl-Up

Action   Start with your head and shoulders off the floor, arms crossed on your chest, and knees slightly bent (a). The greater the flexion of the knee, the more difficult the curl-up. Now curl up to about 30° (**abdominal crunch** — illustration b) or curl up all the way (**bent-leg curl-up** — illustration c), then return to the starting position without letting the head or shoulders touch the floor or allowing the hips to come off the floor. If you allow the hips to raise off the floor and the head and shoulders to touch the floor, you most likely will "swing up" on the next crunch or curl-up, which minimizes the work of the abdominal muscles. If you cannot curl up with the arms on the chest, place the hands by the side of the hips or even help yourself up by holding on to your thighs (illustrations d and e). Do not perform the curl-up exercise with your legs completely extended, as this will strain the lower back. For additional resistance during the abdominal crunch, have a partner add slight resistance to your shoulders as you "crunch up."

Muscles Developed   Abdominal muscles and hip flexors

NOTE: The bent-leg curl-up exercise should be used only by individuals of at least average fitness without a history of lower back problems. New participants and those with a history of lower back problems should use the abdominal crunch exercise in its place.

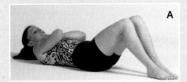
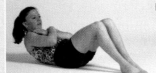
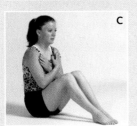
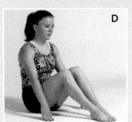
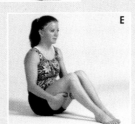
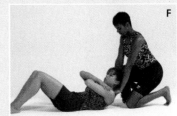

5   Leg Curl

Action   Lie on the floor face down. Cross the right ankle over the left heel (a). Apply resistance with your right foot while you bring the left foot up to 90° at the knee joint (b). Apply enough resistance so the left foot can only be brought up slowly. Repeat the exercise, crossing the left ankle over the right heel.

Muscles Developed   Hamstrings (and quadriceps)

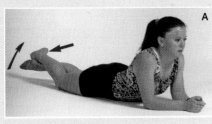
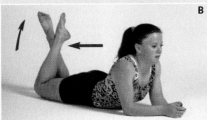

6   Modified Dip

Action   Place your hands and feet on opposite chairs with knees slightly bent (make sure that the chairs are well stabilized). Dip down at least to a 90° angle at the elbow joint, then return to the initial position. To increase the resistance, have someone else hold you down by the shoulders on the way up (see illustration c). You may also perform this exercise using a gymnasium bleacher or box and with the help of a partner, as illustrated in photo d.

Muscles Developed   Triceps, deltoid, and pectoralis major

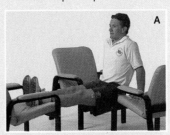
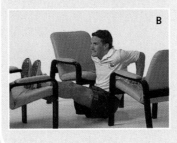
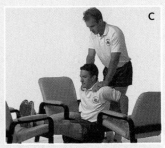

Pull-Up

Action Suspend yourself from a bar with a pronated (thumbs in) grip (a). Pull your body up until your chin is above the bar (b), then lower the body slowly to the starting position. If you are unable to perform the pull-up as described, either have a partner hold your feet to push off and facilitate the movement upward (illustrations c and d) or use a lower bar and support your feet on the floor (e).

Muscles Developed Biceps, brachioradialis, brachialis, trapezius, and latissimus dorsi

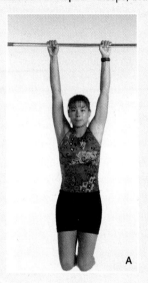
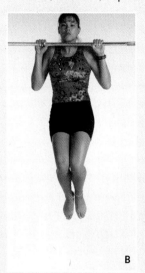
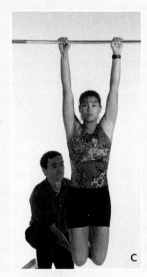
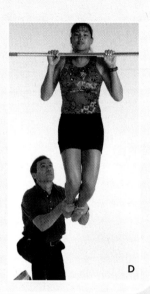

A   B   C   D

Arm Curl

Action Using a palms-up grip, start with the arm completely extended, and with the aid of a sandbag or bucket filled (as needed) with sand or rocks (a), curl up as far as possible, then return to the initial position (b). Repeat the exercise with the other arm.

Muscles Developed Biceps, brachioradialis, and brachialis

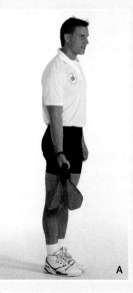
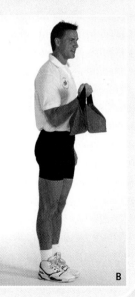

A   B

Heel Raise

Action From a standing position with feet flat on the floor (a), raise and lower your body weight by moving at the ankle joint only (b). For added resistance, have someone else hold your shoulders down as you perform the exercise.

Muscles Developed Gastrocnemius and soleus

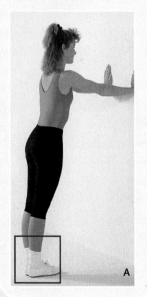
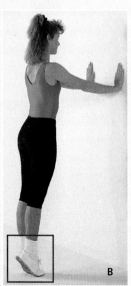

A   B

Leg Abduction and Adduction

Action   Both participants sit on the floor. The person on the left places the feet on the inside of the other person's feet. Simultaneously, the person on the left presses the legs laterally (to the outside — abduction), while the person on the right presses the legs medially (adduction). Hold the contraction for 5 to 10 seconds. Repeat the exercise at all three angles, and then reverse the pressing sequence. The person on the left places the feet on the outside and presses inward, while the person on the right presses outward.

Muscles Developed   Hip abductors (rectus femoris, sartori, gluteus medius and minimus), and adductors (pectineus, gracilis, adductor magnus, adductor longus, and adductor brevis)

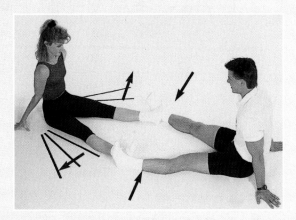

Pelvic Tilt

Action   Lie flat on the floor with the knees bent at about a 90° angle (a). Tilt the pelvis by tightening the abdominal muscles, flattening your back against the floor, and raising the lower gluteal area ever so slightly off the floor (b). Hold the final position for several seconds. The exercise can also be performed against a wall (c).

Areas Stretched   Low-back muscles and ligaments

Areas Strengthened   Abdominal and gluteal muscles

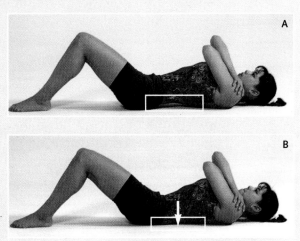

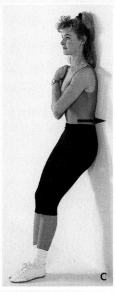

Strength-Training Exercise with Weights

Arm Curl

Action Using a supinated or palms-up grip, start with the arms almost completely extended (a). Curl up as far as possible (b), then return to the starting position.

Muscles Developed Biceps, brachioradialis, and brachialis

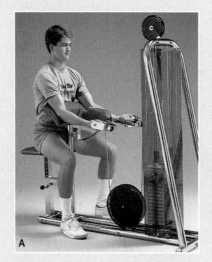
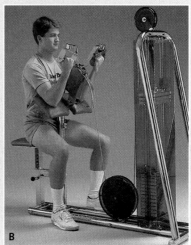

A

B

Bench Press

Action Lie down on the bench with the head by the weight stack, the bench press bar above the chest, and the knees bent so the feet rest on the far end of the bench (a). Grasp the bar handles and press upward until the arms are completely extended (b), then return to the original position. Do not arch the back during this exercise.

Muscles Developed Pectoralis major, triceps, and deltoid

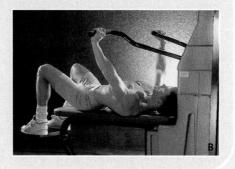

B

Abdominal Crunch and Bent-Leg Curl-Up

See Exercise 4 in this chapter.

Leg Extension

Action Sit in an upright position with the feet under the padded bar and grasp the handles at the sides (a). Extend the legs until they are completely straight (b), then return to the starting position.

Muscles Developed Quadriceps

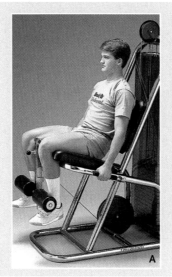
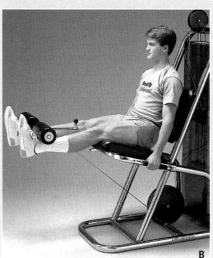

A

B

Leg Curl

Action   Lie with the face down on the bench, legs straight, and place the back of the feet under the padded bar (a). Curl up to at least 90° (b), and return to the original position.

Muscles Developed Hamstrings

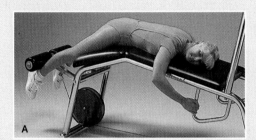
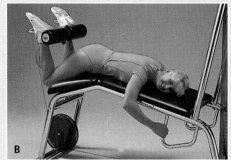

Lat Pull-Down

Action   Starting from a sitting position, hold the exercise bar with a wide grip (a). Pull the bar down until it touches the base of the neck (b), then return to the starting position. (If heavy resistance is used, stabilization of the body may be required either by using equipment as shown or by having someone else hold you down by the waist or shoulders.

Muscles Developed Latissimus dorsi, pectoralis major, and biceps

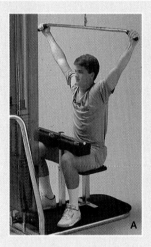
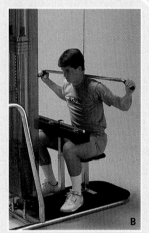

Heel Raise

Action   Start with your feet either flat on the floor or the front of the feet on an elevated block (a), then raise and lower yourself by moving at the ankle joint only (b). If additional resistance is needed, you can use a squat strength-training machine.

Muscles Developed Quadriceps

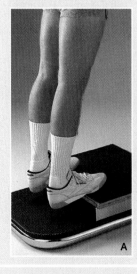
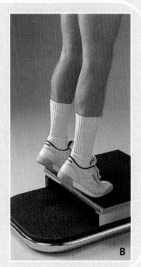

Rowing Torso

Action Sit in the machine with your arms in front of you, elbows bent and resting against the padded bars (a). Press back as far as possible, drawing the shoulder blades together (b). Return to the original position.

Muscles Developed Posterior deltoid, rhomboids, and trapezius

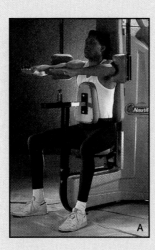
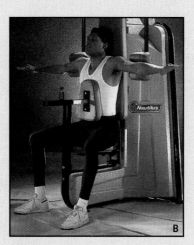

Bent-Arm Pullover

Action Sit back into the chair and grasp the bar behind your head (a). Pull the bar over your head all the way down to your abdomen (b), and slowly return to the original position.

Muscles Developed Latissimus dorsi, pectoral muscles, deltoid, and serratus anterior

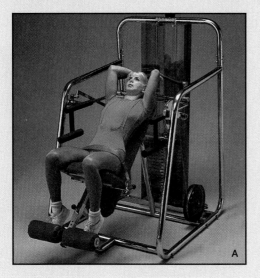
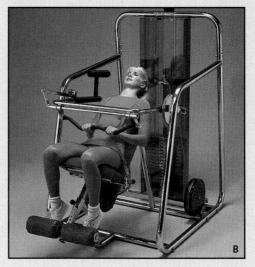

Flexibility Exercises

21 Lateral Head Tilt

Action Slowly and gently tilt the head laterally. Repeat several times to each side.

Areas Stretched Neck flexors and extensors and ligaments of the cervical spine.

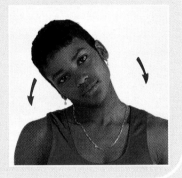

22 Arm Circles

Action Gently circle your arms all the way around. Conduct the exercise in both directions.

Areas Stretched Shoulder muscles and ligaments.

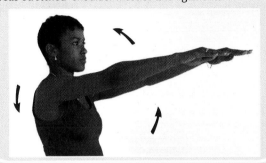

23 Side Stretch

Action Stand straight up, feet separated to shoulder width, and place your hands on your waist. Now move the upper body to one side and hold the final stretch for a few seconds. Repeat on the other side.

Areas Stretched Muscles and ligaments in the pelvic region.

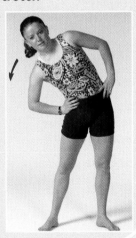

24 Body Rotation

Action Place your arms slightly away from your body, and rotate the trunk as far as possible, holding the final position for several seconds. Conduct the exercise for both the right and left sides of the body. You also can perform this exercise by standing about 2 feet away from the wall (back toward the wall) and then rotating the trunk, placing the hands against the wall.

Areas Stretched Hip, abdominal, chest, back, neck, and shoulder muscles; hip and spinal ligaments.

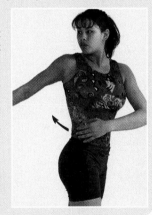

25 Chest Stretch

Action Place your hand on the shoulder of your partner who will in turn push you down by your shoulders. Hold the final position for a few seconds.

Areas Stretched Chest (pectoral) muscles and shoulder ligaments.

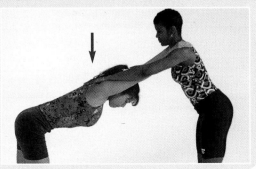

26 Shoulder Hyperextension Stretch

Action Have a partner grasp your arms from behind by the wrists and slowly push them upward. Hold the final position for a few seconds.

Areas Stretched Deltoid and pectoral muscles, and ligaments of the shoulder joint.

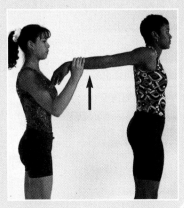

27 Shoulder Rotation Stretch

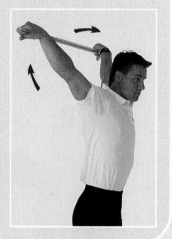

Action With the aid of surgical tubing or an aluminum or wood stick, place the tubing or stick behind your back and grasp the two ends using a reverse (thumbs-out) grip. Slowly bring the tubing or stick over your head, keeping the elbows straight. Repeat several times (bring the hands closer together for additional stretch).

Areas Stretched Deltoid, latissimus dorsi, and pectoral muscles; shoulder ligaments.

28 Quad Stretch

Action Lie on your side and move one foot back by flexing the knee. Grasp the front of the ankle and pull the ankle toward the gluteal region. Hold for several seconds. Repeat with the other leg.

Areas Stretched Quadriceps muscle, and knee and ankle ligaments.

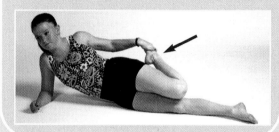

29 Heel Cord Stretch

Action Stand against the wall or at the edge of a step, and stretch the heel downward, alternating legs. Hold the stretched position for a few seconds.

Areas Stretched Heel cord (Achilles tendon), gastrocnemius and soleus muscles.

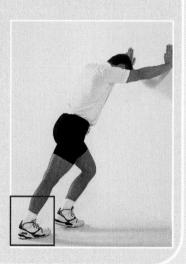

30 Adductor Stretch

Action Stand with your feet about twice shoulder width and place your hands slightly above the knee. Flex one knee and slowly go down as far as possible, holding the final position for a few seconds. Repeat with the other leg.

Areas Stretched Hip adductor

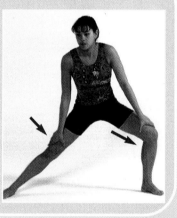

31 Sitting Adductor Stretch

Action Sit on the floor and bring your feet in close to you, allowing the soles of the feet to touch each other. Now place your forearms (or elbows) on the inner part of the thigh and push the legs downward, holding the final stretch for several seconds.

Areas Stretched Hip adductor muscles.

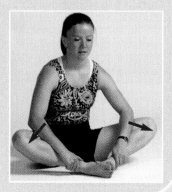

32 Sit-and-Reach Stretch

Action Sit on the floor with legs together and gradually reach forward as far as possible. Hold the final position for a few seconds. This exercise also may be performed with the legs separated, reaching to each side as well as to the middle.

Areas Stretched Hamstrings and lower back muscles, and lumbar spine ligaments.

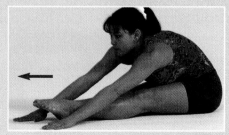

33 Triceps Stretch

Action Place the right hand behind your neck. Grasp the right arm above the elbow with the left hand. Gently pull the elbow backward. Repeat the exercise with the opposite arm.

Areas Stretched Back of upper arm (triceps muscle) and shoulder joint.

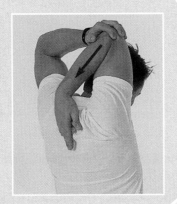

NOTE: Exercises 14 through 20 are also flexibility exercises and can be added to your stretching program.

Exercises for the Prevention and Rehabilitation of Low-Back Pain

34 Single-Knee to Chest Stretch

Action Lie down flat on the floor. Bend one leg at approximately 100° and gradually pull the opposite leg toward your chest. Hold the final stretch for a few seconds. Switch legs and repeat the exercise.

Areas Stretched Lower back and hamstring muscles, and lumbar spine ligaments.

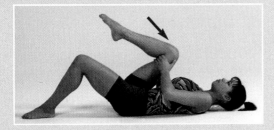

35 Double-Knee to Chest Stretch

Action Lie flat on the floor and then curl up slowly into a fetal position. Hold for a few seconds.

Areas Stretched Upper and lower back and hamstring muscles; spinal ligaments.

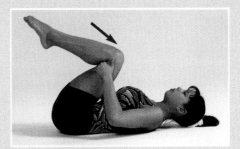

36 Upper and Lower Back Stretch

Action Sit on the floor and bring your feet in close to you, allowing the soles of the feet to touch each other. Holding on to your feet, bring your head and upper chest gently toward your feet.

Areas Stretched Upper and lower back muscles and ligaments

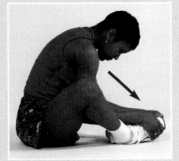

37 Sit-and-Reach Stretch

(see Exercise 32 in this chapter)

38 Back Extension Stretch

Action Lie face down on the floor with the elbows by the chest, forearms on the floor, and the hands beneath the chin. Gently raise the trunk by extending the elbows until you reach an approximate 90° angle at the elbow joint. Be sure the forearms remain in contact with the floor at all times. DO NOT extend the back beyond this point. Hyperextension of the lower back may lead to or aggravate an existing back problem. Hold the stretched position for about 10 seconds.

Areas Stretched Abdominal region.

Additional Benefits Restore lower back curvature.

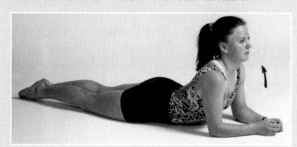

39 Gluteal Stretch

Action Sit on the floor, bend your right leg and place your right ankle slightly above the left knee. Grasp the left thigh with both hands and gently pull the leg toward your chest. Repeat the exercise with the opposite leg.

Areas Stretched Buttock area (gluteal muscles).

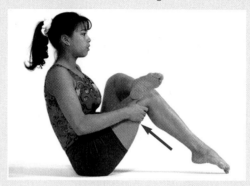

40 Trunk Rotation and Lower Back Stretch

Action Sit on the floor and bend the right leg, placing the right foot on the outside of the left knee. Place the left elbow on the right knee and push against it. At the same time, try to rotate the trunk to the right (clockwise). Hold the final position for a few seconds. Repeat the exercise with the other side.

Areas Stretched Lateral side of the hip and thigh; trunk and lower back.

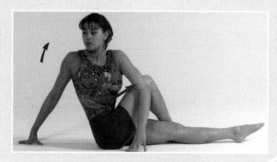

41 Pelvic Tilt

See Exercise 11 in this chapter.

NOTE: This is the most important exercise for use in prevention and treatment of low back pain. This exercise should be incorporated as a part of your daily physical activity and exercise program.

42 Abdominal Crunch and Abdominal Curl-Up

See Exercise 4 in this chapter.

It is important that you do not stabilize your feet when performing either of these exercises, because doing so decreases the work of the abdominal muscles. Also, remember not to "swing up" but rather to curl up as you perform these exercises.

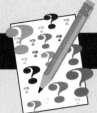

Cardiorespiratory Exercise Prescription

Name _____ Date _____ Grade _____

Instructor _____ Course _____ Section _____

Age _____

NECESSARY LAB EQUIPMENT: None required.

OBJECTIVE: To write your own cardiorespiratory endurance exercise prescription.

Intensity of exercise

1. Estimate your own maximal heart rate (MHR)

    MHR = 220 minus age (220 − age)

    MHR = 22 − _____ = _____ bpm

2. Training intensities (TI) = MHR 3 TI

    60 Percent Ti = _____ × .60 = _____ bpm

    70 Percent Ti = _____ × .70 = _____ bpm

    80 Percent Ti = _____ × .80 = _____ bpm

3. **Cardiorespiratory Training Zone.** The recommended cardiorespiratory training zone is found between the 70% and 90% training intensities. Individuals who have been physically inactive or are in the poor or fair cardiorespiratory fitness categories should use the 60% training intensity during the first few weeks of the exercise program.

    Cardiorespiratory Training Zone: _____ bpm (70% TI) to _____

    Rate of Perceived Exertion (see Figure 7.2, page 162):

    _____ to _____

Mode of Exercise

Select any activity or combination of activities that you enjoy doing. The activity has to be continuous in nature and must get you heart rate up to the cardiorespiratory training zone and keep it there for as long as you exercise. Indicate your preferred mode(s) of exercise:

1. _____ 2. _____ 3. _____

4. _____ 5. _____ 6. _____

Duration and Frequency of Exercise

Please indicate how long each exercise session will last, the days of the week, and the time of day that you will exercise.

Duration: _____ minutes

Select the days of the week and time of day that you will exercise.

____ Monday _____   ____ Tuesday _____   ____ Wednesday _____   ____ Thursday _____

____ Friday _____   ____ Saturday _____   ____ Sunday _____

Exercise Site(s) and Friends

Indicate place(s) where you will exercise: _____

_____

_____

List of friends that will exercise with you: _____

_____

_____

_____

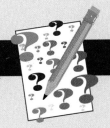

ASSESSMENT 7-2

Muscular Strength/Endurance Prescription

Name _____ Date _____ Grade _____

Instructor _____ Course _____ Section _____

NECESSARY LAB EQUIPMENT: No equipment if the "Strength-Training Exercises Without Weights" program is selected or strength training machines or free weights if "Strength-Training Exercises With Weights" are used.

OBJECTIVE: Write a strength-training exercise program, which may be carried out throughout life.

LAB PREPARATION: Wear exercise clothing and prepare to participate in a sample strength-training exercise session. All of the strength training exercises are illustrated in Chapter 7, pages 180-190.

INSTRUCTIONS: Select one of the two strength-training exercise programs. Perform all of the recommended exercises and, with the exception of the bent- leg curl-up or abdominal crunch exercises, determine the resistance required to do approximately 10 repetitions maximum (for "Strength Training Exercises Without Weights" simply indicate the total number of repetitions performed). For the bent-leg curl-up and abdominal crunch exercises, perform or build up to about 20 repetitions.

I. Strength-Training Exercises Without Weights

Exercise	Repetitions
Step-Up or High Jumper (select and circle one)	_____
Push-Up	_____
Bent-Leg Curl-Up or Abdominal Crunch (select one)	_____
Leg Curl	_____
Modified Dip	_____
Pull-Up or Arm Curl (select one)	_____
Heel Raise	_____
Leg Abduction and Adduction	_____
Pelvic Tilt	_____

II. Strength-Training Exercises With Weights*

Exercise	Repetitions	Resistance
Bench Press	_____	_____
Bent-Leg Curl-Up or Abdominal Crunch (select one)	_____	_____
Leg Extension	_____	_____
Leg Curl	_____	_____
Lab Pulldown	_____	_____
Heel Raise	_____	_____
Rowing Torso	_____	_____
Bent-Arm Pullover	_____	_____

*Most of these exercises can also be performed with free weight

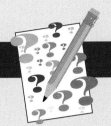

ASSESSMENT 7-3

Muscular Flexibility Prescription

Name _____ Date _____ Grade _____

Instructor _____ Course _____ Section _____

NECESSARY LAB EQUIPMENT: Minor implements such as a chair, a table, an elastic band (surgical tubing or a wood or aluminum stick), and a stool or steps.

OBJECTIVE: To introduce the participant to a sample stretching exercise program that may be carried out throughout life.

INSTRUCTIONS: Wear exercise clothing and prepare to participate in a sample stretching exercise session. All of the flexibility exercises are illustrated in Chapter 10.

Introduction

Perform all of the recommended flexibility exercises given in Chapter 7. Use a combination of slow-sustained and proprioceptive neuromuscular facilitation stretching techniques. Indicate the technique(s) used for each exercise, and, where applicable, the number of repetitions performed and the length of time that the final degree of stretch was held.

Stretching Exercises

Exercise	Stretching Technique[1]	Repetitions	Length of Final Stretch
Lateral Head Tilt	_____	_____	NA[2]
Arm Circles	_____	_____	NA
Side Stretch	_____	_____	NA
Body Rotation	_____	_____	_____
Chest Stretch	_____	_____	_____
Shoulder Hyperextension	_____	_____	
Shoulder Rotation	_____	_____	NA
Quad Stretch	_____	_____	_____
Heel Cord Stretch	_____	_____	_____
Adductor Stretch	_____	_____	_____
Sitting Adductor Stretch	_____	_____	_____
Sit-and-Reach Stretch	_____	_____	_____
Triceps Stretch	_____	_____	_____
Single-Knee to Chest Stretch	_____	_____	_____
Double-Knee to Chest Stretch	_____	_____	_____
Upper and Lower Back Stretch	_____	_____	_____
Back Extension	_____	_____	_____
Gluteal Stretch	_____	_____	_____
Trunk Rotation and Lower Back Stretch	_____	_____	_____

[1]SSS = Slow-sustained stretching, PNF = Proprioceptive neuromuscular facilitation
[2]Not Applicable

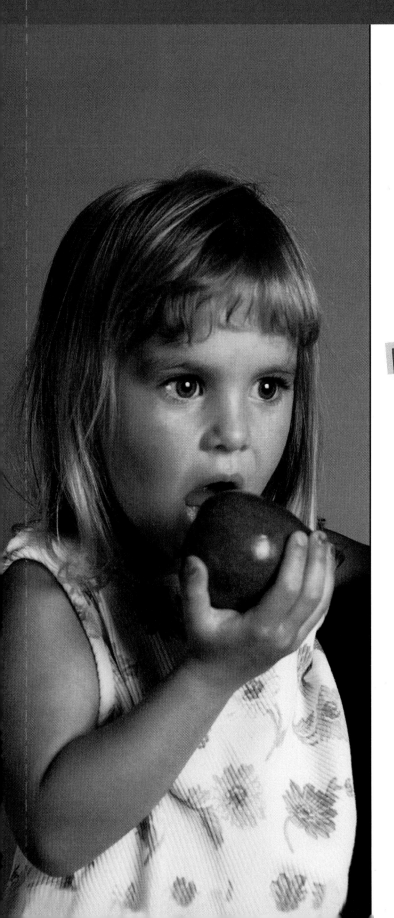

Nutrition and Wellness

OBJECTIVES

- Identify the trends and eating habits of the average American.
- Enumerate the six basic elements of nutrition, their functions and their sources.
- Learn the types of fat and what each does in the body.
- Understand cholesterol and its functions.
- Differentiate the types of carbohydrates and the role of fiber.
- Identify the types of vitamins, their sources and their functions.
- Identify the minerals the body needs, their sources, and their functions.
- List some ways to prevent food-borne diseases.
- Become familiar with the Food Guide Pyramid, the RDA, and Daily Values.
- Learn how to read food labels on packaged products.
- Develop personalized guidelines for a nutritional wellness plan.
- Identify the more common food additives.
- Differentiate food allergies and food sensitivities.

Five decades ago the typical American family was a classic Norman Rockwell vision: Dad in his shirt and tie sat at the head of the table while Mom, complete with a ruffled apron, hurried to bring dinner to her smiling family. It was the age of two-parent, one-career families who sat down to a solid, home-cooked meal three times a day.

As a nation, our eating habits have changed dramatically since then. Dinner is more likely to be a frozen entree popped into the microwave or a hamburger and fries grabbed on the run from a fast-food drive-through. The U.S. Restaurant Association has estimated that approximately 45.8 million people — one-fifth of the U.S. population — eat at a fast-food restaurant every day.

The trends away from agricultural populations and toward single-person households, single-parent families, and women in the workforce had a marked influence on the way we as a nation eat. Fifty years ago, large numbers of Americans grew their own food and ate diets rich in grains, vegetables and fruits. The average diet was significantly lower in fats and refined sugars than our diets are today.

In the decade between 1970 and 1980, the number of fast-food restaurants in the United States more than quadrupled. Today, the United States has more than 175,000 fast-food outlets. Today, few people sit down to breakfast or lunch at home, and as many as a fourth of all Americans eat dinner at a fast-food restaurant. Some estimate that America's

fast-food restaurants serve approximately 200 hamburgers *every second*.

THE SIX BASIC ELEMENTS OF NUTRITION

The six basic elements of **nutrition** — proteins, fats, carbohydrates, vitamins, minerals, and water — provide everything the body needs to maintain itself. These nutrients are transformed into body tissue and functions through **metabolism**. The six basic nutrients fuel metabolism to help the body with:

— growth and the formation of new tissue.

— repair of damaged tissue.

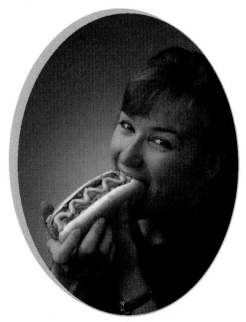

Fast foods should be limited in your diet.

Eating Healthy at Fast-Food Restaurants

If much of your fare comes from fast-food restaurants or cafeterias, that's okay, as long as you make food choices like these:

- Look for chains that offer healthy alternatives such as whole-grain buns, salads, or baked potatoes.
- For breakfast, choose English muffins or pancakes. Avoid fried hash browns, eggs, bacon, sausage, croissants, butter, and Danish rolls.
- If you can, choose a salad bar; lightly sprinkle on cheese and dressing.
- Skip the milk shake or soda; drink juice, low-fat milk, or water instead.
- **Baked potatoes:** A good option, but get a vegetable topping (such as broccoli) if you can instead of butter, sour cream, or cheese.
- **Hamburgers:** Get a single, plain burger; condiments, bacon, and cheese are all high in fat. Better yet, choose roast beef.
- **Chicken:** Order skinless, or take the skin off yourself. Avoid "extra crispy," as the crispness comes from added fat. Avoid chicken nuggets; they usually contain ground-up chicken skin, which is high in fat.
- **Mexican:** Choose chicken tacos or burritos instead of beef; order soft flour tortillas instead of corn tortillas; choose dishes with lots of beans and vegetables and little cheese.
- **Pizza:** Choose vegetable toppings and go light on cheese. Steer away from sausage, pepperoni, olives, extra cheese.

— production of energy.

— conduction of nerve impulses.

— reproduction.

Proteins

Proteins are the body's building blocks, providing the basic materials for cell growth and repair. Protein is composed of carbon, oxygen, hydrogen, and nitrogen. The nitrogen in protein is what gives it the ability to maintain and regulate the body tissues and functions. Protein helps build skin, blood, muscles, and bone; aids in the formation of hormones; regulates the body's chemical processes; forms enzymes; carries nutrients to all body cells; and is a major constituent of the immune system.

Most Americans rely heavily on animal sources of protein, including milk, milk products, eggs, meat, poultry, and fish. Other good plant sources of protein are:

Legumes, grains, and nuts also provide protein to the diet.

- *Legumes,* such as dried beans, dried peas, dried lentils, peanuts, soybeans, and soy products.

- *Grains,* such as oats, rice, barley, cornmeal, and whole-grain breads and pastas.

- *Nuts and seeds,* such as walnuts, cashews, pecans, sunflower seeds, and sesame seeds.

- *Vegetables,* such as broccoli and dark leafy green vegetables.

Proteins derived from both plant and animal sources are made up of about 20 **amino acids.** These enable protein to build and repair tissue, regulate the formation of hormones and enzymes, and maintain the body's chemical balance. Of the 20 amino acids, the body can manufacture 11 itself. The other 9, called **essential amino acids,** must be obtained from the foods we eat.

Complete proteins (chicken and cheddar cheese are examples) contain all of the essential amino acids. **Incomplete proteins** (such as pinto beans and brown rice) contain only some of the essential amino acids. An incomplete protein source can be combined with another food that supplies the missing

essential amino acids. One good combination is peanut butter on whole-grain bread. The best complete protein source is the egg.

Research indicates that amino acids may do more than help rebuild tissues. Certain amino acids trigger the release of neurotransmitters.[1] The amino acid tryptophan triggers serotonin, a neurotransmitter that helps you feel calm, relieves feelings of anxiety, and improves concentration. Found in eggs, poultry, seafood, and dried beans, tyrosine triggers release of the brain chemicals norepinephrine and dopamine, which boost mental energy, improve alertness, and increase motivation.

Only about 12% of the total calories should come from protein. Most Americans eat far too much protein. An American woman, for example, needs only about 46 to 48 grams of protein a day, the equivalent of a cup of low-fat yogurt, a cup of low-fat milk, and 4 ounces of chicken. Protein is essential for the body's growth and repair, but too much can wreak havoc on the body. Excess protein is stored as fat. Too much protein also may accelerate growth of tumors and contribute to heart disease, cancer, and osteoporosis. It causes the body to excrete calcium (needed for strengthening bones and teeth). If a person eats too much protein, the extra nitrogen is excreted in urine, which can strain the kidneys.

Nutrition   The science that studies the relationship between the foods we eat and the functions of the body.

Metabolism   All energy and material transformations that occur within living cells necessary to sustain life.

Proteins   Nutrients that provide the basic materials for cell growth and repair.

Amino acids   Chemical structures that form proteins' ability to build and repair tissue, regulate the formation of hormones and enzymes, and maintain the body's chemical balance.

Essential amino acids   Amino acids that cannot be produced by the body and must be provided by the foods we eat.

Complete protein   A protein source that contains all nine essential amino acids.

Incomplete proteins   Proteins that do not contain all the essential amino acids.

Nutritionist and author Jane Brody said, "Americans excrete the most expensive urine in the world. If it were economical to collect and dry it, tons of nitrogen could be harvested from the nation's toilet bowls each day."[2]

Fats

The most concentrated form of food energy, fat provides 9 calories per gram, more than twice the calories in a gram of carbohydrates or proteins. **Fats** transport fat-soluble vitamins in the body, insulate and protect body organs, regulate hormones, contribute to growth, provide a concentrated source of energy, and are essential for healthy skin. Although the right amount of fat is essential to growth and functioning of the body, too much fat is harmful. Excess dietary fat can lead to high blood pressure, stroke, heart disease, diabetes, and other diseases. Excessive body fat is a leading factor in heart disease (see Chapter 11). It also has been linked to cancers of the colon, breast, uterus, and prostate.

The average American eats much more fat than is recommended or healthy. It is estimated that in a year the average American eats more than 55 pounds of visible fat (salad oil, butter, shortening, for example) and more than 130 pounds of invisible fat (such as the fat in eggs, dairy products, meats, and nuts). The greatest single source of dietary fat in Americans of all ages other than infants is thought to be ground beef. According to the National Research Council, more than half the total fat in the typical American diet comes from milk and milk products, eggs, red meats (beef, pork, veal, and lamb), fish and shellfish, and separated animal fats (such as lard).

The American Heart Association and the U.S. Department of Health and Human Services initially recommended that no more than 30% of the total calories in the diet should come from fat. The American Cancer Society has recommended that 20% or less of the total calories in the diet come from fat for a cancer-prevention diet. On a 30% fat diet, if you eat 1,200 calories a day, you should have no more than 40 grams of fat; for 2,000 calories a day, no more than 67 grams of fat. As a rough indication, figure that 1 teaspoon of fat equals 5 grams.

Of that 30% of calories from fat, less than one-third should come from saturated fats, less than one-third from polyunsaturated fats, and the rest from monounsaturated fats. Table 8.1 lists some common foods and their percent-fat categories.

> *Cholesterol level is not affected as much by the cholesterol you eat as by the overall percentage of fat in the diet.*

A useful guideline to figure out the fat content of individual foods is given in Figure 8.1. All you have to do is multiply the grams of fat by 9 and divide by the total calories in that food. You then multiply that number by 100 to get the percentage. For example, if a food label lists a total of 100 calories and 7 grams of fat, the fat content is 63% of total calories. This simple guideline can help you decrease the fat in your diet. The fat content of selected foods, given in grams and as percent of total calories, is presented in Figure 8.2. The chemical structures of saturated and unsaturated fats are illustrated in Figure 8.3.

Saturated Fats

In pure form **saturated fats** are solid at room temperature, and most come from animal sources. The only exceptions are coconut oil, palm oil, and palm kernel oil (the "tropical oils"), which are highly saturated but still liquid at room temperature. Saturated fats raise the level of low-density lipoproteins (the

Fat Content of Milk

Label	Calories	Total Fat	Saturated Fat
Whole milk	150	8	5
2% milk	120	5	3
1% milk	100	2.5	1.5
Skim* milk	80	0	0

*Also can be called fat-free, nonfat, zero fat.

Source: Food and Drug Administration.

Fat A nutrient that is the most concentrated form of food energy.

Saturated fats Fatty acids with carbon atoms fully saturated with hydrogens, therefore only single bonds link the carbon atoms on the chain. High intake of saturated fats increases the risk for coronary heart disease.

TABLE 8.1 **Percentage of Fat Calories in Common Foods**

Type of Food	Less Than 15% of Calories from Fat	15%-30% of Calories from Fat	30%-50% of Calories from Fat	More Than 50% of Calories from Fat
Fruits and Vegetables	Fruits, plain vegetables, juices, pickles, sauerkraut		French fries, hash browns	Avocados, coconuts, olives
Bread and Cereals	Grains and flours, most breads, most cereals, corn tortillas, pita, matzoh, bagels, noodles and pasta	Corn bread, flour tortillas, oatmeal, soft rolls and buns, wheat germ	Breakfast bars, biscuits and muffins, granola, pancakes and waffles, donuts, taco shells, pastries, croissants	
Dairy Products	Nonfat milk, dry curd cottage cheese, nonfat cottage cheese, nonfat yogurt	Buttermilk, low-fat yogurt, 1% milk, low-fat cottage cheese	Whole milk, 2% milk, creamed cottage cheese	Butter, cream, sour cream, half & half, most cheeses (including part-skim and "lite" cheeses)
Meats		Beef round; veal loin, round, and shoulder; pork tenderloin	Beef and veal, lamb, fresh and picnic hams	All ground beef, spareribs, cold cuts, bacon, sausages, corned beef, hot dogs, pastrami
Poultry Products	Egg whites	Chicken and turkey (light meat without skin)	Chicken and turkey (light meat with skin, dark meat without skin), duck and goose (without skin)	Chicken/turkey (dark meat with skin), chicken/turkey hot dogs and bologna, egg yolks, whole eggs
Seafood	Clams, cod, crab, crawfish, flounder, haddock, lobster, perch, sole, scallops, shrimp, tuna (in water)	Bass and sea bass, halibut, mussels, oyster, tuna (fresh)	Anchovies, catfish, salmon, sturgeon, trout, tuna (in oil, drained)	Herring, mackerel, sardines
Beans and Nuts	Dried beans and peas, chestnuts, water chestnuts		Soybeans	Tofu, most nuts and seeds, peanut butter
Fats and Oils	Oil-free and some "lite" salad dressings			Butter, margarine, all mayonnaise (including reduced-calorie), most salad dressings, all oils
Soups	Bouillons, broths, consomme	Most soups	Cream soups, bean soups, "just add water" noodle soups	Cheddar cheese soup, New England clam chowder
Desserts	Angel food cake, gelatin, some new fat-free cakes	Pudding, tapioca	Most cakes, most pies	
Frozen Desserts	Sherbet, low-fat frozen yogurt, sorbet, fruit ices	Ice milk	Frozen yogurt	All ice cream
Snack Foods	Popcorn (air-popped), pretzels, rye crackers, rice cakes, fig bars, raisin biscuit cookies, marshmallows, most hard candy, fruit rolls	"Lite" microwave popcorn, Scandinavian "crisps," plain crackers, caramels, fudge, gingersnaps, graham crackers	Snack crackers, popcorn (popped in oil), cookies, candy bars, granola bars	Most microwave popcorn, corn and potato chips, chocolate, buttery crackers

FIGURE 8.1

Caloric Value of Food

Sources of Calories

1 gram of carbohydrate ....4 calories
1 gram of protein ....4 calories
1 gram of fat ....9 calories
1 gram of alcohol ....7 calories

Determining % Calories from Fat in Food

Example:
Caloric Distribution for Turkey Breast, 97% Fat Free

Portion size ....1 slice (1 oz)
Calories...........29
Protein ....4 grams × 4 calories = 16 calories
Carbohydrate .....1 gram × 4 calories = 4 calories
Fat ....1 gram × 9 calories = 9 calories
                   Total calories   = 29 calories

Percent Fat Calories =
     (grams of fat × 9) divided by total calories × 100

Percent fat calories in 97% fat free turkey =
          [(1 × 9) ÷ 29] × 100 = 31%

FIGURE 8.2

FAT CONTENT OF SELECTED FOODS

Food *	Calories	% calories from fat	Total fat** (grams)
Coconut oil, 1 tbsp	120	100	13.6
Peanut oil, 1 tbsp	120	100	13.6
Olive oil, 1 tbsp	120	100	13.6
Corn oil, 1 tbsp	120	100	13.6
Canola oil, 1 tbsp	120	100	13.6
Butter, 1 tbsp	102	100	11.5
Margarine, hard, 1 tbsp	102	100	11.4
Margarine, soft, 1 tbsp	77	100	8.6
Ground beef, regular, broiled, 3 oz.	243	66	17.8
Sirloin steak, broiled, 3 oz.	171	36	6.9
Chicken, dark, with skin, baked, 3 oz.	210	57	13.2
Chicken, light, no skin, baked, 3 oz.	139	20	3.0
Salmon, sockeye, broiled, 3 oz.	184	45	9.3
Cod, Atlantic, broiled, 3 oz.	89	7	0.7
Ice cream, 1 cup	269	48	14.3
Cream cheese, 2 tbsp	104	90	10.4
Cheddar cheese, 1 oz.	114	74	9.4
Milk, whole (3.3%), 1 cup	149	49	8.2
Milk, low-fat (1%), 1 cup	102	23	2.6
Cashews, 1/4 cup	187	76	15.7
Peanuts, 1/4 cup	213	76	18.1

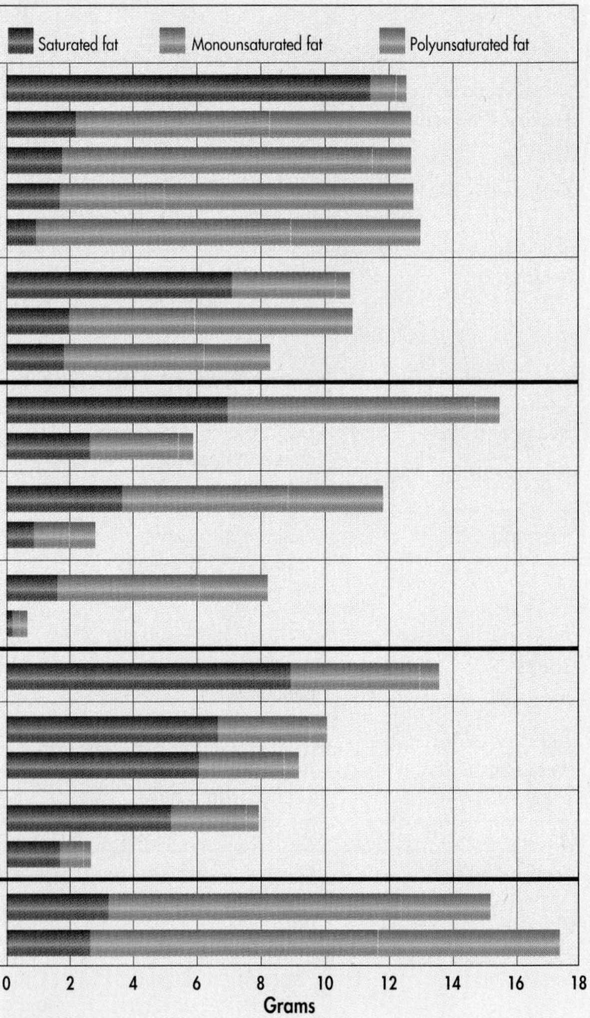

Legend: ■ Saturated fat   ■ Monounsaturated fat   ■ Polyunsaturated fat

(Grams axis: 0 2 4 6 8 10 12 14 16 18)

* Within each group, foods are arranged in order of saturated fat content.
** Total fat exceeds the sum of saturated, monounsaturated, and polyunsaturated fats because it also includes other fatty acids.

Source: *Consumer Reports on Health*, June, 1992.

Saturated fat, monounsaturated fat, and polyunsaturated fat content of selected foods.

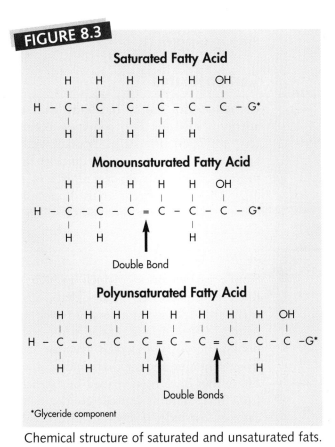

*Glyceride component

Chemical structure of saturated and unsaturated fats.

FIGURE 8.3

most harmful kind of cholesterol) in the bloodstream and have been linked the most strongly to heart disease (Chapter 11) and other degenerative diseases. Examples of foods high in saturated fats are butter, cheese, milk, cream, nondairy cream substitutes, lard, pork, bacon, beef, veal, lamb, poultry skin, hotdogs, luncheon meats, chocolate, and cocoa.

Monounsaturated Fats

Monounsaturated fats, which can accept two more hydrogen atoms, seem to help decrease low-density ("bad") lipoproteins in the bloodstream (see Chapter 11). They are found in peanuts, cashews, olives, and avocados, as well as olive oil, peanut oil, cottonseed oil, and canola oil.

Polyunsaturated Fats

Fats that can accept four more hydrogen atoms, **polyunsaturated fats** lower the level of cholesterol in the bloodstream. They are found in most vegetable oils and, with a few exceptions, are liquid at room temperature. Foods containing polyunsaturated fats include fish, margarine, mayonnaise, walnuts, almonds, pecans, corn oil, safflower oil, sunflower oil, sesame oil, and soybean oil.

Hydrogenated Fats

Some monounsaturated and polyunsaturated fats are **hydrogenated** during manufacturing. During this process, hydrogen is added to the fat to increase shelf life and to make the product harder or more spreadable. Hydrogenated fats are found in shortening, margarine, some crackers, and some nut butters. Eating a vegetable oil that has been hydrogenated may carry as many health risks as eating a saturated fat.

Cholesterol

Cholesterol isn't actually a fat but, rather, is technically a steroid alcohol. Despite its negative publicity, cholesterol does have a beneficial role in the body. It

Omega-3 Oils

A study of traditional Eskimo diets turned up an amazing discovery: Even through the traditional Eskimo diet is about 40% fat, Eskimos have the lowest rate of heart disease in the world. The reason seems to be fish, which are rich in polyunsaturated fats called omega-3 oils. These oils have been shown to reduce cholesterol levels and prevent the build-up of plaque in coronary arteries. In one study, the death rate from heart disease was 50% lower among people who ate at least an ounce of fish every day than those who didn't eat fish.

Taking fish-oil capsules every day isn't as effective as eating fish even once a week. Instead, the diet should include fish rich in omega-3 oils. Tuna, sardines, salmon, mackerel, and herring are best.

Source: Mount Sinai School of edicine.

Monounsaturated fats Fatty acids with only one double bond found along the carbon atom chain.

Polyunsaturated fats Fatty acids with two or more double bonds along the carbon atom chain.

Hydrogenated Hydrogen added to fats to increase shelf life and make the product more spreadable; increases saturation of the fat.

Cholesterol A yellow, waxy, fatlike substance produced naturally by the liver and also ingested in animal tissue.

Trimming the Fat

Instead of This	Try an Equal Amount of This	Save This (Fat Grams)
Chicken breast, fried w/skin, 4 oz.	Chicken breast roasted without skin	11
Extra lean ground beef, 3oz.	Ground breast of turkey	13
Bacon, fried, 1 oz.	Canadian bacon	12
Processed cheese, 3 oz.	Fat-free cheese	27
Whole milk, 1 C.	Skim milk	8
Vegetable oil, 2 T.	Vegetable spray	27
Mayonnaise, 1 T.	Nonfat mayonnaise	11
Margarine, 1 oz.	Diet margarine	12
Italian dressing, 2 T.	Nonfat Italian dressing	14
Guacamole dip	½ C. salsa dip	16
Potato chips, 1 oz.	Pretzels	9
Peanuts, 1 C.	Popcorn	72
Ice cream, 1/2 c.	Nonfat frozen yogurt	7
Danish, doughnut or croissant	Bagel or English muffin with jelly	10

Source: © 1994 Great Performance Inc., 14964 NW Greenbrier Pkwy., Beaverton, OR 97006, (503) 690-9181.

aids in digestion, is a major component of the membranes that protect nerve fibers, aids in production of vitamin D, and helps the body produce the sex hormones estrogen, progesterone, and androgen. Too much cholesterol in the bloodstream, however, places a person at significantly higher risk for developing heart disease.

> *One of the best ways to reduce the production of cholesterol in the body is to reduce the intake of saturated fat.*

The liver produces most of the cholesterol a person needs to stay healthy. The American Heart Association recommends that cholesterol intake be limited to 300 mg or less a day. Plant foods contain no cholesterol. The amount of milk, cheese, dairy products, egg yolks, and meat has to be limited.

Additional information on cholesterol is given in Chapter 11.

Carbohydrates

Carbohydrates supply the body with the energy needed for daily activities. Because they are digested more easily and metabolized more efficiently and quickly than proteins, they are a quicker source of energy. The two different kinds of carbohydrates are simple carbohydrates (sugars) and complex carbohydrates (starches).

Simple Carbohydrates

Simple carbohydrates, which include refined and processed sugars, have given carbohydrates the reputation of being "fattening." They include refined white sugar, honey, sucrose, corn syrup, fructose, dextrose, sorghum, and maltose, among others. Those that have been refined or extracted from their natural sources contain many calories but little, if any, nutritional value — earning them the popular nickname of "empty calories." A diet high in simple carbohydrates can lead to obesity and dental cavities, as well as health problems such as heart disease, diabetes, and hypoglycemia.

Simple carbohydrates are further classified as monosaccharides and disaccharides. These carbohydrates — with *-ose* endings — often take the place of more nutritive foods in the diet.

Monosaccharides. The simplest sugars, **monosaccharides**, are formed by five- or six-carbon skeletons. The three most common monosaccharides are **glucose**, **fructose**, and **galactose**. Both fructose and galactose are converted readily to glucose in the

The average American eats 133 pounds of sugar a year. Most of that is not in the form of sugar we add to foods. An estimated 76 pounds comes from the hidden sugar in a wide array of manufactured and processed foods. For example, an 8-ounce carton of low-fat fruit yogurt contains 7 teaspoons of sugar. A 12-ounce can of cola has 9 teaspoons of sugar.

Source: Mount Sinai School of Medicine.

body. Glucose is used as a source of energy, or it may be stored in the muscles and liver in the form of **glycogen**. Excess glucose in the blood is converted to fat and stored in adipose (fat) tissue. Some of it is eliminated by the kidneys through the urine.

Disaccharides. **Disaccharides** are formed by the linkage of two monosaccharide units, one of which is glucose. The three major disaccharides are **sucrose, lactose, maltose.**

Americans eat an average of 133 pounds of refined sugars a year, about 20% of their total caloric intake.[3] The USDA dietary guidelines for Americans recommend that no more than 10% of total calories come from sugar — about half of the typical intake.

The word *sugar* doesn't always appear on food labels. Instead, manufacturers may list the various kinds of sweeteners separately. The label may have a long list of ingredients including corn syrup, corn starch, sucrose, and honey. These hidden sugars can be deceptive.

> **"** *Jell-O is 83% sugar, and a single 8-ounce can of Coke has approximately 10 teaspoons of sugar.* **"**

Artificial Sweeteners

Artificial sweeteners — some of which are 220 times sweeter than sucrose (table sugar) — actually can increase the craving for sweets. Whereas sugar produces a feeling of fullness or satisfaction, artificial sweeteners do nothing to ease hunger pangs or appease the appetite. People who use artificial sweeteners tend to eat more fats as well.

Complex Carbohydrates

Diets high in **complex carbohydrates** (also called starches) tend to be lower in fat, lower in calories, and higher in dietary fiber than simple carbohydrates. These factors combine to keep the blood sugar at a constant level, stave off malnutrition, and reduce the risks of heart disease, cancer, and other degenerative diseases. The best sources of complex carbohydrates are grains, such as wheat, rice, oats, corn, rye, barley, and millet; potatoes, sweet potatoes, and yams; fruits; vegetables; and legumes, such as soybeans, garbanzo beans, black-eyed peas, kidney beans, butter beans, and peanuts.

Tips For Action

Cutting the Amount of Sugar You Eat

- Substitute water and unsweetened fruit juices for sodas — the number-one source of sugar in the typical American diet.
- Cut back on the number-two source of sugar — processed baked goods such as doughnuts, cookies, cakes, and pies.
- Eat canned fruit packed in its own juice instead of sweetened juices.
- Eat cereals that are low in sugar or contain no sugar.
- Gradually reduce the amount of sugar you add to tea, coffee, and cereal.
- Substitute fresh fruits, raw vegetables, and low-fat crackers for sugar-loaded junk food.
- READ LABELS and cut back on foods that list any type of sugar as one of the first three ingredients.

Carbohydrates   An essential nutrient that is the major source of energy for the human body.

Simple carbohydrates   Carbohydrates that have been refined or extracted from their natural sources, such as white sugar, honey, sucrose, corn syrup, and fructose.

Monosaccharides   The simplest carbohydrates (sugars) formed by five- or six-carbon skeletons. The three most common monosaccharides are glucose, fructose, and galactose.

Glucose   A natural sugar found in food; it also is produced in the body.

Fructose   A sugar that occurs naturally in fruits and honey.

Galactose   A monosaccharide produced from milk sugar in the mammary glands of lactating animals.

Glycogen   Form of carbohydrate (polysaccharide) storage in muscle.

Disaccharides   Simple carbohydrates formed by two monosaccharide units linked together, one of which is glucose. The major disaccharides are sucrose, lactose, and maltose.

Sucrose   Table sugar (glucose plus fructose).

Lactose   A disaccharide consisting of glucose plus galactose.

Maltose   A disaccharide consisting of two units of maltose.

Complex carbohydrates   Also called "starches," nutritionally dense foods that provide excellent sources of energy.

Because they are nutritionally dense, most complex carbohydrate foods are rich in vitamins and minerals. Many contain a significant amount of protein. Complex carbohydrates provide a steady source of energy, making them an excellent choice for physically active people (especially endurance athletes). Complex carbohydrates also are stored in the muscles and the liver as glycogen, which fuels the body when it needs sudden bursts of energy. For most people, nearly half of daily calories come from carbohydrates, at least 80% of which are complex carbohydrates.

One of the "non-nutrients" in complex carbohydrates is **dietary fiber**, formerly called "roughage." It is the part of the plant that is not digested in the small intestine and provides the bulk needed to keep the digestive system running smoothly. **Soluble fiber**, such as gels and pectins, forms a thick, gel-like substance when mixed with water. It isn't digested in the small intestine but instead is absorbed in the large intestine. It helps lower blood cholesterol level, slows emptying of the stomach (prolonging a sense of fullness), and slows the absorption of sugars from the small intestine. It has been shown to reduce the risk of heart disease and diabetes.[4] Good sources of soluble fiber are oats, oat bran, corn bran, apples, pears, prunes, oranges, sweet potatoes, dried beans, and a variety of grains, fruits, and vegetables. The fiber content of selected foods can be found in Table 8.2.

Insoluble fiber, which can't be dissolved in water, is not digested at all and comes mostly from the skins of fruits and vegetables, the seeds of fruits (such as strawberries and raspberries), and the outer tough bran of grains (such as wheat and rice). The best source of insoluble fiber is wheat bran. Other good sources are dried beans and peas, fresh fruits and vegetables eaten with their skins, and most whole grains.

Among the important health benefits of insoluble fiber:[5]

- It speeds the transit time of materials through the intestines.

TABLE 8.2

Fiber Content of Selected Foods (in grams)

	Serving Size	Dietary Fiber
Grains		
Bread, white	1 slice	0.6
Bread, whole wheat	1 slice	1.5
Oat bran, dry	⅓ cup	4.0
Oatmeal, dry	⅓ cup	2.7
Rice, brown, cooked	½ cup	2.4
Rice, white, cooked	½ cup	0.8
Fruits		
Apple, with skin	1 small	2.8
Apricots, with skin	4 fruit	3.5
Banana	1 small	2.2
Blueberries	¾ cup	1.4
Figs, dried	3 fruit	4.6
Grapefruit	½ fruit	1.6
Pear, with skin	1 large	5.8
Prunes, dried	3 medium	1.7
Vegetables		
Asparagus, cooked	½ cup	1.8
Broccoli, cooked	½ cup	2.4
Carrots, cooked, sliced	½ cup	2.0
Peas, green, frozen, cooked	½ cup	4.3
Tomatoes, raw	1 medium	1.0
Legumes		
Kidney beans, cooked	½ cup	6.9
Lima beans, canned	½ cup	4.3
Pinto beans, cooked	½ cup	5.9
Beans, white, cooked	½ cup	5.0
Lentils, cooked	½ cup	5.2
Peas, blackeyed, canned	½ cup	4.7

From James W. Anderson, *Plant Fiber in Foods, 2d Edition*, University of Kentucky, College of Medicine, HCF Nutrition Foundation, P.O. Box 22124, Lexington, KY 40522.

Tips For Action

Boosting Fiber Content in Your Diet

If your diet is low in fiber:

- Substitute brown rice for white rice.
- Substitute whole-wheat products for those made with white wheat.
- Add brown rice, millet, bulgur, or barley to soups, stews, and casseroles.
- Add 100% bran to breakfast cereal or applesauce.
- Sprinkle wheat germ on applesauce, pudding, yogurt, or cottage cheese.
- Eat unpeeled fresh fruits and vegetables.
- Look for whole-grain breads, macaroni, egg noodles, and cereals.

- It stimulates muscles tone in the intestinal walls, softens stools, helps prevent constipation, helps the colon produce more mucus, and has been shown to help prevent cancer of the colon.
- A diet high in insoluble fiber prevents diverticulosis and diverticulitis, disease conditions that occur when the intestine bulges out into "pockets" that can become infected or rupture.

Most Americans eat about 15 grams of fiber a day. The National Cancer Institute recommends doubling that amount, to about 30 grams of fiber a day. The ratio isn't important. Both insoluble and soluble fiber is beneficial.

Vitamins

Vitamins fuel the chemical reactions in the body and enable metabolism to take place, promote growth, and help maintain life and health. They promote good vision, help form normal blood cells, create strong bones and teeth, and enable proper functioning of the heart and the nervous system.

The 13 vitamins fall into two categories.

1. *Fat-soluble vitamins*, including vitamins A, D, E, and K, are stored in the body's fat cells. They are not excreted in the urine and are accumulated in the fat tissues of the body. If you get too many, they can be toxic.

2. *Water-soluble vitamins*, including vitamin C and the B-complex vitamins, dissolve readily in water and are excreted in the urine.

Good sources and important functions of vitamins are given in Table 8.3.

Vitamins C, E, **beta-carotene**, and the mineral selenium are **antioxidants**, preventing oxygen from combining with other substances that it may damage. During metabolism oxygen changes carbohydrates and fats into energy. In this process oxygen is transformed into stable forms of water and carbon dioxide. A small amount of oxygen, however, ends up in an unstable form, referred to as **oxygen-free radicals.**

A free radical molecule has a normal proton nucleus with a single unpaired electron. Having only one electron makes the free radical extremely reactive, and it constantly looks to pair the electron up with one from another molecule. When it steals the second electron from another molecule, that other molecule in turn becomes a free radical. This chain reaction goes on until two free radicals meet to form a stable molecule. Antioxidants help stabilize free radicals so they will not be as reactive until a match can be found. This action is illustrated in Figure 8.4.

Free radicals attack and damage proteins and lipids, in particular the cell membrane and DNA. This damage is thought to play a key role in the development of conditions such as heart disease, cancer, and emphysema.[6] Antioxidants are thought to offer protection by absorbing free radicals before they can cause damage and also by interrupting the sequence of reactions once damage has begun, thwarting certain chronic diseases.

Minerals

Minerals are the inorganic, indestructible substances found in all living cells. They are used in the metabolic process and help form enzymes, hormones, and other chemicals essential to metabolism. Some minerals resemble fat-soluble vitamins: They are not excreted easily by the body, are stored in body cells, and can become toxic if excessive. Other minerals resemble water-soluble vitamins: They don't accumulate in the tissues and are excreted easily by the body.

Of the approximately 31 nutritional minerals, 24 are considered essential for sustaining life. The nutritional minerals fall into two basic categories.

Dietary fiber   The part of the plant that is not digested in the small intestine and that provides the bulk needed to keep the digestive system running smoothly.

Soluble fiber   Fiber that dissolves in water, forming a thick, gel-like substance.

Insoluble fiber   Fiber that can't be dissolved in water or digested.

Vitamins   Nutrients that fuel the chemical reactions in the body and enable metabolism to take place.

Beta-carotene   A precursor to Vitamin A.

Antioxidants   Compounds that prevent oxygen from combining with other substances to which it may cause damage.

Oxygen-free radicals   Substances formed during metabolism which attack and damage proteins and lipids, in particular the cell membrane and DNA; leading to the development of diseases such as heart disease, cancer, and emphysema. Antioxidants are believed to exert a protective effect by absorbing free radicals before they can cause damage and also by interrupting the sequence of reactions once damage has begun.

Minerals   Inorganic substances found in all living cells.

TABLE 8.3 **Major Functions of Vitamins**

Nutrient	Good Sources	Major Functions	Deficiency Symptoms
Vitamin A	Milk, cheese, eggs, liver, and yellow/dark green fruits and vegetables	Required for healthy bones, teeth, skin, gums, and hair. Maintenance of inner mucous membranes, thus increasing resistance to infection. Adequate vision in dim light.	Night blindness, decreased growth, decreased resistance to infection, rough-dry skin.
Vitamin D	Fortified milk, cod liver oil, for salmon, tuna, egg yolk	Necessary for bones and teeth. Needed calcium and phosphorus absorption	Rickets (bone softening), fractures, and muscle spasms
Vitamin E	Vegetable oils, yellow and green leafy vegetables, margarine, wheat germ, whole grain breads and cereals	Related to oxidation and normal muscle and red blood cell chemistry	Leg cramps, red blood cell breakdown
Vitamin K	Green leafy vegetables, cauliflower, cabbage, eggs, peas, and potatoes	Essential for normal blood clotting	Hemorrhaging
Vitamin B$_1$ (Thiamine)	Whole grain or enriched bread, lean meats and poultry, organ fish, liver, pork, poultry, organ meats, legumes, nuts, and dried yeast	Assists in proper use of carbohydrates. Normal functioning of nervous system. Maintenance of good appetite.	Loss of appetite, nausea, confusion, cardiac abnormalities, muscle spasms
Vitamin B$_2$ (Riboflavin)	Eggs, milk, leafy green vegetables, whole grains, lean meats, dried beans and peas	Contributes to energy release from carbohydrates, fats, and proteins. Needed for normal growth and development, good vision, and healthy skin	Cracking of the corners of the mouth, inflammation of the skin, impaired vision.
Vitamin B$_6$ (Pyridoxine)	Vegetables, meats, whole grain cereals, soybeans, peanuts, and potatoes	Necessary for protein and fatty acids metabolism, and normal red blood cell formation	Depression, irritability, muscle spasms, nausea
Vitamin B$_{12}$	Meat, poultry, fish, liver, organ meats, eggs, shellfish, milk, and cheese	Required for normal growth, red blood cell formation, nervous system and digestive tract functioning	Impaired balance, weakness, drop in red blood cell count
Niacin	Liver and organ meats, meat, fish, poultry, whole grains, enriched breads, nuts, green leafy vegetables, and dried beans and peas	Contributes to energy release from carbohydrates, fats, and proteins. Normal growth and development, and formation of hormones and nerve-regulating substances	Confusion, depression, weakness, weight loss
Biotin	Liver, kidney, eggs, yeast, legumes, milk, nuts, dark green vegetables	Essential for carbohydrate metabolism and fatty acid synthesis	Inflamed skin, muscle pain, depression, weight loss
Folic Acid	Leafy green vegetables, organ meats, whole grains and cereals, and dried beans	Needed for cell growth and reproduction and red blood cell formation	Decreased resistance to infection
Pantothenic Acid	All natural foods, especially liver, kidney, eggs, nuts, yeast, milk, dried peas and beans, and green leafy vegetables	Related to carbohydrate and fat metabolism	Depression, low blood sugar, leg cramps, nausea, headaches
Vitamin C (Ascorbic Acid)	Fruits and vegetables	Helps protect against infection; formation of collagenous tissue. Normal blood vessels, teeth, and bones	Slow healing wounds, loose teeth, hemorrhaging, rough-scaly skin, irritability

Reprinted from *Principles & Labs for Physical Fitness & Wellness*. 2d Ed. Werner W. K. Hoeger, & Sharon Hoeger, Morton Publishing Co, 1994.

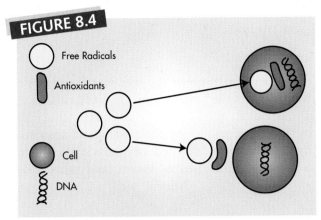

FIGURE 8.4

○ Free Radicals

▮ Antioxidants

● Cell

〰 DNA

Antioxidant protection from oxygen-free radicals.

moderate variety of foods. The one exception is calcium. According to the National Academy of Sciences, 80% of women over age 18 who were surveyed consumed too little calcium, a deficiency that may lead to osteoporosis later in life. The macrominerals, in order of importance to the human body, are calcium, phosphorus, potassium, sulfur, sodium, chloride, and magnesium.

2. **Trace minerals,** those the body needs in very small amounts; 14 are essential to good health. The most abundant, and probably the most important, are iron, zinc, and iodine. Table 8.4 lists selected minerals of both types, along with their sources and functions.

1. The **macrominerals,** or "major" minerals, those the body needs in relatively large amounts. These major minerals constitute as much as 80% of all inorganic material in the human body. Because they are found in so many different foods, deficiencies are not common if people eat even a

Macrominerals   7 minerals the body needs in relatively large amounts.

Trace minerals   14 minerals that the body needs in very small amounts.

TABLE 8.4   Major Functions of Minerals

Nutrient	Good Sources	Major Functions	Deficiency Symptoms
Calcium	Milk, yogurt, cheese, green leafy vegetables, dried beans, sardines, and salmon	Required for strong teeth and bone formation. Maintenance of good muscle tone, heart beat, and nerve function	Bone pain and fractures, periodontal disease, muscle cramps
Iron	Organ meats, lean meats, seafoods, eggs, dried peas and beans, nuts, whole and enriched grains, and green leafy vegetables	Major component of hemoglobin. Aids in energy utilization	Nutritional anemia, and overall weakness
Phosphorus	Meats, fish, milk, eggs, dried beans and peas, whole grains, and processed foods	Required for bone and teeth formation. Energy release regulation.	Bone pain and fracture, weight loss, and weakness
Zinc	Milk, meat, seafood, whole grains, nuts, eggs, and dried beans	Essential component of hormones, insulin, and enzymes. Used in normal growth and development	Loss of appetite, slow healing wounds, and skin problems
Magnesium	Green leafy vegetables, whole grains, nuts, soybeans, seafood, and legumes	Needed for bone growth and maintenance. Carbohydrate and protein utilization. Nerve function. Temperature regulation	Irregular heartbeat, weakness, muscle spasms, and sleeplessness
Sodium	Table salt, processed foods, and meat	Body fluid regulation. Transmission of nerve impulse. Heart action	Rarely seen
Potassium	Legumes, whole grains, bananas, orange juice, dried fruits, and potatoes	Heart action. Bone formation and maintenance. Regulation of energy release. Acid-base regulation	Irregular heartbeat, nausea, weakness
Selenium	Seafood, meat, whole grains	Component of enzyme; functions in close association with vitamin E	Muscle pain, possible heart muscle deterioration; possible hair and nail loss

Can Zinc Cure the Common Cold?

A study at the Cleveland Clinic Foundation, published in *Annals of Internal Medicine*, showed that high doses of zinc (in the form of zinc gluconate lozenges) reduced the duration of many cold symptoms by about 3 days. Of 100 cold-sufferers in the study, half took four to eight zinc gluconate lozenges daily, for a total of 52 to 104 milligrams of zinc a day. They experienced symptom relief in 4 days.

Source: University of California at Berkeley Wellness Letter, 13:2 (Nov. 1996), 1.

Three minerals are especially essential to health and sustaining life. These are calcium, iron, and sodium.

Calcium

Calcium helps regulate the heart, maintain proper fluid balance in the cells, transmit nerve impulses, and clot the blood. Among its other functions, calcium aids in the formation of bones, which is important to people of all ages. Healthy adults replace about one-fifth of their bone tissue every year. This means you need plenty of calcium to help your bones keep pace with what you lose each year. Women have smaller, less dense bones than men and are about eight times more likely to develop osteoporosis.

Bones respond to physical activity by becoming denser and stronger. If you walk a lot, for example, your leg bones will respond by developing more mass. If you use your arms regularly to lift weights or swing a tennis racket, the bones in your arms will grow stronger.

Iron

A deficiency of iron in the diet means too few red blood cells in the bloodstream. This can cause a condition called iron deficiency anemia, characterized by weakness, pallor, shortness of breath, susceptibility to infection, shortened attention span, impaired learning abilities, loss of vision, and other serious physical problems. Women who are menstruating run a particular risk of iron deficiency. As many as 15% of American women of childbearing age may have an iron deficiency because of blood lost during menstruation.

On the other hand, too much iron can cause infections, tissue damage, and severe liver damage, and it also may increase the risk for heart disease. Because the proper balance is so important, you should consult with your doctor before taking any iron

Tips For Action

To Make Sure You Get Enough Calcium:

- Drink plenty of milk. Most adults get about half their calcium from milk. One cup of milk — whether whole milk, 2%, 1%, or skim milk — provides 300 milligrams of calcium.

- Eat foods rich in vitamins A and D; they help your body absorb calcium. Primary sources are milk, broccoli, deep yellow-orange vegetables (carrots, squash, sweet potatoes), and eggs. Although dark leafy vegetables are good sources of vitamin A, they are not good sources of calcium. Many contain an acid that interferes with absorption of calcium.

- Include good nondairy sources of calcium in your diet, such as nuts (especially almonds and hazelnuts), seeds (especially sunflower and sesame), raisins, figs, dried apricots, oranges, soybeans, pinto beans, broccoli, and cauliflower.

- Avoid too much meat and other protein-rich foods as they make your body excrete calcium.

- Cut down on alcohol, caffeine, and phosphates (found in soda) because they leach calcium from the body.

- If you smoke, stop.

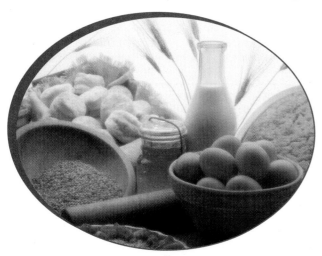

Dairy products are high in calcium, protein, and vitamins A and B$_{12}$; bread is a good source of carbohydrates.

supplement. To make sure your body utilizes the iron you get in your diet:

- Eat foods rich in vitamin C, along with iron-rich foods; vitamin C triples iron absorption.
- Use cast-iron cookware to prepare your food; the body readily uses the iron the food picks up.
- Avoid too much caffeine as it reduces the body's ability to absorb iron. Drink no more than three cups of tea or coffee a day.

Sodium

Sodium, commonly known as salt, is essential to life. Sodium regulates the blood and other body fluids, helps regulate heart activity, and helps transmit nerve impulses. According to the National Academy of Sciences, however, most Americans get as much as 10 times the amount they should. An adult who does not perspire heavily needs only about ¼ teaspoon of salt a day. An estimated 5% to 10% of all people are sensitive to sodium; their blood pressure rises, increasing the risk for stroke, kidney disease and heart disease.

> **An adult who does not perspire heavily needs only about ¼ teaspoon of salt a day.**

Sodium is added to almost all processed foods, and fast-food restaurants add vast amounts of sodium to hamburgers, French fries, and even milk shakes. One fast-food meal of a quarter-pound cheeseburger, fries, and a chocolate shake provides almost 1000 mg more sodium than you should have in an entire day. A single apple pie from McDonald's contains more than 1,000 mg of sodium, twice as much as you need all day. Common condiments, such as ketchup, mustard, barbecue sauce, soy sauce, and MSG, also are significant sources of sodium. You can overload on sodium even if you take certain medications, such as antacids.

Water

Next to air, water is the element most necessary for human survival. You could survive much longer without food than you could without water. Water is the major component of blood, which carries oxygen

Tips For Reducing Salt in Your Diet

About a third of the salt in your diet comes from natural, unprocessed foods you eat. That's probably all you need. The rest comes from processed foods and the salt shaker, which you can safely eliminate. Try these tips:

- Taste food before you salt it. You might even try taking the salt shaker off the table.
- Cut back on the salt you use when cooking. Try other spices instead.
- Avoid salty processed foods, such as bacon, lunch meats, sausage, and ham.
- Remember that "hidden" salt in processed foods — gelatin, instant potatoes, American cheese, and canned fish — are some of the worst offenders.
- Learn to read labels. You should be getting 1100 to 3300 mg of sodium a day, and you can get all, if not most, in unprocessed fruits, vegetables, and meats.

and nutrients to all cells in the body. It helps your body use the other nutrients in your diet, aids your body in getting rid of wastes, helps you digest foods, carries oxygen and nutrients throughout the body, maintains the proper electrolyte balance in the body, lubricates joints, and regulates body temperature — to name just a few functions.

Approximately 60% of your body is made up of water. Some of the denser tissues, such as bones, have less — approximately 20% for bones. Others have more — 75% for brain tissue, for example.

You get some water from the foods you eat. Fruits, for example, are as much as 80% water. Especially good choices are melons and apples. Even foods you don't typically think of as containing much water, such as bread and meat, can be anywhere from 33% to 50% water. In addition to the foods you eat, you should drink eight to ten 8-ounce glasses of water a day — more if you are large,

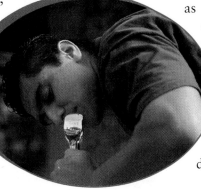
Water is necessary for survival.

physically active, live in a hot climate, or perspire a lot.

You can't always rely on thirst to indicate a water deficit, according to Dr. Barbara Rolls of Johns Hopkins University School of Medicine. A rough indicator is your urine. If it is dark amber color or has a strong odor, you are not drinking enough water. Passing a full bladder of colorless or pale yellow urine at least four times a day means you're getting enough water. In addition to drinking plenty of water:

- Avoid caffeine. It increases the body's need for water while it increases the amount of water the body puts out.

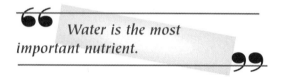

> *Water is the most important nutrient.*

- Avoid alcohol. You need 8 ounces of water to metabolize a single ounce of alcohol.
- Cut down on the amount of sugar you eat. It increases your body's need for water.
- Cut back on protein to a healthy level. The wastes produced from proteins build up in the

kidneys, and you need extra water to flush them out.

- Drink a steady amount of water throughout the day to keep your body well supplied.

FOOD GUIDE PYRAMID

Most Americans eat to much protein, far too much sugar, and too many fats, especially saturated fats. According to the U.S. Senate select committee that issued the original set of dietary goals, the recommended changes are as shown in Figure 8.5, the **Food Guide Pyramid**.

The pyramid conveys three essential elements of a healthy diet:

- *Proportion.* Eat different amounts every day from the basic food groups. The shape of the pyramid tells you at a glance that grains, vegetables, and fruits should make up the bulk of your diet.

Food Guide Pyramid A configuration of daily food choices that stresses the proportion of foods needed for a healthy diet; developed by the U.S. Department of Agriculture.

FIGURE 8.5

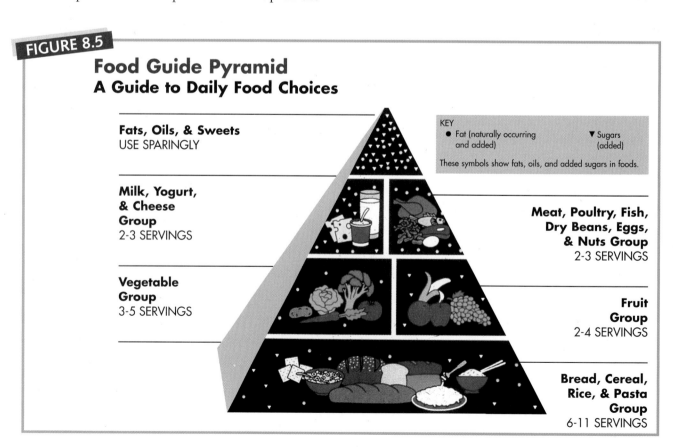

Food Guide Pyramid
A Guide to Daily Food Choices

Fats, Oils, & Sweets
USE SPARINGLY

Milk, Yogurt, & Cheese Group
2-3 SERVINGS

Vegetable Group
3-5 SERVINGS

KEY
● Fat (naturally occurring and added)   ▼ Sugars (added)
These symbols show fats, oils, and added sugars in foods.

Meat, Poultry, Fish, Dry Beans, Eggs, & Nuts Group
2-3 SERVINGS

Fruit Group
2-4 SERVINGS

Bread, Cereal, Rice, & Pasta Group
6-11 SERVINGS

Setting Your Dietary Priorities

More than 300 top nutrition experts in a poll conducted by Medical Consensus Surveys, a research arm of *Prevention* Magazine, were asked to rate 44 nutritional actions (all purported to benefit health) as follows: extremely important, very important, important, not important but may help, or probably worthless. The nutritionists' responses then were compiled and statistically weighted to create a list of dietary "top priorities" for preserving and boosting your health.

Priority/ Ranking	Action
Very High Priority	
79	Control calorie intake to control your weight
76	Reduce all dietary fats
75	Control fat intake to control your weight
High Priority	
71	Increase physical activity to enable greater nutrient intake
71	Enjoy your food
70	Balance your diet among the five food groups
69	Ensure adequate intake of vitamins and minerals to meet the RDAs
65	Replace saturated fats with monosaturated and polysaturated fats
65	If not pregnant or trying to conceive, limit your alcohol intake to one or two drinks per day
63	Replace whole-milk products with low-fat and nonfat dairy products
63	Avoid raw eggs, raw meat, and raw seafood
62	Increase total fiber to at least 20 grams per day
62	Eat more complex carbohydrates, such as grains, rice, beans, potatoes, bread, and pasta
61	Eat more fish in place of meat
59	Ensure adequate intake of soluble fiber
57	Avoid very low calorie diets
56	Cut meat portions to 3 to 4 ounces
55	Reduce dietary cholesterol
54	Ensure adequate intake of insoluble fiber
54	Eat at least five fruits and vegetables per day
54	Eat breakfast
51	Reduce sodium intake
Moderate Priority	
49	Increase intake of cruciferous vegetables, such as broccoli, cauliflower, kale, and others
49	Avoid eating large meals and snacking excessively in the evening when activity levels tend to be low

Priority/ Ranking	Action
48	Switch from butter to margarine
48	Restrict intake of tropical oils
47	Drink six to eight 8-ounce glasses of water (or decaffeinated, low-calorie, and low-fat fluids) every day
47	Avoid nitrates and nitrites (smoked and cured foods)
44	Reduce trans-fatty acids (e.g., stick margarine, hydrogenated vegetable shortening)
43	Reduce sugar intake
41	Eat three square meals a day with a minimum of snacking in between
41	Eat only when you're hungry (regardless of whether it's mealtime or not) and only to satiety
40	Limit your daily caffeine consumption to the amount in 4 cups of coffee
38	Peel or wash fruit before eating to avoid pesticides
37	Increase beta-carotene intake
37	Switch from stick margarine to soft (tub) and liquid margarine
37	Have a regular nutritional assessment
30	Eliminate alcohol from your diet
29	Restrict your intake of phosphorus
Low Priority	
24	Increase intake of vitamin E beyond the RDA without exceeding safe limits
23	Increase intake of vitamin C beyond the RDA without exceeding safe limits
16	Make breakfast the biggest meal of the day
14	Avoid irradiated foods
13	Avoid overgrilled (i.e., charred) or blackened foods

Note: The numbers in the left column represent the relative importance of each positive action, based on a scale of 0 (not important) to 100 (extremely important).

From *Using Foods Wisely.*

Legumes

Legumes contain protein in amounts comparable to other protein-rich foods, and they also are a source of fiber with virtually no fat — healthful qualities that none of the other foods in the meat group have. It doesn't matter where legumes are grouped — with meats or with fruits and vegetables. Just remember to eat them.

- *Moderation.* Use fats and sugars sparingly.
- *Variety.* Choose different foods from each major food group every day. The pyramid doesn't claim that any food is better or worse than another.

Issued by the U.S. Department of Agriculture (USDA), the Food Guide Pyramid replaces the once-standard "basic four food groups" as a nutritional guide. The widest level of the pyramid, at the bottom, indicates the foods you should eat the most of. The top level, indicates the foods you should eat the least of.

What's One Serving?

	Official One Serving
Bagel	2 oz.
Cinnamon roll	2 oz.
Chips	1 oz.
Cookies	1 oz. (small)
French fries	3 oz.
Ice cream	1 scoop
Meat/Chicken/Fish	2 to 3 oz.
Milkshake	8 oz.
Muffins	2 oz.
Pancakes	2 to 3 medium
Pizza	1 or 2 slices
Popcorn	2 to 3 cups
Salad dressing	2 Tbsp.
Soft drinks	8 oz.
Pasta with tomato sauce	1/2 to 1 cup

Source: U.S. Department of Agriculture.

Level 1: Complex Carbohydrates

At the base of the pyramid are the complex carbohydrates: grains, cereals, pastas, and breads. It is recommended that 60% of your daily calorie intake, or 6 to 11 servings a day, come from foods in this group. Within this group, you should focus on whole-grain foods that are lowest in fat and eat refined foods from this group (white bread, white rice, refined cereals) in moderation.

Trying to get as many as 11 servings a day of complex carbohydrates may seem overwhelming until you figure out what the USDA considers to be a *serving*. Some examples of a single serving from the grains, cereals, pastas, and breads group are

- ½ cup of cooked rice
- ½ cup of cooked cereal, or 1 ounce of dry cereal (about one-fourth of a bowl)
- 1 pancake
- 3 pretzels or 6 snack crackers
- 1 tortilla
- ½ of a hamburger bun

Level 2: Vegetables and Fruits

Most vegetables and fruits are naturally low in calories and rich in nutrients. You should eat three to five servings of vegetables a day. A serving of vegetables is considered to be ½ cup of chopped fresh, frozen, or canned vegetables; ¼ cup of dried vegetables; 1 cup of raw leafy vegetables; or ¾ cup of vegetable juice (fresh, frozen, or canned). To save the nutrients in vegetables, they should not be cooked in water or overcooked. Baking, steaming, and microwaving vegetables best preserves the nutrients. Eating them raw, when possible, is best. Eating well-scrubbed skins boosts fiber in the diet, as does eating the skins and edible seeds of fruits (such as those in strawberries, raspberries, and pomegranates).

The USDA recommends at least two to four servings of fresh fruits or fruit juices each day. A serving is considered to be 1 whole fresh fruit (such as a medium banana or medium apple); ½ cup of raw, cooked, or canned fruit; ¼ cup of dried fruit; or ¾ cup of fruit juice (fresh, frozen, or canned).

The best choices are fruits and vegetables that do not have added fat or sodium. For example, raw or cooked cabbage is a good choice, whereas cole slaw made from cabbage and a creamy dressing is not as good. A raw cucumber sliced in a salad is better than pickles (because of the high sodium content).

Level 3: Protein and Dairy

You need fewer servings of protein and dairy, so they fall nearer the top of the pyramid. The USDA recommends two to three servings a day of proteins. The best sources are low in fat: fish, skinless poultry, lean cuts of meat, dried beans, and dried peas, for example.

The key with foods at this level is to serve smaller portions than you probably are accustomed to. A single serving of cooked protein is only 2 to 3 ounces, or about the size of a deck of playing cards.

Quiz

Answer the following questions True or False.

	T	F	
1.	☐	☐	Water is an essential liquid.
2.	☐	☐	Cholesterol is found in egg whites.
3.	☐	☐	All carbohydrates give you energy.
4.	☐	☐	A green salad is always a good low-calorie menu choice.
5.	☐	☐	Women need more calcium and iron than men.

Answers:

1. **TRUE.** Water performs many important functions in the body and we need to drink it daily.

2. **FALSE.** Egg white is almost all protein, while the yolk, or yellow part of an egg, contains about 213 milligrams of cholesterol.

3. **TRUE.** However, simple carbohydrates, like sugar, give you empty calories (no nutritional value). Complex carbohydrates, found in vegetables dried beans and peas, fruits and grains burn slowly and provide energy over a longer period of time. They are high in vitamins, minerals and fiber and low in calories and fat.

4. **TRUE.** A tossed green salad with a selection of vegetables, is a great low-fat nutrition choice. Avoid creamy or oily dressings. Mayonnaise-based salads like potato, chicken, and macaroni are high in calories and fat.

5. **TRUE.** Women lose iron during their monthly menstrual cycles. Women's bones are less dense than men's and as they age, they lose calcium from their bones at a faster rate.

The following non-meat proteins can substitute for 1 ounce of meat:

- 3 ounces of tofu
- 1 egg
- 2 tablespoons of peanut butter
- ½ cup of dried beans or peas, cooked
- ¼ cup nuts

Adults need two servings of dairy products daily. Teenagers and pregnant or breast-feeding women need three servings. Pregnant or breast-feeding teens need four servings. Again, the best of these are low in fat, such as lowfat or skim milk, 1% cottage cheese, and part-skim cheeses (such as ricotta and mozzarella).

A single serving of dairy food consists of 1 cup of milk, 1 cup of yogurt, 2 ounces of processed cheese, 1½ ounces of natural cheese, ½ cup of cottage cheese, or 1½ cups of ice cream or frozen yogurt.

Level 4: Fats and Sugars

The foods at the tip of the pyramid — fats, oils, and sweets — should be eaten sparingly. No recommended servings are given. A diet with too much saturated fat can increase the risk of heart disease. Sugars are high in calories but have no nutritional value. Eating too many sweets fills you up without providing the nutrients you need for a balanced diet.

ENERGY (ATP) PRODUCTION

The energy derived from food is not used directly by the cells. It is transformed into an energy-rich compound called **adenosine triphosphate (ATP)**. The subsequent breakdown of this compound provides the energy used by all energy-requiring processes of the body. ATP must be recycled continually to sustain life and work. It can be resynthesized in three ways:

1. *ATP and ATP-CP system.* The body stores small amounts of ATP and creatine phosphate (CP). These stores are used during all-out activities up to 10 seconds in duration, such as sprinting, long jumping, and weight lifting. The amount of

Adenosine triphosphate (ATP) An energy-rich compound formed by the energy derived from food, in a form the body's cells can use.

stored ATP provides energy for just a few seconds. With all-out efforts, ATP is resynthesized from CP, another high-energy phosphate compound. This is referred to as the ATP-CP or phosphagen system.

Depending on the amount of physical training, the concentration of CP stored in cells is sufficient to allow maximal exertion for up to 10 seconds. Once the CP stores are depleted, the person is forced to slow down or rest to allow ATP to form through anaerobic and aerobic pathways.

2. *Anaerobic or lactic acid system.* During high-intensity (anaerobic) exercise that is sustained between 10 and 180 seconds maximum, ATP is replenished from the breakdown of glucose through a series of chemical reactions that do not require oxygen. In the process, though, lactic acid is produced, which causes muscular fatigue.

Because of the accumulation of lactic acid with high-intensity exercise, the formation of ATP is limited to about 3 minutes. A recovery period then is necessary to allow for the elimination of lactic acid. Formation of ATP through the anaerobic system is possible from glucose (carbohydrates) only.

3. *Aerobic system.* The production of energy during slow-sustained exercise is derived primarily through aerobic metabolism. Both glucose (carbohydrates) and fatty acids (fat) are used in this process. Oxygen is required to form ATP, and under steady-state exercise conditions, lactic acid accumulation is minimal.

Because oxygen is required, a person's capacity to utilize oxygen (maximal oxygen uptake, or VO_{2max} (see Chapter 6) is critical for successful athletic performance in aerobic events. The higher the VO_{2max}, the greater is the capacity to generate ATP through the aerobic system.

DIETARY GUIDELINES FOR NORTH AMERICANS

Based on the available scientific research on nutrition and health and the current dietary habits of the American people, in 1995 the Scientific Committee of the U. S. Department of Health and Human Services and the U.S. Department of Agriculture on diet and health issued the fourth edition of the Dietary Guidelines for healthy American adults and children.

These guidelines potentially can reduce the risk of developing certain chronic diseases. The committee's recommendations are:

- Eat a variety of food. No single food can provide all of the necessary nutrients and other beneficial substances in the amounts the body needs. For good nutrition, you should meet the recommended number of daily servings from each of the five food groups in the Food Guide Pyramid. Within each food group, choose a variety of foods. Food items vary, and each item provides different combinations of nutrients and other substances needed for good health.

- Balance the food you eat with physical activity to maintain or improve your weight. Excessive body weight increases the risk for diseases including heart disease, stroke, diabetes, high blood pressure, and certain cancers. Many people gain weight as adults, and this does not have to be the case. To maintain body weight, you need to balance food intake with the amount of calories the body uses. In ensuing chapters you will find extensive information on weight management and exercise programs to help you balance your energy requirements according to your personal needs.

- Choose a diet with plenty of grain products, vegetables, and fruits. Most of your daily calories should come from these food products. They contain ample amounts of vitamins, minerals, complex carbohydrates, and other substances important for good health.

- Choose a diet low in fat, saturated fat, and cholesterol. Reduce fat intake to 30% or less of total calories. Reduce saturated fatty acid intake to less than 10% of total calories and intake of cholesterol to no more than 300 mg daily. Intake of fat and cholesterol can be lowered by substituting fish, poultry without skin, lean meats, and low or nonfat dairy products for fatty meats and whole-milk dairy products; by choosing more vegetables, fruits, cereals, and legumes; and by limiting oils, fats, egg yolks, and fried and other fatty foods.

- Choose a diet moderate in sugars. Excessive sugar and starch intake can contribute to weight gain and tooth decay. This guideline advises against frequent and large consumption of food items and snacks high in sugar that provide unnecessary calories and few nutrients. The more often that high-sugar foods are consumed, and the longer before brushing the teeth following their consumption, the greater is the risk for tooth decay.

■ Choose a diet moderate in salt and sodium. Limit total daily intake of salt (sodium chloride) to 6 grams or less. This amount represents the equivalent of 2,400 mg of sodium listed in the Daily Value of the Nutrition Label. To decrease your daily sodium intake, limit the use of salt in cooking and do not add it to food at the table. Sparingly consume salty, highly processed, salt-preserved, and salt-pickled foods.

Foods from a wide variety of sources are necessary for a well-balanced diet.

■ If you drink alcoholic beverages, do so in moderation. Alcoholic beverages provide calories but few or no nutrients. Moderate drinking has been linked to a decreased risk for coronary heart disease in some people. High levels of alcohol consumption lead to an increased risk for heart disease, stroke, high blood pressure, certain cancers, cirrhosis of the liver, inflammation of the pancreas, brain damage, birth defects, accidents, violence, suicides, and malnutrition. Limit consumption to the equivalent of less than an ounce of pure alcohol in a single day. This translates into two cans of beer, two small glasses of wine, or two average cocktails. If pregnant, avoid alcoholic beverages altogether.

DAILY VALUES AND FOOD LABELS

Every ten years or so, the National Academy of Sciences issues a new Recommended Dietary Allowance, known simply as the **RDA**, based on a review of the most current research on nutrient needs for healthy people. The RDA provides daily nutrient intake recommendations, set high enough to encompass 97.5% of the healthy population in the United States. Stated another way, the RDA recommendation for any nutrient is well above almost everyone's actual requirement.

Between the late 1960s and the early 1990s, nutrient information on labels was expressed in terms of the U.S. RDA — a set of standard values for the average consumer — derived from the 1968 edition of the RDA. In 1993, the Food and Drug Administration revised food labeling regulations and has replaced the U.S. RDA with *% Daily Values*, based on a 2,000 calorie diet. These require adjustments by the individual depending on daily caloric needs.

In setting the **Daily Values**, the FDA first created two sets of standards: **Reference Daily Intakes (RDI)** and Daily Reference Values (DRV). For FDA purposes, these two sets of standards serve different functions. To avoid consumer confusion in food labeling, however, the FDA combined the RDI and DRV into the Daily Values.

Both the RDA and the Daily Values apply only to healthy people. They are not intended for people who are ill and may require additional nutrients.

Using the food label (Figure 8.6) can help you make healthful food choices. By law, the FDA requires that all the nutrients in a food must be listed on the label *in language the consumer can understand*. By law, every food label also must include the following:

■ The common name of the product.

■ The name and address of the manufacturer, distributor, or packer.

■ The net contents of the package (count, measure, or weight).

■ The ingredients listed in descending order, with the most prominent ingredient listed first.

If the product makes any *nutritional claims*, the law requires that certain nutritional information be listed on the label. By law, the following must be listed under the heading of "Nutritional Information":

■ Serving or portion size.

RDA   Daily nutrient intake recommendations for healthy people issued by the National Academy of Sciences.

Daily Values   Standard nutrition values developed by the Food and Drug Administration (FDA) for use on food labels.

RDI — Reference Daily Intakes — The reference values for protein, vitamins, and minerals.

FIGURE 8.6

Nutrition Facts Title

The new title "Nutrition Facts" signals the new label.

Serving Size

Similar food products now have similar serving sizes. This makes it easier to compare foods. Serving sizes are based on amounts people actually eat.

New Label Information

Some label information may be new to you. The new nutrient list covers those most important to your health. You may have seen this information on some old labels, but it is now required.

Vitamins and Minerals

Only two vitamins, A and C, and two minerals, calcium and iron, are required on the food label. A food company can voluntarily list other vitamins and minerals in the food.

Label Numbers

Numbers on the nutrition label may be rounded for labeling.

Nutrition Facts

Serving Size 1 cup (228g)
Servings Per Container 2

Amount Per Serving

Calories 90   Calories from Fat 30

	% Daily Value*
Total Fat 3g	**5%**
Saturated Fat 0g	**0%**
Cholesterol 0mg	**0%**
Sodium 300mg	**13%**
Total Carbohydrate 13g	**4%**
Dietary Fiber 3g	**12%**
Sugars 3g	
Protein 3g	

Vitamin A	80%	•	Vitamin C	60%
Calcium	4%	•	Iron	4%

*% Daily Values are based on a 2000 calorie diet. Your daily values may be higher or lower depending on your calorie needs:

	Calories	2000	2500
Total Fat	Less than	65g	80g
Sat Fat	Less than	20g	25g
Cholesterol	Less than	300mg	300mg
Sodium	Less than	2400mg	2400mg
Total Carbohydrate		300g	375g
Dietary Fiber		25g	30g

Calories per gram:
Fat 9 • Carbohydrates 4 • Protein 4

Foods that have only a few of the nutrients required on the standard label can use a short label format. What's on the label depends on what's in the food. Small- and medium-sized packages with very little label space also can use a short label.

% Daily Value

% Daily Value shows how a food fits into a 2000-calorie reference diet.

You can use % Daily Value to compare foods and see how the amount of a nutrient in a serving of food fits in a 2000-calorie reference diet.

Daily Values Footnote

Daily Values are the new label reference numbers. These numbers are set by the government and are based on current nutrition recommendations.

Some labels list the daily values for a daily diet of 2000 and 2500 calories. Your own nutrient needs may be less than or more than the Daily Values on the label.

Calories Per Gram Footnote

Some labels tell the approximate number of calories in a gram of fat, carbohydrate, and protein.

Some food packages make claims such as "light," "low fat," and "cholesterol free." These claims can be used only if a food meets strict government definitions. Here are some of the meanings.

Label claim	**Definition***
Calorie-Free	Less than 5 calories
Light or Lite	1/3 fewer calories or 50% less fat; if more than half the calories are from fat, fat content must be reduced by 50% or more
Light in Sodium	50% less sodium
Fat-Free	Less than 1/2 gram fat
Low-Fat	3 grams or less fat**
Cholesterol-Free	Less than 2 milligrams cholesterol and 2 grams or less saturated fat**
Low Cholesterol	20 milligrams or less cholesterol and 2 grams or less saturated fat**
Sodium-Free	Less than 5 milligrams sodium**
Very Low Sodium	35 milligrams or less sodium**
Low-Sodium	140 milligrams or less sodium**
High Fiber	5 grams or more fiber

*Per Reference Amount (standard serving size). Some claims have higher nutrient levels for main dish products and meal products, such as frozen entrees and dinners.

**Also per 50 g for products with small serving sizes (reference amount is 30 g or less or 2 tbsp or less).

Some food packages may now carry health claims. A health claim is a label statement that describes the relationship between a nutrient and a disease or health-related condition. A food must meet certain nutrient levels to make a health claim. Seven types of health claims are allowed. These nutrient-disease relationships include:

A diet:	**And:**
High in calcium	Osteoporosis (brittle bone disease)
High in fiber-containing grain products, fruits, and vegetables	Cancer
High in fruits or vegetables (high in dietary fiber or vitamins A or C)	Cancer
High in fiber from fruits, vegetables, and grain products	Heart disease
Low in fat	Cancer
Low in saturated fat and cholesterol	Heart disease
Low in sodium	High blood pressure

Information on new food label.

■ Servings per container.

■ Calories per serving.

■ Carbohydrates (in grams) per serving.

■ Fats (in grams) per serving.

■ Vitamins, minerals, and proteins (as percentages of the RDA) per serving.

■ The Amount of eight "indicator nutrients" — protein, vitamin A, niacin, thiamin, riboflavin, vitamin C, calcium, and iron.

NUTRIENT SUPPLEMENTATION

According to the U.S. Food and Drug Administration, four of every 10 adults in the United States take nutrient supplements daily, and one in every seven has a nutrient intake almost eight times the RDA. In reality, vitamin and mineral requirements for the body can be met by consuming as few as 1,200 calories per day, as long as the diet contains the recommended servings from the five food groups.

Water-soluble vitamins cannot be stored as long as fat-soluble vitamins. The body readily excretes excessive intakes. Small amounts, however, can be retained for weeks or months in various organs and tissues of the body. Fat-soluble vitamins, on the other hand, are stored in fatty tissue. Therefore, daily intake of these vitamins is not as crucial. Too much vitamin A and vitamin D actually can be detrimental to health.

People should not take megadoses of vitamins. For most vitamins, a megadose is 10 times the RDA or more. For vitamins A and D, it is respectively five and two times the RDA. Mineral doses should not exceed three times the RDA.

No standard percentage above the RDA has been suggested to guide us in determining the level at which a high dose of a given nutrient may cause health problems. For some nutrients, a dose of five times the RDA taken over several months may create problems. For others, it may not pose any threat to human health.

Iron supplementation frequently is recommended for women who have heavy menstrual flow. Some pregnant and lactating women also may require supplements. According to 1990 guidelines by the National Academy of Science, the average pregnant woman who eats an adequate amount of a variety of foods needs to take only a low dose of iron supplement daily. Women who are pregnant with more than one baby may need additional supplements. In all of the above instances, supplements should be taken under a physician's supervision.

Others who may benefit from supplementation are alcoholics and street-drug users who do not have a balanced diet, smokers, strict vegetarians, individuals on extremely low-calorie diets, elderly people who don't eat balanced meals regularly, and newborn infants (usually given a single dose of vitamin K to prevent abnormal bleeding).

For healthy people with a balanced diet, most supplements do not seem to provide additional benefits. They do not help people run faster, jump higher, relieve stress, improve sexual prowess, cure a common cold, or boost energy levels.

Many people who regularly eat fast foods high in fat content or too many sweets think they need vitamin and mineral supplementation to balance their diet. The problem in these cases is not a lack of vitamins and minerals but, instead, a diet too high in calories, fat, and sodium. Supplementation will not offset these poor eating habits.

If you think your diet is not balanced, you first need to determine which nutrients are missing, consulting the Healthy Eating Pyramid and the vitamin and mineral tables in this chapter, then eat more of the foods high in the nutrients deficient in your diet. Nutritional needs do change over the years, too. An adult whose active growth has stopped requires fewer calories than infants, children, or adolescents who are still growing. The rapid growth rate that occurs during the first 12 years and again during various periods of adolescence requires increased calories and nutrients. Except for pregnant women and nursing mothers, adults require progressively fewer calories as they age — but they still have the same nutritional needs. Low-fat foods that are rich in vitamins and minerals are good choices for these adults.

FOOD ADDITIVES

Food additives are chemical agents added to processed foods to help preserve them or to change their appearance (usually color) or enhance their flavor. During the last several decades, considerable controversy arose over the use of artificial colorings after tests on animals showed some to them may cause cancer. Some artificial coloring agents were banned from the market, then reintroduced after inconclusive testing. Even without the risk of cancer, excessive artificial colorings should be avoided, as

Recommended Dietary Allowances*

Category	Age	Weight[b] (lb)	Height[b] (in)	Protein (g)	Vitamin A (mcg RE)[c]	Vitamin D (mcg)[d]	Vitamin E (mg a-TE)[e]	Vitamin K (mcg)	Vitamin C (mg)	Thiamine (mg)
Infants	0-6 months	13	24	13	375	7.5	3	5	30	0.3
	6-12 months	20	28	14	375	10	4	10	35	0.4
Children	1-3	29	35	16	400	10	6	15	40	0.7
	4-6	44	44	24	500	10	7	20	45	0.9
	7-10	62	52	28	700	10	7	30	45	1.0
Males	11-14	99	62	45	1000	10	10	45	50	1.3
	15-18	145	69	59	1000	10	10	65	60	1.5
	19-24	160	70	58	1000	10	10	70	60	1.5
	25-50	174	70	63	1000	5	10	80	60	1.5
	51 plus	170	68	63	1000	5	10	80	60	1.2
Females	11-14	101	62	46	800	10	8	45	50	1.1
	15-18	120	64	44	800	10	8	55	60	1.1
	19-24	128	65	46	800	10	8	60	60	1.1
	25-50	138	64	50	800	5	8	65	60	1.1
	51 plus	143	63	50	800	5	8	65	60	1.0
Pregnant women				60	800	10	10	65	70	1.5
Lactating women	1st 6 months			65	1300	10	12	65	95	1.6
	2nd 6 months			62	1200	10	11	65	90	1.6

[a] The allowances, expressed as average daily intakes over time, are intended to provide for individual variations among most normal persons as they live in the United States under usual environmental stresses. Diets should be based on a variety of common foods in order to provide other nutrients for which human requirements have been less well defined.

[b] Weights and heights of Reference Adults are actual medians for the U.S. population of the designated age. The use of these figures does not imply that the height-to-weight ratios are ideal.

[c] Retinol equivalents. 1 retinol equivalent = 1 mcg retinol or 6 mcg beta carotene. To calculate IU value: for fruits and vegetables, multiply the RE value by ten; for animal-source foods, multiply the RE value by 3.3.

Other Recommended Intakes

The following nutrients have no RDA or Estimated Safe and Adequate Daily Dietary Intake. Instead the daily recommendations listed below are based on guidelines established by various health organizations and experts.

Beta Carotene	5 to 6 milligrams
Cholesterol	no more than 300 milligrams
Dietary Fiber	20 to 30 grams
Potassium	3000 milligrams
Sodium	no more than 2400 milligrams

Ribo-flavin (mg)	Niacin (mg NE)[f]	Vita-min B_6 (mg)	Folate[g] (mcg)	Vita-min B_{12} (mcg)	Cal-cium (mg)	Phos-phorus (mg)	Mag-nesium (mg)	Iron (mg)	Zinc (mg)	Iodine (mcg)	Selen-ium (mcg)
0.4	5	0.3	25	0.3	400	300	40	6	5	40	10
0.5	6	0.6	35	0.5	600	500	60	10	5	50	15
0.8	9	1.0	50	0.7	800	800	80	10	10	70	20
1.1	12	1.1	75	1.0	800	800	120	10	10	90	20
1.2	13	1.4	100	1.4	800	800	170	10	10	120	30
1.5	17	1.7	150	2.0	1200	1200	270	12	15	150	40
1.8	20	2.0	200	2.0	1200	1200	400	12	15	150	50
1.7	19	2.0	200	2.0	1200	1200	350	10	15	150	70
1.7	19	2.0	200	2.0	800	800	350	10	15	150	70
1.4	15	2.0	200	2.0	800	800	350	10	15	150	70
1.3	15	1.4	150	2.0	1200	1200	280	15	12	150	45
1.3	15	1.5	180	2.0	1200	1200	300	15	12	150	50
1.3	15	1.6	180	2.0	1200	1200	280	15	12	150	55
1.3	15	1.6	180	2.0	800	800	280	15	12	150	55
1.2	13	1.6	180	2.0	800	800	280	10	12	150	55
1.6	17	2.2	400	2.2	1200	1200	320	30	15	175	65
1.8	20	2.1	280	2.6	1200	1200	355	15	19	200	75
1.7	20	2.1	260	2.6	1200	1200	340	15	16	200	75

[d] As cholecalciferol. 10 mcg cholecalciferol = 400 IU of vitamin D.

[e] α-tocopherol equivalents. 1 mg d-α tocopherol = 1 α-TE.

[f] t NE (niacin equivalent) is equal to 1 mg of niacin or 60 mg of dietary tryptophan.

[g] Felacin

Estimated Safe and Adequate Daily Dietary Intakes of Selected Vitamins and Minerals[a]

Category	Age	Vitamins		Trace Minerals[b]				
		Biotin (mcg)	Pantho-thenic acid (mg)	Copper (mg)	Man-ganese (mg)	Fluoride (mg)	Chro-mium (mcg)	Molyb-denum (mcg)
Infants	0-6 months	10	2	0.4-0.6	0.3-0.6	0.1-0.5	10-40	15-30
	6-12 months	15	3	0.6-0.7	0.6-1.0	0.2-1.0	20-60	20-40
Children and adolescents	1-3	20	3	0.7-1.0	1.0-1.5	0.5-1.5	20-80	25-50
	4-6	25	3-4	1.0-1.5	1.5-2.0	1.0-2.5	30-120	30-75
	7-10	30	4-5	1.0-2.0	2.0-3.0	1.5-2.5	50-200	50-150
	11 plus	30-100	4-7	1.5-2.5	2.0-5.0	1.5-2.5	50-200	75-250
Adults		30-100	4-7	1.5-3.0	2.0-5.0	1.5-4.0	50-200	75-250

[a] Because there is less information on which to base allowances, these figures are not given in the main table of RDAs and are provided here in the form of ranges of recommended intakes.

[b] Since the toxic levels for many trace elements may be only several times usual intakes, the upper levels for the trace elements given in this table should not be habitually exceeded.

some people have sensitivities to them. Most artificial colorings — in red, yellow, blue, and green — are used to color beverages, candy, gelatin mixes, and baked goods.

In addition to artificial colorings food additives fall into the general categories of antioxidants, emulsifiers, flavorings, preservatives, and sweeteners.

- *Antioxidants.* Antioxidants, such as BA and BHT, are synthetic chemicals used to keep oils and fats from becoming rancid. They often are added to vegetable oils, potato chips, soup base, cereals, meat products, chewing gum, granola, and other foods that contain oils, fats, or nuts. The residue of some antioxidants can be found in body fat, causing concern about these additives.

- *Emulsifiers.* Emulsifiers, such as BIO, are agents used to give a cloudy appearance to citrus-flavored soft drinks. They suspend the flavor oils throughout the drink, improving both flavor and appearance. BIO residues also have been found in body fat.

- *Flavorings.* A number of artificial agents are used in processed foods to enhance flavor. Some — such as sodium nitrate, used in corned beef and bacon as well as other red meats — also are used as coloring agents or preservatives.

- *Preservatives.* Preservatives inhibit bacterial growth, giving processed foods a longer shelf life. Sulfur dioxide and sodium bisulfite — two preservatives that also prevent discoloration in foods such as processed potatoes and dried fruits — have been known to cause severe allergic reactions and are responsible for at least seven deaths.

IRRADIATION

In an attempt to improve the quality of food, some manufacturers have started using **irradiation** to treat both fresh and processed foods. Essentially, foods are exposed to gamma radiation, which lengthens the shelf life of the product and destroys any microorganisms that might have contaminated the food. The FDA has approved irradiation for the following foods.

- Pork (to kill trichinosis, a parasitic worm that infects pork).
- Poultry (to kill salmonella bacteria, which infects a fourth of the nation's chickens).

- Some kinds of seafood (to kill salmonella bacteria and other contaminants).
- Fresh produce and other perishable foods (to lengthen shelf life and reduce waste. Ironically, some fresh produce — such as apples and pears — actually spoil more rapidly *after* irradiation.

The process of irradiation does not make food radioactive. Nevertheless, it does alter the molecular structure of food, resulting in oxygen-free radicals, which may cause cancer and other health problems.

Even though herbs and spices have been irradiated for years, wider-scale irradiation of other foods is fairly recent. As a result, we do not have any data about the long-term results of irradiation.

ALLERGIES AND SENSITIVITIES

According to the National Institute of Allergy and Infectious Disease, only about 1% of all adults in the United States have a true food allergy, in which the body produces antibodies against a certain food. The most common foods involved are wheat, milk, eggs, nuts, shellfish, and soybeans.

Symptoms generally begin within a few minutes after eating the food. In mild cases, this usually consists of a localized rash or hives, often involving the mouth. More serious reactions cause nausea, vomiting, and diarrhea. The most severe reactions can cause irregular heartbeat, difficulty in breathing, changes in blood pressure, and shock. In rare cases, an allergic reaction to food can cause death. In one well-publicized case, a teenager died minutes after eating a candy bar that contained coconut oil.

Few adults actually have food allergies, although many adults become ill after eating certain foods. Those reactions are not caused by allergy. Other reactions to food that can cause illness include the following.

1. *Food sensitivities.* Unlike allergies, which cause distinct reactions within minutes after eating the suspect food, a food sensitivity is a delayed immune reaction. The reaction may set in several hours after eating the food, or after several days. The reaction usually occurs when proteins in the food are not digested completely, triggering an immune reaction. Simply, the immune system fails to recognize the proteins as nutritional substances. Food sensitivities are difficult to diagnose because the symptoms they cause seem unrelated to

a digestive problem. The most common symptoms are headache, joint pain, aching muscles, fluid retention, depression, and fatigue.

2. *Reactions to additives.* An individual may not be allergic to the food itself but instead may react to an additive *in* the food. One additive that causes sensitivity for many is monosodium glutamate (MSG), a flavor enhancer used commonly in Chinese food.

3. *Reactions to naturally occurring substances.* A food reaction may be caused by a substance that occurs naturally in a certain food, such as the caffeine in coffee or chocolate.

4. *Food intolerance.* Some people lack the enzymes needed to digest certain foods. When they eat foods they cannot digest completely, they develop gas, bloating, abdominal pain, diarrhea, and cramping. One of the most common is an intolerance to lactose, sugar found naturally in milk. A person who is lactose-intolerant becomes ill when drinking milk or eating dairy products. This is not an allergy, as it does not produce antibodies.

FOOD-BORNE ILLNESS

Food contaminated with bacteria or parasites can cause food-borne illness, characterized by nausea, vomiting, abdominal pain, bloating, gas, and diarrhea. in 1983, the last year records were kept, 6 million cases of food-borne illness were reported to the Centers for Disease Control; more than 9,000 people died as a result.[7] A well-known example of fatal food-borne illness was the outbreak of *E. coli* infection in the state of Washington, when almost 500 people became ill after eating contaminated hamburgers from a fast-food chain. Three children died during the outbreak. The CDC estimates that currently there are as many as 4 million cases a year of salmonella poisoning and as many as 20,000 cases a year of *E. coli* infection.

The symptoms of food-borne illness most often begin within 5 to 8 hours of eating the contaminated food. Symptoms, however, depend on the type of organism that causes the illness; they may begin as soon as 30 minutes after eating the food or may not develop for as long as several weeks afterward. When symptoms don't develop for days or weeks, the problem often is misdiagnosed because it can't be related readily to a specific food.

Although many cases of food-borne illness can be traced to food served at restaurants, approximately one-third can be traced to careless or unsafe handling and preparation of food in the home. To protect yourself from food-borne illness at home:

- When you shop, put meat, poultry, and fish in separate plastic bags so their drippings don't contaminate your other groceries.

- Check the expiration date on all meat, poultry, and fish before you buy it. When possible, get meat that was put in the cooler that day. Buy only what you can use within the next few days unless you are planning to freeze it. Keep meat, poultry, and fish in the refrigerator no longer than 3 days.

- Never buy meat, poultry, fish, or fresh produce from counters that are not clean.

- Refrigerate perishable foods (including fresh produce) as soon as you get home from the store. Make sure your refrigerator keeps foods at 40°F or cooler; bacteria thrive at temperatures as low as 45°F.

- Never thaw foods on the counter. Foods should be thawed in the refrigerator, in the microwave, or submerged in cold water. Cook food as soon as it is defrosted.

- Wash your hands thoroughly with soap and running hot water before handling any food, after you've touched any raw meat (including poultry and fish), and before you eat.

- Use paper towels to wipe up meat juices, then discard the paper towel. Wash sponges in the dishwasher at least every other day. Wash dishcloths and kitchen towels in hot water, and machine dry. Hang kitchen towels promptly after each use to air-dry and discourage growth of bacteria.

- Wash utensils and cutting boards thoroughly with hot, soapy water after preparing raw meat, poultry, or fish and before using them to prepare foods, such as salad ingredients. When possible, use separate cutting boards.

- If you use a wood cutting board for meat or poultry, never use it to prepare other foods, regardless of how well you wash it. Wood can absorb bacteria, and it is difficult to clean thoroughly.

Irradiation Exposing foods to gamma radiation to prolong shelf-life.

■ Wash cutting boards with soap and hot water after each use, and allow them to air-dry. Wash glass, solid wood, and plastic cutting boards in the dishwasher. Discard a plastic cutting board when it gets excessively cut up.

■ Sanitize cutting boards at least once a week with a solution of 2 teaspoons of chlorine (household) bleach in 1 quart of water. Leave the bleach solution standing on the surface of the cutting board for 5 minutes, rinse well, and allow to air-dry.

■ Avoid eating raw eggs (common in homemade ice cream, homemade mayonnaise, Caesar salad, Hollandaise sauce, and homemade "energy" drinks). Even though fewer than 1% of the nation's eggs are contaminated with *salmonella* bacteria, you should cook eggs until both the yolks and whites are set (not runny).

■ Cook all meat, poultry, and fish thoroughly. An estimated 5% of all meat is contaminated with *E. coli* bacteria, and these bacteria are not destroyed by refrigeration or freezing. Approximately 25% of all chicken marketed in the United States is contaminated with *salmonella* bacteria. The only way to destroy any bacteria in meat is to cook it thoroughly. The juices of pork and chicken should run clear, with no trace of pink in the meat. Cook beef until it is at least medium rare; the more rare the beef, the greater is the risk for food-borne illness. Cook fish until the thickest part is opaque and flakes easily with a fork. Ground meat and poultry pose the greatest risk for contamination, because bacteria on the surface can be mixed into the meat during grinding. Make sure all ground meat is cooked thoroughly, with no traces of pink.

■ Never serve cooked meat on the same plate that held the raw meat.

■ Don't leave cooked foods standing at room temperature for longer than 2 hours; refrigerate leftovers immediately.

Vegetarians

An estimated 1 in 10 American adults eats a **vegetarian** diet, avoiding some or all foods of animal origin. This decision may be based on cultural, religious, moral, ethnic, or health considerations. People who eat animal products sparingly usually realize several health benefits, including reduced risk of heart disease, lower levels of cholesterol and other fats in the blood, lower blood pressure, and lower weight.

The categories of vegetarians, distinguished by the type of food they eat, are:

1. *Semi-vegetarians:* do not eat red meat but do eat fish, poultry, eggs, and dairy products.

2. *Lacto-vegetarians:* avoid all foods of animal origin except milk and milk products.

3. *Ovo-vegetarians:* avoid all foods of animal origin except eggs.

4. *Lacto-ovo-vegetarians:* avoid foods of animal origin except milk, milk products, and eggs.

5. *Pesco-vegetarians:* avoid red meat and poultry but do eat fish, milk, milk products, and eggs.

6. *Vegans:* avoid all foods of animal origin, including dairy products and eggs.

The wide array of available foods allows most vegetarians to get the proper balance of necessary nutrients. Strict vegans do need to make extra effort to get essential amino acids, all necessary macro minerals (especially calcium and iron), and certain vitamins (such as riboflavin and vitamin D), as the best sources of these are milk, eggs, and meat. Good sources of these nutrients include fortified cereals and soy products, tofu, legumes, almonds, asparagus, dark green vegetables, and whole-grain breads.

If you are a vegetarian, consider these suggestions to help avoid nutritional deficiencies:

■ Combine *complementary proteins* to make sure you get complete proteins. In essence, combine vegetables with grains — beans and corn (common in Mexican foods), beans and rice, tofu and rice, black bean and rice soup.

■ Because vegetarian diets usually are low in fat, make sure you get at least 1 gram of fat a day so your body can absorb fat-soluble vitamins.

■ Eat at least one cup of dark green vegetables a day to boost your iron intake. Combine foods rich in vitamin C with foods rich in iron; the vitamin C helps the body absorb iron.

■ If you don't drink milk, eat at least two cups of legumes (dried beans and peas) a day to provide you with adequate calcium.

■ Eat a wide range of foods to better your chances of getting balanced nutrients.

Depending on how strict your diet is, you may need to use a nutritional supplement. Check with your physician or a nutritionist for advice.

DESIGNING A NUTRITIONAL PLAN FOR WELLNESS

The best nutritional plan for you is one that is *personalized* for your situation. The food choices you make depend on how much time you have, where you eat (a dormitory cafeteria? fast-food restaurant? your own kitchen?) and what kinds of foods you *like*. To design a food plan that includes Brussels sprouts, turnip greens, and tuna casserole is senseless if you really dislike those foods.

Designing a nutritional plan involves two fairly simple steps:

1. Consider your lifestyle carefully.
2. Identify the things you need to change.
3. Make some *gradual* changes compatible with your lifestyle. You'll be much more successful if you change things bit-by-bit, allowing yourself time to adjust your habits and tastes.

In general, aim for a good variety of foods from the food groups. Eat lots of complex carbohydrates (fruits, vegetables, whole grains) and only a little protein (meats). Steer away from foods that are high in fats or refined sugars. Make some alternative selections for snacks and desserts — air-popped popcorn, fresh fruits and vegetables, low-fat crackers. Drink soda, tea, coffee, and alcohol in moderation. Drink plenty of water.

If you live in a dormitory, choose low-fat foods that are rich in fiber and high in complex carbohydrates. For example, choose meat that has been broiled rather than fried; choose low-fat yogurt and 1% or skim milk; load up on fresh produce. In fast-food eating, choose salad bars and pasta bars when you can. At salad bars, pile on fresh fruits and vegetables, then use either fat-free dressing, oil and vinegar, or a little lemon juice.

The Healthy Eating Pyramid contained in Figure 8.7 provides simple and sound instructions for nutrition. The pyramid contains five major food groups, along with fats, oils, and sweets, which are to be used sparingly.

If your diet doesn't follow the recommended guidelines, outline the changes you need to make, then design a plan that helps you accomplish those changes.

- Keep a written list for a week or two, and note the foods you eat regularly that don't provide much nutrition. Note the foods, too, that might be bad for you — foods high in saturated fats, refined sugars, salt. The list can serve as a basic blueprint of the things you need to change. You also may use the computer software available with this text for a comprehensive nutrient analysis.

- Little by little, start to substitute nutritious and healthy foods for the things on the list you'd be better off without. If you're eating regular yogurt with fruit and flavorings, opt for nonfat yogurt topped with fresh fruit instead; you'll eliminate a lot of fat and sugar. Or try a halibut or tuna or salmon steak, broiled, in place of beef steak — or a sweet glass of orange juice in place of the cola you normally have between classes.

- Eat a good variety of foods; you're more likely to get the recommended daily allowances of all the essential nutrients that way.

- Whenever you can, eat "natural" or fresh foods. A carrot you slice and steam is the best source of nutrients.

- Start out the day with a good breakfast that provides approximately a third of your daily requirements. You will have more energy, will feel better, and won't suffer that traditional sugar crash mid-morning, when you're tempted to snack on high-fat or sugar-laden foods.

- Make good breakfast choices, including low-fat or skim milk, whole-grain breads and cereals, bagels, bran muffins, nonfat yogurt topped with fresh fruit or sprinkled with wheat germ, fresh fruit, or fruit juice. Steer away from egg yolks, butter, and cream cheese.

- Eat at regular intervals throughout the day: breakfast in the morning, lunch at mid-day, dinner in the early evening, with healthy snacks in between if you need them. You'll have higher energy levels and a better chance of keeping your blood sugar at a constant level.

- Make good lunch choices of salads with low-fat dressing; sandwiches made with whole-grain bread, low-fat spreads, and sliced roasted chicken or turkey; vegetable soup. At the salad bar, load up on fresh vegetables, legumes, and fruits. For the most part, avoid cream soups, predressed pasta salads, cheese, mayonnaise, fried foods, and processed lunch meats.

Vegetarian   Individuals who eat no animal products at all.

FIGURE 8.7

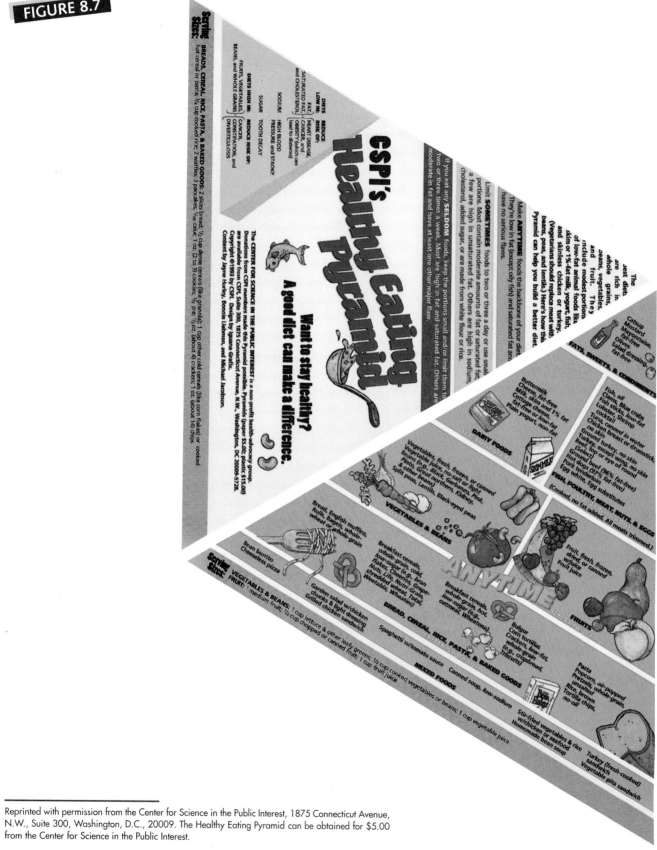

Healthy eating pyramid: A guide to daily food choices.

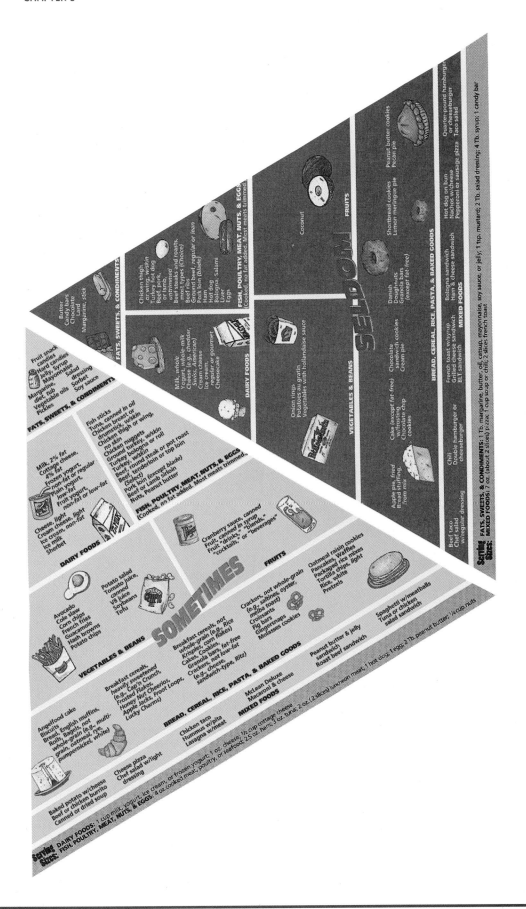

- Include healthy dinner choices such as skinless baked chicken breast; stir-fry foods (these normally emphasize vegetables and use meat only as an accompaniment); pasta; brown rice; whole-grain rolls; steamed vegetables. Top your baked potato with nonfat yogurt instead of butter and sour cream. Use lemon pepper on your vegetables instead of salt and butter.
- When cooking, use less fat. Cook in a nonstick skillet; poach, bake, broil, or roast instead of frying whenever you can; steam or microwave vegetables instead of cooking them in butter.

NOTES

1. Kenneth Davis, "The Effects of Nutrition on the Brain, Nervous System, and Behavior," pp. 640–642 in *Total Nutrition: The Only Guide You'll Ever Need*, Victor Herbert and Genell J. Subak-Sharpe, editors (NY: St. Martin's Press, 1995).
2. Jane Brody, *Jane Brody's Nutrition Book* (NY: Bantam Books, 1987), p. 34.
3. B. Liebman, "The Changing American Diet," *Nutrition Action Healthletter*, May 1990, pp. 8–9.
4. Roberta Larson Duyff, *The American Dietetic Association's Complete Food and Nutrition Guide* (Minneapolis, MN: Chronimed Publishing, 1996), pp. 141–143.
5. Victor Herbert, "Dietary Fiber," pp. 141–143 in *Total Nutrition: The Only Guide You'll Ever Need*, Victor Herbert and Genell J. Subak-Sharpe, editors (NY: St. Martin's Press, 1995).
6. C. A. Rice-Evans and R. H. Burdon, *Free Radical Damage and Its Control* (London: Elsevier, 1994).
7. Rebecca Voelker, "Food-Borne Illness Problems More Than Enteric," *Journal of the American Medical Association* 271:1 (1994), pp. 8–9, 11.

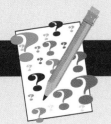

ASSESSMENT 8-1

Test for Fats

Name _____ Date _____ Grade _____

Instructor _____ Course _____ Section _____

True/False

1. Egg yolks contain the "bad" cholesterol called LDL.

2. Mayonnaise made from canola oil has less fat than regular mayonnaise, which is generally made from soybean oil.

3. The more unsaturated fat a food has, the more it will raise blood-cholesterol levels.

4. Polyunsaturated fats are converted to saturated fats when heated, such as in deep-fat frying.

5. A jar of peanut butter labeled as "cholesterol free" is better than regular brands.

6. A label that reads "95% fat free" means the food contains only 5% of its calories from fat.

7. The best way to decrease blood-cholesterol levels is to eat less cholesterol.

8. A third of the average U.S. woman's fat intake comes from salad dressing, margarine, cheese, and beef.

9. A label that reads "low cholesterol" means the food has fewer calories than regular brands and no saturated fat.

10. Veggie burgers are always a low-fat alternative to hamburgers.

Multiple-Choice

Select the best answer to the following questions.

11. A product is labeled as containing only vegetable oils. It would be:
    a. high in only saturated fat
    b. high in only unsaturated fat
    c. high in either saturated fat or unsaturated fat
    d. high in unsaturated fat and might contain some cholesterol

12. A woman has a total blood-cholesterol level of 220 mg/dl and an HDL level of 60 mg/dl. What is this person's ratio of total cholesterol to HDL cholesterol? Is she at high or low risk for heart disease?
    a. 3:7 ratio and low risk
    b. 2:7 ratio and low risk
    c. 7:2 ratio and low risk
    d. 4:5 ratio and high risk

13. A 5-ounce serving of ground beef has how much more fat than the same size serving of skinless chicken breast?
    a. 50%   c. 75%
    b. 65%   d. 95%

14. There are 30 grams of fat and 309 calories in an avocado. What is the percentage of fat calories?
    a. 42%   c. 87%
    b. 62%   d. 97%

15. A food is considered low-fat if it has how many grams of fat per 100 calories?
    a. 3   c. 10
    b. 5   d. 30

16. According to the American Heart Association, people ideally should adopt a low-fat diet that contains no more than 30% fat calories:
    a. starting at birth
    b. at 2 years of age
    c. at puberty
    d. in early adulthood

17. An olive-oil label states that the product is "extra light." This means
    a. it has a lighter color and taste than other olive oils
    b. it weighs less
    c. it has fewer calories
    d. it is lower in saturated fats

From *Facing Fats* by Elizabeth Somer in *SHAPE*, January, 1994.

18. Whole milk gets 48% of its calories from fat. What percentage of calories come from fat in 2% low-fat milk?
    - a. 2%
    - b. 15%
    - c. 25%
    - d. 30%

19. Experts recommend limiting your saturated-fat intake to no more than 10% of total calorie intake. If you eat 2,000 calories per day, your saturated-fat allowance would be
    - a. 10 grams
    - b. 22 grams
    - c. 27 grams
    - d. 36 grams

20. A Taco Bell taco salad contains how many teaspoons of fat?
    - a. 9
    - b. 12
    - c. 15
    - d. 25

Answers:

1. **False.** LDL is a carrier of cholesterol in the blood. It is not found in food.

2. **False.** They contain similar amounts of fat and calories.

3. **False.** The more *saturated* fat in your diet, the more your blood-cholesterol level will be raised.

4. **False.** However, frying does expose these fats to oxygen, and once oxidized, they can increase heart-disease risk.

5. **False.** Cholesterol is found only in animal products.

6. **False.** The label refers only to fat content by weight. The percentage of calories from fat would be much higher. For instance, a 95% fat-free Janet Lee Chopped Ham contains 60% fat calories (2 grams of fat per 30-calorie slice).

7. **False.** Reducing your saturated fat intake is the most important dietary factor for lowering blood cholesterol.

8. **True.** The average woman in the United States gets 9% of her fat from salad dressing, 8% from margarine, 8% from cheese and 7% from beef, for a total of one-third.

9. **False.** A food can be cholesterol-free and still be high in calories and/or saturated fat.

10. **False.** Commercial veggie burgers get anywhere from 6% of 66% of their calories from fat.

11. **c.** Most vegetable oils are high in unsaturated fats. However, manufacturers also use tropical oils, such as palm or coconut oils, which are as saturated as lard.

12. **a.**

13. **d.**

14. **c.**

15. **a.** There are 9 calories per gram of fat, so a food that has 3 grams of fat per 100 calories is 27% fat; a food that is less than 30% fat is considered low-fat.

16. **b.**

17. **a.**

18. **d.**

19. **b.**

20. **c.**

To find your score, total your correct answers.

18 or more: All of that label reading has paid off! You are a bona fide fat sleuth.

15 to 17: You put the average American to shame. If you practice what you know, your diet is probably within the low-fat zone.

12 to 14: You keep company with the majority of Americans and may be confused when it comes to fat. Review the answers and see if you can improve your score.

Less than 12: Oops. It's time to take the fat issue more seriously.

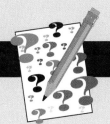

ASSESSMENT 8-2

Personal Diet Quiz

Name _____ Date _____ Grade _____

Instructor _____ Course _____ Section _____

Are You Meeting Your Fiber Quota?

To find out how close you come to meeting your daily fiber quota, keep track of everything you eat for 3 days. Then, take the quiz below and add up your points. This quiz was developed with assistance from nutrition lecturer Liz Applegate, and nutrition professor Judith Stern, both at the University of California, Davis.

1. What type of bread (including rolls and muffins) did you usually eat?

    a. whole-wheat or whole-grain   +4
    b. white or partial whole-wheat   +2

2. How many servings of oat products did you average daily? (1 serving = 1 cup cooked oatmeal or oat bran.)

    a. 2 or more   +4
    b. 1   +3
    c. 1/2   +2
    d. none   0

3. How many times during the last 3 days did you eat beans (legumes), such as kidney beans, pintos, garbanzos, soybeans, lentils, and split peas?

    a. 3 or more   +4
    b. 2   +3
    c. 1   +2
    d. none   0

4. How many times during the 3-day period did you eat high-fiber breakfast cereals?

    a. 3 or more   +4
    b. 2   +3
    c. 1   +2
    d. none   0

5. How many times during the 3-day period did you eat cooked whole-grain side dishes, such as brown rice or barley?

    a. 3 or more   +4
    b. 2   +3
    c. 1   +2
    d. none   0

6. Approximately how many servings of canned or fresh fruits and vegetables did you eat daily? (Use an average from the previous 3 days. 1 serving = 1/2 cup cooked or 1 cup or 1 piece raw.)

    a. 7 or more   +5
    b. 5-6   +4
    c. 3-4   +2
    d. 1-2   +1
    e. none   −2

Scoring: If your overall score is over 20, your fiber intake is probably adequate. If it is lower, try to increase your fiber intake using the foods mentioned above.

Check Your Calcium Intake

If you are not a fan of dairy products, you may be coming up far short of your calcium needs. But even if you are a milk lover, how much calcium your body actually absorbs depends upon your genetic makeup. And how much you retain depends upon your intake of salt and protein. This duo increases the elimination of calcium, causing your body to steal calcium it needs from your bones.

The following quiz was developed with the assistance of Robert P. Heaney, professor of medicine at Creighton University School of Medicine, Omaha, Nebraska. It can tell you how close your diet comes to providing the appropriate amount of bone food. Just check the answer that applies to you.

1. I eat a serving of yogurt (8 ounces), milk (1 cup), or cheese (1 ounce) at least once a day.

    _____ True   +3
    _____ False   −1

2. Dairy products give me gas and bloating, so I avoid them.

    _____ True   −1
    _____ False   +1

3. I make sure I eat one or more of the following nondairy sources of calcium at least 3 times a week: leafy green vegetables (kale, bok choy, or broccoli), shellfish (oysters

or clams), or canned fish with bones (salmon or sardines).

_____ True   +1

_____ False   0

4. I make an effort to slip dairy foods into my diet whenever I can (grating cheese over salads, for example).

_____ True   +1

_____ False   0

5. I eat calcium-enriched forms of products (such as breakfast cereal or fruit juice) whenever possible.

_____ True   +1
_____ False   −1

6. When given a choice, I drink carbonated soft drinks over low-fat dairy drinks or water.

_____ True   −1
_____ False   0

7. I tend to get my protein from meats.

_____ True   −1
_____ False   +1

8. I usually salt food automatically without tasting them.

_____ True   −1
_____ False   +1

Scoring: If you scored between 7 and 9, you are laying the dietary foundation for a rock-solid skeleton. (Remember, though, that even if you scored a perfect 9, you may still have a bone deficit if you are inactive, underweight or postmenopausal, have a family history of osteoporosis, or take aluminum-based antacids or other calcium-robbing drugs.) If you scored between 4 and 6, try to include more low-fat dairy products and go easy on the calcium bandits. If you scored below 4, your skeleton may be becoming perilously porous. Learn to love low-fat yogurt and make friends with skim milk. Ask your doctor about taking a calcium supplement.

Can You Find the Hidden Salt?

If you've already banned the saltshaker from the table and sworn off salty snacks — good for you! But to keep your intake at the recommended one-teaspoon-a-day limit takes a bit more vigilance. Three-fourths of your dietary sodium is hidden in already-prepared foods, experts say. And many salt-laced foods, such as cereal, diet soda and instant pudding don't taste a bit salty.

Just how good are you at avoiding this hidden salt? If you're eating more potassium-rich fresh fruits and vegetables than packaged convenience foods, for example, you're probably doing great. (Potassium helps rid your body of excess sodium.)

Take this quiz to find out where you stand on the hidden salt scale.

1. When barbecuing meat or fish, I'm more likely to brush on herbs or homemade marinara sauce than commercial ketchup, barbecue sauce, or soy sauce.

_____ True   +1
_____ False   −1

2. The fresh fruits and vegetables and lean meats in my grocery cart usually crowd out the canned, frozen, and processed food.

_____ True   +1
_____ False   −1

3. I buy only the low-salt type of margarine.

_____ True   +1
_____ False   −1

4. I usually have dehydrated, instant versions of soups, sauces, salad dressings, oatmeal, or other foods on hand.

_____ True   −1
_____ False   +1

5. I steam, microwave, broil, or stir-fry vegetables rather than boil them.

_____ True   +1
_____ False   −1

6. Processed cheese never passes my lips.

_____ True   +1
_____ False   −1

7. I rinse canned foods such as tuna, ham, and beans before preparing them.

_____ True   +1
_____ False   −1

8. I'm a sucker for deli food — cold cuts, prepared salads, pastrami, ham, smoked fish, and so on.

_____ True   −1
_____ False   +1

9. I usually order my hamburger with the works — cheese, pickles, ketchup, mustard and special sauce.

_____ True   −1
_____ False   +1

10. When dining out, I usually order oil and vinegar dressing for my salad, and ask for gravies and sauces on the side.

_____ True   +1
_____ False   −1

Scoring: 8-10: You're a top-notch salt sleuth. 5-7: There's room for improvement. Scan food labels closely for the key phrases "sodium-free" or "very low sodium." Below 5: You're probably relying on too many prepared condiments and packaged convenience foods. Try to cut down on these.

ASSESSMENT 8-3

Is Osteoporosis in Your Future?

Name _____ Date _____ Grade _____

Instructor _____ Course _____ Section _____

Risk factors you CANNOT control:

	YES	NO
1. Are you female?	☐	☐
2. Do you have a family history of osteoporosis?	☐	☐
3. Are your ancestors from the British Isles, northern Europe, China, or Japan?	☐	☐
4. Are you very fair-skinned?	☐	☐
5. Are you small-boned?	☐	☐
6. Are you over age 35?	☐	☐
7. Have you had your ovaries removed, or did you have an early menopause?	☐	☐
8. Did you breast-feed your baby?	☐	☐
9. Are you allergic to milk and milk products?	☐	☐
10. Have you never been pregnant?	☐	☐
11. Do you have cancer or kidney disease?	☐	☐
12. Do you have to take chemotherapy, steroids, anticonvulsants, or anticoagulants?	☐	☐

Risk factors you CAN control:

	YES	NO
13. Is your daily routine stressful?	☐	☐
14. Do you smoke?	☐	☐
15. Do you drink alcohol?	☐	☐
16. Do you avoid milk and cheese in your diet?	☐	☐
17. Do you get very little exercise?	☐	☐
18. Do you drink a lot of soft drinks?	☐	☐
19. Is your diet high in protein?	☐	☐
20. Do you consume a lot of caffeine (five or more cups of coffee per day or equivalent)?	☐	☐
21. Are you amenorrheic (without a monthly period)?	☐	☐
22. Do you get less than 1,000 mg. of calcium a day?	☐	☐
23. Is your body weight very low?	☐	☐
24. Do you crash diet?	☐	☐
25. Do you have a high sodium (salt) intake?	☐	☐

If you answered "yes" to three (3) of the above questions, you are at risk for osteoporosis and may want to ask your doctor to give you a bone density screening test. The more questions you answered "yes" to, the higher your risk of developing osteoporosis in the future.

Many clinical studies suggest that osteoporosis is a preventable disease. As you can see from the quiz, you can do several things right now to help prevent osteoporosis in your future.

Adapted from *Marion Laboratories, Inc.*

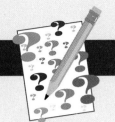

ASSESSMENT 8-4

How's Your Diet?

Name _____ Date _____ Grade _____

Instructor _____ Course _____ Section _____

The 40 questions below will help you focus on the key features of your diet. The (+) or (−) numbers under each set of answers instantly pat you on the back for good habits or alert you to problems you may not even realize you have.

The Grand Total rates your overall diet, on a scale from "Great" to "Arghh!"

The quiz focuses on fat, cholesterol, sodium, sugar, fiber, and vitamins A and C. It doesn't attempt to cover everything in your diet. Also, it doesn't try to measure precisely how much of these key nutrients you eat. What the quiz will do is give you a rough sketch of your current eating habits and, implicitly, suggest what you can do to improve them.

Don't despair over a less-than-perfect score. A healthy diet isn't built overnight.

INSTRUCTIONS: Under each answer is a number with a + or − sign in front of it. Circle the number that is directly beneath the answer you choose. That's your score for the question. (If you use a pencil, you can erase your answers and give the quiz to someone else.)

Circle only one number for each question, unless the instructions tell you to "average two or more scores if necessary."

How to average: In answering question 18, for example, if you drink club soda (+3) and coffee (−1) on a typical day, add the two scores (which gives you +2) and then divide by 2. That gives you a score of +1 for the question. If averaging gives you a fraction, round it to the nearest whole number.

If a question doesn't apply to you, skip it.

Pay attention to serving sizes. For example, a serving of vegetables is 1/2 cup. If you usually eat one cup of vegetables at a time, count it as two servings.

Add up all your + scores and your − scores.

Subtract your − scores from your + scores. That's your GRAND TOTAL.

QUIZ

1. How many times per week do you eat unprocessed red meat (steak, roast beef, lamb or pork chops, burgers, etc.)?
   - (a) never   (b) 1 or less   (c) 2-3
      +3   +2   0
   - (d) 4-5   (e) 6 or more
      −1   −3

2. After cooking, how large is the serving of red meat you usually eat? (To convert from raw to cooked, reduce by 25%. For example, 4 oz. of raw meat shrinks to 3 oz. after cooking. There are 16 oz. in a pound.)
   - (a) 8 oz. or more   (b) 6-7 oz.   (c) 4-5 oz.
      −3   −2   −1
   - (d) 3 oz. or less   (e) don't eat red meat
      0   +3

3. Do you trim the visible fat when you cook or eat red meat?
   - (a) yes   (b) no   (c) don't eat red meat
      +1   −3   0

4. How many times per week do you eat processed meats (hot dogs, bacon, sausage, bologna, luncheon meats, etc.)? (OMIT products that contain 1 gram of fat or less per serving.)
   - (a) none   (b) less than 1   (c) 1-2
      +3   +2   0
   - (d) 3-4   (e) 5 or more
      −1   −3

5. What kind of ground meat or poultry do you usually eat?
   - (a) regular ground beef   (b) lean ground beef
      −3   −2
   - (c) ground round   (d) ground turkey
      0   +1
   - (e) Healthy Choice™   (f) don't eat ground meat
      +2   +3

6. What type of bread do you usually eat?
   (a) whole wheat or other whole grain
      +3
   (b) rye   (c) pumpernickel
      +2   +2
   (d) white, "wheat," French, or Italian
      −2

7. How many times per week do you eat deep-fried foods (fish, chicken, vegetables, potatoes, etc.)?
   (a) none   (b) 1-2   (c) 3-4   (d) 5 or more
      +3   0   −1   −3

8. How many servings of non-fried vegetables do you usually eat per day? *(One serving = 1/2 cup. INCLUDE potatoes.)*
   (a) none   (b) 1   (c) 2   (d) 3   (e) 4 or more
      −3   0   +1   +2   +3

9. How many servings of cruciferous vegetables do you usually eat per week? *(ONLY count kale, broccoli, cauliflower, cabbage, Brussels sprouts, greens, bok choy, kohlrabi, turnip, and rutabaga. One serving = 1/2 cup.)*
   (a) none   (b) 1-3   (c) 4-6   (d) 7 or more
      −3   +1   +2   +3

10. How many servings of vitamin-A-rich fruits or vegetables do you usually eat per week? *(ONLY count carrots, pumpkin, sweet potatoes, cantaloupe, spinach, winter squash, greens, and apricots. One serving = 1/2 cup.)*
    (a) none   (b) 1-3   (c) 4-6   (d) 7 or more
       −3   +1   +2   +3

11. How many times per week do you eat at a fast-food restaurant? *(INCLUDE burgers, fried fish or chicken, croissant or biscuit sandwiches, topped potatoes, and other main dishes. OMIT meals of just plain baked potato, broiled chicken, or salad.)*
    (a) never   (b) less than 1   (c) 1   (d) 2
       +3   +1   0   −1
    (e) 3   (f) 4 or more
       −2   −3

12. How many servings of grains rich in complex carbohydrates do you eat per day? *(One serving = 1 slice of bread, 1 large pancake, 1 cup whole grain cold cereal, or 1/2 cup cooked cereal, rice, pasta, bulgur, wheat berries, kasha, or millet. OMIT heavily-sweetened cold cereals.)*
    (a) none   (b) 1-3   (c) 4-5   (d) 6-8
       −3   0   +1   +2
    (e) 9 or more
       +3

13. How many times per week do you eat fish or shellfish? *(OMIT deep-fried items, tuna packed in oil, shrimp, squid, and mayonnaise-laden tuna salad — a little mayo is okay.)*
    (a) never   (b) 1-2   (c) 3-4   (d) 5 or more
       −2   +1   +2   +3

14. How many times per week do you eat cheese? *(INCLUDE pizza, cheeseburgers, veal or eggplant parmigiana, cream cheese, etc. OMIT low-fat or fat-free cheeses.)*
    (a) 1 or less   (b) 2-3   (c) 4-5   (d) 6 or more
       +3   +2   −1   −3

15. How many servings of fresh fruit do you eat per day?
    (a) none   (b) 1   (c) 2   (d) 3   (e) 4 or more
       −3   0   +1   +2   +3

16. Do you remove the skin before eating poultry?
    (a) yes   (b) no   (c) don't eat poultry
       +3   −3   0

17. What do you usually put on your bread or toast? *(AVERAGE two or more scores if necessary.)*
    (a) butter or cream cheese
       −3
    (b) margarine or peanut butter   (c) diet margarine
       −1   0
    (d) jam or honey   (e) fruit butter   (f) nothing
       −2   +1   +3

18. Which of these beverages do you drink on a typical day? *(AVERAGE two or more scores if necessary.)*
    (a) water or club soda
       +3
    (b) fruit juice   (c) diet soda   (d) coffee or tea
       +1   −1   −1
    (e) soda, fruit "drink," or fruit "ade"
       −3

19. Which flavorings do you add to your foods most frequently? *(AVERAGE two or more scores if necessary.)*
    (a) garlic or lemon juice   (b) herbs or spices
       +3   +3
    (c) salt or soy sauce   (d) margarine
       −2   −2
    (e) butter   (f) nothing
       −3   +3

20. What do you eat most frequently as a snack? *(AVERAGE two or more scores if necessary.)*
    (a) fruits or vegetables   (b) sweetened yogurt
            +3   +2
    (c) nuts   (d) cookies or fried chips   (e) granola bar
        −1   −2   −2
    (f) candy bar or pastry   (g) nothing
              −3   0

21. What is your most typical breakfast? *(SUBTRACT an extra 3 points if you also eat bacon or sausage.)*
    (a) croissant, danish, or doughnut   (b) eggs
              −3   −3
    (c) pancakes or waffles   (d) cereal or toast
              −2   +3
    (e) low-fat yogurt or cottage cheese
              +3
    (f) don't eat breakfast
              0

22. What do you usually eat for dessert?
    (a) pie, pastry, or cake   (b) ice cream
            −3   −3
    (c) fat-free cookies or cakes
            −1
    (d) frozen yogurt or ice milk
            +1
    (e) nonfat ice cream or sorbet   (f) fruit
            +1   +3
    (g) don't eat dessert
            +3

23. How many times per week do you eat beans, split peas, or lentils?
    (a) none   (b) 1   (c) 2   (d) 3 or more
        −2   +1   +2   +3

24. What kind of milk do you drink?
    (a) whole   (b) 2% low-fat   (c) 1% low-fat
        −3   −1   +2
    (d) 1/2% or skim   (e) none
            +3   0

25. What dressings or toppings do you usually add to your salads? *(ADD two or more scores if necessary.)*
    (a) nothing, lemon, or vinegar
            +3
    (b) fat-free dressing
            +2
    (c) low- or reduced-calorie dressing
            +1
    (d) regular dressing   (e) croutons or bacon bits
            −1   −1
    (f) cole slaw, pasta salad, or potato salad
            −1

26. What sandwich fillings do you eat most frequently? *(AVERAGE two or more scores if necessary.)*
    (a) luncheon meat   (b) cheese or roast beef
            −3   −1
    (c) peanut butter   (d) low-fat luncheon meat
            0   +1
    (e) tuna, salmon, chicken, or turkey
            +3
    (f) don't eat sandwiches
            0

27. What do you usually spread on your sandwiches? *(AVERAGE two or more scores if necessary.)*
    (a) mayonnaise   (b) light mayonnaise
            −2   −1
    (c) ketchup, mustard, or fat-free mayonnaise
            0
    (d) nothing
            +2

28. How many egg yolks do you eat per week? *(ADD 1 yolk for every slice of quiche you eat.)*
    (a) 2 or less   (b) 3-4   (c) 5-6   (d) 7 or more
            +3   0   −1   −3

29. How many times per week do you eat canned or dried soups? *(OMIT low-sodium, low-fat soups.)*
    (a) none   (b) 1-2   (c) 3-4   (d) 5 or more
        +3   0   −2   −3

30. How many servings of a rich source of calcium do you eat per day? *(One serving = 2/3 cup milk or yogurt, 1 oz. cheese, 1½ oz. sardines, 3½ oz. salmon, 5 oz. tofu made with calcium sulfate, 1 cup greens or broccoli, or 200 mg of a calcium supplement.)*
    (a) none   (b) 1   (c) 2   (d) 3 or more
        −3   +1   +2   +3

31. What do you usually order on your pizza? *(Vegetable toppings include green pepper, mushrooms, onions, and other vegetables. SUBTRACT 1 point from your score if you order extra cheese.)*
    (a) no cheese with vegetables
            +3
    (b) cheese with vegetables
            +1
    (c) cheese   (d) cheese with meat toppings
            0   −3
    (e) don't eat pizza
            +2

32. What kind of cookies do you usually eat?
    (a) graham crackers or ginger snaps
        +1
    (b) oatmeal   (c) sandwich cookies (like Oreos)
        −1   −2
    (d) choc. coated, choc. chip, or peanut butter
        −3
    (e) don't eat cookies
        +3

33. What kind of frozen dessert do you usually eat? *(SUBTRACT 1 point from your score for each topping you use — whipped cream, hot fudge, nuts, etc.)*
    (a) gourmet ice cream   (b) regular ice cream
        −3   −1
    (c) sorbet, sherbet, or ices
        +1
    (d) frozen yogurt, fat-free ice cream, or ice milk
        +1
    (e) don't eat frozen desserts
        +3

34. What kind of cake or pastry do you usually eat?
    (a) cheesecake, pie, or any microwave cake
        −3
    (b) cake with frosting or filling
        −2
    (c) cake without frosting
        −1
    (d) unfrosted muffin, banana bread, or carrot cake
        0
    (e) angelfood or fat-free cake
        +1
    (f) don't eat cakes or pastries
        +3

35. How many times per week does your dinner contain grains, vegetables, or beans, but little or no animal protein (meat, poultry, fish, eggs, milk, or cheese)?
    (a) none   (b) 1-2   (c) 3-4   (d) 5 or more
        −1   +1   +2   +3

36. Which of the following salty snacks do you typically eat? *(AVERAGE two or more scores if necessary.)*
    (a) potato chips, corn chips, or packaged popcorn
        −3
    (b) reduced-fat potato or tortilla chips
        −2
    (c) salted pretzels
        −1
    (d) unsalted pretzels or baked corn or tortilla chips
        +1
    (e) homemade air-popped popcorn
        +3
    (f) don't eat salty snacks
        +3

37. What do you usually use to saute vegetables or other foods? *(Vegetable oil includes safflower, corn, canola, olive, sunflower, and soybean.)*
    (a) butter or lard
        −3
    (b) more than one tbsp of margarine or veg. oil
        −1
    (c) no more than one tbsp or margarine or veg. oil
        0
    (d) no more than one tablespoon of olive oil
        +1
    (e) water or broth
        +2

38. What kind of cereal do you usually eat?
    (a) whole grain (like oatmeal or shredded wheat)
        +3
    (b) low-fiber (like cream of wheat or corn flakes)
        0
    (c) sugary low-fiber (like frosted flakes)
        −1
    (d) granola
        −2

39. With what do you make tuna salad, pasta salad, chicken salad, etc.?
    (a) mayonnaise   (b) light mayonnaise
        −2   −1
    (c) nonfat mayonnaise   (d) low-fat yogurt
        0   +2
    (e) nonfat yogurt
        +3

40. What do you typically put on your pasta? *(ADD one point if you also add sauteed vegetables. AVERAGE two or more scores if necessary.)*
    (a) tomato sauce
        +3
    (b) tomato sauce with a little parmesan
        +3
    (c) white clam sauce   (d) meat sauce or meat balls
        +1   −2
    (e) Alfredo, pesto, or other creamy sauce
        −3

YOUR GRAND TOTAL

+59 to +116	**GREAT!**	You're a nutrition superstar. Give yourself a big (non-butter) pat on the back.
0 to +58	**GOOD**	Pin your quiz on the nearest wall.
−58 to −1	**FAIR**	Hang in there
−117 to −59	**ARGHH!**	Empty your refrigerator and cupboard. It's time to start over.

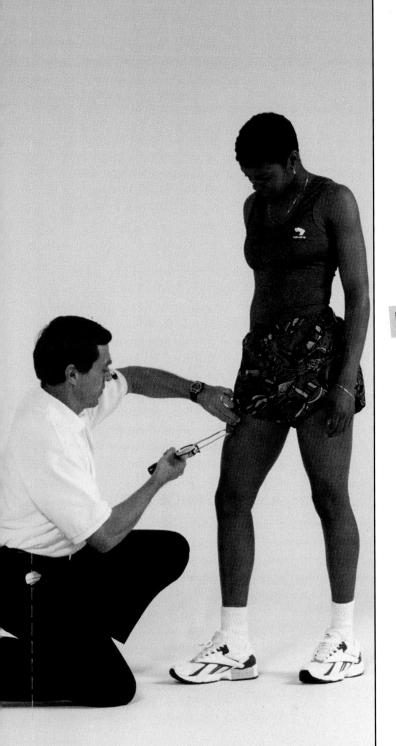

Body Composition Assessment

9

OBJECTIVES

- Define body composition and its relationship to recommended body weight assessment.
- Learn the difference between essential fat and storage fat.
- Understand the methodology used to assess body composition according to skinfold thickness and girth measurements.
- Be able to determine recommended weight according to recommended percent body fat values.
- Understand the importance of waist-to-hip ratio and body mass index.

The term **body composition** is used in reference to the fat and nonfat components of the human body. The fat component usually is called **fat mass** or **percent body fat**. The nonfat component is termed **lean body mass**.

For many years people relied on height/weight charts to determine recommended body weight. We now know, however, that these tables can be highly inaccurate for many people and they fail to identify critical fat values associated with higher risk for disease. The proper way to determine **recommended weight** is through body composition by finding out what percent of total body weight is fat and what amount is lean tissue.

Once the fat percentage is known, recommended body weight can be calculated from recommended body fat. Recommended body weight, also called "healthy weight," is defined as the body weight at which there seems to be no harm to human health. This includes the absence of any medical condition that would improve with weight loss and a fat distribution pattern that is not associated with increased risk for illness.

Although various techniques for determining percent body fat were developed several years ago, many people still are unaware of these procedures and continue to depend on height/weight charts to find out their recommended body weight. The standard height/weight tables were first published in 1912. They were based on average weights (including shoes and clothing) for men and women who obtained life insurance policies between 1888 and 1905. The recommended body weight on these tables is obtained according to gender, height, and frame size. Because no scientific guidelines are given to determine frame size, most people choose their frame size based on the column in which the weight comes closest to their own!

To determine whether people are truly obese or falsely at recommended body weight, body composition must be established. Obesity is related to an excess of body fat. If body weight is the only criterion, an individual easily can be overweight according to height/weight charts, yet not have any excess body fat. Football players, body builders, weight lifters, and other athletes with large muscle size are typical examples. Some of these athletes who appear to be 20 or 30 pounds overweight really have little body fat.

Too Fat?

The inaccuracy of height/weight charts was illustrated clearly when a young man who weighed about 225 pounds applied to join a city police force but was turned down without having been granted an interview. The reason? He was "too fat," according to the height/weight charts. When this young man's body composition later was assessed at a preventive medicine clinic, he was shocked to find out that only 5% of his total body weight was in the form of fat — considerably lower than the recommended standard. In the words of the technical director of the clinic, "The only way this fellow could come down to the chart's target weight would have been through surgical removal of a large amount of his muscle tissue."

At the other end of the spectrum, some people who weigh very little and are viewed by many as skinny or underweight actually can be classified as obese because of their high body fat content. People who weigh as little as 100 pounds but are more than 30% fat (about one-third of their total body weight) are not uncommon. These cases are found more often in sedentary people and those who are always dieting. Physical inactivity and constant negative caloric balance both lead to a loss in lean body mass (see Chapter 10). From these examples, body weight alone clearly does not always tell the true story.

ESSENTIAL AND STORAGE FAT

Total fat in the human body is classified into two types: essential fat and storage fat. **Essential fat** is needed for normal physiological functions, and without it, human health deteriorates. This essential fat constitutes about 3% of the total weight in men and 12% in women. The percentage is higher in women because it includes sex-specific fat, such as that found in the breast tissue, the uterus, and other sex-related fat deposits.

Storage fat is the fat stored in adipose tissue, mostly beneath the skin (subcutaneous fat) and around major organs in the body. This fat serves three basic functions:

1. As an insulator to retain body heat.
2. As energy substrate for metabolism.
3. As padding against physical trauma to the body.

The amount of storage fat does not differ between men and women, except that men tend to store fat around the waist and women more so around the hips and thighs.

TECHNIQUES FOR ASSESSING BODY COMPOSITION

Body composition can be determined through several different procedures. The most common techniques are: (a) hydrostatic or underwater weighing, (b) skinfold thickness, (c) girth measurements, and (d) bioelectrical impedance.

When using the different techniques, slightly different values are obtained. Therefore, when assessing body composition, the same technique should be used for pre- and post-test comparisons.

Hydrostatic Weighing

Hydrostatic weighing has been used as the standard of body composition. Almost all other techniques to determine body composition are validated against hydrostatic weighing. It is the most accurate technique available if it is administered properly and if the individual is able to perform the test adequately. The psychological factor of being weighed while submerged underwater makes hydrostatic weighing difficult to administer to the aqua-phobic.

The person's residual lung volume (the amount of air left in the lungs following complete forceful exhalation) must be measured to accurately determine percent body fat according to hydrostatic weighing. If the residual volume cannot be measured, as is the case in many health/fitness centers, the volume is estimated using predicting equations, which may sacrifice the accuracy of the assessment.

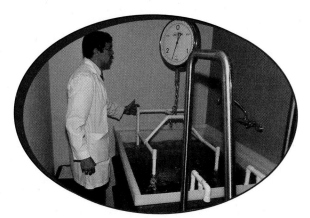

*Hydrostatic weighing technique
for body composition assessment.*

Because of the cost, time, and complexity of hydrostatic weighing, most health and fitness programs prefer **anthropometric measurement** techniques, which correlate quite well with hydrostatic weighing. These techniques, primarily skinfold thickness and girth measurements, allow a quick, simple, and inexpensive estimate of body composition.

Skinfold Thickness

Assessing body composition using skinfold thickness is based on the principle that approximately half of the body's fatty tissue is directly beneath the skin. Valid and reliable estimates of this tissue give a good indication of percent body fat.

The skinfold test is done with the aid of pressure calipers. Several sites must be measured to reflect the total percentage of fat: triceps, suprailium, and thigh skinfolds for women; and chest, abdomen, and thigh

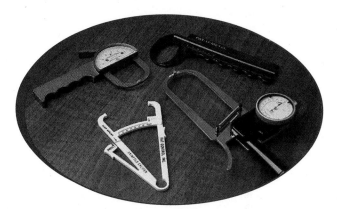

*Various types of skinfold calipers
used to assess skinfold thickness.*

Body composition Term used in reference to the fat and nonfat components of the human body. Body composition is important in the assessment of recommended or "ideal" body weight.

Fat mass Weight of the total amount of fat in the body.

Percent body fat Ratio of fat in the body to total weight; includes both essential and storage fat. Used in body composition assessment.

Lean body mass Body weight without body fat.

Recommended weight Body weight at which there seems to be no harm to human health.

Essential fat Minimal amount of body fat needed for normal physiological functions; constitutes about 3% of total weight in men and 12% in women.

Storage fat Body fat in excess of essential fat; stored in adipose tissue.

Anthropometric measurement Measurement of body girths at different sites.

for men (Figure 9.1). All measurements should be taken on the right side of the body.

Even with the skinfold technique, some training is necessary to obtain accurate measurements. Also, different technicians may produce slightly different measurements from the same person. Therefore, the same technician should take pre- and post-measurements.

Measurements should be done at the same time of the day, preferably in the morning, as changes in water hydration from activity and exercise can increase skinfold girth. The procedure for assessing percent body fat using skinfold thickness is given in Figure 9.2. If skinfold calipers* are available to you, you may proceed to assess your percent body fat with the help of your instructor or an experienced technician.

---

* This instrument is available at most colleges and universities. If unavailable, you can purchase an inexpensive, yet reliable skinfold caliper from: Fat Control Inc., P.O. Box 10117, Towson, MD 21204, Phone 301-296-1993.

FIGURE 9.1

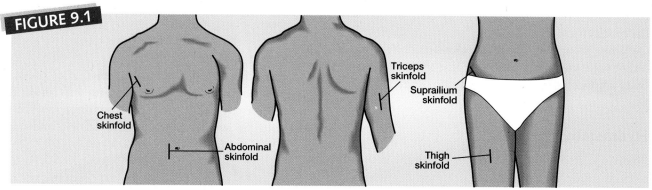

Anatomical landmarks for skinfold measurements.

FIGURE 9.2

Body Fat Assessment According to Skinfold Thickness Technique

1. Select the proper anatomical sites. For men, chest, abdomen, and thigh skinfolds are used. For women, use triceps, suprailium, and thigh skinfolds (*see* Figure 9.1). Take all measurements on the right side of the body with the person standing. The correct anatomical landmarks for skinfolds are:

   Chest: a diagonal fold halfway between the shoulder crease and the nipple.

   Abdomen: a vertical fold taken about one inch to the right of the umbilicus.

   Triceps: a vertical fold on the back of the upper arm, halfway between the shoulder and the elbow.

   Thigh: a vertical fold on the front of the thigh, midway between the knee and hip.

   Suprailium: a diagonal fold above the crest of the ilium (on the side of the hip).

2. Measure each site by grasping a double thickness of skin firmly with the thumb and forefinger, pulling the fold slightly away from the muscular tissue. The calipers are held perpendicular to the fold, and the measurement is taken ½ inch below the finger hold. Each site is measured three times and the values are read to the nearest .1 to .5 mm. The average of the two closest readings is recorded as the final value. The readings should be taken without delay to avoid excessive compression of the skinfold. Releasing and refolding the skinfold is required between readings.

3. When doing pre- and post-assessments, the measurement should be conducted at the same time of day. The best time is early in the morning to avoid water hydration changes resulting from activity or exercise.

4. Percent fat is obtained by adding the three skinfold measurements and looking up the respective values on Table 9.1 for women, Table 9.2 for men under age 40, and Table 9.3 for men over age 40.

   For example, if the skinfold measurements for an 18-year-old female are: (a) triceps = 16, (b) suprailium = 4, and (c) thigh = 30 (total = 50), the percent body fat is 20.6%

Procedure for body fat assessment according to skinfold thickness technique.

TABLE 9.1 Percent Fat Estimates for Women Calculated From Triceps, Suprailium, and Thigh Skinfold Thickness

Sum of 3 Skinfolds	Age to the Last Year								
	Under 22	23 to 27	28 to 32	33 to 37	38 to 42	43 to 47	48 to 52	53 to 57	Over 58
23– 25	9.7	9.9	10.2	10.4	10.7	10.9	11.2	11.4	11.7
26– 28	11.0	11.2	11.5	11.7	12.0	12.3	12.5	12.7	13.0
29– 31	12.3	12.5	12.8	13.0	13.3	13.5	13.8	14.0	14.3
32– 34	13.6	13.8	14.0	14.3	14.5	14.8	15.0	15.3	15.5
35– 37	14.8	15.0	15.3	15.5	15.8	16.0	16.3	16.5	16.8
38– 40	16.0	16.3	16.5	16.7	17.0	17.2	17.5	17.7	18.0
41– 43	17.2	17.4	17.7	17.9	18.2	18.4	18.7	18.9	19.2
44– 46	18.3	18.6	18.8	19.1	19.3	19.6	19.8	20.1	20.3
47– 49	19.5	19.7	20.0	20.2	20.5	20.7	21.0	21.2	21.5
50– 52	20.6	20.8	21.1	21.3	21.6	21.8	22.1	22.3	22.6
53– 55	21.7	21.9	22.1	22.4	22.6	22.9	23.1	23.4	23.6
56– 58	22.7	23.0	23.2	23.4	23.7	23.9	24.2	24.4	24.7
59– 61	23.7	24.0	24.2	24.5	24.7	25.0	25.2	25.5	25.7
62– 64	24.7	25.0	25.2	25.5	25.7	26.0	26.2	26.4	26.7
65– 67	25.7	25.9	26.2	26.4	26.7	26.9	27.2	27.4	27.7
68– 70	26.6	26.9	27.1	27.4	27.6	27.9	28.1	28.4	28.6
71– 73	27.5	27.8	28.0	28.3	28.5	28.8	29.0	29.3	29.5
74– 76	28.4	28.7	28.9	29.2	29.4	29.7	29.9	30.2	30.4
77– 79	29.3	29.5	29.8	30.0	30.3	30.5	30.8	31.0	31.3
80– 82	30.1	30.4	30.6	30.9	31.1	31.4	31.6	31.9	32.1
83– 85	30.9	31.2	31.4	31.7	31.9	32.2	32.4	32.7	32.9
86– 88	31.7	32.0	32.2	32.5	32.7	32.9	33.2	33.4	33.7
89– 91	32.5	32.7	33.0	33.2	33.5	33.7	33.9	34.2	34.4
92– 94	33.2	33.4	33.7	33.9	34.2	34.4	34.7	34.9	35.2
95– 97	33.9	34.1	34.4	34.6	34.9	35.1	35.4	35.6	35.9
98–100	34.6	34.8	35.1	35.3	35.5	35.8	36.0	36.3	36.5
101–103	35.2	35.4	35.7	35.9	36.2	36.4	36.7	36.9	37.2
104–106	35.8	36.1	36.3	36.6	36.8	37.1	37.3	37.5	37.8
107–109	36.4	36.7	36.9	37.1	37.4	37.6	37.9	38.1	38.4
110–112	37.0	37.2	37.5	37.7	38.0	38.2	38.5	38.7	38.9
113–115	37.5	37.8	38.0	38.2	38.5	38.7	39.0	39.2	39.5
116–118	38.0	38.3	38.5	38.8	39.0	39.3	39.5	39.7	40.0
119–121	38.5	38.7	39.0	39.2	39.5	39.7	40.0	40.2	40.5
122–124	39.0	39.2	39.4	39.7	39.9	40.2	40.4	40.7	40.9
125–127	39.4	39.6	39.9	40.1	40.4	40.6	40.9	41.1	41.4
128–130	39.8	40.0	40.3	40.5	40.8	41.0	41.3	41.5	41.8

Body density is calculated based on the generalized equation for predicting body density of women developed by A. S. Jackson, M. L. Pollock, and A. Ward. *Medicine and Science in Sports and Exercise* 12, (1980), pp. 175–182. Percent body fat is determined from the calculated body density using the Siri formula.

TABLE 9.2 Percent Fat Estimates for Men 40 and Under Calculated from Chest, Abdomen, and Thigh Skinfold Thickness

Sum of 3 Skinfolds	Under 19	20 to 22	24 to 25	26 to 28	29 to 31	32 to 34	35 to 37	38 to 40
8– 10	.9	1.3	1.6	2.0	2.3	2.7	3.0	3.3
11– 13	1.9	2.3	2.6	3.0	3.3	3.7	4.0	4.3
14– 16	2.9	3.3	3.6	3.9	4.3	4.6	5.0	5.3
17– 19	3.9	4.2	4.6	4.9	5.3	5.6	6.0	6.3
20– 22	4.8	5.2	5.5	5.9	6.2	6.6	6.9	7.3
23– 25	5.8	6.2	6.5	6.8	7.2	7.5	7.9	8.2
26– 28	6.8	7.1	7.5	7.8	8.1	8.5	8.8	9.2
29– 31	7.7	8.0	8.4	8.7	9.1	9.4	9.8	10.1
32– 34	8.6	9.0	9.3	9.7	10.0	10.4	10.7	11.1
35– 37	9.5	9.9	10.2	10.6	10.9	11.3	11.6	12.0
38– 40	10.5	10.8	11.2	11.5	11.8	12.2	12.5	12.9
41– 43	11.4	11.7	12.1	12.4	12.7	13.1	13.4	13.8
44– 46	12.2	12.6	12.9	13.3	13.6	14.0	14.3	14.7
47– 49	13.1	13.5	13.8	14.2	14.5	14.9	15.2	15.5
50– 52	14.0	14.3	14.7	15.0	15.4	15.7	16.1	16.4
53– 55	14.8	15.2	15.5	15.9	16.2	16.6	16.9	17.3
56– 58	15.7	16.0	16.4	16.7	17.1	17.4	17.8	18.1
59– 61	16.5	16.9	17.2	17.6	17.9	18.3	18.6	19.0
62– 64	17.4	17.7	18.1	18.4	18.8	19.1	19.4	19.8
65– 67	18.2	18.5	18.9	19.2	19.6	19.9	20.3	20.6
68– 70	19.0	19.3	19.7	20.0	20.4	20.7	21.1	21.4
71– 73	19.8	20.1	20.5	20.8	21.2	21.5	21.9	22.2
74– 76	20.6	20.9	21.3	21.6	22.0	22.2	22.7	23.0
77– 79	21.4	21.7	22.1	22.4	22.8	23.1	23.4	23.8
80– 82	22.1	22.5	22.8	23.2	23.5	23.9	24.2	24.6
83– 85	22.9	23.2	23.6	23.9	24.3	24.6	25.0	25.3
86– 88	23.6	24.0	24.3	24.7	25.0	25.4	25.7	26.1
89– 91	24.4	24.7	25.1	25.4	25.8	26.1	26.5	26.8
92– 94	25.1	25.5	25.8	26.2	26.5	26.9	27.2	27.5
95– 97	25.8	26.2	26.5	26.9	27.2	27.6	27.9	28.3
98–100	26.6	26.9	27.3	27.6	27.9	28.3	28.6	29.0
101–103	27.3	27.6	28.0	28.3	28.6	29.0	29.3	29.7
104–106	27.9	28.3	28.6	29.0	29.3	29.7	30.0	30.4
107–109	28.6	29.0	29.3	29.7	30.0	30.4	30.7	31.1
110–112	29.3	29.6	30.0	30.3	30.7	31.0	31.4	31.7
113–115	30.0	30.3	30.7	31.0	31.3	31.7	32.0	32.4
116–118	30.6	31.0	31.3	31.6	32.0	32.3	32.7	33.0
119–121	31.3	31.6	32.0	32.3	32.6	33.0	33.3	33.7
122–124	31.9	32.2	32.6	32.9	33.3	33.6	34.0	34.3
125–127	32.5	32.9	33.2	33.5	33.9	34.2	34.6	34.9
128–130	33.1	33.5	33.8	34.2	34.5	34.9	35.2	35.5

Body density is calculated based on the generalized equation for predicting body density of men developed by A. S. Jackson and M. L. Pollock, *British Journal of Nutrition* 40, (1978) pp. 497–504. Percent body fat is determined from the calculated body density using the Siri formula.

TABLE 9.3 **Percent Fat Estimates for Men Over 40 Calculated from Chest, Abdomen, and Thigh Skinfold Thickness**

Sum of 3 Skinfolds	Age to the Last Year							
	41 to 43	44 to 46	47 to 49	50 to 52	53 to 55	56 to 58	59 to 61	Over 62
8– 10	3.7	4.0	4.4	4.7	5.1	5.4	5.8	6.1
11– 13	4.7	5.0	5.4	5.7	6.1	6.4	6.8	7.1
14– 16	5.7	6.0	6.4	6.7	7.1	7.4	7.8	8.1
17– 19	6.7	7.0	7.4	7.7	8.1	8.4	8.7	9.1
20– 22	7.6	8.0	8.3	8.7	9.0	9.4	9.7	10.1
23– 25	8.6	8.9	9.3	9.6	10.0	10.3	10.7	11.0
26– 28	9.5	9.9	10.2	10.6	10.9	11.3	11.6	12.0
29– 31	10.5	10.8	11.2	11.5	11.9	12.2	12.6	12.9
32– 34	11.4	11.8	12.1	12.4	12.8	13.1	13.5	13.8
35– 37	12.3	12.7	13.0	13.4	13.7	14.1	14.4	14.8
38– 40	13.2	13.6	13.9	14.3	14.6	15.0	15.3	15.7
41– 43	14.1	14.5	14.8	15.2	15.5	15.9	16.2	16.6
44– 46	15.0	15.4	15.7	16.1	16.4	16.8	17.1	17.5
47– 49	15.9	16.2	16.6	16.9	17.3	17.6	18.0	18.3
50– 52	16.8	17.1	17.5	17.8	18.2	18.5	18.8	19.2
53– 55	17.6	18.0	18.3	18.7	19.0	19.4	19.7	20.1
56– 58	18.5	18.8	19.2	19.5	19.9	20.2	20.6	20.9
59– 61	19.3	19.7	20.0	20.4	20.7	21.0	21.4	21.7
62– 64	20.1	20.5	20.8	21.2	21.5	21.9	22.2	22.6
65– 67	21.0	21.3	21.7	22.0	22.4	22.7	23.0	23.4
68– 70	21.8	22.1	22.5	22.8	23.2	23.5	23.9	24.2
71– 73	22.6	22.9	23.3	23.6	24.0	24.3	24.7	25.0
74– 76	23.4	23.7	24.1	24.4	24.8	25.1	25.4	25.8
77– 79	24.1	24.5	24.8	25.2	25.5	25.9	26.2	26.6
80– 82	24.9	25.3	25.6	26.0	26.3	26.6	27.0	27.3
83– 85	25.7	26.0	26.4	26.7	27.1	27.4	27.8	28.1
86– 88	26.4	26.8	27.1	27.5	27.8	28.2	28.5	28.9
89– 91	27.2	27.5	27.9	28.2	28.6	28.9	29.2	29.6
92– 94	27.9	28.2	28.6	28.9	29.3	29.6	30.0	30.3
95– 97	28.6	29.0	29.3	29.7	30.0	30.4	30.7	31.1
98–100	29.3	29.7	30.0	30.4	30.7	31.1	31.4	31.8
101–103	30.0	30.4	30.7	31.1	31.4	31.8	32.1	32.5
104–106	30.7	31.1	31.4	31.8	32.1	32.5	32.8	33.2
107–109	31.4	31.8	32.1	32.4	32.8	33.1	33.5	33.8
110–112	32.1	32.4	32.8	33.1	33.5	33.8	34.2	34.5
113–115	32.7	33.1	33.4	33.8	34.1	34.5	34.8	35.2
116–118	33.4	33.7	34.1	34.4	34.8	35.1	35.5	35.8
119–121	34.0	34.4	34.7	35.1	35.4	35.8	36.1	36.5
122–124	34.7	35.0	35.4	35.7	36.1	36.4	36.7	37.1
125–127	35.3	35.6	36.0	36.3	36.7	37.0	37.4	37.7
128–130	35.9	36.2	36.6	36.9	37.3	37.6	38.0	38.5

Body density is calculated based on the generalized equation for predicting body density of men developed by A. S. Jackson and M. L. Pollock, *British Journal of Nutrition* 40 (1978), pp. 497–504. Percent body fat is determined from the calculated body density using the Siri formula.

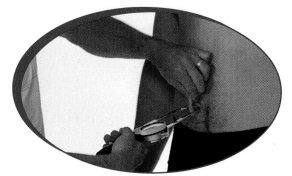

Skinfold thickness technique for body composition assessment.

Girth Measurements

A simpler method to determine body fat is by measuring circumferences at various body sites. All this technique requires is a standard measuring tape, and good accuracy can be achieved with little practice. The limitation is that it may not be valid for athletic individuals (men or women) who participate actively in strenuous physical activity or people who can be classified visually as thin or obese.

The required procedure for girth measurements is given in Figure 9.3. Measurements for women

---

FIGURE 9.3

Body Fat Assessment According to Girth Measurements

Girth Measurements for Women*

1. Using a regular tape measure, determine the following girth measurements in centimeters (cm):

   Upper Arm: Take the measure halfway between the shoulder and the elbow.

   Hip: Measure at the point of largest circumference.

   Wrist: Take the girth in front of the bones where the wrist bends.

2. Obtain the person's age.

3. Using Table 9.4, find the girth measurement for each site and age in the lefthand columns. Look up the constant values in the righthand columns. These values will allow you to derive body density (BD) by substituting the constants in the following formula:

   $$BD = A - B - C + D$$

4. Using the derived body density, calculate percent body fat (%F) according to the following equation:

   $$\%F = (495 \div BD) - 450**$$

   Example: Jane is 20 years old, and the following girth measurements were taken: biceps = 27 cm, hip = 99.5 cm, wrist = 15.4 cm.

Data	Constant
Upper Arm = 27 cm	A = 1.0813
Age = 20	B = .0102
Hip = 99.5 cm	C = .1206
Wrist = 15.4 cm	D = .0971

   $$BD = A - B - C + D$$
   $$BD = 1.0813 - .0102 - .1206 + .0971 = 1.0476$$
   $$\%F = (495 \div BD) - 450$$
   $$\%F = (495 \div 1.0476) - 450 = 22.5$$

Girth Measurements for Men*

1. Using a regular tape measure, determine the following girth measurements in inches (the men's measurements are taken in inches as contrasted with centimeters for women):

   Waist: Measure at the umbilicus (belly button).

   Wrist: Measure in front of the bones where the wrist bends.

2. Subtract the wrist from the waist measurement.

3. Obtain the person's weight in pounds.

4. Look up the percent body fat (%F) in Table 9.5 by using the difference obtained in step 2 above and the person's body weight.

   Example: John weighs 160 pounds, and his waist and wrist girth measurements are 36.5 and 7.5 inches, respectively.

   Waist girth = 36.5 inches
   Wrist girth = 7.5 inches
   Difference = 29.0 inches
   Body weight = 160.0 lbs.
   %F = 22

* Reproduced by permission from R. B. Lambson, "Generalized Body Density Prediction Equations for Women Using Simple Anthropometric Measurements." Unpublished doctoral dissertation, Brigham Young University, August 1987.

** From W. E. Siri, Body Composition From Fluid Spaces and Density, (Berkeley: University of California, Donner Laboratory of Medical Physics, 1956).

*** Table 3.5 reproduced by permission from A. G. Fisher, and P. E. Allsen, Jogging (Dubuque, IA: Wm. C. Brown, 1987). This table was developed according to the generalized body composition equation for men using simple measurement techniques by K. W. Penrouse, A. G Nelson, and A. G. Fisher, Medicine and Science in Sports and Exercise 17:2 (1985) p. 189. © American College of Sports Medicine 1985.

Procedure for body fat assessment according to girth measurements.

TABLE 9.4 Conversion Constants from Girth Measurements to Calculate Body Density for Women

Upper Arm (cm)	Constant A	Age	Constant B	Hip (cm)	Constant C	Hip (cm)	Constant C	Wrist (cm)	Constant D
20.5	1.0966	17	.0086	79	.0957	114.5	.1388	13.0	.0819
21	1.0954	18	.0091	79.5	.0963	115	.1394	13.2	.0832
21.5	1.0942	19	.0096	80	.0970	115.5	.1400	13.4	.0845
22	1.0930	20	.0102	80.5	.0976	116	.1406	13.6	.0857
22.5	1.0919	21	.0107	81	.0982	116.5	.1412	13.8	.0807
23	1.0907	22	.0112	81.5	.0988	117	.1418	14.0	.0882
23.5	1.0895	23	.0117	82	.0994	117.5	.1424	14.2	.0895
24	1.0883	24	.0122	82.5	.1000	118	.1430	14.4	.0908
24.5	1.0871	25	.0127	83	.1006	118.5	.1436	14.6	.0920
25	1.0860	26	.0132	83.5	.1012	119	.1442	14.8	.0933
25.5	1.0848	27	.0137	84	.1018	119.5	.1448	15.0	.0946
26	1.0836	28	.0142	84.5	.1024	120	.1454	15.2	.0958
26.5	1.0824	29	.0147	85	.1030	120.5	.1460	15.4	.0971
27	1.0813	30	.0152	85.5	.1036	121	.1466	15.6	.0983
27.5	1.0801	31	.0157	86	.1042	121.5	.1472	15.8	.0996
28	1.0789	32	.0162	86.5	.1048	122	.1479	16.0	.1009
28.5	1.0777	33	.0168	87	.1054	122.5	.1485	16.2	.1021
29	1.0775	34	.0173	87.5	.1060	123	.1491	16.4	.1034
29.5	1.0754	35	.0178	88	.1066	123.5	.1497	16.6	.1046
30	1.0742	36	.0183	88.5	.1072	124	.1503	16.8	.1059
30.5	1.0730	37	.0188	89	.1079	124.5	.1509	17.0	.1072
31	1.0718	38	.0193	89.5	.1085	125	.1515	17.2	.1084
31.5	1.0707	39	.0198	90	.1091	125.5	.1521	17.4	.1097
32	1.0695	40	.0203	90.5	.1097	126	.1527	17.6	.1109
32.5	1.0683	41	.0208	91	.1103	126.5	.1533	17.8	.1122
33	1.0671	42	.0213	91.5	.1109	127	.1539	18.0	.1135
33.5	1.0666	43	.0218	92	.1115	127.5	.1545	18.2	.1147
34	1.0648	44	.0223	92.5	.1121	128	.1551	18.4	.1160
34.5	1.0636	45	.0228	93	.1127	128.5	.1558	18.6	.1172
35	1.0624	46	.0234	93.5	.1133	129	.1563		
35.5	1.0612	47	.0239	94	.1139	129.5	.1569		
36	1.0601	48	.0244	94.5	.1145	130	.1575		
36.5	1.0589	49	.0249	95	.1151	130.5	.1581		
37	1.0577	50	.0254	95.5	.1157	131	.1587		
37.5	1.0565	51	.0259	96	.1163	131.5	.1593		
38	1.0554	52	.0264	96.5	.1169	132	.1600		
38.5	1.0542	53	.0269	97	.1176	132.5	.1606		
39	1.0530	54	.0274	97.5	.1182	133	.1612		
39.5	1.0518	55	.0279	98	.1188	133.5	.1618		
40	1.0506	56	.0284	98.5	.1194	134	.1624		
40.5	1.0495	57	.0289	99	.1200	134.5	.1630		
41	1.0483	58	.0294	99.5	.1206	135	.1636		
41.5	1.0471	59	.0300	100	.1212	135.5	.1642		
42	1.0459	60	.0305	100.5	.1218	136	.1648		
42.5	1.0448	61	.0310	101	.1224	136.5	.1654		
43	1.0434	62	.0315	101.5	.1230	137	.1660		

(Continued)

TABLE 9.4 Conversion Constants from Girth Measurements to Calculate Body Density for Women (continued)

Upper Arm (cm)	Constant A	Age	Constant B	Hip (cm)	Constant C	Hip (cm)	Constant C	Wrist (cm)	Constant D
43.5	1.0424	63	.0320	102	.1236	137.5	.1666		
44	1.0412	64	.0325	102.5	.1242	138	.1672		
		65	.0330	103	.1248	138.5	.1678		
		66	.0335	103.5	.1254	139	.1685		
		67	.0340	104	.1260	139.5	.1691		
		68	.0345	104.5	.1266	140	.1697		
		69	.0350	105	.1272	140.5	.1703		
		70	.0355	105.5	.1278	141	.1709		
		71	.0360	106	.1285	141.5	.1715		
		72	.0366	106.5	.1291	142	.1721		
		73	.0371	107	.1297	142.5	.1728		
		74	.0376	107.5	.1303	143	.1733		
		75	.0381	108	.1309	143.5	.1739		
				108.5	.1315	144	.1745		
				109	.1321	144.5	.1751		
				109.5	.1327	145	.1757		
				110	.1333	145.5	.1763		
				110.5	.1339	146	.1769		
				111	.1345	146.5	.1775		
				111.5	.1351	147	.1781		
				112	.1357	147.5	.1787		
				112.5	.1363	148	.1794		
				113	.1369	148.5	.1800		
				113.5	.1375	149	.1806		
				114	.1382	149.5	.1812		
						150	.1818		

include the upper arm, hip, and wrist; for men, the waist and wrist.

Bioelectrical Impedance

The bioelectrical impedance technique is much simpler to administer, but it does require costly equipment. In this technique, the individual is hooked up to a machine and a weak electrical current (totally painless) is run through the body to analyze body composition (body fat, lean body mass, and body water). The technique is based on the principle that fat tissue is not as good a conductor of an electrical current as lean tissue is. The easier the conductance, the leaner the individual.

The accuracy of current equations used in estimating percent body fat with this technique is still questionable. More research is required before the equations approach the accuracy of hydrostatic weighing, skinfolds, or girth measurements.

An advantage of bioelectrical impedance is that results are highly reproducible. Unlike other techniques, in which experienced technicians are necessary to obtain valid results, almost anyone can administer bioelectrical impedance. And, although the test results may not be completely accurate, this instrument is valuable in assessing body composition changes over time.

If this instrument or some other type of equipment for body composition assessment is available to you, you can use it to determine your percent body fat. You may want to compare the results with other techniques. Following all manufacturer's instructions will ensure the best possible result.

TABLE 9.5　Estimated Percent Body Fat for Men Obtained from Waist Minus Wrist Girth Measurements (Inches) and Body Weight

Weight	22	22.5	23	23.5	24	24.5	25	25.5	26	26.5	27	27.5	28	28.5	29	29.5	30	30.5	31	31.5	32	32.5	33	33.5	34	34.5	35	35.5	36	36.5	37	37.5	38	38.5	39	39.5	40	40.5	41	41.5	42	42.5	43	43.5	44	44.5	45	45.5	46	46.5	47	47.5	48	48.5	49	49.5	50
120	4	6	8	10	12	14	16	18	20	21	23	25	27	29	31	33	35	37	39	41	43	45	47	49	50	52	54	56	58																											
125	4	6	7	9	11	13	15	17	19	20	22	24	26	28	30	32	33	35	37	39	41	43	45	46	48	50	52	54	56	58																										
130	3	5	7	9	11	13	15	16	18	20	22	23	25	27	29	31	32	34	36	38	39	41	43	45	46	48	50	52	53	55	57																									
135	3	5	7	8	10	12	14	16	18	19	21	23	25	26	28	30	32	33	35	37	38	40	42	44	45	47	49	51	52	54	55	56																							
140	3	5	6	8	10	12	14	15	17	19	21	22	24	26	28	29	31	33	34	36	38	39	41	43	44	46	48	49	51	53	54	55	56																						
145	3	4	6	8	10	11	13	15	17	18	20	22	23	25	27	28	30	32	33	35	37	38	40	42	43	45	47	48	50	52	53	54	55	55																					
150	2	4	6	7	9	11	13	14	16	18	19	21	23	24	26	27	29	31	32	34	35	37	39	40	41	43	44	46	48	49	50	52	53	55	55																			
155	2	4	5	7	9	10	12	14	16	17	19	20	22	24	25	27	29	30	32	33	35	37	38	40	41	43	44	46	47	49	50	52	53	55	55																		
160	2	4	5	7	8	10	12	13	15	17	18	20	22	23	25	26	28	30	31	33	34	36	38	39	41	42	44	45	47	48	50	51	53	54	54																		
165	2	3	5	6	8	10	11	13	15	16	18	19	21	23	24	26	27	29	31	32	34	35	37	39	40	41	43	44	46	47	48	50	52	54	54																	
170	2	3	4	6	7	9	11	13	14	16	17	19	21	22	24	25	27	29	30	32	33	35	36	38	40	41	43	44	45	47	48	50	51	52	54	54																
175	2	3	4	6	7	9	10	12	14	15	17	18	20	22	23	25	26	28	29	31	32	34	35	37	39	40	41	43	44	45	47	48	50	51	52	53																
180	3	4	5	7	8	10	12	13	14	16	18	19	21	22	24	25	27	28	30	31	32	34	35	37	38	40	41	43	44	45	47	48	49	50	52	53	53															
185	3	4	5	6	8	9	11	13	14	15	17	18	20	21	23	24	25	27	28	30	31	33	34	35	37	38	40	41	43	44	45	46	48	49	50	51	53															
190	2	4	5	6	8	9	11	12	14	15	16	18	19	21	22	24	25	26	28	29	31	32	33	35	36	38	39	40	42	43	44	46	47	48	49	50	51	52														
195	2	3	5	6	7	9	11	12	13	15	16	18	19	20	22	23	25	26	27	29	30	31	33	34	35	37	38	40	41	42	44	45	46	48	49	50	51	52														
200	2	3	4	6	7	8	10	11	12	14	15	17	18	19	21	22	24	25	26	28	29	30	31	32	33	35	36	37	38	39	40	41	43	44	45	46	47	48	49	50	51	52												
205	2	3	4	5	7	8	10	11	12	14	15	16	18	19	20	22	23	24	25	27	28	29	30	32	33	34	36	37	38	39	41	42	43	44	46	47	48	49	51	52													
210	2	3	4	5	6	8	9	11	12	13	14	16	17	18	20	21	22	24	25	26	27	29	30	31	32	34	35	36	38	39	40	41	43	44	45	46	47	49	50	51													
215	2	3	4	5	6	8	9	10	11	13	14	15	17	18	19	20	22	23	24	25	27	28	29	30	32	33	34	35	36	38	39	40	42	43	44	45	46	48	49	50	51												
220	2	3	3	5	6	7	8	10	11	12	13	15	16	17	18	20	21	22	23	24	26	27	28	29	30	32	33	34	35	37	38	39	40	41	42	44	45	46	47	48	49	50	51										
225	2	3	3	4	6	7	8	9	10	12	13	14	15	16	18	19	20	21	22	24	25	26	27	28	30	31	32	33	34	35	36	37	38	40	41	42	43	44	45	46	47	48	49	50	51								
230	2	3	3	4	5	7	8	9	10	11	12	14	15	16	17	18	20	21	22	23	24	25	26	28	29	30	31	32	33	34	35	36	37	38	39	40	41	42	43	44	45	46	47	48	49	50	51						
235	2	3	3	4	5	6	7	9	10	11	12	13	14	16	17	18	19	20	21	22	23	25	26	27	28	29	30	31	32	33	34	35	36	37	38	39	40	41	42	43	44	45	46	47	48	49	50	51					
240	2	3	3	4	5	6	7	8	9	11	12	13	14	15	16	17	18	20	21	22	23	24	25	26	27	28	29	30	31	32	33	34	35	36	37	38	39	40	41	42	43	44	45	46	47	48	50						
245	2	3	3	4	5	6	7	8	9	10	11	12	13	15	16	17	18	19	20	21	22	23	24	25	26	27	28	29	30	31	32	33	34	35	36	37	38	39	40	41	42	43	44	45	46	47	48	49	50				
250	2	3	3	4	4	6	7	8	9	10	11	12	13	14	15	16	17	18	19	21	22	23	24	25	26	27	28	29	30	31	31	32	33	34	35	36	37	38	39	40	41	42	43	44	45	46	47	48	49	50			
255	2	3	3	4	4	5	6	7	8	9	10	11	12	13	14	15	16	17	18	20	21	22	23	24	25	26	27	28	29	30	31	32	33	34	35	36	37	38	39	40	41	42	43	44	44	45	46	47	48	49	50		
260	2	3	3	4	4	5	6	7	8	9	10	11	12	13	14	15	16	17	18	19	20	21	22	23	24	25	26	27	28	29	30	31	32	33	34	35	36	37	38	39	40	41	42	43	44	45	46	47	48	49	50		
265	2	3	3	4	4	5	6	7	7	8	9	11	12	13	14	15	16	16	17	18	19	20	21	22	23	24	25	26	27	28	29	30	31	32	33	34	35	36	37	38	39	40	41	42	43	44	45	46	47	48	49		
270	2	3	3	4	4	5	6	6	7	8	9	10	11	12	13	14	15	16	17	18	19	20	21	22	23	24	25	26	27	28	29	30	31	32	33	34	35	36	37	37	38	39	40	41	42	43	44	45	46	47	48		
275	2	3	3	4	4	5	6	6	7	8	9	10	11	12	13	14	14	15	16	17	18	19	20	21	22	23	24	24	25	26	27	28	29	30	31	32	33	34	35	36	37	38	39	40	41	42	43	44	45	46	47		
280	2	3	3	4	4	5	6	6	7	8	9	10	11	11	12	13	14	15	16	17	18	19	20	21	21	22	23	24	25	26	27	28	29	30	31	32	33	34	35	36	37	38	39	40	41	42	43	44	45	45	46		
285	2	3	3	4	4	5	6	6	7	8	9	9	10	11	12	13	14	15	16	16	17	18	19	20	21	22	23	24	25	26	26	27	28	29	30	31	32	33	34	35	36	37	38	39	40	41	42	43	43	44	45		
290	2	3	3	4	4	5	6	6	7	7	8	9	10	11	12	13	14	14	15	16	17	18	19	20	21	22	23	23	24	25	26	27	28	29	30	31	32	33	34	35	36	37	38	39	40	41	41	42	43	44			
295	2	3	3	4	4	5	5	6	7	7	8	9	10	11	12	12	13	14	15	16	17	18	19	20	20	21	22	23	24	25	26	27	28	29	29	30	31	32	33	34	35	36	37	38	39	40	41	42	43				
300	2	3	3	4	4	5	5	6	7	7	8	9	10	11	11	12	13	14	15	16	17	18	18	19	20	21	22	23	24	25	26	27	28	28	29	30	31	32	33	34	35	36	37	38	39	40	41	42	43				

WAIST-TO-HIP RATIO

Scientific evidence suggests that the way people store fat affects the risk for disease. Some individuals tend to store fat in the abdominal area (called the "apple" shape). Others store it primarily around the hips and thighs (gluteal femoral fat or "pear" shape).

Obese individuals with a lot of abdominal fat clearly are at higher risk for coronary heart disease, congestive heart failure, hypertension, adult-onset diabetes (Type II), and strokes than are obese people with similar amounts of total body fat that is stored primarily in the hips and thighs. Relatively new evidence also indicates that among individuals with high abdominal fat, those whose fat deposits are around internal organs (visceral fat) are at even greater risk for disease than those whose abdominal fat is primarily beneath the skin (subcutaneous fat).[1]

Because of the higher risk for disease in individuals who tend to store a lot of fat in the abdominal area, as contrasted with the hips and thighs, a waist-to-hip ratio test was designed by a panel of scientists appointed by the National Academy of Sciences and the Dietary Guidelines Advisory Council for the U.S. Departments of Agriculture and Health and Human Services. The waist measurement is taken at the point of smallest circumference, and the hip measurement is taken at the point of greatest circumference.

The waist-to-hip ratio differentiates the "apples" from the "pears." Men tend to be apples, and women tend to be pears. The panel recommends that men need to lose weight if the waist-to-hip ratio is 1.0 or higher. Women need to lose weight if the ratio is .85 or higher (see Table 9.6). More conservative estimates indicate that the risk starts to increase when the ratio exceeds .95 and .80 for men and women, respectively. For example, the waist-to-hip ratio for a man with a 40-inch waist and a 38-inch hip would be 1.05 (40 ÷ 38). This ratio may indicate higher risk for disease.

TABLE 9.6
Disease Risk According to Waist-to-Hip Ratio

Waist-to-Hip Ratio		
Men	Women	Disease Risk
≤0.95	≤0.80	Very Low
0.96–0.99	0.81–0.84	Low
≥1.00	≥0.85	High

BODY MASS INDEX

Another technique scientists use to determine thinness and excessive fatness is the Body Mass Index (BMI). This index incorporates height and weight to estimate critical fat values at which the risk for disease increases.

BMI is calculated by multiplying your weight in pounds by 705, dividing this figure by your height in inches, and then dividing by the same height again (or weight in kilograms divided by the square of the height in meters). For example, the BMI for an individual who weighs 172 pounds and is 67 inches tall would be 27 (172 × 705 ÷ 67 ÷ 67).

According to BMI, the lowest risk for chronic disease is in the 22 to 25 range (see Table 9.7). Individuals are classified as overweight between 25 and 30. BMIs above 30 are defined as obesity and below 20 as underweight.

TABLE 9.7
Disease Risk According to Body Mass Index (BMI)

BMI	Disease Risk
<20.00	Moderate to Very High
20.00 to 21.99	Low
22.00 to 24.99	Very Low
25.00 to 29.99	Low
30.00 to 34.99	Moderate
35.00 to 39.99	High
≥40.00	Very High

BMI is a useful tool to screen the general population, but, similar to height/weight charts, it fails to differentiate fat from lean body mass or where most of the fat is located (see waist-to-hip ratio). Using BMI, athletes with a large amount of muscle mass (body builders, football players) easily can fall in the moderate or even high-risk categories. Therefore, body composition and waist-to-hip ratios are better procedures to determine health risk and recommended body weight.

DETERMINING RECOMMENDED BODY WEIGHT

After finding out your percent body fat, you can determine your current body composition classification according to Table 9.8. In this table you will find the

TABLE 9.8   **Body Composition Classification According to Percent Body Fat**

Age	Excellent		Good		Moderate	Overweight	Significantly Overweight
MEN							
≤19	12.0		12.1–17.0		17.1–22.0	22.1–27.0	≥ 27.1
20–29	13.0		13.1–18.0		18.1–23.0	23.1–28.0	≥ 28.1
30–39	14.0		14.1–19.0		19.1–24.0	24.1–29.0	≥ 29.1
40–49	15.0		15.1–20.0		20.1–25.0	25.1–30.0	≥ 30.1
≥ 50	16.0		16.1–21.5		21.1–26.0	26.1–31.0	≥ 31.1
WOMEN							
Age	Excellent		Good		Moderate	Overweight	Significantly Overweight
≤19	17.0		17.1–22.0		22.1–27.0	27.1–32.0	≥ 32.1
20–29	18.0		18.1–23.0		23.1–28.0	28.1–33.0	≥ 33.1
30–39	19.0		19.1–24.0		24.1–29.0	29.1–34.0	≥ 34.1
40–49	20.0		20.1–25.0		25.1–30.0	30.1–35.0	≥ 35.1
≥ 50	21.0		21.1–26.5		26.1–31.0	31.1–36.0	≥ 36.1

  ■ High physical fitness standard   ■ Health fitness standard

health fitness and the high physical fitness percent fat standards.

For example, the recommended health fitness fat percentage for a 20-year-old female is 28% or less. The health fitness standard is established at the point at which there seems to be no harm to health in terms of percent body fat. A high physical fitness range for this same woman would be between 18% and 23%.

The high physical fitness standard does not mean you cannot be somewhat below this number. Many highly trained male athletes are as low as 3%, and some female distance runners have been measured at 6% body fat (which may not be healthy).

Although people generally agree that the mortality rate is greater for obese people, some evidence indicates that the same is true for underweight people. "Underweight" and "thin" do not necessarily mean the same thing. A healthy thin person has total body fat around the high fitness percentage, whereas an underweight person has extremely low body fat, even to the point of compromising the essential fat.

The 3% essential fat for men and 12% for women seem to be the lower limits for people to maintain good health. Below these percentages normal physiologic functions can be seriously impaired. Some experts point out that a little storage fat (over the essential fat) is better than none at all.

As a result, the health and high fitness standards for percent fat in Table 9.8 are set higher than the minimum essential fat requirements, at a point beneficial to optimal health and well-being. Finally, because lean tissue decreases with age, one extra percentage point is allowed for every additional decade of life.

Your recommended body weight is computed based on the selected health or high fitness fat percentage for your age and gender. Your decision to select a "desired" fat percentage should be based on your current percent body fat and your personal health/fitness objectives. To compute your own recommended body weight:

1. Determine the pounds of body weight in fat (FW). Multiply body weight (BW) by the current percent fat (%F) expressed in decimal form (FW = BW × %F).

2. Determine lean body mass (LBM) by subtracting the weight in fat from the total body weight (LBM = BW − FW). (Anything that is not fat must be part of the lean component.)

3. Select a desired body fat percentage (DFP) based on the health or high fitness standards given in Table 9.8.

4. Compute recommended body weight (RBW) according to the formula: RBW = LBM ÷ (1.0 − DFP).

As an example of these computations, a 19-year-old female who weighs 160 pounds and is 30% fat would like to know what her recommended body weight would be at 22%:

Gender: female

Age: 19

BW: 160 lbs.

%F: 30% (.30 in decimal form)

1. FW = BW × %F
   FW = 160 × .30 = 48 lbs.

2. LBM = BW − FW
   LBM = 160 − 48 = 112 lbs.

3. DFP: 22% (.22 in decimal form)

4. RBW = LBM ÷ (1.0 − DFP)
   RBW = 112 ÷ (1.0 − .22)
   RBW = 112 ÷ (.78) = 143.6 lbs.

In Assessments 9-1 and 9-2 you will have the opportunity to determine your own body composition, recommended body weight, and disease risk according to waist-to-hip ratio and BMI.

Other than hydrostatic weighing, skinfold thickness seems to be the most practical and valid technique to estimate body fat. If skinfold calipers are available, use this technique to assess percent body fat. If calipers are unavailable, you can estimate your percent fat according to the girth measurements technique or another technique available to you. (You may wish to use several techniques and compare the results.)

IMPORTANCE OF REGULAR BODY COMPOSITION ASSESSMENT

Children do not start with a weight problem. Although a small group struggles with weight throughout life, most are not overweight when they reach age 20 or so.

Current trends indicate that starting at age 25, the average man and woman in the United States gains 1 pound of weight per year. Thus, by age 65, the average American will have gained 40 pounds of weight. Because of the typical reduction in physical activity in our society, however, the average person also loses a half a pound of lean tissue each year. Therefore, over this span of 40 years, there has been an actual fat gain of 60 pounds accompanied by a 20-pound loss of lean body mass[2] (see Figure 9.4).

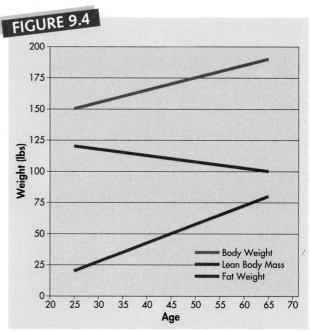

FIGURE 9.4

Typical body composition changes for adults in the United States.

These changes cannot be detected unless body composition is assessed periodically.

If you are on a diet/exercise program, you should repeat the computations about once a month to monitor changes in body composition. This is important because lean body mass is affected by weight reduction programs and amount of physical activity. As lean body mass changes, so will your recommended body weight. To make valid comparisons, the same technique should be used between pre- and post-assessments.

Changes in body composition resulting from a weight control/exercise program were illustrated in a co-ed aerobics course taught during a 6-week summer term. Students participated in aerobic dance routines four times a week, 60 minutes each time. On the first and last days of class, several physiological parameters, including body composition, were assessed. Students also were given information on diet and nutrition, and they basically followed their own weight control program.

At the end of the 6 weeks, the average weight loss for the entire class was 3 pounds (see Figure 9.5). Because body composition was assessed, however, class members were surprised to find that the average fat loss was actually 6 pounds, accompanied by a 3-pound increase in lean body mass.

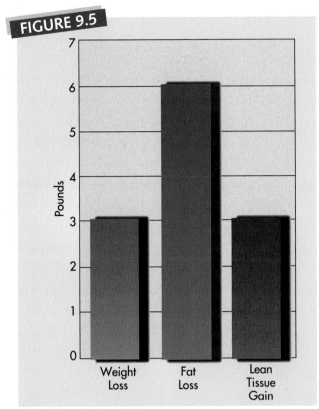

FIGURE 9.5

Effects of a 6-week aerobics program on body composition.

When dieting, body composition should be reassessed periodically because of the effects of negative caloric balance on lean body mass. As is discussed in Chapter 10, dieting alone does decrease lean body mass. This lean body mass loss can be reduced or eliminated by combining a sensible diet with physical exercise.

NOTES

1. *Fat Distribution During Growth and Later Health Outcomes*, edited by C. Bouchard, and F. E. Johnson (New York: Alan R. Liss, 1988).
2. "Exercise and Weight Control: Myths, Misconceptions, and Quackery," lecture given by J.H. Wilmore at annual meeting of American College of Sports Medicine, Indianapolis, June 1994.

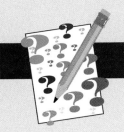

ASSESSMENT 9-1

Body Composition Assessment
and Recommended Body Weight Determination

Name _____ Date _____ Grade _____

Instructor _____ Course _____ Section _____

NECESSARY LAB EQUIPMENT: Skinfold calipers and standard measuring tapes.

OBJECTIVE: To assess percent body fat using skinfold thickness and/or girth measurements and to determine recommended body weight based on percent body fat.

INSTRUCTIONS: If skinfold calipers are available, use the skinfold thickness technique to assess your percent body fat (see Figure 9.2, page 242). If calipers are unavailable, estimate the percent fat according to the girth measurements technique. You may wish to use both techniques and compare the results. Compute your recommended body weight according to your current and recommended percent body fat guidelines provided in Table 9.8, page 251).

I. Percent Body Fat According to Skinfold Thickness

Men		Women	
Chest (mm):	_____	Triceps (mm):	_____
Abdomen (mm):	_____	Suprailium (mm):	_____
Thigh (mm):	_____	Thigh (mm):	_____
Total (mm):	_____	Total (mm):	_____
Percent Fat:	_____	Percent Fat:	_____

II. Percent Fat According to Girth Measurements

Men

Waist (inches):	_____
Wrist (inches):	_____
Difference:	_____
Body Weight:	_____
Percent Fat:	_____

Women

Upper Arm (cm):	_____	Constant A =	_____
Age:	_____	Constant B =	_____
Hip (cm):	_____	Constant C =	_____
Wrist (cm):	_____	Constant D =	_____

BD* = A − B − C + D

BD = _____ − _____ − _____ + _____ = _____

Percent Fat = (495 ÷ BD) − 450 = (495 ÷ _____) − 450 = _____

*Body density

III. Recommended Body Weight Determination

A. Body Weight (BW): _____

B. Current Percent Fat (%F)**: _____

C. Fat Weight (FW) = BW × %F

FW = _____ × _____ = _____

D. Lean Body Mass (LBM) = BW − FW = _____ − _____ = _____

E. Age: _____

F. Desired Fat Percent (DFP − *see* Table 3.7): _____

G. Recommended Body Weight (RBW) = LBM ÷ (1.0 − DFP**)

RBW = _____ ÷ (1.0 − _____) = _____

**Express percentages in decimal form (e.g., 25% = .25)

Weight and Health: Disease Risk Assessment

Name _____ Date _____ Grade _____

Instructor _____ Course _____ Section _____

NECESSARY LAB EQUIPMENT: Scale and standard measuring tapes.

OBJECTIVE: Determine disease risk based on the waist-to-hip ratio and the body mass index (BMI)

INSTRUCTIONS: Determine your height, waist, and hip measurements in inches. Record your body weight in pounds. Compute your waist-to-hip ratio and BMI as indicated below.

I. Waist-to-Hip Ratio

Waist (inches): _____

Hip (inches): _____

Ratio (waist ÷ hip): _____ Disease Risk: _____

Recommended Standards

Waist-to-Hip Ratio		Disease Risk
Men	**Women**	**Disease Risk**
<.95	<.80	Very Low
.96–.99	.81–.84	Low
>1.0	>.85	High

II. Body Mass Index

Weight (pounds): _____

Height (inches): _____

BMI = Weight × 705 ÷ Height 4 Height

BMI = _____ × 705 ÷ _____ ÷ _____

BMI = _____ Disease Risk: _____

Recommended Standards

BMI	Disease Risk
< 20.00	Moderate to Very High
20.00 to 21.99	Low
22.00 to 24.99	Very Low
25.00 to 29.99	Low
30.00 to 34.99	Moderate
35.00 to 39.99	High
≥40.00	Very High

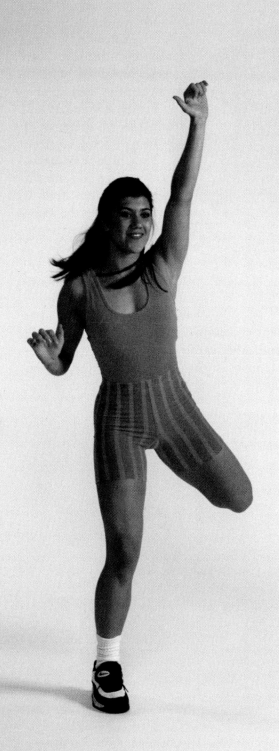

Weight Management, Eating Disorders, and Wellness

OBJECTIVES

- Differentiate overweight and obesity.
- Become familiar with eating disorders and their associated medical problems and behavior patterns.
- Understand the physiology of weight loss, including setpoint theory and the effects of diet on basal metabolic rate.
- Learn about fad diets and other myths and fallacies regarding weight control.
- Recognize the role of a lifetime exercise program in a successful weight loss and maintenance program.
- Learn how to implement a physiologically sound weight reduction and weight maintenance program.
- Learn behavior modification techniques that help a person adhere to a lifetime weight maintenance program.

Achieving and maintaining recommended body weight is a major objective of a physical fitness program. The assessment of recommended body weight was discussed in Chapter 9. Next to poor cardiorespiratory fitness, excessive body fat is the most common problem in fitness and wellness assessments.

Two terms used in reference to people who weigh more than recommended are overweight and obesity. **Overweight** indicates an excess amount of weight against a given standard such as height or recommended percent body fat. **Obesity** is characterized by an excessively high amount of body fat in relation to lean body mass. Obesity levels are established at a point at which the excess body fat can lead to health problems.

Extreme thinness also can lead to life-threatening medical conditions. About 14% of the American population is underweight. Social pressures to attain model-like thinness have contributed to a gradual increase in the number of people who develop eating disorders. Anorexia and bulimia are discussed later in this chapter.

Obesity is a health hazard of epidemic proportions among physically inactive individuals with unhealthy eating practices.

strokes, thromboembolic disease, osteoarthritis, varicose veins, and intermittent claudication.

Data from the Aerobics Research Institute in Dallas confirm that as body fat increases, so do blood cholesterol and triglycerides. As illustrated in Figure 10.1, however, the data also show that the higher the fitness level, the lower the mortality rate, regardless of body weight.[1] This finding is of significance, because aerobically fit/obese men had a lower risk of death than unfit men of normal weight and as low a risk of death as fit men of normal weight. Thus, a lack of physical activity and not the weight problem itself is more likely to be the cause of premature death rates associated with obesity.

Granted, people have genetic differences. Some moderately overweight people do have health problems, but this is not the case for most. Overweight people with diabetes and other cardiovascular risk factors (elevated blood lipids, high blood pressure, physical inactivity, and poor eating habits) benefit from weight

OVERWEIGHT VERSUS OBESITY

Approximately 65 million Americans are overweight or consider themselves to be overweight. Of these, 30 million are obese. About 50% of all women and 25% of all men are on a diet at any given moment. People spend about $40 billion yearly attempting to lose weight. More than $10 billion goes to memberships in weight-reduction centers and another $30 billion to diet food sales.

Most overweight people (an excess of 10 to 20 pounds) are not obese. Although research findings are inconsistent, the health consequences of excessive body weight appear to be exaggerated and may apply primarily to severely overweight individuals.

Obesity has been associated with several serious health problems and is thought to account for 15% to 20% of the mortality rate in the United States each year. Obesity has been viewed as a major risk factor for diseases of the cardiovascular system, including coronary heart disease, hypertension, congestive heart failure, high levels of blood lipids, atherosclerosis,

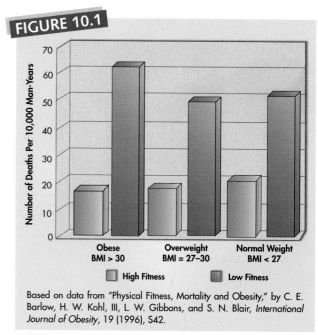

FIGURE 10.1

Based on data from "Physical Fitness, Mortality and Obesity," by C. E. Barlow, H. W. Kohl, III, L. W. Gibbons, and S. N. Blair, *International Journal of Obesity*, 19 (1996), S42.

Relationship between body weight, fitness, and mortality.

loss. Overweight people who otherwise are apparently healthy and are physically active, exercise regularly, and eat a healthy diet do not appear to be at greater risk for early death.

Nonetheless, recommended body composition is a primary objective of overall physical fitness and enhanced quality of life. Individuals at recommended body weight are able to participate in a wide variety of moderate to vigorous activities without functional limitations. These people have the freedom to enjoy most of life's recreational activities to their fullest potential. Excessive body weight does not allow an individual to enjoy vigorous lifetime activities such as basketball, soccer, racquetball, surfing, mountain cycling, and mountain climbing. High fitness and recommended body weight give a person a degree of independence throughout life that the great majority of people in developed nations no longer enjoy.

Recommended body weight is best determined through the assessment of body composition.

Tolerable Weight

Many people want to lose weight so they will look better. That's a noteworthy goal. The problem, however, is that they have a distorted image of what they would really look like if they were to reduce to what they think is their ideal weight. Hereditary factors play a big role, and only a small fraction of the population has the genes for a "perfect body."

As people set their own target weight, they should be realistic. Attaining the excellent percent body fat figure in Chapter 9, Table 9.8, is extremely difficult for some. It is even more difficult to maintain, unless they are willing to make a commitment to a vigorous lifetime exercise program and permanent dietary changes. Few people are willing to do that. The moderate percent body fat category is more realistic for many people.

Are you happy with your weight? Part of enjoying a better quality of life is being happy with yourself. If you are not, you either need to do something about it or learn to live with it!

If you are above the moderate percent body fat category, you should try to come down and stay in this category, for health reasons. This is the category in which there appears to be no detriment to health.

If you are in the moderate category but would like to be lower, you need to ask yourself how badly you want it. Do you want it badly enough to implement lifetime exercise and dietary changes? If you are not willing to change, you should stop worrying about your weight and deem the moderate category as "tolerable" for you.

THE WEIGHT LOSS DILEMMA

For most people, **yo-yo dieting** carries as great a health risk as being overweight and remaining overweight in the first place. Epidemiological data are beginning to show that frequent fluctuations in weight (up or down) markedly increase the risk of dying of cardiovascular disease.

Based on the findings that constant losses and regains can be hazardous to health, quick-fix diets should be replaced by a slow but permanent weight-loss program, as described in this chapter. Individuals reap the benefits of recommended body weight when they get to their recommended body weight and stay there throughout life.

Unfortunately, only about a tenth of all people who begin a traditional weight loss program without exercise are able to lose the desired weight. Worse, only five in 100 are able to keep the weight off. The body is highly resistant to permanent weight changes through caloric restrictions alone.

Traditional diets have failed because few of them incorporate lifetime changes in food selection and exercise as fundamental to successful weight loss. When the diet stops, weight gain begins. The $40 billion diet industry tries to capitalize on the idea that weight can be lost quickly without taking into

Overweight   Indicates an excess amount of weight against a given standard such as height or recommended percent body fat.

Obesity   A chronic disease characterized by an excessively high amount of body fat in relation to lean body mass.

Yo-yo dieting   Constantly losing and gaining weight.

consideration the consequences of fast weight loss or the importance of lifetime behavioral changes to ensure proper weight loss and maintenance.

In addition, people, especially obese people, tend to underestimate their energy intake. Those who try to lose weight but apparently fail to do so are often described as "diet-resistant." A study published by Dr. Steven Lichtman and colleagues[2] found that, while on a "diet," a group of obese individuals with a self-reported history of diet resistance underreported their average daily caloric intake by almost 50% (1,028 self-reported versus 2,081 actual — see Figure 10.2). These individuals also overestimated their amount of daily physical activity by about 25% (1,022 calories self-reported versus 771 actual calories). These differences represent an additional 1304 calories of energy unaccounted for by the subjects in the study. The findings indicate that failing to lose weight often is related to misreports of actual food intake and level of physical activity.

Fad diets continue to appeal to people. These diets deceive people and claim the person will lose weight by following all instructions. Most fad diets are very low in calories and deprive the body of basic nutrients, generating a metabolic imbalance.

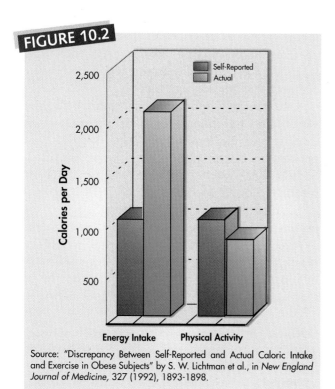

FIGURE 10.2

Source: "Discrepancy Between Self-Reported and Actual Caloric Intake and Exercise in Obese Subjects" by S. W. Lichtman et al., in *New England Journal of Medicine*, 327 (1992), 1893-1898.

Differences between self-reported and actual daily caloric intake and exercise in obese individuals attempting to lose weight.

Under these conditions, a lot of the weight lost is in the form of water and protein, and not fat.

On a crash diet, close to half the weight loss is in lean (protein) tissue. When the body uses protein instead of a combination of fats and carbohydrates as a source of energy, weight is lost as much as 10 times faster.[3] A gram of protein produces half the amount of energy that fat does. In the case of muscle protein, one-fifth of protein is mixed with four-fifths water. Each pound of muscle yields only one-tenth the amount of energy of a pound of fat. As a result, most of the weight loss is in the form of water, which on the scale, of course, looks good.

Some diets allow only certain specialized foods. If people would realize that no magic foods will provide all of the necessary nutrients, and that a person has to eat a variety of foods to be well-nourished, the diet industry would not be as successful. Most of these diets create a nutritional deficiency, which at times can be fatal.

The reason some of these diets succeed is that people eventually tire of eating the same thing day in and day out and start eating less. If they happen to achieve the lower weight but do not make permanent dietary changes, they regain the weight quickly once they go back to their old eating habits.

A few diets recommend exercise along with caloric restrictions — the best method for weight reduction. A lot of the weight lost is because of the exercise, so the diet has achieved its purpose. Unfortunately, if the dieters do not change their food selection and activity level permanently, they gain back the weight once they discontinue dieting and exercise.

EATING DISORDERS

Anorexia nervosa and bulimia arise from physical and emotional problems, thought to develop from individual, family, or social pressures. They are characterized by an intense fear of becoming fat, which does not disappear even after losing extreme amounts of weight. These medical disorders are increasing steadily in most industrialized nations where society encourages low-calorie diets and thinness.

Anorexia Nervosa

Anorexia nervosa is a condition of self-imposed starvation to lose and then maintain very low body weight. Approximately 19 of every 20 anorexics are young women. An estimated 1% of the female population in the United States is anorexic. Anorexic individuals seem to fear weight gain more than death from starvation. Furthermore, they have a distorted image of their body and think of themselves as being fat even when they are emaciated.

Although a genetic predisposition may contribute, the anorexic person often comes from a mother-dominated home, with possible drug addictions in the family. The syndrome may emerge following a stressful life event and uncertainty about the ability to cope efficiently.

Because the female role in society is changing more rapidly, they seem to be especially susceptible. Life experiences such as gaining weight, starting menstrual periods, beginning college, losing a boyfriend, having poor self-esteem, being socially rejected, starting a professional career, or becoming a wife or mother may trigger the syndrome.

These individuals typically begin a diet and at first feel in control and happy about the weight loss, even if they are not overweight. To speed up the weight loss, they frequently combine extreme dieting with exhaustive exercise and overuse of laxatives and diuretics.

Anorexics commonly develop obsessive and compulsive behaviors and emphatically deny their condition. They are preoccupied with food, meal planning, grocery shopping, and unusual eating habits. As they lose weight and their health begins to deteriorate, anorexics feel weak and tired and may realize they have a problem but will not stop the starvation and refuse to consider the behavior as abnormal.

Once they have lost a lot of weight and malnutrition sets in, physical changes become more visible. Some typical changes are **amenorrhea**, digestive problems, extreme sensitivity to cold, hair and skin problems, fluid and electrolyte abnormalities (which may lead to an irregular heartbeat and sudden stopping of the heart), injuries to nerves and tendons, abnormalities of immune function, anemia, growth of fine body hair, mental confusion, inability to concentrate, lethargy, depression, skin dryness, lower skin and body temperature, and osteoporosis.

Many of the changes of anorexia nervosa can be reversed, but treatment almost always requires professional help. The sooner it is started, the better the chances for reversibility and cure. Therapy consists of a combination of medical and psychological

---

Diagnostic Criteria for Anorexia Nervosa

- Refusal to maintain body weight over a minimal normal weight for age and height, e.g., weight loss leading to maintenance of body weight 15% below that expected; or failure to make expected weight gain during period of growth, leading to body weight 15% below that expected.
- Intense fear of gaining weight or becoming fat, even though underweight.
- Disturbance in the way in which one's body weight, size, or shape is experienced; e.g., the person claims to "feel fat" even when emaciated or believes that one area of the body is "too fat" even when obviously underweight.
- In females, absence of at least three consecutive menstrual cycles when otherwise expected to occur (primary or secondary amenorrhea). (A woman is considered to have amenorrhea if her periods occur only following administration of a hormone, such as estrogen.)

Source: American Psychiatric Association, Diagnostic and Statistical Manual of Mental Disorders (Washington, DC, Association, 1987), p. 67.

---

techniques to restore proper nutrition, prevent medical complications, and modify the environment or events that triggered the syndrome.

Unfortunately, anorexics strongly deny their condition. They are able to hide it and deceive friends and relatives quite effectively. Based on their behavior, many of them meet all of the characteristics of anorexia nervosa, but it goes undetected because both thinness and dieting are socially acceptable. Only a well-trained clinician is able to make a positive diagnosis.

> *Anorexics strongly deny their condition. They are able to hide it and deceive friends and relatives quite effectively.*

Bulimia

A pattern of binge eating and purging, **bulimia** is more prevalent than anorexia nervosa. For many

Anorexia nervosa   A condition of self-imposed starvation to lose and then maintain very low body weight.

Amenorrhea   Cessation of regular menstrual flow.

Bulimia   An eating disorder characterized by a pattern of binge eating and purging in an attempt to lose and maintain low body weight.

years it was thought to be a variant of anorexia nervosa, but now it is identified as a separate condition. It afflicts mainly young people. As many as one in every five women on college campuses may be bulimic, according to some estimates. Bulimia also is more prevalent than anorexia nervosa in males.

Bulimics usually are healthy-looking people, well-educated, near recommended body weight, who enjoy food and often socialize around it. In actuality, they are emotionally insecure, rely on others, and lack self-confidence and esteem. Recommended weight and food are important to them.

The binge-purge cycle usually occurs in stages. As a result of stressful life events or the simple compulsion to eat, bulimics engage periodically in binge eating that may last an hour or longer.

With some apprehension, bulimics anticipate and plan the cycle. Then they feel an urgency to begin. First they consume a large amount of food — several thousand calories and up to 10,000 calories in extreme cases — in a brief time. A short period of relief and satisfaction is followed by feelings of deep guilt, shame, and intense fear of gaining weight. Purging seems to be an easy answer, as the binging cycle can continue without fear of gaining weight. The most common form of purging is self-induced vomiting.

Bulimics might ingest strong laxatives and emetics. They often go on near-fasting diets and strenuous bouts of exercise. Medical problems associated

> *Unlike anorexics, bulimics realize their behavior is abnormal and feel great shame about it.*

with bulimia include cardiac arrhythmias, amenorrhea, kidney and bladder damage, ulcers, colitis, tearing of the esophagus or stomach, tooth erosion, gum damage, and general muscular weakness.

Unlike anorexics, bulimics realize their behavior is abnormal and feel great shame about it. Fearing social rejection, they pursue the binge-purge cycle in secrecy and at unusual times of the day.

Bulimia can be treated successfully when the person realizes this destructive behavior is not the solution to life's problems. A change in attitude can prevent permanent damage or death. Treatment is available on most school campuses through the school's counseling center or the health center. Local hospitals also offer treatment for eating disorders. Many communities have support groups, frequently led by professional personnel and usually free of charge.

PHYSIOLOGY OF WEIGHT LOSS

Only a few years ago the principles governing a weight loss and maintenance program seemed to be fairly clear, but now we know the final answers are not in yet. Traditional concepts related to weight control have centered on three assumptions: (a) that balancing food intake against output allows a person to achieve recommended weight, (b) that all fat people just eat too much, and (c) that the human body doesn't care how much (or little) fat it stores. Although these statements contain some truth, they still are open to much debate and research.

Energy-Balancing Equation

The principle embodied in the **energy-balancing equation** is simple: If daily energy requirements could be determined accurately, caloric intake could be balanced against output. This is not always the case, though, because genetic and lifestyle-related individual differences determine the number of calories required to maintain or lose body weight.

Table 10.1 offers some general guidelines for estimating daily caloric intake according to lifestyle patterns. This is only an estimated figure and, as discussed later in the chapter, it serves only as a starting point from which individual adjustments have to be made.

Diagnostic Criteria for Bulimia

- Recurrent episodes of binge eating (rapid consumption of a large amount of food in a discrete period of time).
- A feeling of lack of control over eating behavior during the eating binges.
- Regular practice of either self-induced vomiting, use of laxatives or diuretics, strict dieting or fasting, or vigorous exercise to prevent weight gain.
- A minimum average of two binge eating episodes a week for at least three months.
- Persistent overconcern with body shape and weight.

Source: *American Psychiatric Association, Diagnostic and Statistical Manual of Mental Disorders* (Washington, DC, Association, 1987), p. 68-69.

One pound of fat represents 3,500 calories. Assuming that a person's basic daily caloric expenditure is 2,500 calories, if this person were to decrease the daily intake by 500 calories per day, it should result in a loss of 1 pound of fat in 7 days (500 × 7 = 3,500). But research has shown — and many dieters probably have experienced — that even when they carefully balance caloric input against caloric output, weight loss does not always happen as predicted. Furthermore, two people with similar measured caloric intake and output seldom lose weight at the same rate.

The most common explanation regarding individual differences in weight loss and weight gain has been the variation in human metabolism from one person to another. We are all familiar with people who can eat "all day long" and not gain an ounce of weight, while others cannot even "dream about food" without gaining weight. Because experts did not believe that human metabolism alone could account for such extreme differences, they developed several theories that may better explain these individual variations.

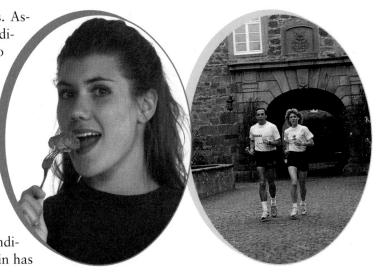

The human body resists weight loss unless healthy behaviors are incorporated in daily lifestyle.

SETPOINT THEORY

Results of several research studies point toward a **weight-regulating mechanism (WRM)** that has a setpoint for controlling both appetite and the amount of fat stored. **Setpoint** is hypothesized to work like a thermostat for body fat, maintaining fairly constant body weight, because it knows at all times the exact amount of adipose tissue stored in the fat cells. Some people have high settings; others have low settings.

If body weight decreases (as in dieting), the setpoint senses this change and triggers the WRM to increase the person's appetite or make the body conserve energy to maintain the "set" weight. The opposite also may be true. Some people have a hard time gaining weight. In this case, the WRM decreases appetite or causes the body to waste energy to maintain the lower weight.

Setpoint and Caloric Input

Every person has his or her own certain body fat percentage (as established by the setpoint) that the body attempts to maintain. The genetic instinct to survive tells the body that fat storage is vital, and therefore it sets an acceptable fat level. This level

remains somewhat constant or may climb gradually because of poor lifestyle habits.

For instance, under strict calorie reduction, the body may make extreme metabolic adjustments in an effort to maintain its setpoint for fat. The basal metabolic rate may drop dramatically against a consistent negative caloric balance, and a person may be on a plateau for days or even weeks without losing much weight. A low metabolic rate compounds a person's problems in maintaining recommended body weight.

These findings were substantiated by research conducted at Rockefeller University in New York.[4] The authors showed that the body resists maintaining altered weight. Obese and lifetime nonobese individuals were used in the investigation. Following a 10% weight loss, in an attempt to regain the lost weight, the body compensated by burning up to 15% fewer calories than were expected for the new reduced weight (after accounting for the 10% loss). The effects were similar in the obese and nonobese

Energy-balancing equation A principle holding that as long as caloric input equals caloric output, the person will not gain or lose weight. If caloric intake exceeds output, the person gains weight; when output exceeds input, the person loses weight.

Weight-regulating mechanism (WRM) Physiologic mechanism located in the hypothalamus of the brain that controls how much the body should weigh (also see Setpoint).

Setpoint The weight control theory that indicates the body has an established weight and strongly attempts to maintain that weight.

participants. These results imply that after a 10% weight loss, a person would have to eat less or exercise more to account for the estimated deficit of about 200 to 300 calories.

In this same study, when the participants were allowed to increase their weight to 10% above their "normal" body weight (pre-weight loss), the body burned 10% to 15% more calories than expected — an attempt by the body to waste energy and return to the pre-set weight. This is another indication that the body is highly resistant to weight changes unless additional lifestyle changes are incorporated to ensure successful weight management. These methods are discussed later in this chapter.

Dietary restriction alone will not lower the setpoint, even though the person may lose weight and fat. When the dieter goes back to the normal or even below-normal caloric intake, at which the weight may have been stable for a long time, he or she regains the fat loss quickly as the body strives to regain a comfortable fat store.

Let's use a practical illustration. A person would like to lose some body fat and assumes that a stable body weight has been reached at an average daily caloric intake of 1,800 calories (no weight gain or loss occurs at this daily intake). In an attempt to lose weight rapidly, this person now goes on a strict low-calorie diet, or even worse, a near-fasting diet. Immediately the body activates its survival mechanism and readjusts its metabolism to a lower caloric balance. After a few weeks of dieting at fewer than 400 to 600 calories per day, the body now can maintain its normal functions at 1,000 calories per day.

Having lost the desired weight, the person terminates the diet but realizes the original intake of 1,800 calories per day will have to be lower to maintain the new lower weight. To adjust to the new lower body weight, the intake is restricted to about 1,500 calories per day. The individual is surprised to find that, even at this lower daily intake (300 fewer calories), weight comes back at a rate of one pound every 1 to 2 weeks. After ending the diet, this new lowered metabolic rate may take several months to kick back up to its normal level.

> *Weight loss should be gradual, not abrupt.*

From this explanation, individuals clearly should never go on very low-calorie diets. Not only will this slow down resting metabolic rate, but it also will deprive the body of basic daily nutrients required for normal function.

Daily caloric intakes of 1,200 to 1,500 calories provide the necessary nutrients if they are distributed properly over the five basic food groups (meeting the daily required servings from each group). Of course, the individual will have to learn which foods meet the requirements and yet are low in fat and sugar.

Under no circumstances should a person go on a diet that calls for below 1,200 and 1,500 calories for women and men, respectively. Weight (fat) is gained over months and years, not overnight. Likewise, weight loss should be gradual, not abrupt.

Lowering the Setpoint

A second way in which the setpoint may work is by keeping track of the nutrients and calories consumed daily. It is thought that the body, like a cash register, records the daily food intake and the brain will not feel satisfied until the calories and nutrients have been "registered."

This setpoint for calories and nutrients seems to work for some people, even when they participate in moderately intense exercise. Some evidence suggests that people do not become hungrier with moderate physical activity. Therefore, people can choose to lose weight either by going hungry or by stepping up their daily physical activity. A greater number of calories burned through physical activity helps to lower body fat.

> *The only practical and sensible way to lower the setpoint is a combination of aerobic exercise and a diet high in complex carbohydrates and low in fat.*

The most common question regarding the setpoint is how it can be lowered so the body will feel comfortable at a lesser fat percentage. At least four factors seem to affect the setpoint directly by lowering the fat thermostat:

1. Aerobic exercise.
2. A diet high in complex carbohydrates.
3. Nicotine.
4. Amphetamines.

New Weight-Loss Drug Redux (dexfenfluramine), Fen-phen

For the first time in 23 years, the U.S. Food and Drug Administration has approved a new anti-obesity drug — *dexfenfluramine* (Redux or fen-phen). It is a distant cousin of Prozac — the drug used by millions for the treatment of depression. Dexfenfluramine works by raising levels of serotonin — a brain chemical that affects mood and satiety.

Unlike many other weight-loss pills, Redux is *not* an amphetamine and it is *not* known to be addictive. However, most health experts do not recommend the use of this drug because of the potential side effects — most significantly, an increase in the risk of primary pulmonary hypertension (blockage of blood vessels in the lungs), a rare lung disease that kills half the people who get it. Other individuals have developed deformity in the heart valve, a condition that can also be fatal.

The Bad News

1. It costs about $2.50 per day.

2. It's *not* a "magic pill" — it's only a "tool." To be effective, the drug must be used in *combination* with a low-calorie diet and regular exercise.

3. Weight loss is *not* dramatic: Patients lose an average of just 7.5 pounds more than dieters who do *not* take the drug. People who do not respond after one month's use will probably never respond.

4. The drug only regulates hunger. If you're like most people, and you eat for reasons *other* than hunger (such as stress, loneliness, boredom), it won't help.

5. Common side effects include lethargy and drowsiness.

6. High doses of the drug cause brain damage in laboratory animals.

7. It *cannot* be used in combination with antidepressants.

8. Recommended candidates are people who are clinically obese.

Sources: U.S. Food and Drug Administration, Dr. Charles Lucas, Chief of the Division of Preventive and Nutritional Medicine, Wiliam Beaumont Hospital, Royal Oak, MI.

The last two are more destructive than the over-fatness, so they are not reasonable alternatives. As far as the extra strain on the heart is concerned, smoking one pack of cigarettes per day is said to be the equivalent of carrying 50 to 75 pounds of excess body fat.

On the other hand, a diet high in fats and refined carbohydrates, near-fasting diets, and perhaps even artificial sweeteners seem to raise the setpoint. Therefore, the only practical and sensible way to lower the setpoint and lose fat weight is a combination of aerobic exercise and a diet high in complex carbohydrates and low in fat.

Because of the effects of proper food management on the body's setpoint, many nutritionists believe the total number of calories should not be the main concern in a weight-control program. Rather, it should be the source of those calories. In this regard, most of the effort is spent in retraining eating habits, increasing the intake of complex carbohydrates and high-fiber foods, and decreasing the consumption of refined carbohydrates (sugars) and fats. In most cases, this change in eating habits will bring about a decrease in total daily caloric intake.

FAT SUBSTITUTES

In 1996 a new fat substitute, **olestra**, was approved by the FDA for use in "savory snacks." According to the University of California at Berkeley *Wellness Letter*,[5] consumers should "just say no" to olestra and not buy products that contain this fat substitute.

Olestra can cause diarrhea and cramping, and it can deplete the body of fat-soluble vitamins, including A, D, E, and K. Vitamin E is a strong antioxidant, and low levels of vitamin K pose a risk for people with bleeding disorders and those on blood-thinning medication. In addition, potential cancer-causing liver-cell changes have been found in animal studies. Although the fat and caloric content of olestra-containing foods is lower than that of foods cooked with natural fats, consuming snacks using this fat substitute not only may pose a risk to good health but also may reinforce unhealthy eating habits.

A NEW APPROACH

A "diet" no longer is viewed as a temporary tool to aid in weight loss but, instead, as a permanent

Olestra Fat substitute made from sugar and fatty acids; provides no calories to the body because it passes through the digestive system without being absorbed.

change in eating behaviors to ensure weight management and better health. The role of physical activity also must be considered, because successful weight loss, maintenance, and recommended body composition seldom are attained without a moderate reduction in caloric intake combined with a regular exercise program.

Fat can be lost by selecting the proper foods, exercising, or restricting calories. When a person tries to lose weight by dietary restrictions alone, lean body mass (muscle protein, along with vital organ protein) always decreases. The amount of lean body mass lost depends entirely on caloric limitation.

When people go on a near-fasting diet, up to half of the weight loss is lean body mass and the other half is actual fat loss (see Figure 10.3).[6] When diet is combined with exercise, close to 100% of the weight loss is in the form of fat, and lean tissue actually may increase.

Loss of lean body mass is never good, because it weakens the organs and muscles and slows down metabolism. Large losses in lean tissue can cause disturbances in heart function and damage to other organs. Equally important is not to overindulge (binge) following very-low-calorie diets. This may cause changes in metabolic rate and electrolyte balance, which could trigger fatal cardiac arrhythmias.

Contrary to some beliefs, aging is not the main reason for the lower metabolic rate. It is not so much that metabolism slows down as that people slow down. As people age, they tend to rely more on the amenities of life (remote controls, cellular telephones, intercoms, single-level homes, riding lawnmowers) that lull a person into sedentary living.

Basal metabolism is related directly to lean body weight. The more the lean tissue, the higher the metabolic rate. As a consequence of sedentary living and less physical activity, the lean component decreases and fat tissue increases. The human body requires a certain amount of oxygen per pound of lean body mass. As fat is considered metabolically inert from the point of view of caloric use, the lean tissue uses most of the oxygen, even at rest. As muscle and organ mass (lean body mass) decrease, so do the energy requirements at rest.

Reductions in lean body mass are common in aging people (because of physical inactivity) and those on severely restricted diets. The loss of lean body mass also may account for a lower metabolic rate (described earlier) and the longer time it takes to kick back up.

Diets with caloric intakes below 1,200 to 1,500 calories cannot guarantee the retention of lean body mass. Even at this intake level, some loss is inevitable unless the diet is combined with exercise. Despite the claims of many diets that they do not alter the lean component, the simple truth is that, regardless of what nutrients may be added to the diet, severe caloric restrictions always prompt a loss of lean tissue. Too many people go on low-calorie diets constantly. Every time they do, the metabolic rate slows down as more lean tissue is lost.

Many people in their 40s and older who weigh the same as they did when they were 20 think they are at recommended body weight. During this span of 20 years or more, these people may have dieted many times without participating in an exercise program. They regain the weight shortly after they terminate each diet, but most of that gain is in fat. Maybe at age 20 they weighed 150 pounds, of which only 15% was fat. Now at age 40, even though they still weigh 150 pounds, they might be 30% fat (see Figure 10.4 and also Figure 9.4 in Chapter 9). At recommended body weight, they wonder why they are eating very little and still having trouble staying at that weight.

EXERCISE: THE KEY TO WEIGHT LOSS AND WEIGHT MAINTENANCE

A more effective way to tilt the energy-balancing equation in your favor is by burning calories

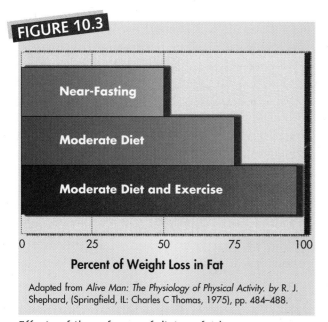

FIGURE 10.3

Near-Fasting

Moderate Diet

Moderate Diet and Exercise

0   25   50   75   100

Percent of Weight Loss in Fat

Adapted from *Alive Man: The Physiology of Physical Activity.* by R. J. Shephard, (Springfield, IL: Charles C Thomas, 1975), pp. 484–488.

Effects of three forms of diet on fat loss.

through physical activity. Exercise also seems to exert control over how much a person weighs.

Starting at age 25, the typical American gains 1 pound of weight per year. This weight gain represents a simple energy surplus of under 10 calories per day. In most cases, the additional weight accumulated in middle age comes from people becoming

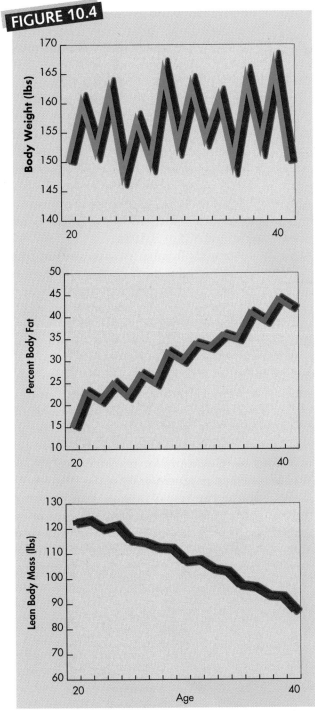

FIGURE 10.4

Effects of frequent dieting without exercise on lean body mass, percent body fat, and body weight.

less physically active and not as a result of increases in caloric intake. Dr. Jack Wilmore, a leading exercise physiologist and expert weight management researcher, stated:

> Physical inactivity is certainly a major, if not the primary, cause of obesity in the United States today. A certain minimal level of activity might be necessary for us to accurately balance our caloric intake to our caloric expenditure. With too little activity, we appear to lose the fine control we normally have to maintain this incredible balance. This fine balance amounts to less than 10 calories per day, or the equivalent of one potato chip.[7]

Exercise is crucial to losing weight and maintaining weight. Not only will exercise maintain lean tissue, but advocates of the setpoint theory say that exercise resets the fat thermostat to a new, lower level. This change may be rapid, or it may take time. A few overweight individuals have exercised faithfully almost daily, 60 minutes at a time, for a whole year before seeing significant weight change. People with a "sticky" setpoint have to be patient and persistent.

> 66 *Physical inactivity is certainly a major, if not the primary, cause of obesity in the United States today.*
> Dr. Jack Wilmore 99

If a person is trying to lose weight, a combination of aerobic and strength-training exercises works best. Aerobic exercise is the best to offset the setpoint, and the continuity and duration of these types of activities cause many calories to be burned in the process. The role of aerobic exercise in successful lifetime weight management cannot be overestimated.

As illustrated in Figure 10.5, greater weight loss is achieved by combining a diet with an aerobic exercise program.[8] Of even greater significance, only the individuals who participated in an 18-month post-diet aerobic exercise program were able to keep the weight off. Those who discontinued exercise gained weight. Furthermore, all those who initiated or resumed exercise during the 18-month follow-up were able to lose weight again. Individuals who only dieted and never exercised regained 60% and 92%

Basal metabolism The lowest level of oxygen consumption and energy requirement necessary to sustain life.

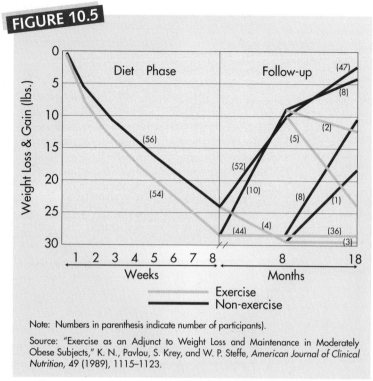

FIGURE 10.5

Note: Numbers in parenthesis indicate number of participants).

Source: "Exercise as an Adjunct to Weight Loss and Maintenance in Moderately Obese Subjects," K. N., Pavlou, S. Krey, and W. P. Steffe, *American Journal of Clinical Nutrition*, 49 (1989), 1115–1123.

Aerobic exercise and weight loss and maintenance in moderately obese individuals.

The aerobic group lost an average of 3½ pounds, 3 of which were fat and the remaining half-pound lean tissue. The combined aerobic and strength-training group lost an average of 8 pounds. Changes in body composition, however, indicated that the latter group actually lost 10 pounds of fat and gained 2 pounds of lean tissue (see Figure 10.6). These findings suggest that a sensible strength-training program is better to lose weight and to maintain or increase muscle mass and metabolic rate.

Another point of interest is that each additional pound of muscle tissue can raise the basal metabolic rate by about 35 calories per day.[10] Thus, an individual who adds 5 pounds of muscle tissue as a result of strength training increases the basal metabolic rate by 175 calories per day (35 × 5), which equals 63,875 calories per year (175 × 365), or the equivalent of 18.25 pounds of fat (63,875 ÷ 3,500).

Strength training is suggested especially for people who think they are at their recommended body weight, yet their body fat percentage is higher than recommended. The number of calories burned during a typical hour-long strength-training session is much less than during an hour of aerobic exercise. Because of the high intensity of strength training, the person needs frequent rest intervals to recover from each set of exercise. The average person actually lifts weights only 10 to 12 minutes in each hour of exercise. In the long run, however, the person enjoys the benefits of gains in lean tissue. Guidelines for developing aerobic and strength-training programs are given in Chapter 7.

Because exercise results in more lean body mass, body weight often remains the same or even increases after beginning an exercise program, while inches and percent body fat decrease. More lean tissue means a higher functional capacity of the human body. With exercise, most of the weight loss becomes apparent after a few weeks of training, after the lean component has stabilized.

Although we now know that a negative caloric balance of 3,500

of their weight loss at the 6- and 18-month follow-up, respectively.

Weight loss may come more rapidly when aerobic exercise is combined with a strength-training program.[9] Two exercise groups — a 30-minute aerobic group and a 15-minute aerobic plus 15-minute strength-training (30 minutes total) group — participated in an 8-week, 3-days-per-week study. Both groups followed a dietary plan consisting of approximately 60% carbohydrates, 20% fats, and 20% proteins.

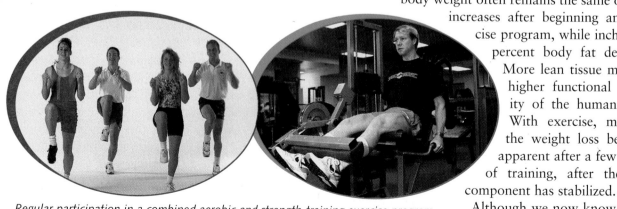

Regular participation in a combined aerobic and strength-training exercise program is the key to successful weight management.

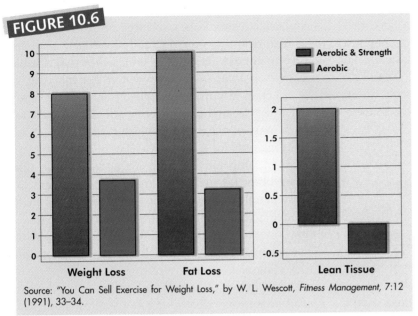

FIGURE 10.6

Source: "You Can Sell Exercise for Weight Loss," by W. L. Wescott, *Fitness Management*, 7:12 (1991), 33–34.

Changes in body composition through aerobic exercise and aerobic/strength-training exercise.

calories does not always result in a loss of exactly one pound of fat, the role of exercise in achieving a negative balance by burning additional calories is significant in weight reduction and maintenance programs.

Sadly, some individuals claim that the amount of calories burned during exercise is hardly worth the effort. They think that cutting their daily intake by some 300 calories is easier than participating in some sort of exercise that would burn the same amount of calories. The problem is that the willpower to cut those 300 calories lasts only a few weeks, and then the person goes right back to the old eating patterns.

Activity	Calories Burned Per Hour
Sitting	80–100
Standing	95–120
Light activity Cleaning house, office work, golf	240–300
Moderate activity Walking briskly (3.5 mph), gardening, cycling (5.5 mph), dancing	370–460
Strenuous activity Jogging (9 min./mile), swimming	580–730
Very strenuous Running (7 min./mile), racquetball, cross-country skiing	740–920

If a person gets into the habit of exercising regularly, say three times a week, running 3 miles per exercise session (about 300 calories burned), this represents 900 calories in one week, about 3,600 in one month, or 46,800 calories per year. This minimal amount of exercise could mean as many as 13.5 extra pounds of fat in one year, 27 in two, and so on.

We tend to forget that our weight creeps up gradually over the years, not just overnight. Hardly worth the effort? And we have not even taken into consideration the increase in lean tissue, possible resetting of the set-point, benefits to the cardiorespiratory system, and, most important, the improved quality of life. The fundamental reasons for overfatness and obesity, few could argue, are lack of physical activity and sedentary living.

> ❝ *Regular activity seems to be the strongest predictor of success in long-term weight management.* ❞

In terms of preventing disease, many of the health benefits people try to achieve by losing weight are reaped through exercise alone, even without weight loss. As indicated earlier in this chapter (see Figure 10.1), exercise offers protection against premature mortality for everyone, including people who already have risk factors for disease. The lack of exercise, not the weight problem itself, possibly is the cause of many of the health risks associated with obesity.

WEIGHT-LOSS MYTHS

Cellulite and **spot reducing** are mythical concepts. Cellulite is nothing but enlarged fat cells that bulge out from accumulated body fat.

Cellulite   Term frequently used in reference to fat deposits that "bulge out." These deposits are nothing but enlarged fat cells from excessive accumulation of body fat.

Spot reducing   Fallacious theory that claims that exercising a specific body part will result in significant fat reduction in that area.

Doing several sets of daily sit-ups will not get rid of fat in the midsection of the body. When fat comes off, it does so throughout the entire body, not just the exercised area. The greatest proportion of fat may come off the biggest fat deposits, but the caloric output of a few sets of sit-ups has practically no effect on reducing total body fat. A person has to exercise much longer to really see results.

> 66
> *You can't "spot reduce."*
> *When you lose fat, you lose it from*
> *all the areas in your body where it is*
> *stored.*
> 99

Other touted means toward quick weight loss — rubberized sweatsuits, steam baths, mechanical vibrators — are misleading. When a person wears a sweatsuit or steps into a sauna, the weight lost is not fat but merely a significant amount of water. Sure, it looks nice when you step on the scale immediately afterward, but this represents a false loss of weight. As soon as you replace body fluids, you gain back the weight quickly.

Wearing rubberized sweatsuits not only hastens the rate of body fluid loss — fluid that is vital during prolonged exercise — but it also raises core temperature at the same time. This combination puts a person in danger of dehydration, which impairs cellular function and in extreme cases can even cause death.

Similarly, mechanical vibrators are worthless in a weight-control program. Vibrating belts and turning rollers may feel good, but they require no effort whatsoever. Fat cannot be shaken off; it is lost primarily by burning it in muscle tissue.

IMPLEMENTING A SOUND AND SENSIBLE WEIGHT-LOSS PROGRAM

Dieting never has been fun and never will be. People who are overweight and are serious about losing weight, however, have to include regular exercise in their life along with proper food management and a sensible reduction in caloric intake.

Some precautions are in order, as excessive body fat is a risk factor for cardiovascular disease. Depending on the extent of the weight problem, a medical examination and possibly a stress ECG (see Abnormal Electrocardiogram in Chapter 11) may be a

good idea before undertaking the exercise program. A physician should be consulted in this regard.

Significantly overweight individuals also may have to choose activities in which they will not have to support their own body weight but that still will be effective in burning calories. Joint and muscle injuries are common in overweight individuals who participate in weight-bearing exercises such as walking, jogging, and aerobics.

Swimming may not be a good exercise either. More body fat makes a person more buoyant, and most people are not at the skill level to swim fast enough to get the best training effect. They tend to just float along, limiting the amount of calories burned as well as the benefits to the cardiorespiratory system.

Some better alternatives are riding a bicycle (either road or stationary), walking in a shallow pool, doing water aerobics,[11] or running in place in deep water (treading water). The latter forms of water exercise are gaining popularity and have proven to be effective in weight reduction without the "pain" and fear of injuries. Through the caloric expenditure based on perceived exertion of the activity (see Table 10.2), you will be able to determine your own daily caloric requirement using Assessment 10-1.

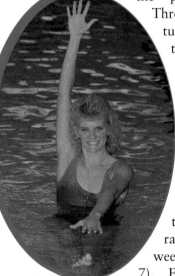

Water aerobics can help lose body fat.

How long should each exercise session last? To develop and maintain cardiorespiratory fitness, 20 to 30 minutes of exercise at the recommended target rate, three to five times per week, is suggested (see Chapter 7). For weight-loss purposes, many experts recommend exercising at least 45 minutes at a time, five to six times a week.

A person should not try to do too much too fast. Unconditioned beginners should start with about 15 minutes of aerobic exercise three times a week, gradually increasing the duration by approximately 5 minutes per week and the frequency by one day per week during the next three to four weeks.

One final benefit of exercise for weight control is that it allows fat to be burned more efficiently. Both carbohydrates and fats are sources of energy. When the glucose levels begin to drop during prolonged exercise, more fat is used as energy substrate.

Equally important is that fat-burning enzymes increase with aerobic training. Fat is lost primarily by burning it in muscle. Therefore, as the concentration of the enzymes increases, so does the ability to burn fat.[12]

In addition to exercise and adequate food management, sensible adjustments in caloric intake are recommended. Most research finds that a negative caloric balance is required to lose weight. Perhaps the only exception is in people who are eating too few calories. A nutrient analysis (see Chapter 8) often reveals that faithful dieters are not consuming enough calories. These people actually need to increase their daily caloric intake (combined with an exercise program) to get their metabolism to kick back up to a normal level.

The reasons for prescribing a lower caloric figure to lose weight are:

1. Most people underestimate their caloric intake and are eating more than they should be eating.

2. Developing new behaviors takes time, and some people have trouble changing and adjusting to new eating habits.

3. Many individuals are in such poor physical condition that they take a long time to increase their activity level enough to offset the setpoint and burn enough calories to aid in loss of body fat.

4. Some dieters have difficulty succeeding unless they can count calories.

5. A few people simply will not alter their food selection. For those who will not change their food selection (which will still increase the risk for chronic diseases), a large increase in physical activity, a negative caloric balance, or a combination of the two is the only solution for successful weight loss.

The daily caloric requirement can be estimated by consulting Tables 10.1 and 10.2 and Assessment 10-1. As this is only an estimated value, individual adjustments related to many of the factors discussed in this chapter may be necessary to establish a more precise value. Nevertheless, the estimated value does offer a beginning guideline for weight control or reduction.

The average daily caloric requirement without exercise is based on typical lifestyle patterns, total body weight, and gender. Individuals who hold jobs that require heavy manual labor burn more calories during the day than those who have sedentary jobs such as working behind a desk.

To find your activity level, refer to Table 10.1 and rate yourself accordingly. The number given in Table 10.1 is per pound of body weight, so you should multiply your current weight by that number. For example, the typical caloric requirement to maintain body weight for a moderately active male who weighs 160 pounds is 2,400 calories (160 lbs × 15 calories per pound).

The second step is to determine the average number of calories you use daily as a result of physical activity. To get this number, figure out the total number of minutes you exercise weekly, and then figure the daily average exercise time. For instance, a person exercising somewhat hard, five times a week, 30 minutes each time, exercises 150 minutes per week (5 × 30). The average daily exercise time is 21 minutes (150 ÷ 7). Round off to the lowest unit.

Next, from Table 10.2, find the energy requirement for the activity (or activities) based on its perceived exertion. In the case of a somewhat hard intensity, the requirement is .070 calories per pound of body weight per minute of activity (cal/lb/min). With a body weight of 160 pounds, this man uses 11.2 calories each minute (body weight × .070, or 160 × .070). In 21 minutes, he uses approximately 235 calories (21 × 11.4).

The fourth step is to obtain the estimated total caloric requirement, with exercise, needed to maintain body weight. To do this, add the typical daily requirement (without exercise) and the average calories used through exercise. In our example, it is 2,635 calories (2,400 + 235).

TABLE 10.1

Average Caloric Requirement Per Pound of Body Weight Based on Lifestyle Patterns and Gender

	Calories Per Pound	
	Men	Women*
Sedentary — limited physical activity	13.0	12.0
Moderate physical activity	15.0	13.5
Hard Labor — strenuous physical effort	17.0	15.0

*Pregnant or lactating women add 3 calories to these values.

TABLE 10.2

Estimated Caloric Expenditure Based on Perceived Exertion of Physical Activity

Perceived Exertion		Caloric Expenditure (Cal/lb/min)
Very, very light	(7)*	0.030
Very light	(9)	0.040
Fairly light	(11)	0.050
Somewhat hard	(13)	0.070
Hard	(15)	0.090
Very hard	(17)	0.100
Very, very hard	(19)	0.110

* Numbers in parenthesis indicate the rate of perceived exertion (RPE), see Figure 7.2, Chapter 7.

Adapted from "Caloric Expenditure of Selected Physical Activities," contained in W. W. K. Hoeger and S. A. Hoeger, *Lifetime Physical Fitness & Wellness* (Englewood: Morton Publishing, 1998), p. 54.

If a negative caloric balance is recommended to lose weight, this person has to consume fewer than 2,635 daily calories to achieve the objective. Because of the many factors that play a role in weight control, the previous value is only an estimated daily requirement. Furthermore, to lose weight, a person can't predict that exactly 1 pound of fat will be lost in 1 week by reducing daily intake by 500 calories (500 × 7 = 3,500 calories, or the equivalent of 1 pound of fat).

The estimated daily caloric figure provides only a target guideline for weight control. Periodic readjustments are necessary because individuals differ, and the estimated daily cost changes as you lose weight and modify your exercise habits.

The recommended number of calories to be subtracted from the daily intake to obtain a negative caloric balance depends on the typical daily requirement. The best recommendation is to decrease the daily intake moderately, never below 1,200 calories for women and 1,500 for men.

A good guideline to follow is to restrict the intake by no more than 500 calories if the daily requirement is below 3,000 calories. For caloric requirements in excess of 3,000, as many as 1,000 calories per day may be subtracted from the total intake. The daily distribution should be approximately 60% carbohydrates (mostly complex carbohydrates), less than 30% fat, and about 12% protein.

Many experts believe a person may take off weight more efficiently by reducing the amount of

daily fat intake to 10% to 20% of the total daily caloric intake. Because 1 gram of fat supplies more than twice the amount of calories that carbohydrates and protein do, the general tendency is not to overeat.

Further, it takes only 3% to 5% of ingested calories to store fat as fat, whereas it takes approximately 25% of ingested calories to convert carbohydrates to fat. Other research points to the fact that if people eat the same amount of calories as carbohydrate or fat, those on the fat diet will store more fat. Successful weight-loss programs allow only small amounts of fat in the diet.

Many people have trouble adhering to a 10%- to 20%-fat-calorie diet. During weight loss periods, however, you are strongly encouraged to do so. Start

Substitution Chart

Butter	Powdered butter flavoring, reduced-calorie margarine
Cooking oil	Vegetable cooking spray, broth, wine
Mayonnaise	Low-calorie salad dressing; reduced-calorie, low-fat mayonnaise
Eggs	Egg substitute or egg whites
Salad dressing	Oil-free or reduced-calorie dressing; flavored vinegars
Sour cream	Plain low-fat or nonfat yogurt, low-fat or nonfat sour cream
Cream cheese	Low-fat cream cheese, Neufchâtel cheese
Whole milk	Skim milk or 1%
Evaporated milk	Evaporated skim milk
Microwave popcorn (pre-bagged)	Air-popped or microwave-popped without fats
Ground beef	Ground chicken or turkey
Bacon and ham	Turkey ham

Moves to Help You Lose

1. Hold walking meetings instead of business lunches.
2. Leave an extra pair of walking shoes in the car and office.
3. Swap coffee breaks for stretch breaks to beat midday blahs.
4. Take the stairs instead of the elevator.
5. Get a long extension cord for the phone so you can walk while you talk.
6. Don't drive distances less than ½ mile.
7. Do stretching exercises while watching TV.
8. Feel the beat and dance around the house.
9. Wash and wax the car yourself.
10. Go dancing instead of sitting at the movies.

© 1994 Great Performance Inc., 14964 NW Greenbrier Pkwy., Beaverton, OR 97006, (503) 690-9181.

with a 20% fat-calorie diet. Refer to Table 10.3 to aid you in determining the grams of fat at 10%, 20%, and 30% of the total calories for selected energy intakes. Also, use the form provided in Assessment 10-2 to monitor your daily fat intake.

The time of day when food is consumed also may play a part in weight reduction. A study conducted at the Aerobics Research Center in Dallas, Texas, indicated that, when a person is on a diet, weight is lost most effectively if most of the calories are consumed before 1:00 p.m. and not during the evening meal. The Center recommends that, when a person is attempting to lose weight, intake should consist of a minimum of 25% of the total daily calories for breakfast, 50% for lunch, and 25% or less at dinner.

Other experts have reported that if most of the daily calories are consumed during one meal, the body may perceive that something is wrong and will slow down the metabolism so it can store a greater amount of calories in the form of fat. Eating most of the calories in one meal also causes a person to go hungry the rest of the day, making the diet more difficult to follow.

Consuming most of the calories earlier in the day seems helpful in losing weight, and also in managing atherosclerosis. The time of day when most of the fats and cholesterol are consumed can influence blood lipids and coronary heart disease. Peak digestion time following a heavy meal is about 7 hours after that meal. If most lipids are consumed during the evening meal, digestion peaks while the person is sound asleep, when the metabolism is at its lowest rate. Consequently, the body may not metabolize fats and cholesterol as well, leading to a higher blood lipid count and increasing the risk for atherosclerosis and coronary heart disease.

To monitor daily progress, you may use a form such as the one given in Assessment 10-2. Meeting the basic requirements from each food group should get top priority. The caloric content for each food is given in the Nutritive Value of Selected Foods list, Appendix A. For a more precise record, the information should be recorded immediately after each meal. According to the person's progress, adjustments can be made in the typical daily requirement or the exercise program, or both.

TABLE 10.3

Grams of Fat as a Percentage of Total Calories for Selected Caloric Intakes

Caloric Intake	Grams of Fat		
	10%	20%	30%
1,200	13	27	40
1,300	14	29	43
1,400	16	31	47
1,500	17	33	50
1,600	18	36	53
1,700	19	38	57
1,800	20	40	60
1,900	21	42	63
2,000	22	44	67
2,100	23	47	70
2,200	24	49	73
2,300	26	51	77
2,400	27	53	80
2,500	28	56	83
2,600	29	58	87
2,700	30	60	90
2,800	31	62	93
2,900	32	64	97
3,000	33	67	100

ADHERING TO A WEIGHT MANAGEMENT PROGRAM

Achieving and maintaining recommended body composition is by no means impossible, but this does require desire and commitment. If weight management is to become a priority in life, people must realize they have to retrain their behavior to some extent.

Modifying old habits and developing new positive behaviors take time. Individuals have applied the following management techniques to change detrimental behavior successfully and adhere to a positive lifetime weight-control program. In developing a retraining program, people are not expected to incorporate all of the strategies listed but should note the ones that apply to them.

1. *Make a commitment to change.* The first ingredient of behavior modification is the desire to change. The reasons for change must be more compelling than those for continuing present lifestyle patterns. You must accept the fact that you have a problem and decide by yourself whether you really want to change. If you have a sincere commitment, your chances for success are enhanced already.

2. *Set realistic goals.* Most people with a weight problem would like to lose weight in a relatively short time but fail to realize that the weight problem developed over several years. A sound weight reduction and maintenance program can be accomplished only by establishing new lifetime eating and exercise habits, both of which take time. In setting a realistic long-term goal, you also should plan short-term objectives. The long-term goal may be to decrease body fat to 20% of total body weight. The short-term objective may be to decrease body fat 1% each month. Objectives like these allow for regular evaluation and help maintain motivation and renewed commitment to attain the long-term goal.

3. *Incorporate exercise into the program.* Choose enjoyable activities, places, times, equipment, and people to exercise with. This will help you adhere to an exercise program.

4. *Develop healthy eating patterns.* Plan to eat three regular meals per day consistent with the body's nutritional requirements. Learn to differentiate hunger from appetite. **Hunger** is the actual physical need for food. **Appetite** is a desire for food, usually triggered by factors such as stress, habit, boredom, depression, food availability, or just the thought of food itself. Eat only when you have a physical need. In this regard, developing and sticking to a regular meal pattern helps control hunger.

5. *Avoid automatic eating.* Many people associate certain daily activities with eating. For example, people eat while cooking, watching television, reading, talking on the telephone, or visiting with neighbors. Most of the time, the foods consumed in these situations lack nutritional value or are high in sugar and fat.

6. *Do not engage in psychological overeating.* Psychological overeaters fall into various categories. The questionnaire provided in Assessment 10-3 will help you become aware of these categories, and knowing when, why, and where you overeat can help you overcome this habit.

7. *Stay busy.* People tend to eat more when they sit around and do nothing. Occupying the mind and body with activities not associated with eating helps take away the desire to eat. Try walking, cycling, playing sports, gardening, sewing, or visiting a library, a museum, a park. Develop other skills and interests, or try something new and exciting to break the routine.

8. *Plan your meals ahead of time.* Sensible shopping is required to accomplish this objective (by the way, shop on a full stomach, because hungry shoppers tend to buy unhealthy foods impulsively and then snack on the way home). Include whole-grain breads and cereals, fruits and vegetables, low-fat milk and dairy products, lean meats, fish, and poultry.

9. *Cook wisely.* Use less fat and refined foods in food preparation. Trim all visible fat from meats, and remove skin from poultry before cooking. Skim the fat off gravies and soups. Bake, broil, and boil instead of frying. Sparingly use butter, cream, mayonnaise, and salad dressings. Avoid coconut oil, palm oil, and cocoa butter. Prepare plenty of bulky foods. Add whole-grain breads and cereals, vegetables, and legumes to most meals. Try fruits for dessert. Beware of soda pop, fruit juices, and fruit-flavored drinks. In addition to sugar, cut down on other refined carbohydrates such as corn syrup, malt sugar, dextrose, and fructose. Drink plenty of water — at least eight glasses a day.

10. *Do not serve more food than you should eat.* Measure the food portions and keep serving dishes away from the table. This means you will eat less, have a harder time getting seconds, and have less appetite because food is not visible. People should not be forced to eat when they are satisfied (including children after they have already had a healthy, nutritious serving).

11. *Learn to eat slowly and at the table only.* Eating is one of the pleasures of life, and we need to take time to enjoy it. Eating on the run is not good because the body doesn't have enough time to "register" nutritive and caloric consumption and people overeat before the body perceives the signal of fullness. Always eating at the table also forces people to take time out to eat, and it deters snacking between meals, primarily because of the extra time and effort required to sit down and eat. When done eating, do not sit around the table. Clean up and put away the food to keep from unnecessary snacking.

12. *Avoid social binges.* Social gatherings commonly entice self-defeating behavior. Plan ahead and visualize yourself in that gathering. Do not feel pressured to eat or drink, and don't rationalize in these situations. Choose low-calorie foods, and entertain yourself with other activities such as dancing and talking.

13. *Beware of raids on the refrigerator and the cookie jar.* When you find yourself in these tempting situations, take control. Stop and think what is happening. If you have the propensity for raids, try environmental management. Do not bring high-calorie, high-sugar, or high-fat foods into your home. If they are already there, store them where they are hard to get to or see. If they are out of sight or not readily available, the temptation is less. Keeping food in inaccessible places tends to discourage people from taking the time and effort to get them. By no means should you have to eliminate treats completely. Do all things in moderation.

14. *Avoid eating out.* Most meals served at restaurants (especially fast-food restaurants) are high in calories and fat. People who eat out regularly often have a difficult time managing their weight. When eating out, plan your choices by selecting low-fat and low-calorie meals, or go to a restaurant noted for healthful menus.

15. *Practice stress management techniques.* Many people snack and increase food consumption in stressful situations. Eating is not a stress-releasing activity and actually can aggravate the problem if weight control is an issue. Several stress-management techniques are set forth in Chapter 3.

16. *Monitor changes and reward accomplishments.* Feedback on fat loss, lean tissue gain, and weight loss is a reward in itself. Awareness of changes in body composition also helps reinforce new behaviors. Being able to exercise without interruption for 15, 20, 30, 60 minutes, cycling a certain distance, running a mile — all these accomplishments deserve recognition. Meeting objectives calls for rewards — but not related to eating. Buy new clothing, a tennis racquet, a bicycle, exercise shoes, or something else that is special and you would not have acquired otherwise.

17. *Think positive.* Avoid negative thoughts on how difficult changing your past behaviors might be. Instead, think of the benefits you will reap, such as feeling, looking, and functioning better, plus enjoying better health and improving your quality of life. Attempt to stay away from negative environments and people who will not be supportive. Avoid those who do not have the same desires and who encourage self-defeating behaviors.

There is no simple and quick way to take off excessive body fat and keep it off for good. Weight management is accomplished by making a lifetime commitment to physical activity and proper food selection. When taking part in a weight (fat) reduction program, people also have to decrease their caloric intake moderately and implement strategies to modify unhealthy eating behaviors.

During the process, relapses into past negative behaviors are almost inevitable. The three most common reasons for relapse are:

1. Stress-related factors (major life changes, depression, job changes, illness).

2. Social reasons (entertaining, eating out, business travel).

3. Self-enticing behaviors (placing yourself in a situation to see how much you can get away with

Hunger The actual physical need for food.

Appetite Desire for food, usually triggered by factors such as stress, habit, boredom, depression, food availability, or just the thought of food itself.

("One small taste won't hurt," leading to "I'll eat just one slice," and finally, "I haven't done so well, so I might as well eat some more").

Making mistakes is human and does not necessarily mean failure. Failure comes to those who give up and do not use previous experiences to build upon and, in turn, develop skills that will prevent self-defeating behaviors in the future. Where there's a will, there's a way, and those who persist will reap the rewards.

NOTES

1. C. E. Barlow, H. W. Kohl, III, L. W. Gibbons, and S. N. Blair, "Physical Fitness, Mortality, and Obesity," *International Journal of Obesity*, 19 (1995), S41-S44.
2. "Discrepancy Between Self-Reported and Actual Caloric Intake and Exercise in Obese Subjects," *New England Journal of Medicine*, 327 (1992), 1893–1898.
3. D. Remington, A. G. Fisher, and E. A. Parent, *How to Lower Your Fat Thermostat* (Provo, UT: Vitality House International, 1983).
4. R. L. Leibel, M. Rosenbaum, and J. Hirsh, "Changes in Energy Expenditure Resulting from Altered Body Weight," *New England Journal of Medicine*, 332 (1995), 621–628.
5. "Olestra: Just Say No," *University of California at Berkeley Wellness Letter* (Palm Coast, FL: Editors, February, 1996).
6. R. J. Shepard. *Alive Man: The Physiology of Physical Activity* (Springfield, IL: Charles C Thomas, 1975), pp. 484–488.
7. "Exercise, Obesity, and Weight Control," *Physical Activity and Fitness Research Digest* (Washington DC: President's Council on Physical Fitness & Sports, May 1994).
8. K. N. Pavlou, S. Krey, and W. P. Steffe, "Exercise as an Adjunct to Weight Loss and Maintenance in Moderately Obese Subjects," *American Journal of Clinical Nutrition*, 49 (1898), 1115–1123.
9. W. L. Wescott, "You Can Sell Exercise for Weight Loss," *Fitness Management*, 7:12 (1991), 33–34.
10. W. W. Campbell, M. C. Crim, V. R. Young, and W. J. Evans, "Increased Energy Requirements and Changes in Body Composition with Resistance Training in Older Adults," *American Journal of Clinical Nutrition*, 60 (1994), 167–175.
11. W. W. K. Hoeger, T. Spitzer-Gibson, J. R. Moore, and D. R. Hopkins, "A Comparison of Selected Training Responses to Water Aerobics and Low-Impact Aerobic Dance," *National Aquatics Journal*, 9 (1993), 13–16.
12. Remington.

ASSESSMENT 10-1

Estimation of Daily Caloric Requirement

Name _____ Date _____ Grade _____

Instructor _____ Course _____ Section _____

NECESSARY LAB EQUIPMENT: Tables 10.1 (page 273) and 10.2 (page 274)

OBJECTIVE: To determine an estimated daily caloric requirement with exercise for weight maintenance and/or reduction.

Computation Form for Daily Caloric Requirement

A. Current body weight   _____

B. Caloric requirement per pound of body weight (use Table 10.1)   _____

C. Typical daily caloric requirement without exercise to maintain
    body weight (A × B)   _____

D. Selected physical activity (e.g., jogging)[1]   _____

E. Number of exercise sessions per week   _____

F. Duration of exercise session (in minutes)   _____

G. Total weekly exercise time in minutes (E × F)   _____

H. Average daily exercise time in minutes (G ÷ 7)   _____

I. Caloric expenditure per pound per minute (cal/lb/min) based on
    perceived exertion of physical activity (use Table 10.2)   _____

J. Total calories burned per minute of physical activity (A × I)   _____

K. Average daily calories burned as a result of the exercise program (H × J)   _____

L. Total daily caloric requirement with exercise to maintain body weight (C + K) _____

M. Number of calories to subtract from daily requirement to achieve
    a negative caloric balance[2]   _____

N. Target caloric intake to lose weight (L − M)   _____

---

[1] If more than one physical activity is selected, you will need to estimate the average daily calories burned as result of each additional activity (steps D through K) and add all of these figures to L above.

[2] Subtract 500 calories if the total daily requirement with exercise (L) is below 3,000 calories. As many as 1,000 calories may be subtracted for daily requirements above 3,000 calories.

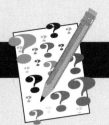

ASSESSMENT 10-2

Daily Nutrition Food Log

Name _____Date _____Grade _____

Instructor _____Course _____Section _____

Age _____   Weight _____   Number of days to be analyzed _____

Sex _____Male   _____Female (Pregnant – P Lactating – L, Neither – N)

Activity Rating: Sedentary (limited physical activity)   = 1
                    Moderate physical activity   = 2
                    Hard labor (strenuous physical activity) = 3

ASSIGNMENT: This laboratory experience should be carried out as homework assignment to be completed over the next seven days.

LAB RESOURCES: Food Guide Pyramid (Figure 8.5, page 212) and list of "Nutritive Value of Selected Foods" (Appendix A).

OBJECTIVE: To meet the minimum daily required servings of the basic food groups and monitor total daily fat intake.

INSTRUCTIONS: Keep a 7-day record of your food consumption using the Food Guide Pyramid and the form provided on the next page. Make additional copies of this form as needed (at least 3 days are recommended). Whenever you have something to eat, record the food code from the Nutritive Value of Selected Foods list contained in Appendix A, the number of calories, grams of fat, and the servings in the corresponding spaces provided for each food group. If a food item is not listed in the Nutritive Value of Selected Foods list, the information can be obtained from the food container itself or from some of the references given at the end of the list of foods in Appendix A.

Record all information immediately after each meal, because it will be easier to keep track of foods and the amounts eaten. If twice the amount of a particular serving is eaten, the calories and grams of fat must doubled and two servings should be recorded under the respective food group.

At the end of the day, the diet is evaluated by checking whether the minimum required servings for each food group were met, and by the total amount of fat consumed. If you have met the required servings, you are well on your way to achieving a well-balanced diet. Additionally, fat intake should not exceed 30% of the total daily caloric consumption. If you are on a diet, you may want to reduce fat intake to less than 20% of total daily calories (see Table 10.3, page 275). You may also use the information in this form (food codes and amounts are required) to run the computer nutrient analysis that is available to course instructors through the Morton Publishing Company.

Name: _____

No.	Code*	Food	Amount	Calories	Fat (gm)	Bread, Cereal, Rice & Pasta	Vegetable	Fruit	Milk, Yogurt & Cheese	Meat, Poultry, Fish, Dry Beans, Eggs, & Nuts
1										
2										
3										
4										
5										
6										
7										
8										
9										
10										
11										
12										
13										
14										
15										
16										
17										
18										
19										
20										
21										
22										
23										
24										
25										
26										
27										
28										
29										
30										
Totals										
Recommended Amount				**	***	6–11	3–5	2–4	2–3	2–3
Deficiencies										

Food Groups (servings)

*See list of nutritive value of selected foods in Appendix A.

**Compute using Table 10.1, page 273.

***Multiply the recommended amount of calories by .30 (30%) and divide by 9 to obtain the recommended amount of grams of fat (if on a diet, multiply by .20 or .10 — see Table 10.3, page 275).

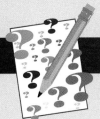

Are You A Psychological Overeater?

Name _____ Date _____ Grade _____

Instructor _____ Course _____ Section _____

NECESSARY LAB EQUIPMENT: None required.

OBJECTIVE: To determine if you are a psychological overeater?

INSTRUCTIONS: Psychological overeaters generally fall into several distinct categories. Finding yourself in one of these categories is no cause for panic. Becoming aware of when, why, and where you overeat can help you avoid the triggers that lead to nonstop nibbling. To find out where you fit in, answer the questions below as follows:

    0 = never   **1 = once in a while**   **2 = fairly often**   **3 = regularly**

The category with the highest score gives you your basic overeating style.

Nervous Night Eater

☐ I often skimp on meals until nightfall, then I stuff my face non-stop.

☐ I crave sweet, salty, or high-fat snacks.

☐ I often munch in front of the TV starting with the evening news on through the late show.

☐ I often conduct midnight raids on the refrigerator.

☐ I have trouble getting to sleep or staying asleep.

☐ I drink more than three cups of coffee a day.

☐ On a scale of 1 to 10, I'd say my stress level rates a 9 or 10.

☐ I've been called a worrywart.

Compulsive Eater

☐ I often skip sit-down meals and usually eat on the run.

☐ I'm rarely without some type of food in my mouth.

☐ I'd rather eat food — even when I'm not hungry — than waste it.

☐ I crave foods that are sweet, starchy, and soft (but I'll eat anything).

☐ I usually sneak food when no one is around to see me eat it.

☐ My favorite beverage is diet soda — lots of it.

☐ I'm cheery on the outside, but inside I feel lonely and blue.

☐ My love life is either stressful or nonexistent.

Closet Binge Eater

☐ About three times a month, I suddenly pig out uncontrollably.

☐ When I binge, I gobble food fast and steadily, easily polishing off an entire bag of cookies.

☐ I binge in private and usually at night.

☐ My binges usually are triggered when I'm upset or stressed out.

☐ Immediately after bingeing I feel calm, but later ashamed and furious at myself.

☐ After a binge, I often fast or crash diet.

☐ Often after bingeing, my stomach aches or I have trouble sleeping.

☐ I often feel angry and depressed but don't know why.

Hand-Me-Down Eater

☐ My family devours king-size portions of rich food at every meal.

☐ My parents and siblings are overweight.

☐ My family frequently snacks together in front of the TV.

☐ The most exercise my family gets is reaching for seconds on pie.

☐ Both my mother and I love to cook.

☐ Having a well-stocked pantry makes me feel secure and loved.

☐ My mother always serves an extravagant dinner with rich desserts.

☐ My family celebrates even minor occasions with lavish feasts.

Thin/Fat

☐ I was overweight as a teenager and now am deathly afraid of gaining weight.

☐ It's a never-ending battle to stay thin.

☐ I eat nothing but low-calorie meals.

☐ I nag those close to me if they gain even a pound or two because I detest fat people.

☐ My life would be ruined if I were to gain weight.

☐ I can tell you the fat and calorie count of nearly every food.

☐ Fat people are weak and have no will power.

☐ Bingeing is the furthest thing from my mind.

Chronic Dieter

☐ I've tried all the latest diets and read all the diet books, but none of them are any good.

☐ Within a few months of losing weight, I'm back to my former fat self.

☐ I often crash-diet before a party or important social event.

☐ I know more than most people about diets, nutrition, and psychological causes for weight gain.

☐ I can tell you exactly how and why I lost and re-gained every pound.

☐ I've memorized the calorie count for foods from A to Z.

☐ Weight-loss groups and doctors have all failed me.

☐ I'm into quick and easy weight loss.

Environmental Eater

☐ I can't resist the aromas emanating from a bakery.

☐ Just reading about luscious dessert recipes makes me drool.

☐ TV food commercials send me to the refrigerator.

☐ Eating food goes along with the territory of my job — power lunches, social dinners, etc.

☐ I eat more than most people at meals.

☐ When dining out, I rarely pass up the pastry dessert cart.

☐ I've begun to develop love handles on my waist and batwings under my arms.

☐ I rarely turn down an extra helping or a meal, even if I'm not hungry — if it's there, I'll eat it.

Couch Potato

☐ I prefer curling up with a bag of chips to physical activity.

☐ The most exercise I get these days is lifting a fork to my mouth.

☐ It takes fewer and fewer calories to maintain the same weight.

☐ I wouldn't be caught dead in workout gear.

☐ Walking to stores at the mall is an effort.

☐ I'm stressed and anxious most of the time.

☐ I sit behind a desk all day.

☐ Once I could have danced all night, but since I've gained weight, I can barely shuffle to the TV.

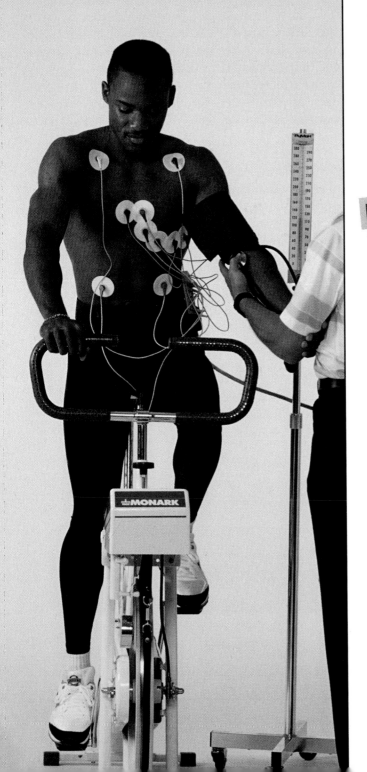

Cardiovascular Wellness

OBJECTIVES

- Define cardiovascular disease and coronary heart disease.
- Explain the differences in HDL, LDL, and VLDL.
- Identify the types of fat and differentiate them.
- Describe the importance of a healthy lifestyle in the prevention of cardiovascular disease.
- List the major risk factors that lead to the development of coronary heart disease.
- Identify the guidelines for cardiovascular disease prevention.

At the beginning of the 20th century, the most common health problems in the United States were infectious diseases such as tuberculosis, diphtheria, influenza, kidney disease, polio, and other diseases of infancy. Progress in the field of medicine largely eliminated these diseases. Nevertheless, as the American people started to enjoy the "good life" (sedentary living, alcohol, fatty foods, excessive sweets, tobacco, drugs), a parallel increase was seen in chronic diseases including cancer, diabetes, emphysema, cirrhosis of the liver — and, in particular, diseases of the cardiovascular system. As the incidence of chronic diseases grew, people began to realize that good health is largely self-controlled and that the leading causes of premature death and illness in the United States could be prevented by adhering to positive lifestyle habits.

INCIDENCE OF CARDIOVASCULAR DISEASE

Cardiovascular disease is the leading cause of death in the United States, accounting for 42.1% of the total mortality rate in 1993. The disease encompasses all pathological conditions that affect the heart and blood vessels. Some examples are coronary heart disease, peripheral vascular disease, congenital heart disease, rheumatic heart disease, atherosclerosis, strokes, hypertension (high blood pressure), and congestive heart failure.

Although heart and blood vessel disease is still the number-one health problem in the United States, the incidence declined by 36% between 1960 and 1990 (see Figure 11.1). The main reasons for this dramatic decrease are health education and better treatment modalities. More people now are aware of the risk factors for cardiovascular disease and are changing their lifestyles to lower their own potential risk for this disease. Further work remains to be done, however, as studies show that the risk of death from cardiovascular disease is greater for the least-educated than the most-educated people.

According to 1997 estimates by the American Heart Association,[1] more than 60 million Americans were afflicted by diseases of the cardiovascular system, including 50 million with hypertension and 13.5 million with coronary heart disease. Many of these individuals have more than one type of cardiovascular disease.

In addition, the yearly estimated cost of heart and blood vessel disease exceeds $151 billion. Heart attacks alone cost American industry approximately 132 million workdays annually, including $22 billion in lost productivity because of physical and emotional disability.

CORONARY HEART DISEASE

The major form of cardiovascular disease is **coronary heart disease (CHD)**, a condition in which the arteries that supply the heart muscle with oxygen and nutrients are narrowed by fatty deposits such as cholesterol and triglycerides. Narrowing of the coronary arteries diminishes the blood supply to the heart muscle, which can precipitate a heart attack (see Figure 11.2).

CHD is the single leading cause of death in the United States, accounting for approximately a third of all deaths and more than half of all cardiovascular deaths. Almost all of the risk factors for CHD are preventable and reversible. Individuals can control them by modifying their lifestyle.

Approximately 1.5 million people have heart attacks each year, more than half a million of whom die as a result. About half the time, the first symptom of coronary heart disease is the heart attack itself, and most of these people die within the first 24

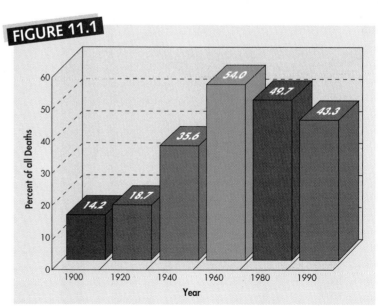

FIGURE 11.1

Incidence of cardiovascular disease in United States for selected year: 1900–1990.

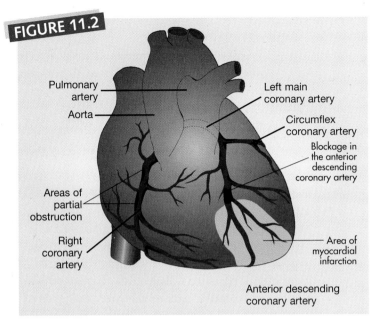

FIGURE 11.2

Pulmonary artery
Aorta
Left main coronary artery
Circumflex coronary artery
Blockage in the anterior descending coronary artery
Areas of partial obstruction
Right coronary artery
Area of myocardial infarction
Anterior descending coronary artery

Heart attack as a result of acute reduction in blood flow through anterior descending coronary artery.

Studies have documented further that multiple interrelations usually exist between risk factors. Physical inactivity, for instance, often contributes to an increase in (a) body weight (fat), (b) cholesterol, (c) triglycerides, (d) tension and stress, (e) blood pressure, and (f) risk for diabetes. The interrelationships among leading cardiovascular risk factors are depicted in Figure 11.3.

Cardiovascular disease The array of conditions that affect the heart and the blood vessels.

Coronary heart disease (CHD) Condition in which the arteries that supply the heart muscle with oxygen and nutrients are narrowed by fatty deposits such as cholesterol and triglycerides.

hours. In one of every five cardiovascular deaths, sudden death is the initial symptom.

About 38% of the people who die are in their most productive years, below age 75. The American Heart Association estimates that more than $700 million a year in the United States is spent in replacing employees who have had heart attacks.

The leading risk factors contributing to CHD are:

- Physical inactivity
- Low HDL-cholesterol
- Elevated LDL-cholesterol
- Smoking
- High blood pressure
- Abnormal stress or resting electrocardiogram
- Family history of heart disease
- Personal history of heart disease
- Diabetes
- Excessive body fat
- Elevated triglycerides
- Tension and stress
- Age

Although genetic inheritance plays a role in CHD, the most important determinant is personal lifestyle. With the exception of age, family history of heart disease, and certain electrocardiogram (ECG) abnormalities, the risk factors are preventable and reversible.

Facts on Coronary Heart Disease

Coronary heart disease (heart attack) caused 487,490 deaths in the United States in 1994 — 1 of every 4.7 deaths.

- Heart attack is the single largest killer of American males and females.
- About every 20 seconds an American will have a heart attack, and about every minute someone will die from one.
- This year as many as 1,500,000 Americans will have a new or recurrent heart attack, and about one-third of them will die.
- At least 250,000 people a year die of heart attack within 1 hour of the onset of symptoms and before they reach a hospital.
- 13,670,000 people alive today have a history of heart attack, angina pectoris (chest pain) or both. This breaks down to 6,930,000 males and 6,750,000 females.
- 5% of all heart attacks occur in people under age 40, and 45% occur in people under age 65.
- About 80% of coronary heart disease mortality in people under age 65 occurs during the first attack.
- 48% of men and 63% of women who died suddenly of coronary heart disease had no previous symptoms of this disease.

Source: *1997 Heart and Stroke Statistical Update*, American Heart Association.

Physical Inactivity

Physical inactivity is responsible for low levels of cardiorespiratory endurance, previously defined as the ability of the lungs, heart, and blood vessels to deliver enough oxygen to the cells to meet the demands of prolonged physical activity. Improving cardiorespiratory endurance through aerobic exercise may have the greatest impact in reducing overall risk for heart disease. Although specific recommendations can be followed to improve each risk factor, a regular aerobic exercise program helps control most of the major risk factors that lead to heart disease.

Aerobic exercise:

— increases cardiorespiratory endurance
— decreases and controls blood pressure
— reduces body fat
— lowers blood lipids (cholesterol and triglycerides)
— improves HDL-cholesterol
— helps control diabetes
— increases and maintains good heart function, sometimes improving certain ECG abnormalities
— motivates toward smoking cessation
— alleviates tension and stress
— counteracts a personal history of heart disease.

The significance of physical inactivity in contributing to cardiovascular risk was clearly shown in 1992, when the American Heart Association added physical inactivity as one of the four major risk factors for cardiovascular disease. (The other three factors are smoking, a poor cholesterol profile, and high blood pressure.) Based on the overwhelming amount of scientific data in this area, evidence of the benefits of aerobic exercise in reducing heart disease is far too impressive to be ignored.

FIGURE 11.3

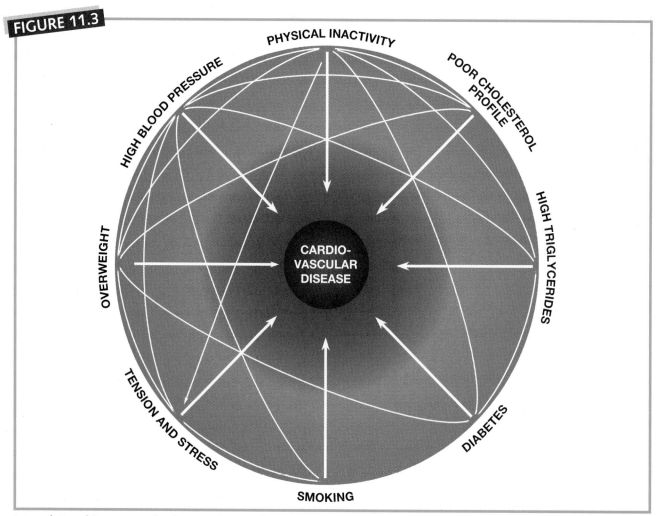

Interrelationships among leading cardiovascular risk factors.

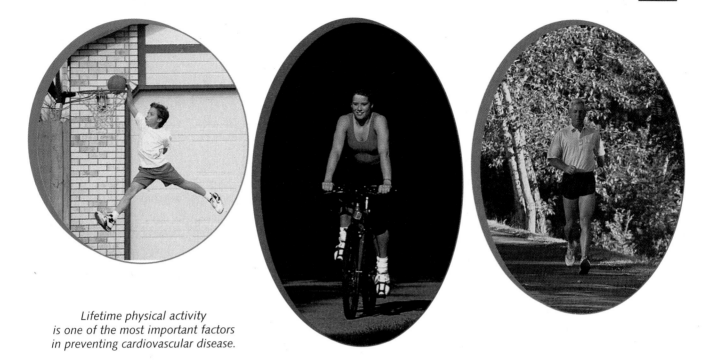

Lifetime physical activity is one of the most important factors in preventing cardiovascular disease.

Research at the Institute for Aerobics Research in Dallas, Texas,[2] clearly shows the tie between cardiorespiratory fitness and mortality, regardless of age and other risk factors (see Figure 11.4). A higher level of physical fitness benefits even those who have other risk factors such as high blood pressure and serum cholesterol, cigarette smoking, and a family history of heart disease. In most cases, unfit people in the study (group 1) without these risk factors had higher death rates than fit people (groups 4 and 5) with these same risk factors.

Although the findings show that the higher the level of cardiorespiratory fitness, the longer the life, the largest drop in premature death is seen between the unfit and the moderately fit groups. Even small improvements in cardiorespiratory endurance greatly decrease the risk for cardiovascular mortality. Most adults who become physically active and engage in moderate-intensity activities can attain these fitness levels easily.

Research published in 1993 substantiated the importance of exercise in preventing CHD.[3] Dr. Ralph Paffenbarger and his colleagues indicated that the benefits to previously inactive adults of starting a moderate to vigorous physical activity program were as important as quitting smoking, managing blood pressure, and controlling cholesterol. The increase in physical activity led to the same decrease as giving up cigarette smoking in relative risk for death from CHD.

Even though physically active individuals have a lower incidence of cardiovascular

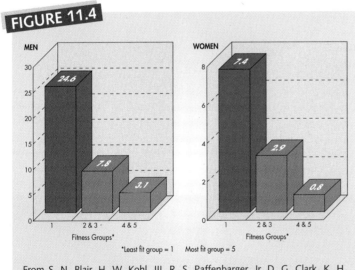

FIGURE 11.4

From S. N. Blair, H. W. Kohl, III, R. S. Paffenbarger, Jr, D. G. Clark, K. H. Cooper, and L. W. Gibbons, "Physical Fitness and All-Cause Mortality: A Prospective Study of Healthy Men and Women." *Journal of the American Medical Association*, 262 (1989), 2395–2401.

Age-Adjusted Cardiovascular Death Rates per 10,000 Person-Years of Follow-up (1970–1985) by Physical Fitness Groups in the Aerobics Center Longitudinal Study, Dallas, Texas (one person-year indicates one person followed up one year later).

disease, a regular physical activity program by itself does not guarantee a lifetime free of cardiovascular problems. Poor lifestyle habits, such as smoking, eating too many fatty/salty/sweet foods, being overweight, and having high stress levels increase cardiovascular risk and will not be eliminated completely through physical activity.

Overall management of the risk factors is the best way to lower the risk for cardiovascular disease. Still, physical activity is one of the most important factors in preventing and reducing cardiovascular problems. The basic principles for cardiorespiratory exercise are given in Chapter 7.

Abnormal Cholesterol Profile

Cholesterol is a waxy substance, technically a steroid alcohol, found only in animal fats and oil. This fatty substance is essential for specific metabolic functions in the body, but an abnormal cholesterol profile contributes to atherosclerotic plaque, a build-up of fatty tissue in the walls of the arteries. As the plaque accumulates, it blocks the blood vessels that supply the heart muscle (myocardium) with oxygen and nutrients, and these obstructions can trigger a myocardial infarction or heart attack (see Figures 11.2 and 11.5).

Cholesterol is carried in the bloodstream by molecules of protein known as high-density lipoproteins (HDLs), low-density lipoproteins (LDLs), and very low-density lipoproteins (VLDLs). Although subcategories of these lipoproteins have been identified, the discussion here focuses only on these major categories.

Cholesterol has received much attention because direct relationships have been established between high total cholesterol, high LDL-cholesterol and low HDL-cholesterol, and the rate of CHD in both men and women. Unfortunately, the heart disguises its problems quite well and typical symptoms of heart disease, such as angina pectoris or chest pain, do not start until the arteries are about 75% blocked. In many cases, the first symptom is sudden death.

The general recommendation by the National Cholesterol Education Program (NCEP) given in Table 11.1, is to keep total cholesterol levels below 200 mg/dl. Other health professionals recommend that total cholesterol in individuals age 30 and younger should not be higher than 180 mg/dl, and for children the level should be below 170 mg/dl. Cholesterol levels between 200 and 239 mg/dl are borderline high, and levels of 240 mg/dl and above indicate high risk for disease.

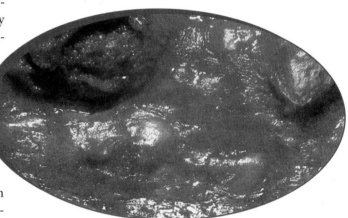

Fatty plaque collects on inner lining of an artery as a result of atherosclerosis.

FIGURE 11.5

THE ATHEROSCLEROTIC PROCESS

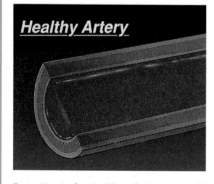
Healthy Artery

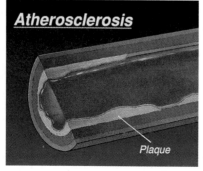
Atherosclerosis

Plaque

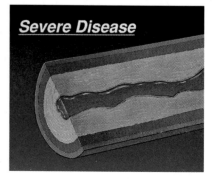
Severe Disease

From *Heart of a Healthy Life.* Courtesy of the American Heart Association, © 1992.

TABLE 11.1 Cholesterol Guidelines

	Amount	Rating
Total Cholesterol	<200 mg/dl	Desirable
	200–239 mg/dl	Borderline high
	≥240 mg/dl	High risk
LDL-Cholesterol	<130 mg/dl	Desirable
	130-159 mg/dl	Borderline high
	≥160 mg/dl	High risk
HDL-Cholesterol	≥45 mg/dl	Desirable
	36–44 mg/dl	Moderate risk
	≤35 mg/dl	High risk

Cholesterol is transported primarily in the form of LDL and HDL. Low-density molecules tend to release cholesterol, which then may penetrate the lining or inner membrane of the arteries and speed up the process of atherosclerosis. The NCEP guidelines state that an **LDL-cholesterol** value below 130 mg/dl is desirable, between 130 and 159 mg/dl is borderline-high, and 160 mg/dl and above carries high risk for cardiovascular disease. VLDL molecules only transport about 10% of the total cholesterol, so not much risk for CHD is attributed to VLDL-cholesterol.

HDL-cholesterol, on the other hand, is the "good cholesterol" and offers some protection against heart disease. In a process known as **reverse cholesterol transport**, HDLs act as scavengers, carrying cholesterol to be metabolized and secreted, thereby preventing plaque from forming in the arteries.

The strength of HDL is in the protein molecules in their coatings. When HDL comes in contact with cholesterol-filled cells, these protein molecules attach to the cells and take their cholesterol. The more HDL-cholesterol, the better.

Evidence suggests that low levels of HDL-cholesterol could be the best predictor of CHD and may be more significant than the total value. Substantial research supports the evidence that a low level of HDL-cholesterol has the strongest relationship to CHD at all levels of total cholesterol, including levels below 200 mg/dl.[4] The recommended HDL-cholesterol value to minimize the risk for CHD is 45 mg/dl or higher. (Guidelines for the various types of cholesterol are given in Table 11.1.)

For the most part, HDL-cholesterol is determined genetically. Generally, women have higher values than men. This is one of the reasons heart disease is less common in women. Black children and adult black men have higher values than caucasians. HDL-cholesterol also decreases with age.

Increasing HDL-cholesterol improves the cholesterol profile and decreases the risk for CHD. Habitual aerobic exercise, weight loss, and quitting smoking all have been shown to raise HDL-cholesterol.[5] Beta-carotene[6] and certain prescription drugs may also promote higher HDL-cholesterol levels.

HDL-cholesterol and a regular aerobic exercise program (intensity level above 6 METs — see Chapter 6) are clearly related. Individual responses to aerobic exercise differ but, generally, the more the exercise, the higher the HDL-cholesterol level.

> " *Generally, the more the exercise, the higher the HDL-cholesterol level.* "

The antioxidant effect of vitamins C and E and beta-carotene also can lower the risk for CHD.[7] Antioxidants prevent oxygen from combining with other substances it may damage. During metabolism, oxygen is used to convert carbohydrates and fats into energy. In doing so, oxygen is transformed into stable forms of water and carbon dioxide. A small amount of oxygen, however, ends up in an unstable form, called **oxygen free radicals**. These free radicals attack and damage proteins and lipids — in particular, the cell membrane and DNA.

Free radicals are thought to play a key role in the development of conditions such as heart disease,

Cholesterol A waxy substance, technically a steroid alcohol, found only in animal fats and oil; used in making cell membranes, as a building block for some hormones, in the fatty sheath around nerve fibers, and in other necessary substances.

LDL-cholesterol Cholesterol-transporting molecules in the blood (bad cholesterol).

HDL-cholesterol Cholesterol-transporting molecules in the blood (good cholesterol).

Reverse cholesterol transport A process in which HDL molecules attract cholesterol and carry it to the liver, where it is changed to bile and eventually excreted in the stool.

Oxygen free radicals Substances formed during metabolism which attack and damage proteins and lipids, in particular the cell membrane and DNA, leading to the development of diseases such as heart disease, cancer, and emphysema.

cancer, and emphysema. Researchers believe antioxidants offer protection by absorbing free radicals before they can cause damage and also by interrupting the sequence of reactions once damage has begun, thwarting certain chronic diseases.

Vitamin C seems to inactivate free radicals, and vitamin E protects LDL from oxidation. Beta-carotene not only absorbs free radicals, keeping them from causing damage, but it also seems to increase HDL levels in some people.

Certain cholesterol-lowering drugs also may help raise HDL levels. Clinical data have shown an improvement when HDL-cholesterol is increased with colestipol plus niacin and the diet is low in fat and saturated fat.

Although the average American consumes between 400 and 600 mg of cholesterol daily, the body actually manufactures more than that. Approximately 1,000 mg of cholesterol per day is produced from saturated fats.[8] Saturated fats are found mostly in meats and dairy products and seldom in foods of plant origin. Poultry and fish contain less saturated fat than beef does, but they should be eaten in moderation (about 3 to 6 ounces per day). Unsaturated fats are mainly of plant origin and cannot be converted to cholesterol.

Because of individual differences, a few people can have higher-than-normal intakes of saturated fats and still maintain normal cholesterol levels. Conversely, some people with a lower intake can have abnormally high cholesterol levels.

If LDL-cholesterol is higher than recommended, it can be lowered by losing body fat, manipulating the diet, and taking medication. A diet low in fat, saturated fat, and cholesterol and high in complex carbohydrates and fiber is recommended to decrease LDL-cholesterol.

The NCEP recommends replacing saturated fat with monounsaturated and polyunsaturated fat (for example, olive, canola, peanut, and corn oils), because these fats do not cause a reduction in HDL-cholesterol. When unsaturated fats replace saturated fats in the diet, the former tend to stimulate the liver to clear cholesterol from the blood.

Earlier studies had suggested that polyunsaturated fats also seemed to cause reduction of the "good" (HDL) cholesterol. Additional research, however, does not support these negative effects on HDL-cholesterol. At typical levels found in the diet, polyunsaturated and monounsaturated fats appear to have similar effects on blood cholesterol.

Many experts believe that to have a significant effect in lowering LDL-cholesterol, total fat consumption must be significantly lower than the current 30% of total daily caloric intake guideline. Consumption of saturated fat ideally should be less than 10% of the total daily caloric intake, and average cholesterol consumption should be much lower than 300 mg per day. Research on the effects of a 30%-fat diet have shown that it has little or no effect in lowering cholesterol, and CHD actually continues to progress in people who have the disease.

The good news comes from a 1991 study in which the participants followed a 10% or less fat-calorie diet combined with a regular aerobic exercise program, primarily walking.[9] In the diet, cholesterol intake was limited to less than 25 mg/day. The participants lowered their cholesterol by an average of 23% in only 3 weeks. The author of the study concluded that the exact percent fat guideline (10% or 15%) is unknown but that 30% total fat calories is definitely too much when attempting to lower cholesterol level.

A daily 10%-total-fat diet requires that the person limit fat intake to an absolute minimum. Some health care professionals contend that a diet like this is difficult to follow indefinitely. People with high cholesterol levels may not have to follow that diet indefinitely but should adopt the 10%-fat diet while attempting to lower cholesterol. Thereafter, eating a 30%-fat diet may be adequate to maintain recommended cholesterol levels. By way of comparison, current fat consumption in the United States averages about 37% of total calories.

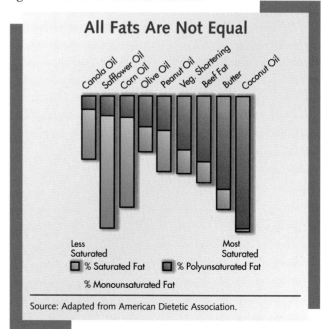

All Fats Are Not Equal

Canola Oil, Safflower Oil, Corn Oil, Olive Oil, Peanut Oil, Veg. Shortening, Beef Fat, Butter, Coconut Oil

Less Saturated — Most Saturated

□ % Saturated Fat   ■ % Polyunsaturated Fat

% Monounsaturated Fat

Source: Adapted from American Dietetic Association.

High Triglycerides

Triglycerides also are known as **free fatty acids**. In combination with cholesterol, they speed up formation of plaque. Fatty acids are carried in the bloodstream primarily by VLDLs and **chylomicrons**.

Triglycerides are found in poultry skin, lunch meats, and shellfish. Primarily, however, they are manufactured in the liver, from refined sugars, starches, and alcohol. High intake of alcohol and sugars (including honey) raises triglyceride levels. They can be lowered by cutting down on these foods along with reducing weight (if overweight) and doing aerobic exercise. An optimal blood triglyceride level is less than 125 mg/dl (see Table 11.2).

Some people consistently have slightly elevated triglyceride levels (above 140 mg/dl) and HDL-cholesterol levels below 35 mg/dl. About 80% of these individuals have a genetic condition called LDL phenotype B (approximately 40% of the U.S. population falls in this category). Although the blood lipids may not be notably high, these people are at higher risk for atherosclerosis and CHD.[10]

People who never have had a blood chemistry test should do so. An initial test always is useful to establish a baseline for future reference. The blood test should include the HDL-cholesterol component.

Although no definite guidelines have been set, after a person has an initial normal baseline test no later than age 20, and keeps recommended dietary and exercise guidelines, a blood analysis every 5 years prior to age 40 should suffice. After age 40, individuals should have a blood lipid test every year, in conjunction with a regular preventive medicine physical examination.

High Blood Pressure (Hypertension)

Blood pressure is a measure of the force exerted against the walls of the blood vessels by the blood flowing through them. Blood pressure is assessed using a sphygmomanometer and a stethoscope. The **sphygmomanometer** consists of an inflatable bladder contained within a cuff and a mercury gravity manometer or an aneroid manometer from which the pressure is read. The pressure is measured in milliliters of mercury (mm Hg) and usually expressed in two numbers. Ideal blood pressure should be 120/80 or below (see Table 11.3). The higher number reflects the pressure exerted during the forceful contraction of the heart or systole and is called the **systolic pressure**. The lower pressure is taken during the heart's relaxation, or diastolic phase, when no blood is being ejected, and is termed **diastolic pressure**.

Based on current American Heart Association estimates, about 50 million people in the United States are hypertensive. **Hypertension** has been viewed as the point at which the pressure doubles the mortality risk, about 160/96. Because statistical evidence clearly indicates that blood pressure readings above 140/90 increase the risk of disease and premature death, however, the American Heart Association considers all blood pressures above 140/90 as hypertension.

Many experts believe that the lower the blood pressure, the better. Even if the pressure is around 90/50, as long as individuals do not have any symptoms of low blood pressure or hypotension, they do

TABLE 11.3   Blood Pressure Guidelines

Rating	Systolic	Diastolic
Ideal	≤120	≤80 mmHg
Borderline high	121–139	81–89 mmHg
Hypertension	≥140	≥90 mmHg

Triglycerides   Fats formed by glycerol and three fatty acids. Also known as free fatty acids.

Free fatty acids (FFA)   Fats formed by glycerol and three fatty acids. Also know as triglycerides.

Chylomicrons   Triglyceride-transporting molecules in the blood.

Blood pressure   A measure of the force exerted against the walls of the vessels by the blood flowing through them.

Sphygmomanometer   An inflatable bladder contained within a cuff and a mercury gravity manometer (or an aneroid manometer) from which the pressure is read.

Systolic pressure   Pressure exerted by the blood against the walls of the arteries during the forceful contraction (systole) of the heart.

Diastolic pressure   Pressure exerted by the blood against the walls of the arteries during the relaxation phase (diastole) of the heart.

Hypertension   Chronically elevated blood pressure.

TABLE 11.2   Triglycerides Guidelines

Amount	Rating
<125 mg/dl	Desirable
126–499 mg/dl	Borderline high
≥500 mg/dl	High risk

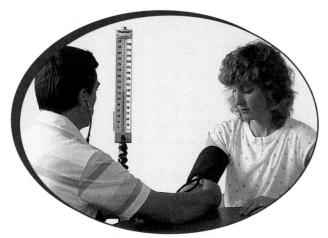

Blood pressure assessment using a mercury gravity manometer.

not need to be concerned. Typical hypotension symptoms are dizziness, lightheadedness, and fainting.

Blood pressure may fluctuate during a regular day. Many factors affect blood pressure, and one single reading may not be a true indicator of your real pressure. For example, physical activity and stress increase blood pressure, whereas rest and relaxation decrease it. Consequently, several measurements should be taken before diagnosing elevated pressure.

As a disease, hypertension has been called the silent killer. It does not hurt, it does not make you feel sick, and unless you check it, years may go by before you even realize you have a problem. High blood pressure is a risk factor not only for CHD but also for congestive heart failure, strokes, and kidney failure.

Smoking

Cigarette smoking is the single largest preventable cause of illness and premature death in the United States. When considering all related deaths, tobacco is responsible for more than 400,000 unnecessary deaths per year. About 50,000 of those who die are nonsmokers who were exposed to second-hand smoke. Smoking has been linked to cardiovascular disease, cancer, bronchitis, emphysema, and peptic ulcers. In relation to coronary disease, smoking speeds up the process of atherosclerosis, and it increases the risk of sudden death following a myocardial infarction (heart attack) threefold.

Smoking prompts the release of nicotine and another 1,200 toxic compounds or so into the bloodstream. Similar to hypertension, many of these substances destroy the inner membrane that protects the walls of the arteries. Once the lining has been damaged, cholesterol and triglycerides can be deposited readily in the arterial wall. As the plaque builds up, it obstructs blood flow through the arteries.

Furthermore, smoking encourages the formation of blood clots, which can completely block an artery already narrowed by atherosclerosis. In addition, carbon monoxide, a byproduct of cigarette smoke, decreases the blood's oxygen-carrying capacity. A combination of obstructed arteries, nicotine, and less oxygen in the heart muscle heightens the risk for a serious heart problem.

Smoking also increases heart rate, raises blood pressure, and irritates the heart, which can trigger fatal **cardiac arrhythmias**. Another harmful effect is a decrease in the "good" HDL-cholesterol that helps control blood lipids. Smoking actually presents a much greater risk of death from heart disease than from lung disease.

> *Smoking actually presents a much greater risk of death from heart disease than from lung disease.*

Pipe and cigar smoking and chewing tobacco also increase the risk for heart disease. Even if no smoke is inhaled, toxic substances are absorbed through the membranes of the mouth and end up in the bloodstream.

Personal and Family History

Individuals who have had cardiovascular problems are at higher risk than those who never have had a problem. People with this history should control the other risk factors as much as they can. Because most risk factors are reversible, this will greatly decrease the risk for future problems. The more time that has passed since the cardiovascular problem occurred, the lower is the risk for recurrence.

Genetic predisposition toward heart disease has been demonstrated clearly and seems to be gaining in importance. All other factors being equal, a person with blood relatives who have or had heart disease before age 60 runs a greater risk than someone who has no such history. The younger the age at which the incident happened to the relative, the greater is the risk for the disease.

In many cases, we have no way of knowing whether a person's true genetic predisposition or simply poor lifestyle habits led to a heart problem. A person may have been physically inactive, overweight, smoked, and had bad dietary habits, leading to a heart attack. Because we cannot differentiate these factors reliably, a person with a family history of cardiovascular problems should watch all other factors closely and maintain as low a risk level as possible. In addition, an annual blood chemistry analysis is recommended strongly to make sure the body is handling blood lipids properly.

Diabetes

Diabetes mellitus is a condition in which blood glucose is unable to enter the cells because the pancreas totally stops producing insulin or does not produce enough to meet the body's needs or the body cannot use insulin properly. As a result, glucose absorption by the cells and the liver is low, leading to high glucose levels in the blood.

The incidence of cardiovascular disease and death in the diabetic population is quite high. Over 80% of people with diabetes mellitus die from cardiovascular disease. People with chronically elevated blood glucose levels also may have problems in metabolizing fats, which can make them more susceptible to atherosclerosis, increase the risk for coronary disease, and lead to other conditions such as vision loss and kidney damage.

Fasting blood glucose levels above 120 mg/dl may be an early sign of diabetes and should be brought to the attention of a physician. Many health care practitioners consider blood glucose levels around 150 to 160 mg/dl as borderline diabetes (see Table 11.4).

The two major types of diabetes are **Type I**, or insulin-dependent diabetes, and **Type II**, or non-insulin-dependent diabetes. Type I also is called juvenile diabetes because it is found mainly in young people. In insulin-dependent diabetes, the pancreas produces little or no insulin. In non-insulin-dependent (Type II) diabetes, often referred to as adult-onset diabetes, the insulin-producing cells function adequately but the body is unable to use insulin properly.

Although there is a genetic predisposition to diabetes, adult-onset diabetes is related closely to overeating, obesity, and lack of physical activity. In most cases, this condition can be corrected through a special diet, a weight-loss program, and a regular exercise program.

A diet high in water-soluble fibers (found in fruits, vegetables, oats, and beans) is helpful in treating diabetes. An aerobic exercise program — walking, cycling, or swimming four to five times per week — often is prescribed because it increases the body's sensitivity to insulin. Individuals who have high blood glucose levels should consult a physician to decide on the best treatment.

According to research, aerobic exercise helps prevent diabetes in middle-aged men.[11] The protective effect is even greater in those with risk factors such as obesity, high blood pressure, and family propensity.

This preventive effect is attributed to lowered body fat and better sugar and fat metabolism through a regular exercise program. At 3,500 calories expended per week through exercise, the risk was cut in half when compared to sedentary men. The preventive effect, the study suggests, should hold for women, too.

Excessive Body Fat

Body composition is the ratio of lean body weight to fat weight. If the body contains too much fat, the person is considered obese. Although some experts recognize obesity as an independent risk factor for CHD, the risks attributed to obesity actually may be caused by other risk factors that usually accompany excessive body fat. Risk factors such as high blood lipids, hypertension, and diabetes usually improve with increased physical activity. As discussed in Chapter 10, overweight people who are physically active do not seem to be at increased risk for premature death.

Attaining recommended body composition helps people reach a better state of health and wellness. People who have a weight problem and desire to achieve recommended weight can do so by

— increasing their physical activity

TABLE 11.4	Blood Glucose Guidelines	
Amount	**Rating**	
≤120	Desirable	
121–159	Borderline high	
≥160	High	

Cardiac arrhythmias   Irregular heart rhythms.

Type I diabetes   Initially occurs primarily in young people. A condition in which the pancreas produces little or no insulin. Also called juvenile diabetes.

Type II diabetes   A condition in which the body is unable to use insulin properly.

— consuming a diet low in fat and refined sugars and high in complex carbohydrates and fiber

— reducing their total caloric intake moderately while still providing all of the necessary nutrients to sustain normal body functions.

Recommendations for weight management are discussed in Chapter 10.

Tension and Stress

Tension and stress (the topic of Chapter 3) have become a normal part of life. Everyone has to deal daily with goals, deadlines, responsibilities, pressures. Almost everything in life (whether positive or negative) is a source of stress. The stressor itself is not what creates the health hazard but, rather, the individual's response to it.

The human body responds to stress by producing more catecholamines (hormones) to prepare the body for fight or flight. These hormones elevate heart rate, blood pressure, and blood glucose levels, enabling the person to take action. If the person "fights or flees," the higher levels of catecholamines are metabolized and the body is able to return to a normal state. If, however, a person is under constant stress and unable to take action (such as with the death of a close relative or friend, loss of a job, trouble at work, financial insecurity), the catecholamines remain elevated in the bloodstream.

People who are unable to relax put constant low-level strain on the cardiovascular system that might manifest itself in heart disease. In addition, when a person is in a stressful situation, the coronary arteries that feed the heart muscle constrict, reducing the oxygen supply to the heart. If the blood vessels are significantly blocked by atherosclerosis, abnormal heart rhythms or even a heart attack may follow.

Age

Age is a risk factor because of the greater incidence of heart disease in older people. This tendency may be induced partly by other factors stemming from changes in lifestyle as we get older (less physical activity, poor nutrition, obesity, and so on).

Young people should not think they will escape heart disease. The process begins early in life. This was clearly shown in American soldiers who died during the Korean and Vietnam conflicts. Autopsies conducted on soldiers killed at 22 years of age and younger revealed that approximately 70% had early stages of atherosclerosis. Other studies have found elevated blood cholesterol levels in children as young as 10 years old.

Even though the aging process cannot be stopped, it certainly can be slowed. Physiological versus chronological age is an important concept in preventing disease. Some individuals in their 60s or older have the body of a 20-year-old. And 20-year-olds often are in such poor condition and health that they almost seem to have the body of a 60-year-old. Risk factor management and positive lifestyle habits are the best ways to slow down the natural aging process.

PREVENTING CARDIOVASCULAR DISEASE

As should be clear by now, most cardiovascular risk factors are preventable and reversible. Overall risk factor management is the best guideline to lower the risk. A regular aerobic exercise program in combination with proper nutrition, avoidance of tobacco, blood pressure control, stress management, and weight control are the key elements in preventing disorders of the cardiovascular system.

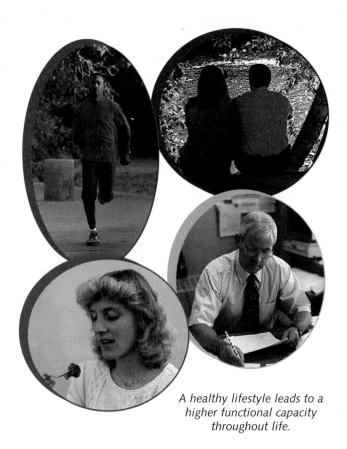

A healthy lifestyle leads to a higher functional capacity throughout life.

Lifetime Physical Activity

An active lifestyle combined with a systematic aerobic exercise program is one of the most important means of preventing and reducing the risk of cardiovascular problems. The basic principles for cardiorespiratory exercise are given in Chapter 7.

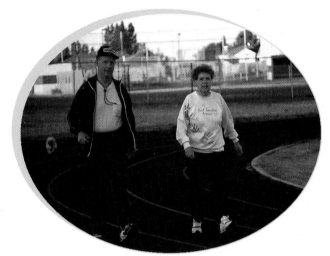

A moderate aerobic exercise program greatly reduces the risk for premature cardiovascular death.

Although greater benefits are obtained at higher intensity levels, even a moderate-intensity aerobic exercise program can reduce cardiovascular risk considerably.[12] A simple 40-minute walking (or equivalent) program, six to seven times per week, seems to have a strong inverse relationship with premature cardiovascular mortality. The minimum amount of exercise recommended for adults to achieve moderate fitness is presented in Table 11.5.

Nutrition Recommendations

Nutrition is the topic of Chapter 8. Here, we specifically relate nutrition to prevention of cardiovascular

Tips For Action — Lowering Cholesterol

To lower LDL-cholesterol levels:

- Consume fewer than three eggs per week.
- Eat red meats (3 ounces per serving) fewer than three times per week, and no organ meats (such as liver and kidneys).
- Do not eat commercially baked foods.
- Drink low-fat milk (1% or less fat, preferably) and eat low-fat dairy products.
- Do not use coconut oil, palm oil, or cocoa butter.
- Eat fish instead of red meat.
- Bake, broil, grill, poach, or steam food instead of frying.
- Refrigerate cooked meat before adding to other dishes. Remove fat hardened in the refrigerator before mixing the meat with other foods.
- Avoid fatty sauces made with butter, cream, or cheese.
- Maintain recommended body weight.

disease. In this regard, the diet should contain ample amounts of fruits, vegetables, and grains. Because of their antioxidant effect, foods high in vitamins C and E and beta-carotene should be a regular part of the diet. Foods high in sugar and salt should be avoided. Alcohol should be consumed in moderation.

The combination of a healthy diet, a sound aerobic exercise program, and weight control is the best prescription for controlling blood lipids. If this does not work, a physician can administer a blood test to

TABLE 11.5	Minimum Aerobic Exercise for Moderate Fitness			
	Activity	Distance (miles)	Time (min.)	Frequency (days/week)
Women				
Program I:	Walking	2 or more	30 or less	3 or more
Program II:	Walking	2	30–40	5–6
Men				
Program I:	Walking	2	27 or less	3 or more
Program II:	Walking	2	30–40	6–7

From *Fitness and Mortality* by S. N. Blair (Dallas: Aerobics Research Center, 1991).

break down the lipoproteins into their various sub-categories. Most U.S. laboratories do not conduct these tests, but the American Heart Association has established six Lipid Disorder Training Centers that administer comprehensive blood tests. Your local American Heart Association can provide further information.

Smoking Cessation

Cigarette smoking, low levels of fitness, a poor cholesterol profile, and high blood pressure are the four major risk factors for CHD. Nonetheless, the risk for cardiovascular disease and cancer starts to decrease the moment you quit smoking. The risk approaches that of a lifetime nonsmoker 10 and 15 years, respectively, after cessation.

Quitting cigarette smoking is no easy task. Only about 20% of smokers who try to quit for the first time succeed each year. The addictive properties of nicotine and smoke make quitting difficult. Smokers have physical and psychological withdrawal symptoms when they stop smoking. Even though giving up smoking can be extremely difficult, it is by no means impossible.

The most crucial factor in quitting cigarette smoking is the person's sincere desire to do so. More than 95% of the successful ex-smokers have been able to quit on their own, either by quitting cold turkey or by using self-help kits available from organizations such as the American Cancer Society, the American Heart Association, and the American Lung Association. Only 3% of ex-smokers have quit as a result of formal "stop smoking" programs.

Blood Pressure Control

Of all hypertension, 90% has no identifiable cause. This **essential hypertension** is treatable. Aerobic exercise, weight reduction, a low-sodium/high-potassium diet, stress reduction, no smoking, a diet designed to decrease blood lipids, lower caffeine and alcohol intake, and antihypertensive medication all have been used effectively to treat essential hypertension. The other 10% of hypertension is caused by pathological conditions such as narrowing of the kidney arteries, glomerulonephritis (a kidney disease), tumors of the adrenal glands, and narrowing of the aortic artery. With this type of hypertension, the pathological cause has to be treated before attacking the blood pressure problem.

A factor contributing to high blood pressure in about half of all hypertensive people is too much sodium in the diet (salt, or sodium chloride, contains approximately 40% sodium). With high sodium intake, the body retains more water, which increases the blood volume and, in turn, drives up blood pressure. Although sodium is essential for normal body functions, only 200 mg, or one-tenth of a teaspoon of salt, is required daily. Even under strenuous conditions of job and sports participation that produce heavy perspiration, the amount of sodium required is seldom more than 3,000 mg per day. Yet, sodium intake in the typical American diet ranges between 6,000 and 20,000 mg per day!

When treating high blood pressure (unless it is extremely high), many physicians suggest trying a combination of aerobic exercise, weight loss, smoking cessation (if the person smokes), and reduced sodium before they recommend medication. In most instances, this treatment brings blood pressure under control.

Several well-documented studies have indicated that nearly 90% of hypertensive patients who begin a moderate aerobic exercise program can expect a notable decrease in blood pressure after only a few weeks of training. The research data also show that exercise, not weight loss, is the major contributor to lower blood pressure. If aerobic exercise is discontinued, these changes are not maintained.

The best advice is to take a preventive approach. Keeping blood pressure under control is easier than trying to bring it down once it is high. Blood pressure should be checked regularly, regardless of whether it is or is not elevated. Regular physical exercise, weight control, a low-salt diet, no smoking, and stress management are the basic means of blood pressure control.

Stress Management

Individuals who are under a lot of stress and do not cope well with it need to take measures to counteract the effects of stress in their lives. First they should try to identify the sources of stress and learn how to cope with them. People need to take control of themselves, examine and act upon the things that are most important in their lives, and ignore less meaningful details. Relaxation techniques for stress management are presented in Chapter 3.

Physical exercise is one of the best ways to relieve stress. When a person takes part in physical activity, the body metabolizes excess catecholamines and is able to return to a normal state. Exercise also steps up muscular activity, which leads to muscular relaxation after completing the physical activity. Many executives prefer the evening hours for their physical activity programs, stopping after work at a health or fitness club. By doing this, they are able to "burn up" the excess tension accumulated during the day and enjoy the evening hours.

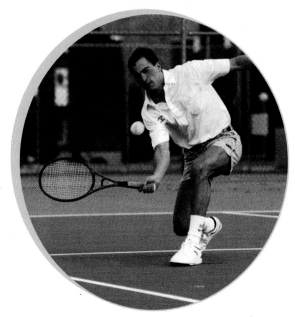

Physical activity is an excellent tool to control stress.

Resting and Stress Electrocardiograms

The electrocardiogram (introduced in Chapter 7) provides a valuable measure of the heart's function. The ECG records the electrical impulses that stimulate the heart to contract. In reading an ECG, five general areas are interpreted: heart rate, heart rhythm, the heart's axis, enlargement or hypertrophy of the heart, and myocardial infarction (heart attack).

On a standard 12-lead ECG, 10 electrodes are placed on the person's chest. From these 10 electrodes, 12 "pictures" or leads of the electrical impulses are studied from 12 different positions as they travel through the heart muscle (myocardium).

By looking at ECG tracings, abnormalities in heart functioning can be identified. Based on the findings, the ECG may be interpreted as normal, equivocal, or abnormal. An ECG does not always identify problems, so a normal tracing is not an absolute guarantee. Likewise, an abnormal tracing does not necessarily signal a serious condition.

Criteria for Stress ECG

Not every adult who wishes to start or continue in an exercise program needs a stress ECG. The following criteria can be applied to determine when this type of test should be administered:

- Men over age 40 and women over age 50.
- A total cholesterol level above 200 mg/dl, or an HDL-cholesterol below 35 mg/dl.
- Hypertensive and diabetic patients.
- Cigarette smokers.
- Individuals with a family history of CHD, syncope, or sudden death before age 60.
- Hypertensive and diabetic patients.
- Cigarette smokers.
- People with an abnormal resting ECG.
- All individuals with symptoms of chest discomfort, dysrhythmias, syncope, or chronotropic incompetence (a heart rate that increases slowly during exercise and never reaches maximum).

ECGs are taken at rest, during the stress of exercise, and during recovery. An **exercise ECG** also is known as a graded exercise stress test or a maximal exercise tolerance test. Similar to a high-speed road test on a car, a stress ECG reveals the heart's tolerance to moderate- and high-intensity exercise. It is a much better test to discover CHD than is a resting ECG.

Stress ECGs also are used to assess cardiorespiratory fitness levels, to screen individuals for preventive and cardiac rehabilitation programs, to detect abnormal blood pressure response during exercise, and to establish actual or functional maximal heart rate for exercise prescription.

At times the stress ECG has been questioned as a reliable predictor of CHD. Even so, it remains the

Essential hypertension   Persistent high blood pressure, having no known cause.

Exercise ECG   An exercise test during which workload is increased gradually (until the subject reaches maximal fatigue) with blood pressure and 12-lead electrocardiographic monitoring throughout the test.

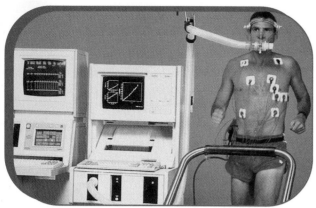

Graded treadmill exercise tolerance test with electrocardiographic monitoring (exercise stress test).

results also are found for people at high risk for cardiovascular disease, in particular men over age 40 and women over age 50 with a poor cholesterol profile, high blood pressure, or a family history of heart disease. Test protocols, number of leads, electrocardiographic criteria, and the skill of the technicians administering the test also affect its sensitivity. Despite its limitations, a stress ECG test is a useful tool in identifying people at high risk for exercise-related sudden death.

most practical, inexpensive, noninvasive procedure available to diagnose latent (undiagnosed/unknown) CHD. The test is accurate in diagnosing CHD about 65% of the time. Part of the problem is that many times those who administer stress ECGs do it without clearly understanding the test's indications and limitations.

The sensitivity of a stress test increases along with the severity of the disease. More accurate

A FINAL WORD

Most of the risk factors for CHD are reversible and preventable. The fact that a person has a family history of heart disease and possibly some of the other risk factors because of neglect in lifestyle does not mean this person is doomed. A healthier lifestyle — free of cardiovascular problems — is something over which you have much control. Willpower and commitment are necessary to develop patterns that eventually will turn into healthy habits and contribute to your total well-being.

NOTES

1. American Heart Association, *Heart and Stroke Facts: 1997 Statistical Supplement* (Dallas: AHA, 1996).
2. S. N. Blair, H. W. Kohl III, R. S. Paffenbarger, Jr, D. G. Clark, K. H. Cooper, and L. W. Gibbons, "Physical Fitness and All-Cause Mortality: A Prospective Study of Healthy Men and Women," Journal of the American Medical Association, 262 (1989), 2395–2401.
3. R. S. Paffenbarger, Jr, R. T. Hyde, A. L. Wing, I. Lee, D. L. Jung, and J. B. Kampert, "The Association of Changes in Physical-Activity Level and Other Lifestyle Characteristics with Mortality Among Men," *New England Journal of Medicine*, 328 (1993), 538–545.
4. P. A. Romm, M. K. Hong, and C. E. Rackley, "High-Density-Lipoprotein Cholesterol and Risk of Coronary Heart Disease," *Practical Cardiology*, 16 (1990), 28–40.
5. C. J. Gluek, "Nonpharmacologic and Pharmacologic Alteration of High Density Lipoprotein Cholesterol: Therapeutic Approaches to Prevention of Atherosclerosis," *American Heart Journal*, 110 (1985), 1107–1115.
6. J. M. Gaziano and C. H. Hennekens, "A New Look at What Can Unclog Your Arteries," *Executive Health Report*, 27:8 (1991), 16.
7. Gaziano and Hennekens.
8. American Heart Association.
9. R. J. Barnard, "Effects of Lifestyle Modification on Serum Lipids," *Archives of Internal Medicine*, 151 (1991), 1389–1394.
10. R. Superko, *Platelets and Lipid Interaction with a Vessel Wall*, presented in symposium at American College of Sports Medicine Annual Meeting, 1991.
11. S. P. Helmrich, D. R. Ragland, R. W. Leung, and R. S. Paffenbarger, "Physical Activity and Reduced Occurrences of Non-Insulin-Dependent Diabetes Mellitus," *New England Journal of Medicine*, 325 (1991), 147–152.
12. Blair et al.

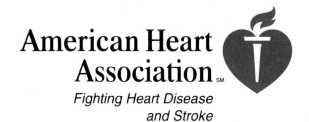

American Heart
Association ₛₘ
*Fighting Heart Disease
and Stroke*

RISKO
A Heart Health Appraisal

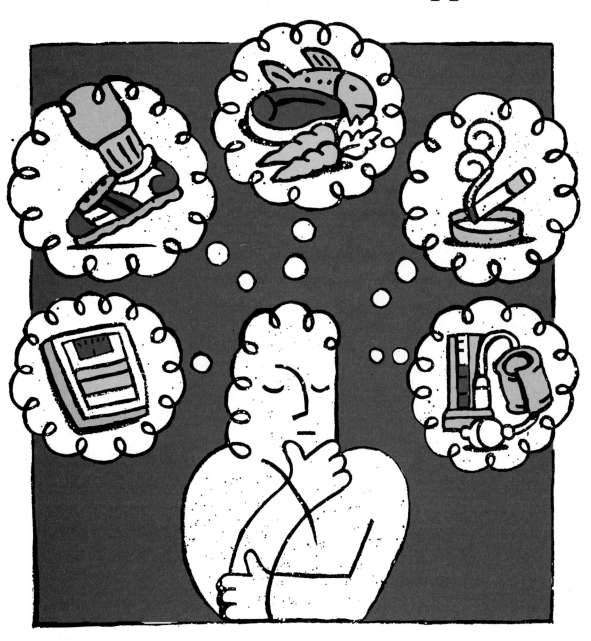

Understanding Heart Disease

Estimates are that almost 500,000 Americans die of coronary heart disease every year. It's the single leading cause of death in the United States – as well as in many other countries.

Scientists have identified certain factors linked with an increased risk of developing coronary heart disease. Some of these factors are unavoidable, like increasing age, being male or having a family history of heart disease. However, many other risk factors can be changed to lower the risk of heart disease. High blood pressure, high blood cholesterol, cigarette smoking and physical inactivity are the four major modifiable risk factors; obesity is a contributing risk factor. Diabetes also strongly influences the risk of heart disease.

This RISKO brochure is a way for you to evaluate your risk of coronary heart disease based upon your risk factors. RISKO scores are based on blood pressure, cholesterol, smoking and weight. Physical inactivity is also an important risk factor but was not part of the statistical base from which RISKO was derived.

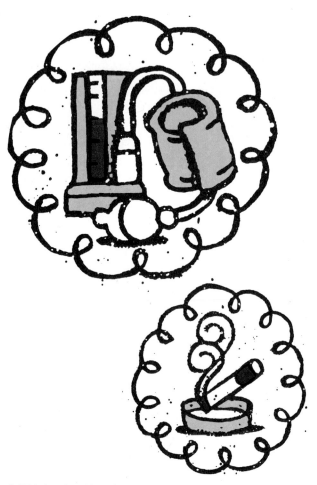

© 1994, American Heart Association

MEN

1. Systolic Blood Pressure

If you **are not** taking anti-hypertensive medications and your blood pressure is...

124 or less	0 points
between 125 and 134	2 points
between 135 and 144	4 points
between 145 and 154	6 points
between 155 and 164	8 points
between 165 and 174	10 points
between 175 and 184	12 points
between 185 and 194	14 points
between 195 and 204	16 points
between 205 and 214	18 points
between 215 and 224	20 points

If you **are** taking anti-hypertensive medications and your blood pressure is...

120 or less	0 points
between 121 and 127	2 points
between 128 and 135	4 points
between 136 and 143	6 points
between 144 and 153	8 points
between 154 and 163	10 points
between 164 and 175	12 points
between 176 and 190	14 points
between 191 and 204	16 points
between 205 and 214	18 points
between 215 and 224	20 points

SCORE

2. Blood Cholesterol

Locate the number of points for your total and HDL cholesterol in the table below.

		HDL 25	30	35	40	50	60	70	80
	140	4	2	0	0	0	0	0	0
	160	5	3	2	0	0	0	0	0
	180	6	4	3	1	0	0	0	0
	200	7	5	4	3	0	0	0	0
	220	7	6	5	4	1	0	0	0
TOTAL	240	8	7	5	4	2	0	0	0
	260	8	7	6	5	3	1	0	0
	280	9	8	7	6	4	2	0	0
	300	9	8	7	6	4	3	1	0
	340	9	9	8	7	6	4	2	1
	400	10	9	9	8	7	5	4	3

SCORE

3. Cigarette Smoking

If you...

do not smoke	0 points
smoke less than a pack a day	2 points
smoke a pack a day	5 points
smoke two or more packs a day	9 points

SCORE

4. Weight

Locate your weight category in the table below. If you are in...

weight category A	0 points
weight category B	1 point
weight category C	2 points

FT	IN	A	B	C
5	1	up to 162	163-250	251+
5	2	up to 167	168-257	258+
5	3	up to 172	173-264	265+
5	4	up to 176	177-272	273+
5	5	up to 181	182-279	280+
5	6	up to 185	186-286	287+
5	7	up to 190	191-293	294+
5	8	up to 195	196-300	301+
5	9	up to 199	200-307	308+
5	10	up to 204	205-315	316+
5	11	up to 209	210-322	323+
6	0	up to 213	214-329	330+
6	1	up to 218	219-336	337+
6	2	up to 223	224-343	344+
6	3	up to 227	228-350	351+
6	4	up to 232	233-368	359+
6	5	up to 238	239-365	366+
6	6	up to 241	242-372	373+

SCORE

TOTAL SCORE

WOMEN

1. Systolic Blood Pressure

SCORE

If you **are not** taking anti-hypertensive medications and your blood pressure is...

125 or less	0 points
between 126 and 136	2 points
between 137 and 148	4 points
between 149 and 160	6 points
between 161 and 171	8 points
between 172 and 183	10 points
between 184 and 194	12 points
between 195 and 206	14 points
between 207 and 218	16 points

If you **are** taking anti-hypertensive medications and your blood pressure is...

117 or less	0 points
between 118 and 123	2 points
between 124 and 129	4 points
between 130 and 136	6 points
between 137 and 144	8 points
between 145 and 154	10 points
between 155 and 168	12 points
between 169 and 206	14 points
between 207 and 218	16 points

2. Blood Cholesterol

SCORE

Locate the number of points for your total and HDL cholesterol in the table below.

TOTAL	HDL 25	30	35	40	50	60	70	80
140	2	1	0	0	0	0	0	0
160	3	2	1	0	0	0	0	0
180	4	3	2	1	0	0	0	0
200	4	3	2	2	0	0	0	0
220	5	4	3	2	1	0	0	0
240	5	4	3	3	1	0	0	0
260	5	4	4	3	2	1	0	0
280	5	5	4	4	2	1	0	0
300	6	5	4	4	3	2	1	0
340	6	5	5	4	3	2	1	0
400	6	6	5	5	4	3	2	2

3. Cigarette Smoking

SCORE

If you...

do not smoke	0 points
smoke less than a pack a day	2 points
smoke a pack a day	5 points
smoke two or more packs a day	9 points

4. Weight

SCORE

Locate your weight category in the table below. If you are in...

weight category A	0 points
weight category B	1 point
weight category C	2 points
weight category D	3 points

FT	IN	A	B	C	D
4	8	up to 139	140-161	162-184	185+
4	9	up to 140	141-162	163-185	186+
4	10	up to 141	142-163	164-187	188+
4	11	up to 143	144-166	167-190	191+
5	0	up to 145	146-168	169-193	194+
5	1	up to 147	148-171	172-196	197+
5	2	up to 149	150-173	174-198	199+
5	3	up to 152	153-176	177-201	202+
5	4	up to 154	155-178	179-204	205+
5	5	up to 157	158-182	183-209	210+
5	6	up to 160	161-186	187-213	214+
5	7	up to 165	166-191	192-219	220+
5	8	up to 169	170-196	197-225	226+
5	9	up to 173	174-201	202-231	232+
5	10	up to 178	179-206	207-238	239+
5	11	up to 182	183-212	213-242	243+
6	0	up to 187	188-217	218-248	249+
6	1	up to 191	192-222	223-254	255+

TOTAL SCORE

What Your Score Means

Note: If you're diabetic, you have a greater risk of heart disease. Add 7 points to your total score.

0-2 — You have a low risk of heart disease for a person of your age and sex.

3-4 — You have a low-to-moderate risk of heart disease for a person of your age and sex. That's good, but there's room for improvement.

5-7 — You have a moderate-to-high risk of heart disease for a person of your age and sex. There's considerable room for improvement in some areas.

8-15 — You have a high risk of developing heart disease for a person of your age and sex. There's lots of room for improvement in all areas.

16 & Over — You have a very high risk of developing heart disease for a person of your age and sex. You should act now to reduce all your risk factors.

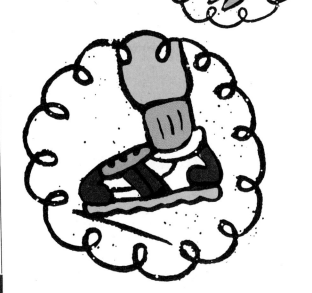

Some Words of Caution

- RISKO is a way for adults who don't have signs of heart disease now to measure their risk. If you already have heart disease, it's very important to work with your doctor to reduce your risk.

- RISKO is not a substitute for a thorough physical examination and assessment by your doctor. It's intended to help you learn more about the factors that influence the risk of heart disease, and thus to reduce your risk.

- If you have a family history of heart disease, your risk of heart disease will be higher than your RISKO score shows. If you have a high RISKO score and a family history of heart disease, taking action now to reduce your risk is even more important.

- If you're a woman under 45 years old or a man under 35 years old, your real risk of heart disease is probably lower than your RISKO score.

- If you're overweight, have high blood pressure or high blood cholesterol, or smoke cigarettes, your long-term risk of heart disease is higher even if your risk of heart disease in the next several years is low. To reduce your risk, you should eliminate or control these risk factors.

How To Reduce Your Risk

- **Quit smoking for good.** Many programs are available to help.

- **Have your blood pressure checked regularly.** If your blood pressure is less than 130/85 mmHg, have it rechecked in two years. If it's between 130-139/85-89, have it rechecked in a year. If your blood pressure is 140/90 or higher, you have high blood pressure and should follow your doctor's advice. If blood pressure medication is prescribed for you, remember to take it.

- **Stay physically active.** Physical inactivity, besides being a risk factor for heart disease, contributes to other risk factors including obesity, high blood pressure and a low level of HDL cholesterol. To condition your heart, try to get 30-60 minutes of exercise 3-4 times a week.

  Activities that are especially beneficial when performed regularly include:
  - brisk walking, hiking, stair-climbing, aerobic exercise and calisthenics;
  - jogging, running, bicycling, rowing and swimming;
  - tennis, racquetball, soccer, basketball and touch football.

  Even low-intensity activities, when performed daily, can have some long-term health benefits. Such activities include:
  - walking for pleasure, gardening and yard work;
  - housework, dancing and prescribed home exercise.

- **Lose weight if necessary.** For many people, losing weight is one of the most effective ways to improve their blood pressure and cholesterol levels.

- **Reduce high blood cholesterol through your diet.** If you're overweight or eat lots of foods high in saturated fats and cholesterol (whole milk, cheese, eggs, butter, fatty foods, fried foods), then make changes in your diet. Look for *The American Heart Association Cookbook* at your local bookstore; it can help you.

- **Visit or write your local American Heart Association for more information and copies of free pamphlets.**
  Some subjects covered include:
  Reducing your risk of heart attack and stroke.
  Controlling high blood pressure.
  Eating to keep your heart healthy.
  How to stop smoking.
  Exercising for good health.

Your contributions to the American Heart Association will support research that helps make publications like this possible.

For more information, contact your local American Heart Association or call 1-800-AHA-USA1 (1-800-242-8721).

American Heart Association ℠

Fighting Heart Disease and Stroke

National Center
7272 Greenville Avenue
Dallas, Texas 75231

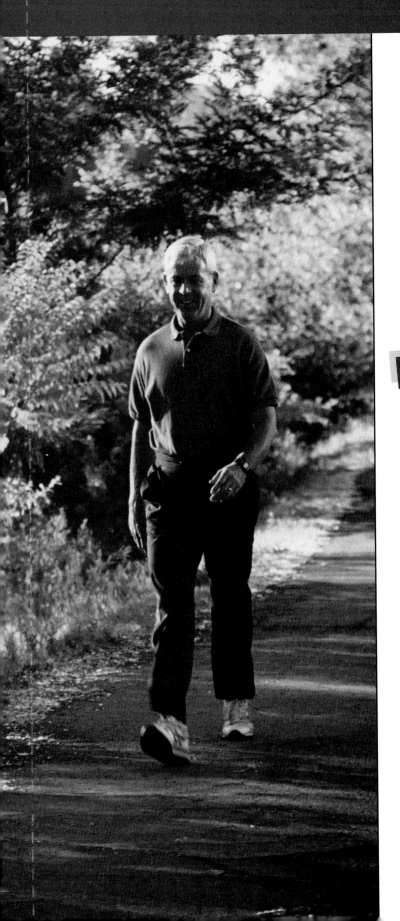

12

Cancer Prevention and Wellness

OBJECTIVES

- Know the differences in characteristics of benign and malignant tumors.
- Differentiate the major types of cancer.
- Recognize precancerous conditions and warning signs of cancer.
- Identify the three basic kinds of skin cancers.
- Learn about the gender-specific cancers, their incidence, and their risk factors.
- List guidelines for preventing cancer, including dietary guidelines.
- Understand the role of self-examinations (and how to conduct these) and examination by physicians.

Although cancer is second only to heart disease as the leading killer in the United States, the cancer death rate is decreasing for the first time since cancer statistics began to be kept in the 1930s.[1] This decline of about 2% a year is attributed to improved prevention and treatment, most markedly a reduction in cigarette smoking.

From 1991 to 1995:

- Deaths from lung cancer among men declined 6.7% (though it increased 6.4% among women).
- Colorectal cancer deaths fell 7% in men and 4.8% in women.
- Prostate cancer deaths dropped 6.3%.
- Breast cancer deaths fell 6.3%, and deaths from ovarian cancer declined by 4.8%.

Although the decline in deaths is certainly good news, American Cancer Society Medical Director Harmon Eyre says that we need to redouble our efforts to get people to stop smoking and to eat a healthier diet.

DEVELOPMENT OF CANCER

Cancer starts when an *initiator* alters DNA, the cell's basic genetic material, in a way that allows the cell to dictate its own rate of growth. The alteration can occur in minutes or days. Initiators include radiation, chemicals, and viruses. Having a cell with altered DNA, however, does not guarantee cancer. Fortunately, special enzymes travel up and down the DNA to repair breaks and changes in it.

Anything that speeds up the rate of cell division lessens the chance that repair enzymes will find the altered part of the DNA in time. Once a cell multiplies and incorporates its newly altered DNA into its genetic instructions, the cell no longer realizes its DNA has been changed.

Compounds that increase cell division are called *promoters*. They are thought to promote cancer either by reducing the time available for repair enzymes to act or by encouraging cells with altered DNA to develop and grow. Development and growth of these altered cells may take up to 20 years. Common promoters are thought to be estrogen, alcohol, and dietary fat in excess.

Even after an altered cell has multiplied, cancer does not necessarily result. First, a cell mass must grow large enough to affect body metabolism. During this initial stage of growth, the immune system

may find the altered cells and destroy them. Or the cancer cells themselves may be so defective that their own DNA limits their ability to grow, and they die anyway.

Actually, most of us probably have cancerous or **precancerous** cells in our bodies at some time. Many of them die because of mutation. Many more are destroyed by a healthy immune system. Occasionally, though, the immune system is unable to dominate, and cancer develops.

Benign and **malignant** tumors differ in a number of ways.

1. Benign tumors resemble the normal tissues that surround them; malignant tumors do not.
2. The cells of benign tumors do not break off and metastasize; the cells of malignant tumors do.
3. Benign tumors do not invade surrounding tissues; malignant tumors do.
4. Benign tumors can be controlled by normal methods used to control any tissue growth; malignant tumors cannot.
5. Almost all benign tumors are encased (contained) in a fibrous capsule; very few malignant tumors are.
6. Benign tumors are not dangerous unless they interfere with blood flow; malignant tumors are fatal if untreated.

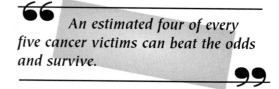

> *An estimated four of every five cancer victims can beat the odds and survive.*

Survival depends on how early the cancer is diagnosed, the tissues involved, strength of the immune system, and potential treatment options. Cures have been discovered for some kinds of cancer. An estimated four of every five cancer victims can beat the odds and survive and 5 million Americans who have had cancer are still alive today. Approximately 3 million of them are considered cured — having survived 5 years or longer without any further signs of the cancer.

INCIDENCE OF CANCER

Someone in the United States dies of cancer every minute. It strikes people of all ages and is the leading killer of children between ages 3 and 14. More than half a million people in the United States die from cancer each year, and more than a million are diagnosed each year. One of every five deaths from any cause in the United States is from cancer.[2]

The incidence of cancer varies slightly between men and women. The most common cancers in men are prostate, lung, colon/rectal, and urinary/bladder, in that order. The most common cancers in women are breast, lung, colon/rectal, uterine, and ovarian. Leading sites and deaths from cancer in men and women are shown in Figure 12.1.

RISK FACTORS

In more than half of all diagnosed cases, the cancer has metastasized, making treatment more difficult. The American Cancer Society estimates that two of every five people who die from cancer could have been saved if they had been diagnosed sooner. We can go a long way toward preventing cancer by changing our behaviors.

The probable causes of cancer are many. We know that cancer is caused by certain substances in the environment. We also know that cigarette smoking and dietary factors play a role. So do heredity (the inherited tendency for certain kinds of cancers), and race. Some cancers can be caused by viruses. Viruses that increase the risk for cancer include Epstein-Barr, human papilloma, Hepatitis B, and T-cell leukemia/lymphoma. Although some controversy still surrounds the notion, increasing evidence suggests that attitudes and emotions might increase

Cancer   A group of more than a hundred diseases in which cells grow at an uncontrolled rate, mature in an abnormal way, and spread to invade nearby tissues.

Precancerous   A condition in which a benign (noncancerous) condition has the potential to become cancerous.

Benign   Noncancerous.

Malignant   Cancerous.

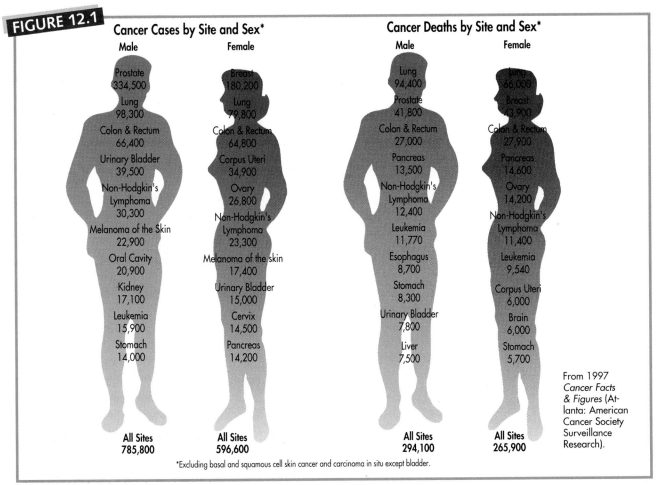

FIGURE 12.1

Cancer Cases by Site and Sex*

Male — All Sites 785,800

Prostate 334,500
Lung 98,300
Colon & Rectum 66,400
Urinary Bladder 39,500
Non-Hodgkin's Lymphoma 30,300
Melanoma of the Skin 22,900
Oral Cavity 20,900
Kidney 17,100
Leukemia 15,900
Stomach 14,000

Female — All Sites 596,600

Breast 180,200
Lung 79,800
Colon & Rectum 64,800
Corpus Uteri 34,900
Ovary 26,800
Non-Hodgkin's Lymphoma 23,300
Melanoma of the skin 17,400
Urinary Bladder 15,000
Cervix 14,500
Pancreas 14,200

Cancer Deaths by Site and Sex*

Male — All Sites 294,100

Lung 94,400
Prostate 41,800
Colon & Rectum 27,000
Pancreas 13,500
Non-Hodgkin's Lymphoma 12,400
Leukemia 11,770
Esophagus 8,700
Stomach 8,300
Urinary Bladder 7,800
Liver 7,500

Female — All Sites 265,900

Lung 66,000
Breast 43,900
Colon & Rectum 27,900
Pancreas 14,600
Ovary 14,200
Non-Hodgkin's Lymphoma 11,400
Leukemia 9,540
Corpus Uteri 6,000
Brain 6,000
Stomach 5,700

From 1997 *Cancer Facts & Figures* (Atlanta: American Cancer Society Surveillance Research).

*Excluding basal and squamous cell skin cancer and carcinoma in situ except bladder.

1997 cancer incidence and deaths by site and sex.

susceptibility to cancer and could cause physiological changes in the body that can lead to the development of cancer.

Table 12.1 shows the probability of developing invasive cancers. You can't control some causes of cancer — heredity and race, for instance — but you can actively reduce many identified risk factors and help beat the odds of developing cancer. Proven risk factors are discussed in the following pages.

Tobacco

Cigarette smoking has been called the number-one preventable cause of death in the United States. It is estimated to directly cause approximately 30% of all cancers in the United States and approximately 87% of all lung cancers among Americans. It also is a leading cause of bladder cancer.[3]

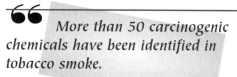

> More than 50 carcinogenic chemicals have been identified in tobacco smoke.
> — *Your Patient and Fitness, 9:1*

Smoking — which also contributes to other serious diseases including emphysema, heart disease, and stroke — introduces carbon monoxide and lethal **carcinogens** into the body. Your chance of getting cancer as a result of cigarette smoking is related to how long you have smoked, how many packs a day you smoke, and how deeply you inhale the smoke.

Smokeless tobacco also poses significant risk for cancer, despite the persistent myth that it's okay to "chew" as long as you don't smoke. Smokeless or chewing tobacco is a leading cause of cancer of the mouth, throat, esophagus, and larynx.

Also of concern is **secondhand smoke**. Children are at particular risk for lung disease such as bronchitis.[4] Nonsmokers who live with smokers have been found to develop lung cancer at a higher rate than other nonsmokers.

Diet

Diet is estimated to be a major factor in 60% of cancers in women and 40% of cancers in men.[5] Some scientists believe the role of diet may be equivalent to cigarette smoking in boosting the risk of developing cancer. A diet high in saturated fats increases the risk for cancer. Specific culprits are tropical oils (such as coconut oil and palm oil) and animal fats (fatty meats, whole milk, cheese, and other animal-source foods). The cancer risk increases substantially if more than 30% of daily calories comes from fat and more than 10% comes from saturated fats.

Also, if the diet doesn't contain enough fiber, the risk of certain kinds of cancers, especially cancer of the colon, increases dramatically. Other dietary factors that increase the risk of cancer include:

- foods cured or pickled with salt or nitrites, such as luncheon meats.
- smoked foods.
- charcoal-broiled foods.
- foods containing cyclamates (a type of artificial sweetener).
- vitamin and mineral deficiency.
- excessive alcohol consumption.

Environmental Carcinogens

Carcinogens include atmospheric agents ranging from electromagnetic radiation and radon gas to chemicals such as vinyl chloride and arsenic. In most cases, the risk of cancer is related to the dose. One-time massive exposure to a carcinogen may cause cancer, as can prolonged, long-term exposure to small amounts.

As carcinogens are identified, policies are instituted to protect the public from exposure. For example, strict building codes now ban the use of asbestos. Accidental exposure still occurs however, in demolishing or remodeling old buildings. Schools, in particular, have to take extreme measures to prevent children from being exposed to the asbestos formerly used to fireproof the structures.

TABLE 12.1 Developing Invasive Cancers

Site	Sex	Birth to 39 Years	40 to 59 Years	60 to 79 Years	Ever (Birth to Death)
All sites	Male	1 in 58	1 in 13	1 in 3	1 in 2
	Female	1 in 52	1 in 11	1 in 4	1 in 3
Breast	Female	1 in 217	1 in 26	1 in 15	1 in 8
Colon and Rectum	Male	1 in 1,667	1 in 108	1 in 23	1 in 16
	Female	1 in 2,000	1 in 137	1 in 30	1 in 17
Prostate	Male	<1 in 10,000	1 in 103	1 in 8	1 in 6

Source: CA — A Cancer Journal for Clinicians, 45:1.

The chemicals in the water we drink, the hydrocarbons emitted in automobile exhaust, and the agents in some insecticides and pesticides have been shown to cause cancer at certain levels. Even though few people are exposed to a high level of these pollutants, the effects of chronic, low-level exposure are being studied.

Medical Substances

Cancer can follow exposure to certain medical substances such as drugs, agents used in chemotherapy, medications used to suppress the

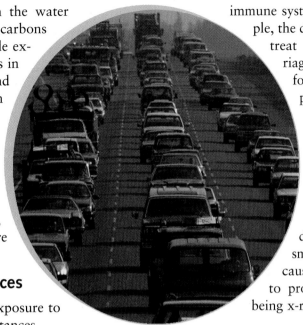

Automobile exhaust was a leading source of environmental carcinogens before the advent of catalytic converters.

immune system, hormones, and x-rays. For example, the drug diethylstilbestrol (DES) — used to treat complications and prevent miscarriages until the mid 1960s — has been found to cause cancer of the female reproductive organs in the daughters of women who took the drug.

Cancer caused by x-rays is rare, but it can happen from exposure to large doses of radiation. Precise calibration of x-ray equipment has helped prevent accidental exposure to large doses in most cases. The effects of radiation are cumulative, so repeated small doses over a long period may be a cause for concern. Lead shields are used to protect parts of the body that are not being x-rayed from accidental exposure.

Viruses

The first virus known to cause cancer was identified in 1911 by a scientist who injected it into chickens, causing cancerous tumors. Since that time, exhaustive research has been conducted in the attempt to identify viruses that may cause cancers in humans.

One group of viruses — three variants of the human papilloma virus (HPV), which causes genital warts — is suspected of causing cervical cancer and other genital malignancies. These cancer-causing viruses can be sexually transmitted.[6]

Approximately 2% of all cancers in the United States may be related to viruses. In some cases the virus may be responsible for causing or initiating the cancer; once the disease takes hold, the virus no longer is in the picture. In other situations, the viruses may not actually cause the cancer but may increase the risk of developing cancer.

Scientists also have identified a particular kind of virus called **retroviruses**. The human immunodeficiency virus (HIV), which causes AIDS, is a retrovirus.

Controversy still surrounds the notion of cancer-causing viruses. Most scientists conclude that certain

Possible Carcinogens (Cancer-Causing Substances)

- Aflatoxins (in rotting peanuts)
- Alcohol
- Alkylating agents
- Anabolic steroids
- Arsenic
- Asbestos
- Benzene
- Benzo(a)pyrene (in tobacco smoke)
- Beryllium
- Betel nuts
- Cadmium
- Chlornaphazine
- Chrome ores
- Chrysene (in tobacco smoke)
- Coke (a type of coal)
- Creosote oil
- Cyclamates
- Diethylstilbestrol (DES)
- Estrogen (synthetic)
- Ionizing radiation
- Immunosuppressive drugs
- Isopropyl oil
- Mesothorium
- Nickel carbonyl
- Nickel ores
- Nitrates
- Nitrites
- Nitrosamines
- Oral contraceptives
- Paraffin oil (crude)
- Penacetin
- Radiation
- Radium
- Radioactive dust/gas
- Radon
- Soots
- Tars
- Tar fumes
- Tobacco
- Ultraviolet light
- Vinyl chloride
- Wood dust
- X-rays

Carcinogens   Cancer-causing substances.

Secondhand smoke   A mixture of smoke exhaled by smokers and smoke from the burning end of a cigarette, pipe, or cigar.

Retroviruses   Viruses that invade a cell's genetic structure and are passed on to each succeeding generation of cells as the cells divide.

viruses may cause cancer only under certain circumstances. For example, Epstein-Barr virus (EBV), which causes mononucleosis in the United States, causes a cancer called *Burkitt's lymphoma* among children in Africa. Scientists now are researching the possibility that EBV, or similar viruses responsible for herpes, may sharply increase the risk of Hodgkin's disease, cervical cancer, and some forms of leukemia.

Heredity

Heredity is a factor in an estimated 10% of all cancers in the United States. Approximately 14 million Americans are at risk because they inherited the tendency for certain malignancies.[7] Cancers caused by hereditary factors often begin in childhood and can increase the likelihood of developing the cancer by as much as 30 times normal odds.

> *Heredity is a factor in an estimated 10% of all cancers in the United States.*

Certain genetic markers called **oncogenes** can be used to predict cancer in some cases. Cancer also can be predicted if **suppressor genes**, which protect against cancer, are missing from certain genetic material.

In a few cases, the cancer itself is inherited. One example is retinoblastoma, a cancer of the eye that occurs in infants and young children. More often, what is inherited is not the actual cancer but, rather, the predisposition for that cancer, the tendency to develop that cancer. Exciting new research has identified, for example, a gene that predisposes its carriers to cancer of the colon. Once the gene is identified, a person carrying the gene can take certain precautions and undergo aggressive early screening to improve the odds of preventing or successfully treating the disease.

The risk for certain leukemias can be genetically passed from parent to child. The tendency for lung, colon, breast, uterine, prostate, bone, brain, stomach, and adrenal gland cancers also can be inherited.

Stress

An individual's response to stress has been linked to the risk for developing cancer, as well as certain other diseases, such as heart disease. Chronic stress and the hormones it unleashes on the body interfere

Signs of Inherited Cancer

Four patterns generally identify hereditary cancers.
1. Many family members develop the same kind of cancer.
2. The cancer strikes victims at an earlier age than usual. (Breast cancer, for example, typically occurs in the 60s but may strike a woman in her 40s who inherited the tendency.)
3. The cancer strikes more than once (in both breasts, for example, or in two different places in the liver).
4. The person has an unusual gender pattern. (For example, a cancer unusual in women will affect all the women in a family.)

with the immune system's ability to recognize cancerous cells and destroy them.

Joseph G. Courtney of the University of California, Los Angeles, School of Public Health and his co-workers joined forces with researchers in Sweden and their large database on Stockholm-area patients with colorectal cancer. Courtney's team confirmed that on-the-job aggravation seems to put people at higher risk for developing colon and rectal cancers. Those who reported a history of workplace problems over the past 10 years faced 5.5 times the colorectal cancer risk as adults who reported no such problems.[8]

Although controversy still surrounds the idea, researchers have identified a "cancer-prone" personality, a collection of traits that seem to occur in people who later develop cancer. Called the Type C personality, it is characterized by unusual compliance and the tendency to internalize conflict. It also is marked by the individual's inability to deal with stress in a healthy way.

Chronic Irritation

Evidence indicates that chronic irritation of cells or tissues can lead to the development of cancer. Linked to certain kinds of cancers and increased risk for cancer are:

— chronic low-grade infections.
— repeated bladder infections.
— repeated ulceration of tissues.

— chronic infection of scar tissue.

— constant irritation of a mole or other benign growth.

— certain kinds of injuries.

— long-term irritation of gallstones against the gallbladder.

Estrogen-Replacement Therapy

When the level of estrogen, normally produced by the ovaries, tapers off as a woman reaches menopause, physicians often prescribe estrogen-replacement therapy to ease or delay the troublesome symptoms of menopause. Evidence shows that estrogen-replacement therapy also helps to prevent osteoporosis, a loss of bone tissue that affects mostly older women. Estrogen-replacement therapy, however, increases the risk of endometrial cancer (a cancer of the lining of the uterus) and may increase the risk of breast cancer.

The risk factors just discussed are general risk factors for cancer. Knowing the specific risk factors for certain kinds of cancers can help you reduce the odds of developing one of the more common cancers.

TYPES OF CANCER

Cancers have been classified according to six general types:

1. *Carcinomas.* Spread through the *bloodstream and lymph system*, carcinomas — the most common kind of cancers — affect the tissues that line most body cavities and cover body surfaces. Examples are lung cancer, breast cancer, skin cancer, colon cancer, and uterine cancer. (If the cancer occurs in a gland, it is called an *adenocarcinoma.*)

2. *Sarcomas.* Spread through the *bloodstream*, sarcomas affect the connective tissues of the body, such as the muscles, bones, and cartilage. Sarcomas are not as common as carcinomas, but they grow and spread more quickly and form more solid tumors.

3. *Lymphomas.* Spread through the *lymph system*, lymphomas are cancers of the lymphatic, or infection-fighting, cells. Lymph nodes in the groin, armpits, and neck can be affected. An example of lymphoma is Hodgkin's disease.

4. *Melanomas.* Spread through the *bloodstream*, melanomas affect the skin. They generally begin as a mole that later becomes cancerous. They grow and spread rapidly.

The Seven Warning Signs of Cancer

1 A change in bowel or bladder habits.

2 A sore that does not heal.

3 Unusual bleeding or discharge.

4 Thickening or a lump in the breast or elsewhere.

5 Indigestion or difficulty in swallowing.

6 An obvious change in a wart or mole.

7 A nagging cough or hoarseness.

5. *Leukemias.* Spread through the *bloodstream*, leukemias affect the tissues that manufacture blood, especially the spleen and the bone marrow.

6. *Neuroblastomas.* Spread through the *bloodstream*, neuroblastomas affect the nervous system or the adrenal glands. Relatively uncommon, they occur most often in children under age 10.

CANCER SITES

Some common cancer sites are discussed in the following pages, and Table 12.2 summarizes pertinent data on these cancers.

Skin Cancer

More than 800,000 Americans are diagnosed with some form of skin cancer every year. Skin cancer is probably the most underrated type of cancer: it accounts for approximately 40% of all cancers, and is the fastest-growing type of cancer in men over 50.[9] The sharp increase in the incidence of skin cancer is alarming. Over the past decade, it has increased 93%. At current rates of increase, one in 90 Americans will have skin cancer by the year 2000.

Oncogenes Pieces of genetic material that serve as markers to predict later mutation and development of certain cancers, probably by encouraging mutation of related cells.

Suppressor genes Pieces of genetic material that are part of a cell's normal protective mechanism against development of cancer.

TABLE 12.2 Common Cancers

	Risk Factors	Warning Signals	Early Detection	Treatment	5-Year Survival with Treatment
Lung cancer (est. 170,000 new cases a year; 149,000 deaths)	Cigarette smoking for 20 or more years; exposure to certain industrial substances, particularly asbestos; secondhand smoke; radiation; radon.	Persistent cough, sputum streaked with blood, chest pain, recurring bronchitis or pneumonia.	Difficult to detect early. Diagnosis based on chest x-ray, sputum testing, fiberoptic bronchoscopy (direct examination of the lungs by means of a specially lighted tube).	Surgery, radiation therapy, chemotherapy.	The leading cause of cancer death among both men and women.
Breast cancer (est. 183,000 new cases a year; 46,300 deaths)	Over age 50, personal or family history of breast cancer, no children, first child after age 30, dense breast tissue, obesity, high fat intake, alcohol, estrogen replacement therapy after menopause.	Breast changes: lumps, thickening, swelling, puckering, dimpling, skin irritation, nipple distortion, scaliness, discharge, pain, tenderness.	Monthly breast self-examination. Professional breast exam every 3 years for women ages 20-40 and every year over age 40. Yearly mammography for all women over 50, every 1 or 2 years for women 40-49; baseline mammogram for those 35-39. Tissue biopsy confirms diagnosis.	Surgery, from lumpectomy (local removal of tumor) to a modified radical mastectomy (removal of breast and lymph glands, leaving underlying muscle intact); radiation; chemotherapy; or all three. For metastatic breast cancer, autologous bone marrow transplantation.	Until recently, the leading cause of cancer death in women; now surpassed by lung cancer.
Uterine and cervical cancer (46,000 new cases a year, 10,100 deaths)	For cervical cancer: early age of first intercourse, multiple sex partners, genital herpes, human papilloma virus infection, significant exposure to secondhand smoke. For uterine cancer: infertility, failure to ovulate, prolonged estrogen therapy, obesity.	Unusual vaginal bleeding or discharge.	Pap smear every 3 years after two initial negative tests 1 year apart.	Surgery, radiation, or a combination of the two. In precancerous stages, cervical cells may be destroyed by extreme cold or intense heat. Precancerous endometrial changes are treated with the hormone progesterone.	Cervical cancer mortality has declined 70% during the last 40 years with wider application of the Pap smear. Postmenopausal women with abnormal bleeding should be checked.
Ovarian cancer (est. 20,700 new cases a year)	Family history of ovarian cancer; personal history of breast cancer; obesity; infertility (because the abnormality that interferes with conception may also play a role in cancer development); low levels of transferase, an enzyme involved in metabolism of dairy foods.	Often no obvious symptoms until advanced stages. Painless swelling of abdomen; irregular bleeding; lower abdominal pain; digestive and urinary abnormalities; fatigue; backache; bloating; weight gain.	Women with family history: annual pelvic and abdominal exams; blood test for a tumor marker called CA125 every 6 months; annual pelvic ultrasound. (In cases of very high risk, some oncologists recommend prophylactic removal of ovaries no later than age 35.)	Surgery, sometimes in combination with chemotherapy or radiation.	85% if detected and treated early; 23% in advanced cases.

Type	Who's at risk	Warning signals	Detection	Treatment	Comments
Colon and rectum cancer (est. 152,000 new cases a year; 57,000 deaths)	Personal or family history of colon and rectal cancer or polyps (growths) in the colon or rectum; inflammatory bowel disease; high-fat, low-fiber diet.	Unusual bleeding from rectum, blood in stool, a change in bowel habits.	Digital rectal exam (once a year after age 40); stool-blood slide test that detects blood in feces (every year after age 50); proctosigmoidoscopy, a rectal exam using a hollow, lighted tube (every 3-5 years after age 50, following 2 consecutive normal annual exams). Diagnosis may require a colonoscopy (viewing the entire colon) or a barium enema.	Surgery, sometimes in combination with chemotherapy or radiation.	Considered a highly curable disease when digital and proctoscopic examinations are included in routine checkups.
Skin cancer (melanoma) (est. 32,000 new cases a year; 6,800 deaths)	Excessive exposure to sun, fair complexion, occupational exposure to carcinogens. (Inherited skin disorders, such as xeroderma pigmentosum and familial atypical multiple mole melanoma, account for 10% of cases.)	Unusual skin condition, especially a change in size or color of a mole; appearance of a darkly pigmented growth or spot; oozing, scaliness, bleeding; appearance of a bump; change in sensation, itchiness, tenderness, or pain.	Examine moles on your skin once a month.	Surgery, radiation, electrodesiccation (tissue destruction by heat); cryosurgery (tissue destruction by cold), or a combination of therapies.	Melanoma is readily detected by observation and diagnosed by simple biopsy.
Oral cancer (including pharynx) (est. 29,800 new cases a year; 7,700 deaths)	Heavy smoking of cigarettes, cigars, pipes; excessive drinking; use of chewing tobacco.	A sore that bleeds easily and doesn't heal; a lump or thickening; a reddish or whitish patch; difficulty chewing, swallowing, or moving the tongue or jaws.	Regular exams by your dentist or primary-care physician.	Surgery and radiation.	Many more lives should be saved because the mouth is easily accessible to visual examination by physicians and dentists.
Leukemia (est. 29,300 new cases a year; 18,600 deaths)	Down syndrome and other inherited abnormalities; excessive exposure to radiation and to certain chemicals, such as benzene.		Difficult to detect early because its symptoms are often similar to those of less serious conditions, such as flu. Diagnosis is based on blood tests and bone-marrow biopsy.	Chemotherapy, drugs, blood transfusions, and antibiotics; bone-marrow transplants.	Leukemias are cancers of blood-forming tissues and are characterized by the abnormal production of immature white blood cells. Acute leukemia strikes mainly children and is treated by drugs that have extended life from a few months to as much as 10 years. Chronic leukemia strikes usually after age 25 and progresses less rapidly.
Testicular cancer (6,100 new cases a year)	Young men under age 35.		Testicular self-examinations.	Surgical removal of the diseased testis, radiation therapy, chemotherapy, removal of nearby lymph nodes.	96% if the cancer is localized; 89% overall.
Prostate cancer (est. 165,000 new cases a year; 35,000 deaths)	Risk increases with age, black men more susceptible than whites. Suspected risk factors: family history, high-fat diet, exposure to heavy metal cadmium, high number of sexual partners, history of frequent STDs.	Frequent urination, difficulty urinating, blood in the urine, lower back pain.	Rectal exam; new blood test available.	Surgical removal of prostate, conventional radiation, or implanting "seeds" of radioactive iodine in the prostate; hormone therapy.	Occurs mainly in men over 60; can be detected by digital rectal exam at annual checkup.

Adapted from the American Cancer Society, *Cancer Facts and Figures*, 1993.

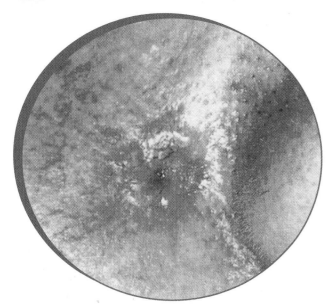

Basal cell carcinoma.

The three basic kinds of skin cancers are:

1. *Basal cell carcinoma.* This is the most common, and least serious, of the skin cancers. It usually does not spread, and it grows slowly. Most basal cell carcinomas occur on the face, neck, and hands — areas of frequent exposure to the sun.

2. *Squamous cell carcinoma.* This type of cancer grows faster than the basal cell type and involves deeper layers of skin, but it rarely spreads to other parts of the body.

Precancerous Skin Conditions

Precancerous conditions are those in which a benign, or noncancerous, condition becomes cancerous for one reason or another. Generally, physicians recommend that the following precancerous skin conditions be surgically removed or repaired to prevent their becoming cancerous, regardless of how low the risk may be:

- Benign tumors
- Chronic scaly patches on the skin
- Brown or black warts
- Moles subject to chronic irritation (such as those on the waist that are constantly rubbed by a waistband or belt)
- A lump on the lip, tongue, or inside the cheek
- A scaly patch on the inside of the cheek

Skin Types

A fair-skinned person (Type 1) in the sun at noon and at an elevation of about 5000 feet stands a good chance of beginning to burn within 10 minutes. The times are determined by multiplying the sun-protection factor (SPF) number by 10 minutes. For example, SPF 15 x 10 min. = 150 min. = 2 hrs. 30 min. To determine how long a given SPF will protect your skin, this 6-point standard scale used by dermatologists gives guidelines for your exposure limits.

Type 1
Fair skin with blue or green eyes and light blond or red hair; typical time for skin to burn: 10–20 minutes.

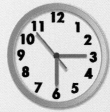

Type 2
Fair skin with deep blue, hazel or brown eyes and ash blond, deep red, or light brown hair; typical burn time: 15–30 minutes.

Type 3
Medium skin with brown eyes and brown hair; typical burn time: 20–40 minutes.

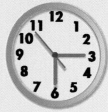

Type 4
Light to medium brown skin with dark brown eyes and hair; typical burn time: 25–50 minutes.

Type 5
Light to golden brown skin with dark brown eyes and black hair; typical burn time: 30–60 minutes.

Type 6
Brown to deepest brown skin with dark brown eyes and black hair; typical burn time: 40–75 minutes.

3. *Malignant melanoma.* This rapidly growing cancer is the most dangerous skin cancer and almost always spreads to other organs. Of the 8,000 people who die from skin cancer each year, approximately 6,000 succumb to malignant melanoma. It is the number-one cancer killer of American women ages 25 to 29 and number two for women ages 30 to 34.

Basal and squamous cell carcinomas are detected and treated quite easily. Malignant melanoma can be treated successfully if it is diagnosed and treated early. If not treated early, **metastasis** makes treatment extremely difficult.

The risk factors for skin cancer include:

— sun exposure (most dangerous are ultraviolet B rays, at their strongest between 10 a.m. and 2 p.m.).

— fair skin that burns easily and rarely tans.

— blonde and red hair.

— artificial sources of ultraviolet rays, such as tanning booths and sunlamps.

— history of one or more severe sunburns.

— a dark brown or black wart.

— birthmarks and congenital moles (although these do not always become cancerous, they should be watched closely and removed if they begin to grow or change in appearance).

— moles that are irritated chronically (moles at the waistline, bra line, or other areas where clothing rubs them constantly).

— occupational exposure to creosote, coal tar, pitch, arsenic, or radium.

Danger signs of skin cancer are given in Figure 12.2.

Metastasis The process that occurs when cancer cells from one growth break off, enter the bloodstream or lymph system, and are carried to a distant part of the body, where they cause another cancerous growth to begin.

FIGURE 12.2

Danger Signs of Skin Cancer

The American Academy of Dermatology advises: Know your spots and do a spot check. Also, have your skin checked by a doctor for any changes once a year. If you notice one of the following changes in your skin, you should see your family doctor or dermatologist immediately:

- **Basal-cell or squamous-cell carcinomas:** any lesion that is new, starts growing, starts changing, bleeds, is scabby, or doesn't heal.

- **Melanoma:**

  A. *Asymmetry:* One half of a mole or lesion doesn't look like the other half.

B. *Border:* A mole has an irregular, scalloped, or not clearly defined border.

C. *Color:* The color varies or is not uniform from one area of a mole or lesion to another, whether the color is tan, brown, black, white, red, or blue.

D. *Diameter:* The lesion is larger than 6 millimeters or larger than a pencil eraser.

- **Actinic keratosis:** a precancerous skin lesion that is dry, scaly, reddish, and slightly raised.

Melanoma Warnings

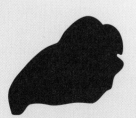

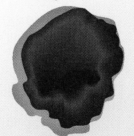
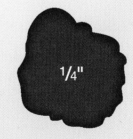

| Asymmetrical | Border irregular | Color varied | Diameter larger than ¼" |

Adapted from *FDA Consumer*, May 1991.

Danger signs of skin cancer.

Lung Cancer

The leading cancer killer among both men and women, lung cancer caused an estimated 157,400 deaths in 1995. Lung cancer occurs almost exclusively among cigarette smokers. According to the U.S. Department of Health and Human Services, the cellular changes and tissue damage that lead to lung cancer have been observed in 93% of active smokers and 6% of former smokers but only 1% of those who have never smoked. Researchers estimate that close to 90% of all lung cancer could be eliminated if people did not smoke.[10]

Once a disease affecting men predominantly, lung cancer in women has risen along with higher smoking rates among women. Today, lung cancer is decreasing steadily in men while increasing steadily in blacks, teenagers, and women. Lung cancer now outnumbers breast cancer as the leading cause of cancer deaths in women.

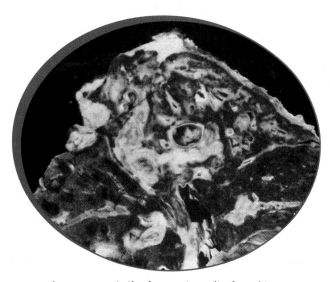

Lung cancer is the frequent result of smoking.

Lung cancer spreads rapidly, and it is rarely detected early, as it usually does not cause symptoms or show up on an x-ray until it is quite advanced. By that time, the damage usually is too extensive to treat successfully. The 5-year survival rate of lung cancer patients is only about 13%.

When symptoms do arise, they might be manifested by persistent hoarseness, a nagging cough, repeated bouts of pneumonia or bronchitis, or spitting up blood. Treatment consists of surgery for localized cancers, combined with radiation treatment and chemotherapy for lung cancer that has spread.

The number-one risk factor for lung cancer is cigarette smoking. Most at risk are those who have smoked more than 20 years. Secondhand smoke inhaled by nonsmokers who live or work with smokers also increases the risk of lung cancer significantly. The Centers for Disease Control and Prevention estimate that 3,000 nonsmokers die each year from lung cancer caused by secondhand tobacco smoke. Other risk factors for lung cancer include:

— exposure to asbestos.
— high-level air pollution.
— exposure to carcinogenic chemicals.
— exposure to certain metals (cadmium, cobalt, chromium, silver, nickel, steel).
— exposure to arsenic or radioactive ores.
— exposure to radon gas.

All other risk factors for lung cancer are much more marked if the individual also smokes.

Colon and Rectal Cancer

Cancer of the colon and rectum — also called *colorectal cancer* — is the third leading cancer killer in the United States among both men and women. About 155,000 new cases are diagnosed each year, and almost 60,000 Americans die of colorectal cancer annually. If detected early, colorectal cancer usually can be treated successfully because it grows and spreads quite slowly. Treatment usually consists of radiation or surgery.

Changes in bowel habits and bleeding from the rectum not attributable to hemorrhoids are the most common signs of colorectal cancer. Bright red blood in the stools that is not attributable to hemorrhoids is another sign. Risk factors include:

— a personal or family history of polyps (benign growths) in the colon or rectum.
— a family history of colorectal cancer.
— a diet high in fats and low in fiber.
— inflammatory bowel problems, such as colitis.

Age also is considered a risk factor. The risk for colorectal cancer increases sharply after age 40. Researchers believe that at least half, and possibly *all*, cases of colorectal cancer can be attributed to a genetic tendency for polyps in the colon or rectum combined with a high-fat, low-fiber diet.

The American Cancer Society recommends a colon exam called a *flexible sigmoidoscopy* for men and women beginning at age 50. The test should be started at age 40 for those with a family history of colorectal cancer or ulcerative colitis.

Breast Cancer

The second leading killer of women, breast cancer kills almost 50,000 American women each year. Approximately 182,000 women in the United States are diagnosed with breast cancer every year. American Cancer Society estimates are that one in 8 American women will develop breast cancer at some time in her life.

Early detection is the key. With early detection and treatment, the 5-year survival rate for breast cancer can be as high as 93%. Heightened awareness of the disease, together with breast self-examination and regular mammograms beginning at a younger age have improved survival rates because cancers are being diagnosed earlier.

General symptoms of breast cancer include a thickening or lump in the breast, distortion or dimpling of a breast, swollen lymph nodes under the arm, or retraction, pain, discharge, or scaliness of the nipple. General risk factors for breast cancer include:

— a grandmother, mother, or sister with breast cancer.
— early onset of menstruation (before age 12).
— delayed onset of menopause (after age 55).
— first pregnancy after age 30.
— obesity.
— a woman who has never been pregnant.
— a woman who has never breastfed.
— age (dramatic increase after age 50).

A report from the Utah Population Database suggests that 17% to 19% of breast cancer cases may be attributable to a family history of the disease. Also, women with a first-degree relative with colon cancer had a 30% increase in risk for breast cancer. A family history of breast cancer, however, does not necessarily affect the prognosis or outcome adversely.

Hormone replacement therapy (HRT), usually for post-menopausal women, may be associated with a higher risk, although the available data are difficult to interpret. Some researchers believe the progestin component of HRT may have a greater impact on risk than the estrogen component. The studies of oral contraceptives, which contain the same hormones, show no significant increase in risk. Because of the remaining uncertainty, though, some gynecologists advise against long-term use of oral contraceptives in young women who have not borne children.

Despite earlier findings that a high-fat diet raises the risk, more recent studies have found little support for a role of dietary fat in the onset of breast cancer. Evidence is mounting that daily alcohol consumption does increase the risk, however. Daily consumption of vitamin A — as little as one carrot or less — may reduce the risk.

Exercise also may reduce the risk of breast cancer. Some researchers think exercise may change the proportions of estrogen and progesterone produced during the menstrual cycle, which may affect the risk.

Other studies reveal interesting findings, but these have not been confirmed yet. According to one of these, the longer a woman breastfeeds and the more babies she nurses, the less is her risk for breast cancer.[11] Diethylstibestrol (DES) taken during pregnancy increases a woman's risk for breast cancer later in life, but this risk probably is small and does not increase with time. Environmental factors — specifically, pesticide residues in food — also have been implicated, but this is difficult to study systematically.

> **The American Cancer Society estimates that only 5%–10% of breast cancer is inherited.**

Many factors probably contribute to a woman's risk of developing breast cancer, but the known risk factors account for only a small percentage of breast cancer cases. The majority of patients (60%–70%) have no known risk factors for the disease except older age. Thus, age is the most influential known risk factor.

Cervical Cancer

More than half of all uterine cancers start in the cervix, the neck of the uterus that protrudes into the top end of the vagina. The death rate from cancer of the cervix has decreased more than 70% during the past four decades because of early detection, mainly in the form of Pap smears (especially among younger women) and regular gynecological examinations.

Today, approximately 60,000 women are diagnosed with invasive cervical cancer each year in the

United States. With early diagnosis, treatment usually is successful because the cancer has not spread. Unusual vaginal bleeding or discharge is often an early symptom. Risk factors for cervical cancer can be:

— early age at first intercourse.
— multiple sex partners.
— a history of viral genital infections, especially herpes and the human papilloma virus.
— cigarette smoking.

Uterine Cancer

Uterine cancer, which involves the endometrium, or lining, of the uterus, strikes approximately 48,000 women in the United States each year. Because of improved early detection, the death rate from uterine cancer has fallen dramatically. Only about 4,000 deaths a year in this country are attributed to uterine cancer. With early detection, treatment generally is successful. Symptoms of uterine cancer might be unusual vaginal discharge, unusual vaginal bleeding, or bleeding between menstrual periods. Risk factors for uterine cancer include:

— late onset of menopause.
— history of infertility/failure to ovulate.
— prolonged estrogen replacement therapy.
— obesity.
— diabetes.

Ovarian Cancer

Although ovarian cancer claims a relatively few 14,500 American women each year, it is a particularly difficult cancer because it typically reveals no symptoms until in its latest stages and it can be difficult to diagnose. The survival rate 5 years after diagnosis averages 40%. Late symptoms include abdominal swelling or bloating (the most common sign), persistent abdominal gas, and unexplained stomachaches or indigestion.

Age is a factor. The risk increases with age and is highest for women in their 60s. For unknown reasons, the rates are higher in Jewish women. This form of cancer also strikes Americans, Scandinavians, and Scots at three times the rate it hits Japanese women.

Other risk factors include:

— a grandmother, mother, or sister with ovarian cancer.
— never had children (doubles the risk).
— use of oral contraceptives.

— occurrence of colorectal, breast, or uterine cancer (doubles the risk).
— early onset of ovulation.

A diet high in fat may be a risk factor for ovarian cancer, though more research is needed.

Prostate Cancer

The leading cancer in American men and the second leading cause of cancer death in men (after lung cancer), prostate cancer strikes more than 244,000 men in the United States every year. More than 40,000 die from it.

Prostate cancer often is detected early because it generally provokes an array of symptoms fairly early in its development. The symptoms, however, can be mistaken for signs of other, more common ailments, such as an enlarged prostate or bladder infection. If detected early, prostate cancer can be treated successfully about 84% of the time. A new blood test that measures the amount of prostate-specific antigen (PSA) in the blood can be used to help diagnose prostate cancer. The test is recommended for men beginning at age 50.

Signs and symptoms of prostate cancer include pain in the pelvis, lower back, or upper thighs; blood in the urine or semen; pain or burning during urination; frequent urination; and weak or interrupted urine, difficulty starting or stopping the flow of urine, or inability to urinate.

The risk of prostate cancer increases with age. For that reason, the American Cancer Society recommends an annual prostate exam beginning at age 40. At highest risk are men over age 65, in whom more than 80% of all prostate cancers are diagnosed. Another substantial risk factor is race: Black men in the United States have the highest rate of prostate cancer in the world (30% higher than for whites). Oddly enough, the cancer is relatively rare in Africa and is much more common in North America and northwest Europe than it is in Central and South America or the Near East.

Other risk factors include:

— a family history of prostate cancer.
— occupational exposure to cadmium.
— a high-fat diet.

Testicular Cancer

Although testicular cancer is not one of the most common types of cancer in the United States, it is the most common cancer in young men between ages 17 and 34. Of all cancer deaths in that age group, 12% are from testicular cancer. For unknown reasons, the incidence of testicular cancer in this age group has been increasing steadily. If this cancer is found in its early stages, the chances for cure are nearly 100%.

Early detection is the key to successful treatment. Many men discover the cancer themselves through self-examination. The major warning sign is an often painless thickening or hard lump in the testicle. Other signs include pain or a sensation of heaviness in the affected testicle, an accumulation of fluid or blood in the scrotum, and a dull ache in the groin that may involve the lower abdomen. Although the exact cause of testicular cancer is not known, identified risk factors for testicular cancer include:

— an undescended testicle (risk can be 40 times as high).
— a testicle that did not descend until after age 6 (risk can be 40 times as high).
— a grandfather, father, or brother with testicular cancer.

Bladder Cancer

Approximately 50,000 new cases of bladder cancer are diagnosed each year in the United States, and close to 10,000 Americans die from it each year. If the cancer is detected while it is still confined to the bladder — before it has metastasized to involve other organs — almost nine in 10 can be cured. A new test called *flow cytometry* currently is being evaluated as an early detection tool for bladder cancer.

The most common signs of bladder cancer are more frequent urination and blood in the urine. The cancer is four times more common in men than in women. Other risk factors include:

— cigarette smoking (smoking is believed to cause almost half the bladder cancers in men and approximately 40% of the bladder cancers in women).
— occupational exposure to leather and rubber.
— occupational exposure to dyes.
— living in an urban area.

Pancreatic Cancer

Although pancreatic cancer is not one of the most common cancers, its incidence has more than doubled in the past two decades, making it the fourth most common cancer killer in American men

and the fifth most common cancer killer among American women.

Almost 30,000 new cases are diagnosed in the United States each year, and more than 27,000 Americans die each year of pancreatic cancer. The survival rate from pancreatic cancer is low because the disease spreads rapidly. Few patients with pancreatic cancer survive more than 3 years. In addition, pancreatic cancer is a "silent" disease, usually progressing without symptoms until extremely advanced stages.

The risk for pancreatic cancer increases with age. The highest risk is between ages 65 and 79. More men die of pancreatic cancer each year, but women are diagnosed in higher numbers. Blacks are at higher risk than people of other races. Other risk factors include:

— smoking cigarettes.
— consuming alcohol.
— eating a high-fat diet.
— being exposed to gasoline and some chemical cleaners on the job.

Oral Cancer

Oral cancer has increased substantially over the past two decades, which correlates with the popularity of smokeless tobacco, or chewing tobacco. Twice as many men as women get oral cancer. More than 30,000 Americans are diagnosed with oral cancer each year, and approximately 8,500 die.

Oral cancer can develop anywhere in the oral cavity. Most often it develops on the lining of the cheeks, the lips, the gums, and the floor of the mouth. Signs of oral cancer generally include a sore that fails to heal or that bleeds easily; a whitish patch that does not go away (called *leukoplakia*); a lump or thickening in the cheek, tongue, or lips; and difficulty chewing or swallowing.

The most common risk factor is the use of smokeless tobacco (chewing tobacco). Other risk factors are smoking cigarettes, cigars, or a pipe, and excessive alcohol consumption.

Leukemia

Leukemia, a cancer of the blood-forming tissues (such as the spleen and the bone marrow, can strike people of all ages. Though most people believe it is more common among children, it actually strikes 12 times more adults than children. Approximately 28,000 people (2,500 of them children) are diagnosed with leukemia each year in the United States.

With advances in treatment, survival rates have improved dramatically over the past three decades.

Leukemia can be chronic or acute, and it has a number of varieties. Two of the known risk factors for leukemia are excessive exposure to radiation and exposure to benzenes and other hydrocarbons.

Many forms of leukemia develop slowly and cause few, if any, symptoms. As the immature white blood cells progressively crowd out the red blood cells, normal white blood cells, and platelets, symptoms begin to develop. Leukemia often is misdiagnosed in adults because the most common initial symptom is fatigue, which is a symptom of a number of conditions. Leukemia usually is diagnosed much more quickly in children because additional symptoms — such as weight loss, paleness, frequent nosebleeds, easy bruising, and repeated infections — tend to develop suddenly and rapidly in children.

GUIDELINES FOR PREVENTING CANCER

As much as 85% of all cancer is related to lifestyle and environmental factors over which we have control. By changing your lifestyle and taking control over your environment, you have a pretty good chance of beating the odds of getting cancer. Your general risk for cancer can be cut dramatically by

— avoiding substances known to cause cancer, such as tobacco and overuse of alcohol.

> 66 *As much as 85% of all cancer is related to lifestyle and environmental factors over which we have control.* 99

— avoiding overexposure to sunlight.
— avoiding overeating and eating an anti-cancer diet.
— doing appropriate self-examinations and getting regular checkups to boost your chances of early detection.

Table 12.3 summarizes major preventive measures.

Smoking Cessation

According to former U.S. Surgeon General C. Everett Koop, the single best thing you can do to lower your risk for cancer is to stop smoking. Smoking causes 85% of all lung cancers and three of 10 cancers overall. If you don't smoke, don't start. If you're smoking now, stop. That holds true for any tobacco in any form, not just cigarette smoking.

Your lungs will start to heal as soon as you stop smoking. Your risk will be slightly higher than if you never smoked, but eventually the risk can be the same as nonsmokers. A smoking cessation program is presented in Chapter 13.

Even if you don't smoke yourself, you should limit the amount of cigarette smoke you are exposed to. Nonsmokers who are forced to breathe the cigarette smoke of others run an increased risk of developing cancer.

Limited Sun Exposure

The major cause of skin cancer is too much sun, so if you want to lower your risk for developing skin cancer, limit your exposure to the sun. Sunscreens protect against the ultraviolet rays of the sun. The sun protection factor (SPF) tells you the protection you're getting. An SPF of 10, for example, lets you stay in the sun 10 times as long as you normally would without burning. If your skin normally starts to redden after 20 minutes, a sunscreen with an SPF of 10 lets you stay in the sun 200 minutes before you start to burn. After that time, you'll begin to burn. You can't simply apply more and expect longer protection.

Always use a sunscreen if you're going outside for longer than 15 minutes, even if you think you won't be getting that much sun exposure. Choose a sunscreen that provides adequate protection for your skin type. Choose a broad-spectrum sunscreen that protects against both UVA and UVB radiation. Apply it at least 30–45 minutes before exposure to the sun. Apply the sunscreen frequently if you're in and out of the water (look for a waterproof or water-resistant sunscreen). Apply the screen heavily to areas where your skin is thin, such as your nose, face, neck, and hands. Use sunscreen even on cloudy days (clouds don't block the ultraviolet rays) and during the winter when you're outside. Sunscreen is especially important the closer you are to the equator and if you're at a high altitude, which affords less protection from UV rays.

To further cut your risk for overexposure to the sun:

■ Even when using a sunscreen, avoid being in the sun between 10 a.m. and 3 p.m., when UV rays are at their most intense. If your shadow is shorter than your height, the sun is strong enough to quickly burn your skin. You can burn even if you're sitting in the shade. Plan outdoor activities during the early morning or early evening hours, when sun is less intense and temperatures are cooler.

- Even if you are using a sunscreen, avoid long sun exposure whenever possible.

- If you have to stay outside for long periods, wear protective clothing — long pants, a long-sleeved shirt, a hat with a brim or visor. Wear tightly woven cottons, and avoid white or thin fabrics. Don't sit in the sun in wet clothing.

Tanning poses a risk for skin cancer from overexposure to ultraviolet rays of the sun.

- Don't assume that because your skin isn't red, it isn't getting burned. A sunburn becomes most evident 6 to 24 hours after being in the sun.

- Avoid surfaces that reflect the sun's rays more intensely: concrete, snow, expanses of metal, expanses of sand.

- Stay out of the sun or take extra precautions if you are taking antibiotics (especially penicillin or tetracycline), birth control pills, insulin (especially oral insulin), diuretics, and some medications used to lower blood pressure. They increase the damage from ultraviolet rays.

- Don't drink alcohol if you will be exposed to sunlight. Alcohol, too, increases the damage from ultraviolet rays.

TABLE 12.3 Preventing Cancer

Smoking	Cigarette smoking is responsible for 85% of lung cancer cases among men and 75% among women — about 83% overall. Smoking accounts for about 30% of all cancer deaths. Those who smoke two or more packs of cigarettes a day have lung cancer mortality rates 15 to 25 times greater than nonsmokers.
Sunlight	Almost all of the more than 600,000 cases of nonmelanoma skin cancer diagnosed each year in the United States are considered to be sun-related. Sun exposure is a major factor in the development of melanoma, and the incidence increases for those living near the equator and at high altitudes.
Alcohol	Oral cancer and cancers of the larynx, throat, esophagus, and liver occur more frequently among heavy drinkers of alcohol.
Smokeless tobacco	Use of chewing tobacco or snuff increases risk of cancer of the mouth, larynx, throat, and esophagus and is highly habit-forming.
Estrogen	For mature women, estrogen treatment to control menopausal symptoms increases risk of endometrial cancer. Estrogen use by menopausal women calls for careful discussion between the woman and her physician.
Radiation	Excessive exposure to ionizing radiation can increase cancer risk. Most medical and dental x-rays are adjusted to deliver the lowest dose possible without sacrificing image quality. Excessive radon exposure in homes may increase risk of lung cancer, especially in cigarette smokers. If levels are found to be too high, remedial actions should be taken.
Occupational hazards	Exposure to several different industrial agents (nickel, chromate, asbestos, vinyl chloride, etc.) increases risk of various cancers. Risk from asbestos is greatly increased when combined with cigarette smoking.
Nutrition	Risk for colon, breast, and uterine cancers increases in obese people. High-fat diets may contribute to the development of cancers of the colon, and prostate. High-fiber foods may help reduce risk of colon cancer. A varied diet containing plenty of vegetables and fruits rich in vitamins A and C may reduce risk for a wide range of cancers. Salt-cured, smoked, and nitrite-cured foods have been linked to esophageal and stomach cancer. Heavy use of alcohol, especially when accompanied by cigarette smoking or chewing tobacco, increases risk of cancers of the mouth, larynx, throat, esophagus, and liver.

Adapted from the American Cancer Society.

■ Don't patronize tanning salons or booths, and don't use a sunlamp. Tanned skin is damaged skin. There is no such thing as a "safe" tan.

Most important, do whatever you can to avoid a sunburn. The risk of skin cancer from exposure to sunlight is cumulative. Each time you are unprotected and exposed to sunlight, some amount of damage accrues. With increasing damage, you also increase your risk of developing skin cancer. Sunburns are especially dangerous. Experts say that even one bad sunburn during childhood can double your risk for getting skin cancer later on.

Anti-Cancer Diet

The first specific recommendations relating to an "anti-cancer diet" were published 15 years ago, when the National Academy of Sciences issued a report stating that certain changes in diet could reduce the risk of cancer. Since then, the National Institutes of Health, the U.S. Surgeon General, the U.S. Department of Agriculture, and the U.S. Department of Health and Human Services have joined the National Academy of Sciences in continuing research on the link between diet and cancer. They conclude that at least 35% of cancer deaths are caused by what people eat.

Food affects the risk of cancer in at least three ways.

1. Some foods *protect* against cancer. These foods contain chemicals and other compounds that actually can stop or reverse steps in the development of cancer. These chemicals also boost the body's natural defenses against various carcinogens.

2. Some foods (such as smoked foods) contain carcinogens. Others contain chemicals (such as nitrite) that are converted into carcinogens during the digestive process.

3. Eaten regularly for long periods, certain foods, especially those high in fat, provide an environment in which cancer cells can grow more readily.

Based on research by the U.S. Surgeon General and a variety of scientific agencies, the American Institute for Cancer Research has issued a four-part dietary guideline to reduce the risk of cancer:

1. Reduce total dietary fat to no more than 30% of total calories. In particular, reduce saturated fat (fat that is solid at room temperature) to less than 10% of total calories.

2. Eat more fruits, vegetables, and whole grains.

3. Eat salt-cured, salt-pickled, and smoked foods rarely.

4. Drink alcoholic beverages in moderation or not at all.

The American Cancer Society and the National Academy of Science have jointly released the following detailed dietary guidelines for reducing cancer risk:

■ *Maintain a normal weight.* A 12-year study involving almost a million Americans showed that those who were overweight — especially those who were 40% or more overweight — ran substantially higher risks for cancer. According to the study, those who are obese run a one-and-a-half times greater risk for cancer of the breast and colon, two times higher risk for cancer of the prostate, three times greater risk for cancer of the gallbladder, and five times greater risk for uterine cancer. The American Cancer Society recommends limiting calories and increasing exercise to maintain recommended weight.

■ *Reduce the amount of fat you eat.* Major sources of fat in the American diet are visible fats (the fats we add to foods, such as butter, mayonnaise, and salad dressings) and the less visible fats that are found in eggs, dairy foods, meats, and baked goods. Cut down on foods high in fats, such as red meats, whole milk and whole milk products, cheeses, butter, pastries, candies, and oils. Trim all visible fat from your meat before cooking it,

The UV Index

The Ultraviolet Index is a measure of the sun's damaging ultraviolet rays during the hottest part of the day. This chart can help you interpret the UV Index the next time you see one:

Solar-hazard Rating	Health Risk	Time to Burn*
0–2	Very low	More than 30 minutes
3–4	Low	15 to 90 minutes
5–6	Moderate	10 to 60 minutes
7–9	High	7 to 35 minutes
10 & over	Very high	5 to 30 minutes

*The "time to burn" ranges are based on the amount of time it takes for a person to sunburn and varies widely by skin type.

and remove skin and fat from chicken before cooking. Instead of frying foods, use low-fat methods of cooking such as broiling, steaming, baking). Use less cooking oil than a recipe calls for. Skim all visible fats from soups, stews, and gravies; if you can, refrigerate them overnight, then remove the hardened fat that rises to the surface. Cut back on the use of cream, butter, margarine, shortening, mayonnaise, and salad dressing. Substitute foods naturally low in fat, such as whole grains, legumes, fruits, and vegetables.

- *Eat a wide variety of more high-fiber foods*, such as whole-grain cereals, whole-grain breads, bran cereals, legumes (including kidney beans), lima beans, pinto beans, rice, popcorn, and brown rice. Leave well-scrubbed skins on fruits and vegetables. Eat foods with visible hulls, seeds, and textured skins, such as strawberries, raspberries, and peaches.

- *Eat food rich in vitamins A and C every day.* Good sources of vitamin A are fresh foods that are dark green or deep yellow in color: spinach, broccoli, carrots, sweet potatoes, squash, apricots, and peaches. Good sources of vitamin C are citrus fruits (such as oranges, grapefruit, and tangerines), strawberries, cantaloupes, tomatoes, and green peppers. Many of these foods also are rich in beta-carotene.

- *Eat cruciferous vegetables* such as cabbage, broccoli, cauliflower, Brussels sprouts, and kohlrabi.

- *Cut down on salt-cured, smoked, and nitrite-cured foods.* Nitrites in salt-cured and salt-pickled foods become carcinogenic during the digestive process. Limit the amount of bacon, ham, hot dogs, beef jerky, smoked fish, smoked meats, and salt-cured fish you eat. If you barbecue often, cook food at lower temperatures or a greater distance from the flame so food doesn't get charred.

- *If you drink, use alcohol in strict moderation.* Alcohol significantly increases your risk for a number of cancers, especially if you also smoke cigarettes. Besides the harmful effects of the alcohol itself, alcohol can interfere with eating a healthy, balanced diet.

In addition to these guidelines, the following dietary suggestions can further reduce your risk of cancer:

- *Get plenty of calcium.* It seems to help neutralize carcinogenic substances in the digestive tract. Early studies indicate calcium may help prevent colon cancer. Low-fat milk and nonfat milk and dairy products are good sources, as are dark-green vegetables, and foods that have been fortified with calcium.

- *Avoid foods that have been treated heavily with chemicals or pesticides* or processed with large amounts of additives. Wash fruits and vegetables well before you eat them.

- *Refrigerate foods* that need it, especially fruits and vegetables. Fruits and vegetables naturally produce nitrites, a process that refrigeration slows down.

Table 12.4 summarizes the dietary measures that may lower your risk for cancer. The key seems to be variety and moderation.

Appropriate Self-Exams

One of the keys to successful cancer treatment is early detection. You should examine yourself regularly for skin and breast or testicular cancer.

Skin Self-Exams

One of the easiest and quickest self-exams is a brief survey to detect possible skin cancers (see Figure 12.3). A simple skin self-exam can reduce deaths from melanoma by as much as 63%, saving as many as 4,500 lives in the United States each year.

- Make a drawing of yourself. Include a full front view, a full back view, and close-up views of your head (both sides), the soles of your feet, the tops of your feet, and the backs of your hands.

- After you get out of the bath or shower, examine yourself closely in a full-length mirror. On your sketch make note of any moles, warts, or other skin marks you find anywhere on your body. Pay particular attention to areas that are exposed to the sun constantly, such as your face, the tops of your ears, and your hands.

- Briefly describe each mark on your sketch: its size, color, texture, and so on.

- Repeat the exam about once a month. Watch for changes in the size, texture, or color of moles, wart, or other skin mark. If you notice any difference, contact your physician. You also should contact a doctor if you have a sore that does not heal.

Breast Self-Exams

Early detection of breast cancer is vital to successful treatment, and a woman who performs regular

TABLE 12.4 Anti-Cancer Dietary Measures

Substance	Associated Cancers	Comments	Steps to Take
Fiber	May *decrease* risk of colorectal cancer.	Different types of fiber may affect cancer risk differently. Benefits also may be due to lower fat intakes usually associated with high-fiber diets.	Eat 4 to 5 servings a day of a variety of vegetables, fruits, whole-grain cereals, and legumes. Maximize fiber in vegetables and fruits by eating them unpeeled.
Fruits and vegetables	May *decrease* risk of colorectal and breast cancers.	Eat good sources of fiber (see above). Cruciferous vegetables, such as broccoli, cabbage, and Brussels sprouts, also - contain indoles — nitrogen compounds that, in some studies, have knocked out carcinogens that can lead to breast cancer.	To maximize indole intake, eat vegetables raw, steamed, or microwaved; boiling leaches up to half the indoles.
Fat	May *increase* risk of breast, colon, and prostate cancers.	Lowering fat intake will almost automatically lower caloric intake and boost fiber intake — steps that also will lower cancer risk.	Decrease calories from fat to 25% to 30% of total daily calories. (Current average intake is 40% of total calories.)
Alcohol	Heavy use *increases* risk of cancers of the oral cavity, larynx, and esophagus; moderate use may *increase* breast cancer risk.	Cigarette smoking in conjunction with alcohol drinking greatly increases cancer risk. Alcohol use also can cause liver cirrhosis, which may lead to liver cancer.	Drink only occasionally and sparingly.
Salt-cured, smoked, barbecued and nitrite-preserved foods	May *increase* risk of stomach, esophageal, and lung cancers.	Smoking and charcoal-grilling foods produces tars that are similar to those in cigarette smoke, and are absorbed by the food. Manufacturers have substantially decreased nitrites used in meat preservation.	Opt for other cooking methods; limit intake of salt-cured and nitrite-preserved foods.
Beta-carotene and antioxidant vitamins (A, C, and E)	Inconclusive	Vitamin E and beta-carotene have been associated with lower rates of cancer in humans; a lesser effect has been noted with the other antioxidant nutrients. More research is needed.	Eat a balanced and varied diet to ensure that you get the RDA for all vitamins; do not take megadose vitamin supplements.
Selenium	Inconclusive	Limited evidence shows this trace element may protect against breast and colon cancers; however, it is highly toxic in high doses.	Taking selenium supplements can be dangerous; you get all the selenium you need from a varied diet.
Artificial sweeteners	Inconclusive	High levels of saccharin cause bladder cancer in rats, but no evidence of this in humans. Long-term effects of aspartame are unknown.	Moderate use poses no risk.
Coffee and caffeine	None	Both coffee and caffeine have received a clean bill of health.	Moderate use of coffee and caffeine does not appear to be a risk.
Food additives	None	Chemical additives found to be carcinogenic in animals have been banned; insufficient evidence that additives currently in use have any cancer risk or benefit.	None

Reprinted with permission of the *Johns Hopkins Medical Letter Health After 50*, © MedLetter Associates, 1992.

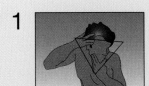

1 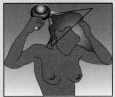 Examine your face, especially the nose, lips, mouth, and ears – front and back. Use one or both mirrors to get a clear view.

2 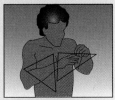 Thoroughly inspect your scalp, using a blow dryer and mirror to expose each section to view. Get a friend or family member to help, if you can.

3 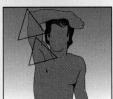 Check your hands carefully: palms and backs, between the fingers, and under the fingernails. Continue up the wrists to examine both front and back of your forearms.

4 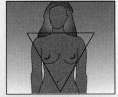 Standing in front of a full-length mirror, begin at the elbows and scan all sides of your upper arms. Don't forget the underarms.

5 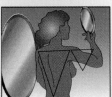 Next focus on the neck, chest, and torso. Women should lift breasts to view the underside.

6 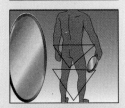 With your back to the full-length mirror, use the hand mirror to inspect the back of your neck, shoulders, upper back, and any part of the back of your upper arms you could not view in step 4.

7 Still using both mirrors, scan your lower back, buttocks, and backs of both legs.

8 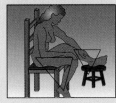 Sit down; prop each leg in turn on another stool or chair. Use the hand mirror to examine the genitals. Check front and sides of both legs, thigh to shin; ankles, tops of feet, between toes, and under toenails. Examine soles of feet and heels

Reprinted with permission from *Family Practice Recertification*, Vol. 14, No. 3, March, 1992.

Self-exam for skin cancer.

monthly self-exams has a much better chance of detecting changes that could indicate problems. When you're doing self-exams regularly, you can detect a growth when it's about the size of a pea; a physician doing a breast exam probably won't detect it until it's two to three times that size.

Perform the exam on both breasts regularly, once a month. A week after your menstrual period is the best time, as your breasts won't be subject to the swelling that sometimes precedes menstruation, and it will be a regular reminder. If you don't have periods, pick a day you can remember easily (such as the first day of the month). See Figure 12.4.

The key to breast self-examination is to do the exam regularly. Cancer is detected soonest when you notice a change from one month to the next. Immediately report to your doctor any changes or anything unusual. And don't forego your yearly medical exam.

Testicular Self-Exam

Testicular cancer detected early can be treated successfully a good deal of the time. The key to early detection is a simple, 3-minute self-exam done once a month. Choose a day each month (the first day usually is easy to remember), and do the exam as soon as you get out of a warm bath or shower, as your testicles and scrotal skin are most relaxed then. You need to examine both testicles, one at a time as demonstrated in Figure 12.5.

- Using both hands, roll the testicle gently between your thumbs and fingers. You'll feel a rope-like structure toward the back of the testicle. That's the epididymis, and it's normal. Most cancers occur toward the front of the testicle, and they will feel like a pea-sized lump or hard knot.

- Repeat the exam on the other testicle.

- Immediately report to your doctor any nodules or lumps.

Age-Appropriate Checkups

In addition to self-exams you do at home, your physician can do examinations and tests to enable early detection of cancer. The exams in Table 12.5 are the final weapon in your arsenal against cancer.

If you are at high risk for a certain cancer, you should have screening tests more often. Check with your physician. Sexually active women should have annual Pap smears and pelvic exams as soon as sexual activity begins. Women also should have a mammography. Recent findings indicate that mammograms should begin while a woman is in her 40s — not in her 50s, as has been recommended routinely by federal agencies since 1993. One of the advantages of earlier mammograms is that almost half the breast cancers in women under age 50 are noninvasive forms that are virtually 100% curable if detected early. Left undetected and untreated, these cancers progress into invasive cancers that are more difficult to cure.

To get the best reading from your mammogram, make sure the x-ray technician is certified by the American Registry of Radiological Technologists or a state licensing board; that the technician has mammogram training; and that the facility is accredited by the American College of Radiology (ACR).

New guidelines by the American Cancer Society recommend mammograms every 1 to 2 years between ages 40 and 49, and annual mammograms beginning at age 50. In addition to monthly breast self-exams, the ACS recommends a breast exam by a physician every 3 years for women ages 20 to 40 and annual exams by a physician every year beginning at age 40.

NOTES

1. National Cancer Institute.
2. American Cancer Society, *Cancer Facts and Figures, 1977.*
3. American Cancer Society.
4. American Lung Association.
5. National Academy of Sciences.
6. R. Lowry, D. Holtzman, B. I. Truman, L. Kann, J. L. Collins, and L. J. Kolbe, "Substance Use and HIV-Related Sexual Behaviors Among U.S. High School Students," *American Journal of Public Health,* 84:1116–1120 (1994).
7. American Cancer Society, *Cancer Facts & Figures — 1994* (Atlanta: American Cancer Society, 1994).
8. *Epidemiology,* (Sept. 1993)
9. American Cancer Society, *Cancer Facts & Figures — 1994.*
10. American Cancer Society, *Cancer Facts & Figures — 1994*, p. 22.
11. American Cancer Society, *Cancer Facts & Figures — 1994.*

FIGURE 12.4

1 Raising one arm at a time over your head, use the fingertips of the opposite hand to check for any changes, lumps, or thickening.

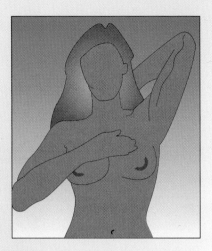

2 Start near the nipple and work outward in widening circles.

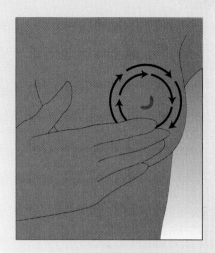

3 Visually examine your breasts in a mirror with your arms at your sides.

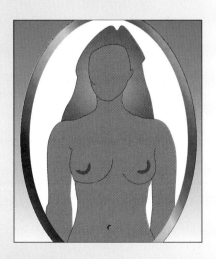

4 Visually examine your breasts in a mirror with your arms raised above your head.

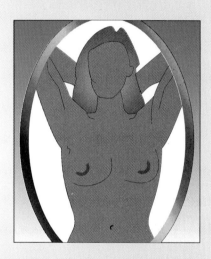

5 Check your nipples by squeezing them gently. Unless you have recently had a baby, any discharge is abnormal.

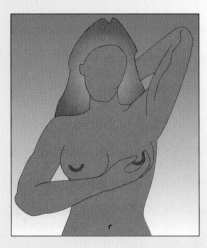

6 Place a pillow under your shoulder and your arm under your head. With your other hand, feel your breast and armpit for lumps, thickening, or other changes.

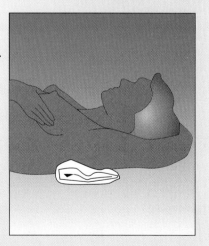

Adapted from *Family Practice Recertification* 14(3), March 1992. Used by permission.

Breast self-exam.

FIGURE 12.5

How do I do this examination?

Here's how to go about it: Roll each testicle between your thumb and first three fingers until you have felt the entire surface (see Figure below). The testicles should feel round and smooth, like hard-boiled eggs.

These are the things you have to be on the lookout for:

- Lumps
- Irregularities
- A change in the size of the testicle
- Pain in the testicle
- A dragging or heavy sensation.

How often do I have to do this exam?

Do it at least once a month. It helps to pick a regular day of the month — the day of your birthday, the first of the month, the first Sunday, or some other day that's easy for you to remember. You can do the exam more often if you like.

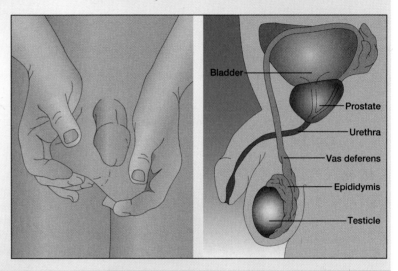

Testicular self-exam.

TABLE 12.5 Medical Checkups

Examination	Age and Frequency
Cancer-related checkup (skin, thyroid gland, mouth, lymph glands, ovaries, prostate gland, testicles)	- Age 20 to 40: every 3 to 4 years - Beginning at age 40: once a year
Breast	- Ages 20 to 40: physician exam every 3–4 years - Ages 35–39: one baseline mammogram - Ages 40–50: exam and mammogram every 2 years - Age 50 and older: exam and mammogram annually
Colon and rectum	- Ages 40 and up: digital rectal exam annually - Ages 50 and up: stool blood test annually - Ages 50 and up: proctology exam every 2 years after two negative annual exams
Uterus	- Ages 20 to 40: pelvic exam every 3 years - Ages 40 and up: pelvic exam annually
Cervix	- Ages 20 to 40: pelvic exam and Pap smear once every 2 years after two consecutive negative tests - Age 40 and up: annual exams regardless of age; if sexually active with more than one partner
Prostate	- Ages 40 and up: digital exam annually and PSA protein test

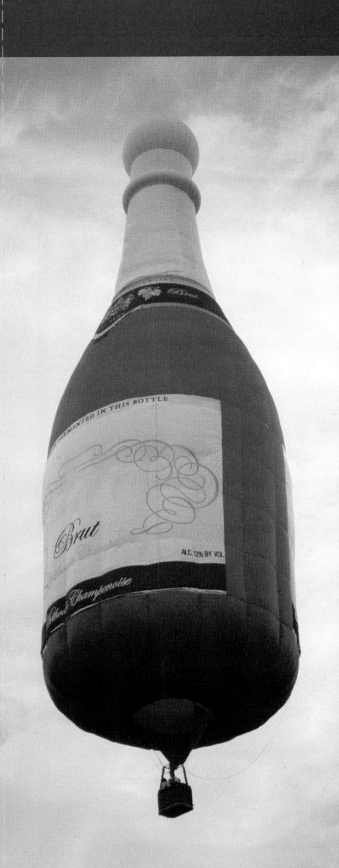

Addictive Behavior and Wellness

Hello

We all have habits. You might have the habit of flopping down in front of the television as soon as you get home every day, or biting your nails when you're bored. Most habits are harmless, but when a habit escalates into an addiction, it threatens wellness. Broadly defined, an **addiction** is an abnormal or disordered relationship with an object (such as tobacco or alcohol) or an event or behavior (such as shoplifting or gambling). Continued involvement with the object or activity has harmful consequences. Addiction is a process that evolves over time. It almost always begins as a pleasurable, voluntary activity but ends by causing continuous disruption in an addict's life.

Typical characteristics of addictive behavior are

— a compulsive need to do something

— loss of control of actions

— repeating the action even though the results are harmful.

Most people with addictions deny they have a problem. They can't see it even though people around them see it clearly.

To be addictive, a substance must be able to produce a positive change in mood. Drugs produce the most powerful addiction because of their ability to change mood. Addiction, however, goes far beyond dependence on drugs. People also can become addicted to computers, exercise, television, work, cleanliness, or over-the-counter medications. A person may switch addictions from one object or behavior to another.

Addiction threatens all five dimensions of wellness — physical, emotional, social, intellectual, and spiritual.

1. *Physical wellness.* People who are addicted to an object or an event typically fail to take good care of themselves because they are preoccupied with the addictive behavior. They might not get enough sleep, may skip meals, and could even put themselves in dangerous situations. Certain addictive behaviors damage the body itself. As examples, bulimia damages the throat and alcoholism damages the liver. The stress accompanying some addictions can injure virtually every organ and system in the body.

2. *Emotional wellness.* Addictive behavior lowers self-esteem. The addict usually feels guilty, anxious, angry, depressed, and ashamed. Many addicts have unexplained mood swings or episodes of rage and violence.

3. *Social wellness.* Other than the interaction the addiction requires, an addict usually is a loner who gradually cuts off relationships with family members, friends, colleagues, or classmates. Addiction brings with it a powerful preoccupation that takes priority over people, places, and events outside of the addictive behavior.

Signs of Addictive Behavior

- No matter how much you get, it's never enough. You're frustrated constantly by the need to do more or get more. (That frustration, incidentally, is much different from the motivation that stems from challenge and determination.)

- You don't get pleasure from the behavior. It doesn't contribute to an overall sense of well-being.

- The behavior becomes predictable. You know you'll do a certain thing a certain way. The pattern doesn't change.

- You become inflexible about the behavior. For example, you run 2 miles before class every morning, and balk at a friend's suggestion that you play tennis instead. If your friend won't run with you, you run anyway — either before you play tennis or instead of playing tennis.

- You have a lower sense of self-worth or self-esteem because of what you're doing, but you can't seem to stop.

- Even if you don't enjoy the behavior, you feel driven to do it anyway. For example, you might be disgusted by your obsession to look at pornographic magazines and might think it's a dirty habit, but you can't seem to stop. Your behavior even might make you sick, but you can't seem to change.

- You stay locked in the behavior as a way of escaping demands or stresses, not because you see the behavior as an exhilarating challenge.

- The behavior dulls your senses, provides an escape, or otherwise helps you get away from stress, unhappiness, boredom, or frustration. Whenever you get a chance for challenge or reward, you resort to the addictive behavior instead of taking a chance on some other behavior.

4. *Mental wellness.* Addiction impairs reasoning, judgment, and logic. Things that used to provide intellectual challenge or stimulation — course-work in a graduate class, exploration of nearby geological sites, debates over a current topic — no longer matter.

5. *Spiritual wellness.* Because of the time and energy demands of an addiction, addicts have difficulty maintaining the same priorities and values they once had. Addicts gradually lose a sense of self and a feeling of being connected to the people and the world around them. They can't focus on something greater than self, nor can they appreciate themselves in a meaningful way.

6. *Occupational wellness*, which some models also consider a sixth dimension. All of the addict's focus is on the addictive behavior, leaving little time for school or a job. Absenteeism increases; quality takes a dive; relationships with professors, other students, colleagues, and supervisors suffer.

THE ADDICTIVE PERSONALITY

The notion of an addictive personality is controversial. One school of thought flatly believes there is no such thing as an addictive personality. Another believes no set of personality traits leads to addiction but has identified a constellation of traits that disposes someone to addiction. The more of these characteristics a person has, and the stronger each trait or condition is, the more vulnerable that person is to addiction.

The Nonaddictive Personality

Some traits of people who are *not* likely to have addictive behavior are as follows.

- They have the ability to face problems head-on with optimism and realism, and they work to overcome their problems. They recognize their own limitations and pace themselves accordingly to maximize their ability to cope.

- They are able and eager to look at their circumstances realistically. They set realistic goals and work toward achieving their goals in a structured, reasonable way. They escape the frustration and disappointment that come with unreached goals.

- They aren't too hard on themselves. They recognize their limitations and weaknesses and also appreciate their strengths and good qualities. They structure their lives so they can maximize their strengths without having to shed their weaknesses.

- They have a keen interest in other people, allow others the freedom to pursue their own interests, and have at least a few deep relationships with other people. They have the ability to love and be loved and consider others' feelings, desires, and needs as they fashion their own behavior. They are not controlled by others but at the same time are sensitive to others.

- They are happy, spontaneous, creative, and like to try new things.

- They see plenty of positive things in life and are eager to discover more. They appreciate things in their lives and have a fresh sense of humor that allows them to retain some perspective about what happens to them.

Traits That Make People Prone to Addiction

The objects, events, or behaviors involved in addiction aren't necessarily bad, but an addict has an unhealthy or abnormal relationship with those objects, events, or behaviors. For example, food provides us with nutrition and energy, but food addicts eat compulsively and endanger their health. Sex provides intimacy, but a sex addict becomes preoccupied with pornography or an ever-expanding gamut of sexual partners. Drugs can cure disease, but drug addicts harm themselves by abusing the substance. The addictive personality is one who has learned not to trust people, does not have healthy relationships, and never has learned to connect to other people, his or her own emotions, and the surrounding world.[1]

Despite controversy surrounding the notion of an "addictive personality," most professionals agree that the following traits make individuals vulnerable to addictive behavior:

- A genetic factor may predispose a person to addictive behavior. This factor seems especially prevalent with the tendency for alcohol and drug abuse.

- They have low self-esteem and lack confidence.

Addiction   An abnormal or disordered relationship with an object, event, or behavior.

- They feel powerless and victimized by their surroundings. An addictive behavior can engender a feeling of strength or aggression they can't cultivate on their own.

- They fear personal criticism and constantly seek approval from others. They are overly concerned with how others think of them.

- They display antisocial behavior and have a strong sense of alienation from other people. They are unable to communicate well and are unable to seek comfort from others.

- They are particularly susceptible to peer pressure.

- They are less mature and are not able to deal maturely with situations as their counterparts. They tend to become dependent, conforming, and compliant, even when they think their own needs are being compromised.

- They do anything possible to avoid conflict, are extremely fearful of being criticized, and try desperately to please others.

- They *seem* outgoing and sociable but have a great deal of trouble developing any kind of interpersonal relationship. They fear deep involvement, usually because they feel incapable of handling relationships.

- They have a need for instant gratification.

- They recognize problems, but instead of tackling them head-on, they feel overwhelmed and incapable. They lack problem-solving skills. They deny the problem, hide from the problem, or run away from the problem.

- When threatened by a problem, they try to escape — sometimes through fantasy or daydreaming but always through something that helps them forget about the problem.

- They don't have the ability to set realistic, reasonable goals and go about achieving them systematically. Instead, they set unrealistic or even impossible goals, then drive toward those goals erratically. When they don't achieve their goals, they sink into depression.

- They worry about their own capabilities and fear the future and what it might hold, feel unsure about their ability to measure up, and dread what lies ahead.

- They do not deal well with stress. They allow stress to build up without knowing how to cope with it, and when things get really tough, the addictive behavior seems like the only way out.

- They don't deal well with frustration. Much of that stems from deep feelings of inferiority. They usually have felt inferior since early childhood and have been unable to meet problems head-on. With a constant fear of being overwhelmed, embarrassed, or compromised, they turn to addictive behavior to escape or to get a false sense of power over their environment.

- They lack normal levels of spontaneity, creativity, and eagerness for life. As a result, they get bored and turn to an addiction to relieve the boredom.

- They often come from high-risk backgrounds. Higher rates of addictive behavior, especially drug and alcohol abuse, are found in populations of the economically disadvantaged, latchkey children, abuse victims, people with physical or mental handicaps, school dropouts, pregnant teenagers, runaways, the homeless, and children of alcoholics.

- They often are risk-takers who are impulsive and have unusually high levels of energy. They look for excitement and stimulation and turn to an addictive behavior to get it.

RISK FACTORS OF ADDICTION

Addictive behavior covers a wide spectrum — eating disorders, compulsive gambling, shoplifting, compulsive spending, alcoholism, sexual addiction, to name a few. Factors leading to addiction include the following:

- The behavior is reinforced.

- The addiction is an attempt to meet basic human needs, such as physical needs, the need to feel safe, the need to belong, the need to feel important, or the need to reach one's potential.

- The addiction relieves stress.

- The addiction can be present within the person's value system (a person whose values wouldn't let him or her shoot heroine may be able to rationalize compulsive eating or obsessive television watching, for example).

- A serious physical illness is present, and the addiction provides escape from pain or the fear of disfigurement.

- There is pressure to perform or succeed.

- The person hates himself or herself.

- Brain activity may vary. Some addictions may be attributable to intense brainwave speed.

- Society allows addiction. Advertising even encourages it (you can sleep better with a pill, beer helps you enjoy sports more fully, parties are more fun with alcohol, and so on).

Most people with addictions deny their problem. Even when the addiction is clear to people around them, they continue to deny that the addiction exists. Instead, they:

- Get angry when someone tries to talk about the behavior.
- Make excuses for their actions.
- Blame others for the problem.
- Put distance between themselves and the problem by focusing on a bigger problem.
- Admit the problem, but fail to take any steps to change.

The same general traits and behaviors are involved in all kinds of addictions, whether they involve food, sex, gambling, shopping, or drugs. Most common, however, are addictions to caffeine, tobacco, alcohol, marijuana, and cocaine.

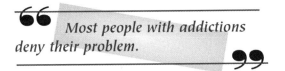

> *Most people with addictions deny their problem.*

CAFFEINE

Caffeine is probably the most widely used drug in the United States. An estimated 82%–92% of Americans consume caffeine regularly, and almost half of all Americans drink coffee every day.[2] Caffeine is found in coffee, tea, cocoa, chocolate, colas, a variety of soft drinks (including orange, lemon lime, and root beer), and a number of prescription and over-the-counter drugs. Caffeine is a common ingredient in nonprescription drugs for cold and allergy relief, pain relief, weight control, alleviation of fluid retention, and alertness. Caffeine occurs naturally in coffee, tea, and chocolate, and it is added to other products during manufacturing. Many who use it do not consider it to be a drug. Table 13.1 shows the caffeine content of various substances.

Regular coffee drinkers are at greater risk for heart disease, coronary artery disease, and heart attack. One study showed that drinking five cups of coffee a day may increase the risk of heart attack.[3]

TABLE 13.1 Caffeine Content

Beverage/Food	Avg. Mg. Caffeine	Range
Caffeine Content		
Coffee (5-oz. cup)		
Brewed, drip method	115	60–180
Brewed, percolator	80	40–170
Instant	65	30–120
Decaffeinated, brewed	3	2–5
Decaffeinated, instant	2	1–5
Tea		
Brewed, U.S. brands (5 oz.)	40	20–90
Brewed, imported brands (5 oz.)	60	25–110
Instant (5 oz.)	30	25–50
Iced (12 oz.)	70	67–76
Cocoa (5 oz.)	4	2–20
Chocolate milk (8 oz.)	5	2–7
Milk chocolate (1 oz.)	6	1–15
Dark chocolate, semisweet (1 oz.)	20	5–35
Baker's chocolate (1 oz.)	26	26
Chocolate-flavored syrup (1 oz.)	4	4

Another study found that women who drink one-half to four cups of tea a day are twice as likely to have premenstrual syndrome (PMS).[4] Much more moderate amounts of caffeine — sometimes no more than the amount in one cup of coffee — may pose a risk in some individuals, too.

> *One Excedrin or two Anacin contain as much caffeine as two cups of instant coffee.*

The effects of caffeine are felt within 15 to 45 minutes of ingestion. Caffeine can cause the following:

- Increase in heart rate, blood pressure, and blood cholesterol levels.
- Increase in metabolism and the amount of oxygen the body's cells require.
- Increase in urinary output.
- Impairment of fine-motor control.
- Dizziness.
- Headaches.

- Wakefulness (insomnia).
- Irritability, anxiety, agitation, nervousness.
- Feelings of panic.
- Increased appetite.
- Clammy hands/sweating.
- Nausea or indigestion, and occasional heartburn.
- Diarrhea.

As the effects of caffeine wear off, a user might feel mentally or physically depressed, let down, weak, and fatigued. A person addicted to caffeine will get a severe headache within 4 hours if he or she stops using caffeine.

Chronic use of caffeine can lead to **caffeinism**. Symptoms include rapid breathing and heart rate, involuntary muscle twitches, agitation, nausea, loss of appetite, and chronic insomnia. In some cases it can cause convulsions and hallucinations.

TOBACCO

Tobacco products — cigarettes, cigars, pipes, smokeless tobacco — all contain the addictive drug **nicotine**. People who smoke only pipes and cigars seem to have fewer health risks from smoking than those who smoke cigarettes, but they still run a much higher risk than people who don't smoke at all.

Prevalence and Demographics of Smoking

The percentage of the U.S. population that smokes has declined over the last 2½ decades, although the ratio of male-to-female smokers has narrowed. The death rate reflected in Figure 13.1 attests to the toll that smoking-related disease has taken over the years.

Adults with less than a 12th-grade education are more than twice as likely to smoke as are those with a college degree. Also counterbalancing the overall decrease in smoking in the adult population, smoking by teens is increasing. At present, about 35% of students in grades 9–12 smoke cigarettes, whereas only 25% of adults smoke.[5] Figure 13.2 breaks down student cigarette use by grade level.

Health Risks

Besides the risk of earlier death, the proven health risks of smoking, shown in Figure 13.3, include:

- Lung cancer; according to the American Cancer Society, approximately 90% of all lung cancer is caused directly by cigarette smoking, and of the

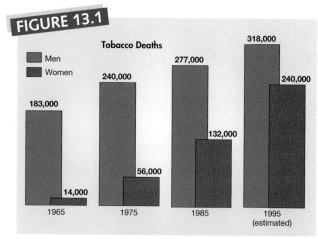

FIGURE 13.1

Tobacco Deaths

- Men
- Women

1965: 183,000 / 14,000
1975: 240,000 / 56,000
1985: 277,000 / 132,000
1995 (estimated): 318,000 / 240,000

Annual smoking-attributed deaths in the United States.

10% that occurs in nonsmokers, one in five results from inhaling secondary cigarette smoke. The particulates in tobacco smoke are 500,000 times greater than the most heavily polluted air in the world. Lung cancer is the leading cause of cancer death in the United States, killing more than 153,000 Americans every year.

- Exposure to carbon monoxide, which reduces the ability of red blood cells to carry oxygen. The concentration of carbon monoxide in tobacco smoke is 800 times higher than the level considered safe by the U.S Environmental Protection Agency (EPA). Filtered cigarettes deliver even greater concentrations of carbon monoxide.
- Oral cancer (cancer of the mouth, palate, larynx, pharynx, and esophagus in cigarette smokers; and cancer of the lip, tongue, and jaw in pipe smokers). An estimated 70% of all oral cancer cases are caused by cigarettes or chewing tobacco.

Clove Cigarettes

Some people smoke clove cigarettes, believing that they are made entirely of ground cloves and carry none of the risk of tobacco. Clove cigarettes, however, are about 40% ground cloves and 60% tobacco. They actually may be more dangerous than regular cigarettes because they contain more nicotine, tar, and carbon monoxide than regular tobacco, and the numbing effect of the eugenol in cloves anesthetizes the throat and causes the smoke to be inhaled much more deeply.

FIGURE 13.2

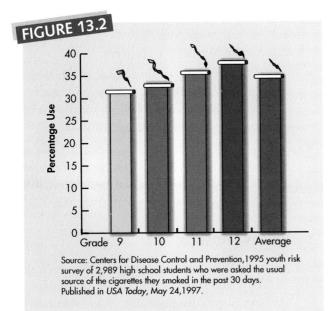

Source: Centers for Disease Control and Prevention,1995 youth risk survey of 2,989 high school students who were asked the usual source of the cigarettes they smoked in the past 30 days. Published in *USA Today*, May 24,1997.

Cigarette use by high school students under age 18 by grade level.

- Cancer of the pancreas (the risk increases by 70% in smokers).
- Cancer of the bladder (smoking is the greatest risk factor in bladder cancer; more than half of all men who get cancer of the bladder are cigarette smokers).
- Cervical cancer (the risk is highest for women under age 30).

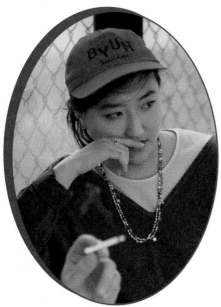

Legislation to protect nonsmokers' rights is being stepped up.

- Chronic obstructive pulmonary disease (emphysema, asthma, and chronic bronchitis; an estimated 90% of all cases are smokers, and smokers run 25 times higher risks).
- Damage to the respiratory system, increasing the risk of pneumonia, influenza, and colds. Smoke

Facts About Second-hand Tobacco Smoke

Every year in America, an estimated 3,000 nonsmokers die from lung cancer caused by second-hand tobacco smoke. If you breathe it regularly, you're probably at risk.

- Exposure to second-hand smoke causes 30 times as many lung cancer deaths as all regulated air pollutants combined.
- Second-hand smoke leads to coughing, phlegm, chest discomfort, reduced lung function, and reddening, itching, and watering of your eyes.
- More than 4,000 chemical compounds have been identified in tobacco smoke; at least 43 are known to cause cancer in humans or animals.
- Exposure to second-hand smoke contributes up to 300,000 infections annually in children younger than 18 months. Infections include potentially serious conditions such as pneumonia and bronchitis. Between 7,500 and 15,000 children are hospitalized as a result of these infections.
- Second-hand smoke triggers 8,000 to 26,000 new cases of asthma in children and worsens symptoms in 400,000 to 1 million asthmatic children.
- Infants are three times more likely to die from Sudden Infant Death Syndrome (SIDS) if their mothers smoke during and after pregnancy.
- There is no safe level of exposure to second-hand cigarette smoke.

From Centers for Disease Control and Prevention, Atlanta, GA, and Environmental Protection Agency.

Caffeinism A toxic condition resulting from chronic use of caffeine.

Nicotine A poisonous, addictive component of tobacco, inhaled when smoking or absorbed through the lining of the mouth when chewing it.

destroys the air sacs in the lungs, reducing their ability to absorb oxygen and eliminate carbon dioxide. Smokers are 18 times more likely than nonsmokers to die of lung disease.

- Heart attacks, strokes, and coronary artery disease, including damage to the inner surface of coronary arteries. Smoking reduces the amount of oxygen that gets to the heart, weakening it. Smokers are twice as likely to have a stroke. Smoking also adds an estimated 10 years of aging to the arteries. More than a quarter of a million deaths from heart disease each year (half of those who die from heart disease) are attributed directly to cigarette smoking. Smokers have a 70% higher death rate from heart disease; heavy smokers, a 200% higher death rate than moderate smokers.

- Peptic ulcer. Death rates from peptic ulcer are much higher in smokers because the condition is much harder to treat for smokers.

- Risk of miscarriage, stillbirths, death during infancy, and low birthweight babies (children born to women who smoke are still physically and socially underdeveloped at the age of 7).

- Increase in risk for sudden infant death syndrome (SIDS) among babies born to mothers who smoke and higher rates of asthma and middle-ear infections among children of smoking parents.

Smokeless Tobacco

Because many users erroneously consider smokeless tobacco (chew and snuff) to be a safer alternative, its use has increased dramatically over the past 2

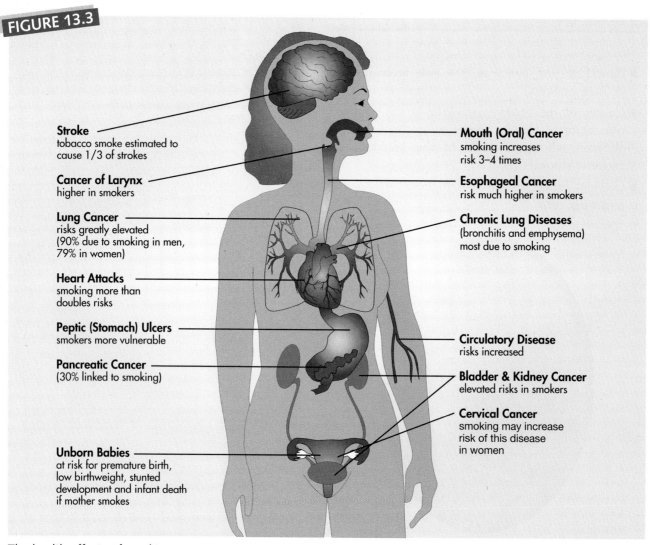

FIGURE 13.3

Stroke
tobacco smoke estimated to cause 1/3 of strokes

Cancer of Larynx
higher in smokers

Lung Cancer
risks greatly elevated (90% due to smoking in men, 79% in women)

Heart Attacks
smoking more than doubles risks

Peptic (Stomach) Ulcers
smokers more vulnerable

Pancreatic Cancer
(30% linked to smoking)

Unborn Babies
at risk for premature birth, low birthweight, stunted development and infant death if mother smokes

Mouth (Oral) Cancer
smoking increases risk 3–4 times

Esophageal Cancer
risk much higher in smokers

Chronic Lung Diseases
(bronchitis and emphysema) most due to smoking

Circulatory Disease
risks increased

Bladder & Kidney Cancer
elevated risks in smokers

Cervical Cancer
smoking may increase risk of this disease in women

The health effects of smoking.

decades. Each year, doctors see 30,000 new cases of oral cancer in the United States.[6] Nearly a third of the nation's 10 million users are under age 21. One in five U.S. high school males uses spit tobacco.

Tobacco leaves are treated with molasses and other flavorings. A plug of the tobacco is placed between the lower lip and the gums, where it is sucked to release the nicotine. A dip of chewing tobacco contains two to three times more nicotine than a cigarette. An average-sized dip held in the mouth for 30 minutes is the equivalent of smoking four cigarettes. Someone who uses two cans of chewing tobacco a week

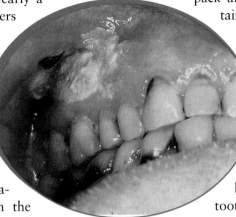

Oral cancer (white growth) and gum and teeth damage caused by smokeless tobacco.

gets as much nicotine as someone who smokes a pack and a half every day. It also contains cancer-causing nitrosamines at levels higher than foods may legally contain. Snuff is even more dangerous because powdered tobacco releases more of its chemicals in the mouth.

Smokeless tobacco causes oral cancer as well as a variety of mouth and gum diseases, including loss of taste, bad breath, gingivitis, pyorrhea, tooth loss, unusual wear on tooth surfaces, tooth decay, receding gums, damage to the jawbone, and leukoplakia (precancerous thick, rough, leathery, white patches on the tongue, gums, or inner cheek). One in five people who develop leukoplakia is eventually diagnosed with oral cancer. Smokeless tobacco also has been shown to increase blood pressure and to interfere with the body's ability to use the nutrients in food effectively.

If a person quits, the benefits start almost immediately, and 15 years after quitting smoking, the risk of death and disease will be no higher than if the person had never smoked at all (assuming the person is not already ill when quitting). The risk of dying of heart attack is cut in half after only 1 year of not smoking. Some think that nothing else a person can do for health can have such immediate, far-reaching dividends as quitting smoking.

ALCOHOL

Alcohol is the most widely used recreational drug in the United States. An estimated 70% of all Americans drink alcohol regularly.[7] Of those, 10% are heavy drinkers, and that 10% drinks more than half of all the alcohol consumed in the United States. Approximately 85% of America's college students drink alcoholic beverages and 25% abuse alcohol. Alcohol use becomes abuse when it interferes with family, work, school, or social life or when it involves any violation of the law (including drunk driving).

A problem of particular concern on America's college campuses is **binge drinking**. Binge drinkers use alcohol for the sole purpose of getting intoxicated.

Binge drinking Imbibing at least five alcoholic beverages in one sitting for men and four for women.

Healthy People 2000 Objectives For Tobacco Use

The U.S. Department of Health and Human Services has listed these goals for tobacco use in the United States by the year 2000:

- Reduce cigarette smoking to less than 15 percent of all adults (special target groups are blue-collar workers, adults who have not graduated from high school, military personnel, pregnant women and women of reproductive age, Blacks, Hispanics, Native Americans, Alaska natives, and southeast Asian men)

- Reduce cigarette smoking among children so less than 15 percent go on to smoke as adults

- Have at least half the adult smokers stop for at least one day a year

- Have at least 60 percent of women who smoke cigarettes stop while they are pregnant

- Expose no more than 20 percent of children aged 6 and under to cigarette smoke at home

- Have no more than 6 percent of males aged 12 to 24 use smokeless tobacco

- Establish all elementary, middle, and secondary schools as tobacco-free environments and include tobacco prevention in all curricula

- Establish smoke-free environments in 75 percent of the nation's workplaces

- Enact comprehensive clean indoor air acts that prohibit smoking in all 50 states

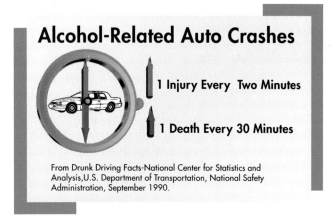

Alcohol-Related Auto Crashes

1 Injury Every Two Minutes

1 Death Every 30 Minutes

From Drunk Driving Facts-National Center for Statistics and Analysis, U.S. Department of Transportation, National Safety Administration, September 1990.

Alcohol is thought to be the cause of more than half of all fatal automobile accidents in the United States.[8] Someone is injured every minute, and someone dies every 23 minutes from an alcohol-related accident. One in every two of us is projected to be involved in an alcohol-related accident at some time in our lives. Our entire society suffers the consequences of alcohol abuse in terms of crimes, medical expenses, and emotional health. Figure 13.4 graphically shows the role of alcohol in many societal problems.

Alcohol poses a tough dilemma. It is socially acceptable among many people who use alcohol to celebrate a victory, ease tension in a difficult situation, bring on relaxation after a hard day, or even inspire a little romance. Almost half of all sixth-graders have tried wine coolers, yet only a fifth of those surveyed knew that wine coolers contained alcohol. And even though the legal drinking age is 21 in all 50 states, more than 90% of all high school seniors drink at least some alcohol; more than a third reported having 5 or more drinks in one sitting during the previous 2 weeks, and 4% drink every day.

People drink for many reasons, but what has fascinated researchers are the reasons people are able to avoid having problems with alcohol. According to

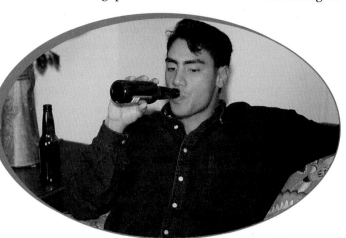

About 84% of college students are drinkers.

the National Institute on Alcohol Abuse and Alcoholism, a lot depends on how they were exposed to alcohol as they grew up. You're least likely to have a problem with alcohol if your parents had responsible drinking habits and the following attitudes:

■ Alcohol is a food and should be used in small quantities at mealtimes.

FIGURE 13.4

Societal Costs of Alcohol Abuse

Percent Alcohol-related

	Percent
On-the-job accidents	75
Drowning	70
Murders	60
Suicide	55
Highway fatalities	50
Rape	50
Child Abuse	49
Pedestrian fatalities	40

Percent of common problems that are related to alcohol.

Teens and Alcohol

■ 88% of American kids between ages 16 and 18 say that alcohol is a critical problem in their schools.

■ 78% of older teens say alcohol is always available at the parties they attend.

■ First use of alcohol typically begins at about age 13.

■ Up to two-thirds of teen and collegiate sexual assault and date rape cases are linked to alcohol.

- Alcohol is a beverage; it is not the focus of a group activity.

- Drinking doesn't prove you're more grown up or "more of a man."

- Getting drunk is not acceptable.

- No one has to drink. Abstinence is a legitimate choice.

An obvious problem associated with drinking is intoxication. The "morning after" usually is marred by fatigue, weakness, nausea, vomiting, dehydration, extreme sensitivity to light and sound, severe headache, bloodshot eyes, and the inability to remember part or all of what went on while you were drunk.

Health Risks

Long-term risks associated with alcohol, depicted in Figure 13.5, include:

- Permanent damage to brain cells and small brain size. Alcohol abuse can cause Korsakoff's syndrome (loss of memory, psychosis, learning loss, and degeneration of brain matter) and Wernicke's syndrome (visual impairment and confusion).

- Nerve damage and interference with neurotransmitters, causing loss of sensation.

- Damage to muscle fibers.

- Alcoholic cardiomyopathy (degeneration of the heart muscle).

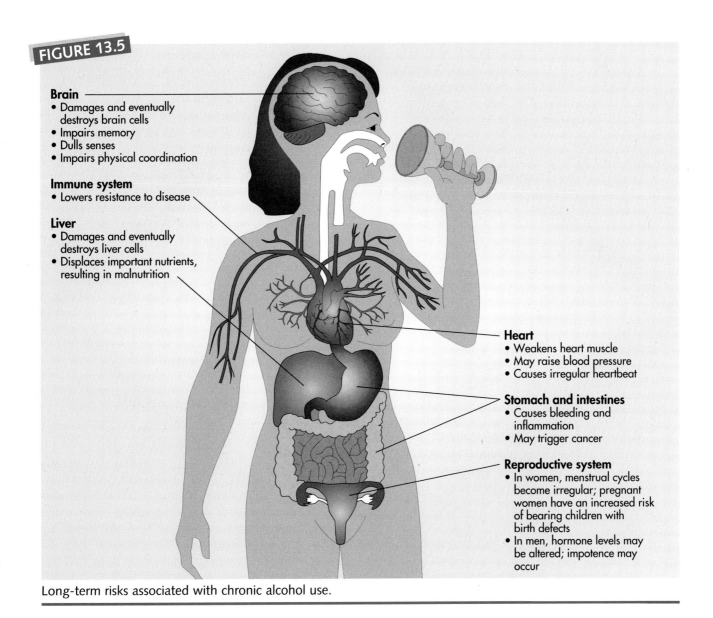

FIGURE 13.5

Brain
- Damages and eventually destroys brain cells
- Impairs memory
- Dulls senses
- Impairs physical coordination

Immune system
- Lowers resistance to disease

Liver
- Damages and eventually destroys liver cells
- Displaces important nutrients, resulting in malnutrition

Heart
- Weakens heart muscle
- May raise blood pressure
- Causes irregular heartbeat

Stomach and intestines
- Causes bleeding and inflammation
- May trigger cancer

Reproductive system
- In women, menstrual cycles become irregular; pregnant women have an increased risk of bearing children with birth defects
- In men, hormone levels may be altered; impotence may occur

Long-term risks associated with chronic alcohol use.

- High blood pressure, heart attack, damage to coronary arteries, irregular heartbeat, disruption of blood flow to the heart, and angina (chest pain, usually on exertion). Though the National Heart, Lung, and Blood Institute suggests that moderate alcohol consumption can reduce the risk of heart disease, you should not use alcohol as a preventive for heart disease as alcohol use has too many other harmful effects.

- Anemia.

- Greater risk for pneumonia, emphysema, tuberculosis, and other lung diseases.

Healthy People 2000 Objectives For Alcohol Use

The U.S. Department of Health and Human Services has the following goals for the year 2000:

- Reduce deaths from alcohol-related motor vehicle accidents to 8.5 per 100,000 people.

- Reduce deaths from cirrhosis to no more than six per 100,000 people.

- Have less than 28% of high school seniors and less than 32% of college students engage in episodes of heavy drinking.

- Reduce average annual alcohol consumption to less than 2 gallons of alcohol per adult (it's 2.5 gallons now).

- Establish alcohol and drug treatment programs for traditionally underserved people in all 50 states.

- Establish drug and alcohol policies in at least 60% of the workplaces with 50 or more employees.

- Establish effective driver's license suspension or revocation laws in all 50 states for people caught driving under the influence of alcohol or drugs.

- Establish laws that more effectively limit access to alcohol by minors in all 50 states.

- Restrict promotion of alcoholic beverages to young audiences in at least 20 states.

- Establish laws in all 50 states that reduce legal blood alcohol concentration to .04% in adults and .00% in those younger than 21.

- Establish routine drug/alcohol screening and referrals for treatment among at least 75% of the nation's primary health care providers.

- Cirrhosis of the liver, cancer of the liver, fibrosis of the liver (in which the liver begins to fill with scar tissue), or chronic enlargement of the liver.

- Breast cancer. Women who drink between three and nine drinks a week have a 30% increased risk for breast cancer. Women who have three drinks a day run a 100% higher risk.

- Cancer of the mouth, tongue, pharynx, esophagus, stomach, and intestines.

- Esophageal varices (varicose veins in the esophagus; death can come rapidly if the varices rupture).

- More risk for peptic ulcers or bleeding of the stomach lining from irritation.

- Inflammation of the pancreas or interference with its ability to produce insulin.

- Malnutrition (because the small intestine may be unable to absorb nutrients).

- Less immunity and ability to fight infection.

- Increased risk for all cancer, especially cancer of the liver, esophagus, stomach, mouth, and tongue. Men who have only one drink a day increase their cancer risk by 23%; with two drinks a day, the risk jumps to 123%.

- Damage to the gastrointestinal system, including chronic stomach irritation, chronic inflammation of the pancreas, chronic diarrhea, and inflammation of the esophagus. Alcohol also interferes with the absorption of nutrients in the small intestine. Alcohol interferes particularly with the absorption of calcium, increasing the risk for osteoporosis.

Fetal Alcohol Syndrome

Women who drink throughout pregnancy run the risk of giving birth to a baby with **fetal alcohol syndrome (FAS)**, the second leading cause of mental retardation in the United States and the third most common birth defect. An estimated 2.7 in 1,000 babies born in the United States has FAS.[9] Three to four times that number have fetal alcohol effects (FAE), which occurs when babies are exposed to alcohol in the womb but do not have the classic signs of fetal alcohol syndrome. Some experts now think even a few drinks during the entire term of a pregnancy or one episode of heavy drinking can be harmful to the fetus.

Tests show the blood alcohol content is much higher in the fetus than in the mother who drank the alcohol. The greatest harm probably is done during the first 3 months of pregnancy, when the fetus is most susceptible, but alcohol at any time during fetal development can cause damage. Generally, drinking during the first trimester damages organ development; during the last trimester, it damages development of the central nervous system.

FAS is characterized by low birthweight, small head size, mental retardation, poor motor development, long-term developmental disabilities, and a distinctive set of facial malformations (short eye openings, low nasal bridge, thin upper lip, and absence of a groove above the upper lip).

MARIJUANA

After a period of decline beginning in the late 1970s, marijuana use by teens is rising dramatically.[10] Made from the dried, crushed leaves and flowers of the *cannabis sativa* plant, marijuana — which looks a lot like tobacco — most often is rolled into papers and smoked like cigarettes. Some users pack it firmly into a pipe or smoke it through a water pipe. Less often, it is brewed into tea or baked in brownies. Although marijuana is a chemically complex plant, with more than 400 identified substances, the one that has made marijuana popular is its chief psychoactive agent, **THC** (delta-9-tetrahydrocannabinol).

The flowering top of Cannabis sativa.

The marijuana that today's college students smoke is much more potent than what earlier generations smoked. It is estimated that the plants cultivated today have three times the amount of THC as those cultivated just 10 years ago.

Marijuana is fat-soluble, stored in the fatty tissues of the brain, body, and reproductive organs. The immediate effects of marijuana intoxication are felt within 10 to 30 minutes and usually last several hours, and marijuana actually stays in the system as long as a month. The body has difficulty completely eliminating the marijuana, and the effects are cumulative, building up over time. What this means is that if you smoke a joint every weekend, which may not seem all that bad, your body is constantly permeated with the drug.

Marijuana has been on a roller coaster as far as the media are concerned. Publicity has ranged from virtual scare tactics about the monstrous effects of the drug to a casual attitude that marijuana is not that bad. The truth lies somewhere in between. Immediate effects are bloodshot eyes, dry mouth and throat, coughing, mild muscular weakness, and lowered blood pressure. As far as researchers can tell, marijuana use has the following risks and long-term effects:

- Inhibited brain and motor functions.
- Changes in cell membranes, especially those in the brain and reproductive tracts, interfering with cells' ability to absorb energy.
- Interference with immunity, compromising the ability to fight infection.
- Faster heart rate and heightened blood pressure, leading to long-term cardiac damage (this is a problem particularly for people who already have arteriosclerosis, angina, or some other heart disease).
- Lung damage as much as four times that caused by cigarette smoking and the same amount of tobacco smoke. Marijuana is higher in tars and contains more carcinogens.
- Impaired oxygen and carbon dioxide exchange in the lungs.
- Depressed sex drive and impotence.
- Impaired male fertility because of lowered sperm count, reducing sperm motility (movement) and damaging sperm (causing irregularly shaped sperm).
- Reduced female fertility by inhibiting ovulation.
- Birth defects in babies born to mothers who smoke it during pregnancy (especially low birthweight, prematurity, and congenital deformities similar to those of fetal alcohol syndrome).

Fetal alcohol syndrome   A set of mental and physical characteristics in a newborn caused by moderate to heavy alcohol drinking during pregnancy.

THC   The psychoactive ingredient in marijuana.

Inconclusive research indicates that marijuana may cause breaks in both the ova and the sperm, resulting in birth defects.

Perhaps one of the most serious risks from marijuana use is its status as a gateway drug. Those who use marijuana regularly are much more likely to try other, more dangerous drugs, such as cocaine.

> *Perhaps one of the most serious risks from marijuana use is its status as a gateway drug.*

COCAINE

Also commonly known as "coke" and "snow," cocaine is a crystalline powder extracted from the leaves of the coca plant grown in Central and South America. Cocaine is not related to cocoa plants. It probably is the most powerfully addictive of any of the illicit drugs and can be injected, smoked (**freebasing**), or inhaled through the nose. Figure 13.6 shows the forms of cocaine. It acts as both a powerful local anesthetic and a central nervous system stimulant. In fact, mixtures of novocaine and caffeine have been sold on the street as cocaine. Cocaine use has been generally declining. Figure 13.7 shows the trends in cocaine use.

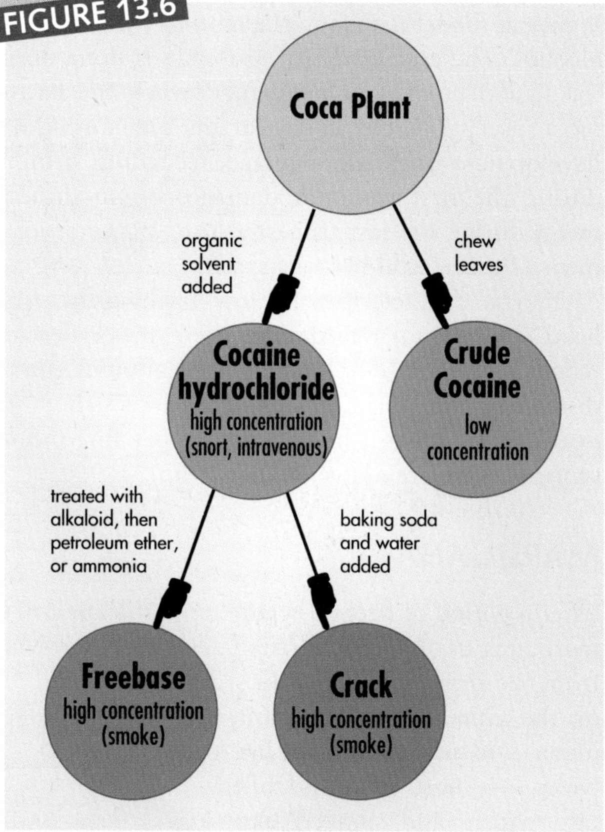

The effects of cocaine can be immediate and devastating. Cocaine that is snorted reaches the brain within 3 minutes; when smoked or injected, it reaches the brain within seconds. Powdered cocaine that is snorted can destroy the sense of smell, damage the mucous membranes and destroy the septum of the nose, and cause sinusitis. Smoking cocaine causes lung and liver damage, weight loss, and an increase in blood pressure and heart rate. Injecting cocaine can damage the linings of the arteries, damage the heart, and cause skin infections. More than 200,000 drugs were involved in cases admitted to hospital emergency rooms during a recent year. Of those cases, 26% involved cocaine.[11] Cocaine has been

FIGURE 13.6

Forms of cocaine.

Powdered cocaine.

known to cause sudden death. In a well-known case, Boston Celtics star Len Bias collapsed and died from cocaine shortly after being signed to the team.

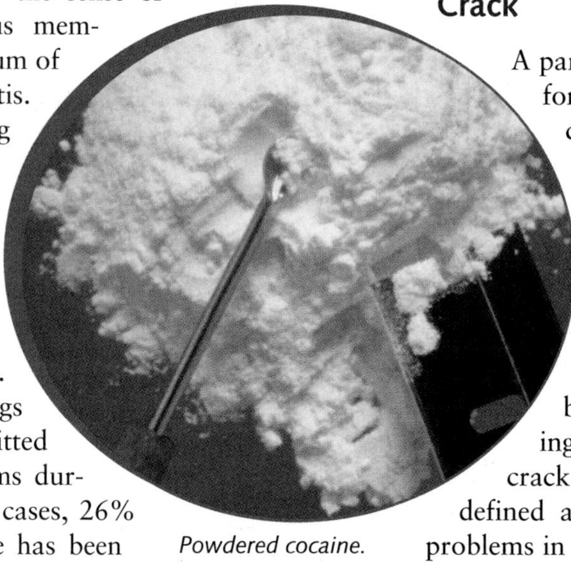

Crack

A particularly dangerous and addictive form of cocaine is **crack**, which derives its name from a popping or crackling sound that happens when it is smoked. Crack is manufactured by mixing cocaine with ammonia, baking soda, and water, then heating it until the hydrochloride evaporates. Crack cocaine reaches the brain within 4 to 6 seconds, creating intense euphoria. Addiction to crack is so powerful that it has been defined as one of the most serious drug problems in the country.

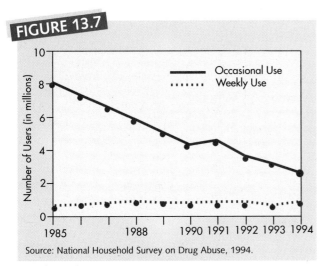

Number of new cocaine users per year.

Health Effects

Health effects of cocaine include the following:

- Rapid increase in heart rate and blood pressure (can cause strokes or bleeding in the brain, even in young, healthy people).
- Increased breathing rate.
- Heart and respiratory failure, including fluid buildup in the lungs.
- Raised body temperature.
- Lowered immune system response.
- Damaged upper respiratory system (if inhaled).
- Less appetite (can lead to malnutrition).
- Liver damage.
- Impotence.
- "Cocaine psychosis," characterized by paranoia, delusions, and violence.

Babies born to cocaine users have incurred significant developmental problems before birth. Cocaine crosses the placenta, exposing the fetus to the drug. In addition, fluctuations in the mother's blood pressure cause blood vessels in the baby's brain to deteriorate, eventually resulting in strokes. Babies who are born cocaine-addicted have the following health effects.

- Signs of withdrawal at birth (including jitteriness, inability to sleep, irritability).

- Longlasting emotional and social problems — difficult to console and comfort, unable to relate and react to people in a normal way.
- Brain damage.
- Heart defects.
- Kidney damage.
- Possible malformed head, arms, fingers.
- Increased risk for sudden infant death syndrome (SIDS).

OTHER ADDICTIVE DRUGS AND CAUTIONS

Other drugs, legal and illegal, carry risk factors as well. The relative use of legal and illegal drugs in the United States is depicted in Figure 13.8. We will not delve into each of these in this book except to mention the **synergistic effect**. If you're taking any kind of medication — even over-the-counter drugs such as a cold medicine — you could get into serious trouble if you drink. Alcohol blocks the actions of some drugs and vastly increases the effects of many others, resulting in something similar to a severe overdose. We cannot list all the drugs here, but be especially cautious if you're taking:

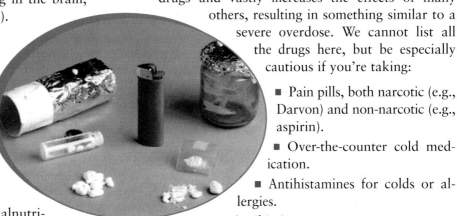

Two types of homemade crack pipes.

- Pain pills, both narcotic (e.g., Darvon) and non-narcotic (e.g., aspirin).
- Over-the-counter cold medication.
- Antihistamines for colds or allergies.
- Antibiotics.
- Sleeping pills.
- Diet pills.
- Tranquilizers.
- Medication for depression.

Freebasing Smoking cocaine that has been separated from its hydrochloric salt by mixing it with a volatile chemical.

Crack A particularly dangerous and addictive form of cocaine manufactured by mixing cocaine with ammonia, baking soda, and water, then heating it to evaporate the hydrochloride.

Synergistic effect A phenomenon in which the effects of using more than one drug simultaneously are different and greater than using any of the drugs alone.

Natural Versus Unnatural Highs

In contrast to natural and healthy highs, unnatural highs result from self-imposed attempts to escape; upon returning to normal functioning, an increasing disappointment with normal day-to-day living occurs. The heaviest impact in being involved in unnatural highs, however, is on relationships.

The most basic relationship that any of us have as adults is with ourselves. Father John Powell has discussed a three-step process toward maturity that begins with our relationship with ourselves. The three steps in this process generally occur in the following order to ensure integrated growth toward maturity:

- Accept yourself.
- Be yourself.
- Forget yourself.

These steps can be viewed as part of an upward-pointing spiral with gradually widening cycles representing growth as we continue to more fully accept ourselves, learn to truly be ourselves, and forget ourselves in the service of others. This, in turn, allows us to accept ourselves more deeply and continue with the cycle. Natural highs can occur at any point in the cycle and provide support and encouragement to continue the growth.

Let's briefly examine the destructive nature of chemical dependency as it relates to this process of growth. Carl Jung once described alcoholism to Alcoholics Anonymous founder, Bill Wilson, as "a spiritual disease which has at its base a drive for wholeness. . . ." Chemical dependency might be understood as an attempt to be happy with who we are, to feel whole and complete, and to accept ourselves.

The first use of chemicals for most people occurs as part of an attempt to be accepted. Once individuals accept themselves as okay just the way they are, they are more capable of truly being themselves in their own uniqueness.

Harry Guntrip has described mental health as the capacity to live life to the fullest in ways that enable us to realize our own natural potentialities and that unite us with, rather than divide us from, all the human beings who make up our world. He has said, "Nothing is more sad than to see a human being facing his basic withdrawnness, and complaining with a terrible sense of frustration that he cannot express himself, cannot get in touch with other people, and cannot love." Father Joseph Martin, well known for his films and lectures on chemical dependency, states, "An alcoholic is a creature who is cut off from the very purpose for which he was created to love and to be loved" (from his video presentation, "Alcoholism and the Family").

Chemical highs give people a superficial sense of acceptance in such a way as to not allow true self-acceptance to take place. In consequence, there is no foundation for truly being oneself and developing one's own talents. In fact, the process is hindered through decreased mental and physical capacity and an increased narrowing of interests. As chemical dependency progresses unchecked, it eventually will cause huge losses in all areas of life — and eventually the loss of life itself.

An AA poem clearly illustrates the destructive nature of the misguided, however well-intentioned, use of alcohol and other drugs.

We drank for happiness
and became unhappy.
We drank for joy
and became miserable.
We drank for sociability
and became argumentative.
We drank for friendship
and made enemies.
We drank for sleep
and awakened without rest.
We drank for strength
and felt weak.
We drank "medicinally"
and acquired health problems.
We drank for relaxation
and got the shakes.
We drank for bravery
and became afraid.
We drank to make conversation easier
and slurred our speech.
We drank to feel heavenly
and ended up feeling like hell.
We drank to forget
and were forever haunted.
We drank for freedom
and became slaves.
We drank to erase problems
and saw them multiply.
We drank to cope with life
and invited death.

Viktor Frankl has described happiness as an experience that cannot be sought directly but can come only as a byproduct of serving others.

Chemical dependency treatment assists individuals to begin to experience growth and satisfaction by replacing unhealthy dependence on chemicals with healthy and more mature understanding and appreciation of the interdependence among themselves, others, and a higher power. Through abstinence, and involving themselves in the process of accepting themselves, being themselves, and forgetting themselves, natural highs begin to occur. Thoreau stated it beautifully: "Sometimes we are clarified and calmed healthily, as we never were before in our lives, not by an opiate, but by some unconscious obedience to the all-just laws, so that we become like a still lake of purest crystal, and without an effort our depths are revealed to ourselves. All the world goes by and is reflected in our deeps."

From *Professional Counselor*, December 1993.

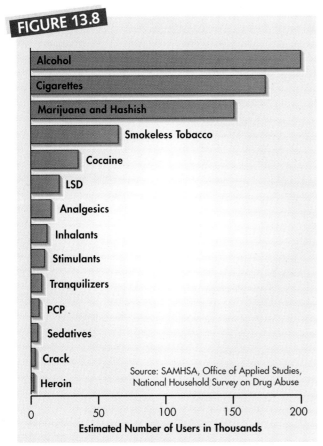

FIGURE 13.8

Estimated Number of Users in Thousands

Source: SAMHSA, Office of Applied Studies, National Household Survey on Drug Abuse

Estimated numbers of lifetime users of illicit drugs, alcohol, and tobacco in the United States population, aged 12 and older: 1995.

Alcohol also can have serious, even fatal, consequences if you drink while you're taking the medications commonly prescribed for high blood pressure, water retention, epilepsy, diabetes, hemophilia, or heart disease. To be safe, it's best to abstain from alcohol completely. If you don't, talk to your doctor or pharmacist about possible drug-alcohol interactions *before* you have a drink.

MANAGING ADDICTIVE BEHAVIOR

When attempting to manage addictive behavior, people go through five basic steps.[12]

1. *Precontemplation*, in which people have no intention of making a change in the near future. Although others are aware of the problem, addicted people may not see that they have a problem. People in this stage who agree to therapy or a treatment program usually do so because they are being pressured (by family members, an employer, the court). While pressure is on, they appear to be changing. As soon as the pressure is off, they return to their old behaviors.

 For the fourth consecutive year, drug arrests in 1995 increased dramatically on U.S. college campuses.

— *Chronicle of Higher Education*

2. *Contemplation*, in which people realize they have a problem and are thinking seriously about trying to change but have not yet made a commitment to change. People in this stage know where they want to go, but they aren't quite ready to go there yet. Typically, people in this stage struggle: they want to overcome the addiction, but they are put off by the amount of time and effort it will require. People usually stay at this stage for a long time, an average of 2 years or so. Many people who try to change addictive behavior stay in the contemplation stage and never actually make the change.

The Return of Heroin

Heroin, the scourge of the 1960s and the 1970s, has returned. The drug is so prevalent, potent, and cheap that it has expanded from the streets and underground to the middle class. The Drug Enforcement Agency says about 600,000 hard-core heroin addicts are now living in the USA. The number of individuals treated for heroin addiction at the Betty Ford Center in California doubled in 1997.

Estimated number of people in the USA age 12 and older who have used heroin:

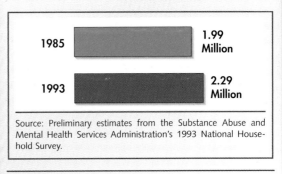

| 1985 | 1.99 Million |
| 1993 | 2.29 Million |

Source: Preliminary estimates from the Substance Abuse and Mental Health Services Administration's 1993 National Household Survey.

Source: "Heroin Returns as an Upscale Drug of Choice," by Karen Thomas, USA Today.

How Different Drugs Affect the Body

	Alcohol	Amphetamines ("Speed," "Bennies," "Black Beauties," "Uppers")	Cocaine ("Crack")	LSD (and other hallucinogens)
Type of Drug (Chemical)	■ *ethyl alcohol* (ethanol), a clear liquid (in beer, wine, spirits); ■ made from gain, fruit, vegetables or synthetically ■ favored for its relaxing, intoxicating properties since antiquity ■ beers contain about 5% alcohol, wines to 12% and spirits about 40% (about 13.6 g per drink) ■ a sedative-hypnotic and central nervous system (CNS) depressant	■ synthetically produced: *amphetamine* (Speed), *dextroamphetamine* (Dexedrine), *methylamphetamine* or "Ice," *methylphenidate* (Ritalin), etc. ■ used as pills, inhaled or injected (Speed) ■ CNS stimulants that resemble action of adrenaline (natural body hormone)	■ derived from South American coca bush (still chewed in Andes to offset fatigue) ■ crack is mixture of cocaine and baking soda • *cocaine hydrochloride* is white powder ("coke," "C," "flake," "snow") ■ formerly used in many medicines (until 1920) ■ stimulant action — like amphetamine, but now legally classed as a narcotic	■ derived from mushrooms (*psilocybin*) or cactus (*mescaline*) or synthetically — e.g., *lysergic acid* (LSD) or "acid" and *phencyclidine* (PCP) — "hog," "angel dust" ■ structures resemble *catecholamines* — normal brain neurotransmitters ■ hallucinogens can distort reality and produce severe delusions
Short Term Effects (after a single dose)	■ effects vary with size, sex, and amount of food in stomach; ■ initial relaxation and loss of inhibitions ■ increased sociability ■ impaired coordination ■ slowing down of reflexes and mental processes ■ attitude changes, increased risk-taking and bad judgment/danger in driving car, operating machinery ■ sleepiness	■ nervous system briefly stimulated ■ reduces appetite ■ increases energy, offsets fatigue ■ talkative restlessness, greater alertness ■ faster breathing ■ rise in heart rate and blood pressure (with risk of burst blood vessels and heart failure) ■ temperature raised, mouth dry, skin sweaty ■ pupils dilated ■ alleviates nose-stuffiness (original medicinal use)	■ short-acting, powerful CNS stimulant, also a local anesthetic ■ effects vary depending whether drug is "snorted" (inhaled), injected, put in mouth, rectum or vagina, or smoked (as crack) ■ transient euphoria and increased energy ■ appetite-loss ■ rise in heart-rate and breathing ■ dilated pupils ■ agitated, restless talkativeness ■ brief rise in sex drive	■ unpredictable effects — at first like amphetamine ■ excitation, arousal ■ temperature raised ■ altered sense of smell, shape, size, color, distance ■ exhilaration, "mind-expansion" or anxiety — depending on user ■ rapid pulse, dilated pupils, blank stare ■ exaggerated power sense with possibly violent behavior ■ later — dramatic perceptual distortions ■ occasionally convulsions
With Larger Doses and Longer Use	■ blackouts (memory loss) ■ facial flushing; slurred speech ■ staggering gait, stupor ■ rise in blood pressure ■ pancreatitis, hepatitis, stomach ulcers, injuries (broken bones) ■ effects magnified by other depressants (e.g., opiates, barbiturates, tranquilizers, antihistamines, sleep aids, cold remedies) ■ alone or combined with other drugs can increase accident rates ■ overdose may be fatal, from respiratory distress	■ bizarre behavior, talkativeness, restlessness, tremors, excitability ■ sense of power, superiority, aggression ■ illusions and hallucinations ■ some users become paranoid, suspicious, panicky, violent ■ raised blood pressure ■ insomnia	■ permanently stuffy nose (if snorted) and risk of perforated nasal septum ■ brief euphoric effect followed by "crash" — depression ■ anesthetic effect can depress brain function ■ bizarre, erratic, perhaps violent actions ■ paranoid "psychosis" (disappears if drug is discontinued) ■ sensation of "crawling under the skin" ■ convulsions, disturbed heart action, even death	■ anxiety, panic attacks, paranoid delusions, occasionally psychosis (like schizophrenia) ■ injury or accidents due to drug-induced delusions or distance misjudgment ■ increased risk of fetal abnormalities ■ tolerance develops rapidly but also disappears fast with renewed drug sensitivity ■ with PCP, high fever, muscle spasm, erratic behavior, psychosis lasting weeks or more
Long-Term Effects (prolonged repeated use)	■ harms many body organs: pancreas, GI tract, blood circulation, heart, liver, kidney, brain ■ may produce liver cirrhosis, ulcers, memory loss, impotence ■ increased risk of cancers (mouth, larynx, throat, maybe breast) ■ vitamin depletion ■ damages offspring ■ dependence frequent	■ malnutrition, emaciation (owing to appetite loss) ■ anxiety states ■ "amphetamine-psychosis" (with schizophrenia-like hallucinations) ■ kidney damage ■ susceptibility to infection ■ sleep disorders • *psychological* dependence	■ weight loss, malnutrition ■ destroyed nose tissues (if sniffed) ■ restlessness, mood swings, insomnia, *extreme* excitability, suspiciousness/paranoia, delusions ("psychosis") ■ depression ■ impotence ■ risk of heart attacks ■ strong *psychological* dependence	■ long-term medical effects not known ■ may include muscle tenseness, "flashbacks" — brief, spontaneous recurrence of prior LSD (hallucinogenic) experiences ■ prolonged, profound depression ■ panic attacks ■ no *physical* dependence
Withdrawal Symptoms	■ insomnia, headache ■ nausea ■ shakiness, tremors ■ sweating, seizures	■ long sleep, chills ■ ravenous hunger ■ depression	■ little or no withdrawal sickness; sleepiness ■ extreme exhaustion ■ possibly "cocaine blues" (depression)	■ few withdrawal effects, possible "flashbacks," anxiety

Adapted from *Health News*, May 1990.

Nicotine	Caffeine	Cannabis (marijuana, "pot," "grass," hashish)	Narcotic (Opioid) analgesics (painkillers)	Solvents (Inhalants)
▪ derived from tobacco ▪ used medicinally in South America ▪ tobacco smoke contains 4,000 chemicals but nicotine is the most addictive ▪ a typical Canadian cigarette contains one mg nicotine but amount absorbed varies with smoker ▪ stimulates central nervous system	▪ derived from tea, coffee beans, kola nuts, chocolate ▪ used in many medicines (e.g., with painkillers, cold/cough, pain remedies, antihistamines) ▪ average cup of coffee contains 60-75 mg caffeine, colas about 35 mg (per 250 ml) ▪ CNS stimulant	▪ derived from *cannabis sativa* or hemp plant; preparations vary in potency; "hash" most potent, marijuana least ▪ smoked in "joints" or chewed (sometimes with food) ▪ medicinally used for epilepsy, glaucoma, against nausea ▪ classed as hallucinogen	▪ poppy derivatives (opium, codeine, morphine, heroin) and synthetics (Demerol, Methadone, Dilaudid, Percodan) ▪ smoked, eaten, or injected ▪ ancient painkillers used medicinally ▪ deaden pain, produce euphoria and drowsiness	▪ volatile organic hydro-carbons from petroleum and natural gas (e.g., gasoline, toluene, hexane, chloroform, carbon tetrachloride, nail polish remover or acetone, lighter fluid, paint thinners, cleaning fluid, airplane cement, plastic glue) ▪ hallucinogenic effects
▪ speeds pulse ▪ stimulates, then reduces brain and nervous system activity ▪ blood pressure rises ▪ sense of relaxation ▪ reduced urine output ▪ impairs cleansing action of lung's cilia (hairs) ▪ greater alertness and concentration abilities (claimed)	▪ stimulates brain, speeds nerve-cell transmission ▪ elevates mood and alertness ▪ stimulates mental activity ▪ speeds up breathing, metabolism ▪ enhances mental performance ▪ postpones fatigue ▪ shortens sleep ▪ more urine output ▪ rise in blood fats ▪ increases stomach acidity ▪ decreases appetite	▪ produces dreamlike euphoria, laughter, relaxation ▪ alters sense of space, time ▪ increases heart rate ▪ reddens eyes ▪ dreamy, "stoned" look ▪ at later stages, users are quiet, reflective, sleepy ▪ combined with alcohol, increased effects, distorted behavior ▪ impairs short-term memory, thinking, and ability to drive car or perform complex tasks	▪ briefly stimulate, then de-press higher brain centers ▪ give quick pleasure surge (for few minutes) then stupor (which mutes hunger, pain, sex-drive) ▪ taken by mouth, effects slower, no initial pleasure surge ▪ pupils tiny, body warm, limbs heavy ▪ mouth dry, skin itchy ▪ users may "nod" off, alternately awake or asleep, oblivious to surroundings	▪ exhilaration, light-headed-ness, excitability, disorientation ▪ confusion, slurred speech, dizziness ▪ distorted perception ▪ visual and auditory hallucinations ▪ muscular control impaired ▪ possible nausea, increased saliva, sneezing ▪ reflexes dampened ▪ recklessness, feelings of power, invincibility
▪ lung damage ▪ damaged blood circulation ▪ slowed wound-healing ▪ vitamin C depletion ▪ shortness of breath ▪ more upper respiratory infections ▪ cancer-formation risks	▪ nervousness, hand tremors ▪ delayed sleep onset, reduces "depth" of sleep, insomnia ▪ abnormally rapid heartbeat ▪ jitteriness ▪ mild delirium possible ▪ convulsions (rare) ▪ suspected cancer-causing agent	▪ slowed digestive (gastrointestinal) activity ▪ time misjudgment ▪ sharpened or distorted sense of color, sound ▪ thinking slow and confused ▪ apathy, loss of motivation/drive ▪ large doses can produce severe confusion, panic attacks ▪ hallucinations (even psychosis)	▪ extremities heavy ▪ permanent drowsiness ▪ pupils become pinpoints ▪ skin cold, moist, bluish ▪ progressively slower breathing ▪ depressed breathing ▪ *supervised pain-killing doses* let people remain quite clear-headed and safe ▪ dangers increase with alcohol intake	▪ drowsiness and possible unconsciousness ▪ severe disorientation ▪ risks increase with fume concentration ▪ irregular heartbeat, heart action disturbed ▪ large doses may cause heart failure — e.g., "sudden sniffing death" (especially with spot removers or airplane cement)
▪ narrowed blood vessels, risk of heart attack, stroke ▪ bronchitis, emphysema ▪ raised risk of cancers of mouth, lung, larynx, throat, bladder, pancreas, possibly cervix ▪ stomach ulcers ▪ impairs fetal growth ▪ strong dependence	▪ raised blood cholesterol level ▪ risk of stomach ulcers ▪ suspected cancer-inducing agent ▪ *possible* damage to unborn baby ▪ regular coffee use (more than 5 cups daily) can lead to dependence (getting "hooked" on drug)	▪ loss of drive, reduced energy ▪ regular heavy use increases risk of — bronchitis, lung cancer — reduced sex hormones — impaired learning — memory loss — possible decrease in immunity ▪ *psychological* dependence	▪ constipation ▪ moodiness ▪ risk of endocarditis (heart infection) and other infections (AIDS) from needle-sharing ▪ hormone upsets (menstrual irregularities) ▪ liver damage ▪ damaged offspring ▪ strong dependence	▪ pallor, thirst, nose, eye, mouth sores ▪ irritability, hostility, forget-fulness ▪ may damage liver, kidney and brain ▪ nosebleeds, impaired blood cell formation ▪ depression, weight-loss ▪ other drugs compound damage ▪ dependence possible
▪ anxiety, jitteriness ▪ inability to concentrate ▪ increased appetite	▪ severe headache ▪ irritability ▪ tiredness	▪ withdrawal symptoms mild — possible nausea, insomnia, anxiety, irritability	▪ striking withdrawal effects (4-5 hours after last dose), sweating, anxiety, diarrhea, "gooseflesh," shivering, tremors	▪ restlessness, anxiety, irri-tability, headaches ▪ stomach upsets ▪ delirium (rare)

3. *Preparation*, in which people intend to change and actually make small progress toward change. This is the stage in which people make a firm decision to change. For example, a person who decides to quit smoking may prepare by cutting down from a pack a day to only five cigarettes a day.

4. *Action*, in which people actually make the changes necessary to overcome the addiction. This step is most visible and receives the greatest recognition from others. Action, however, does not imply that the behavior has actually *changed* — only that the person has *started* changing. A person who has decided to quit smoking is not taking action by cutting down to five low-nicotine cigarettes a day. That's preparation. The action stage means the person no longer smokes at all.

5. *Maintenance*, in which people work to prevent a relapse. Maintenance actually is a continuation of change. It may last a lifetime. A person is considered to be in the maintenance stage if he or she has maintained the behavior change for at least 6 months. If the change has been maintained for less than 6 months, the person is still in the action stage.

Most people are unsuccessful in changing addictive behavior on their first attempt. Relapse is the rule, not the exception. Relapse can cause people to feel embarrassed, guilty, and ashamed. Instead of picking up where they left off in the action stage, some revert to the precontemplative stage. Most go back to the contemplation or preparation stages and start again to make concrete plans.

How successful a person is in overcoming an addiction depends on which stage he or she is in when the change process begins.

General Suggestions

Five general suggestions can help a person committed to change:

1. *Watch yourself.* Changing an addiction requires you first to know what you're up against. Define your addiction and where it fits into your life. This requires some self-watching. Keep a "behavioral diary" a few weeks, recording the times you engage in the behavior, the circumstances surrounding it, and your emotions at the time.

2. *Manage yourself.* Study your diaries, looking for patterns. Does a specific time of day cause problems for you? Do your emotions play a critical role? Do certain activities cause you to indulge your addiction? Analyze what you've learned, and devise a plan.

Change the consequences of your behavior. If you indulge to relax, for example, your addiction provides *positive* reinforcement. Instead, decide to give up something you enjoy — watching a favorite television show, going out to eat with friends Friday night — for every time you relapse.

Visualize what you're going to be like (or look like) if your addiction continues. Using your imagination, get into some really vivid scenes. Now visualize how you'll look, feel, or be if you can conquer your addictive behavior.

3. *Face reality.* You can't play games your whole life. Eventually you'll have to face reality, expose yourself to temptation, and overcome it.

Start by going cold turkey. Completely avoid the addictive substance. After about a month, when you feel ready, start facing small temptations. As you face smaller ones successfully, you'll be ready for the larger ones. This kind of practice takes time. Go at it slowly, one step at a time. Keep reading your diaries and watching yourself, identifying the things that act as cues or signals, then figure out which are the most dangerous for you. Begin with the least dangerous, and expose yourself to it. Keep practicing until you've mastered that step, then move on.*

4. *Develop alternative pleasures.* You probably get some pleasure from your addiction — a feeling of euphoria, an escape from stress, or entertainment. Figure out what it is. Then figure out a new, positive way of getting the same thing. Make a list of positive things you can do that will bring you pleasure — reading a good book, roller blading with friends, taking a weekend trip. You will have an easier time breaking away from your addictive behavior if you have something pleasant to replace it with.

5. *Prevent relapse.* Realize you could fall back into your addictive behavior. Stay on guard. Plan ahead. If you know you'll be in a situation that will be difficult, develop some strategies. If you

---

*If your addiction involves drugs, alcohol, or any health- or life-threatening behavior, abstain completely; don't try to "condition" yourself.

can, avoid the people, places, and things that spell trouble for you. If you do slip, don't give up. See it as a temporary mistake, and stick to your plans for success.

Specific techniques and suggestions can help you overcome an addiction to tobacco and can help you establish responsible behavior when it comes to alcohol.

Overcoming Tobacco Addiction

To quit smoking is extremely difficult. A smoker not only must overcome the addiction to nicotine but also must break the habit of reaching for a cigarette at certain times. Further, nicotine withdrawal can be unpleasant, causing nausea, vomiting, restlessness, irritability, and an intense craving for tobacco.

No one method of quitting works for everyone. Your reasons for smoking and your habits are unique to you. So are your life circumstances. Some suggest that if you are severely depressed, going through a major life crisis, or having severe emotional problems, you should reduce the number of cigarettes you smoke instead of quitting completely until you are back on track. If you smoke two or more packs

Aids in Quitting Smoking

The Food and Drug Administration has approved a new nicotine spray, Nicotrol NS. This product is projected to be a big help to smokers in general, and specifically to *heavier* smokers.

Nicotine *gum* (available over-the-counter) and nicotine *patches* (available by prescription) have been on the market for several years.

The advantage of the spray over the gum and patch is that the nicotine hits the bloodstream faster. This means the spray provides more immediate relief from nicotine cravings. One squirt up each nostril equals 1 mg of nicotine.

Source: McNeil Consumer Products.

of cigarettes a day, you might do better by first trying to cut down the number of cigarettes you smoke, then gradually stopping the habit completely.

Some of the following techniques or suggestions may help in smoking cessation:

■ There are no safe cigarettes and no safe way to smoke. While you are quitting, though, choose a

Strategies for Dealing with Why You Smoke

	Why You Smoke	Substitutes
Stimulation	You smoke to keep from slowing down, for a lift, to pep you up.	Find something else to pep you up — a hobby, brisk walks, simple exercises
Handling	You like the ritual of smoking, to have something in your hands and mouth.	Pick something else to handle: coins, pen or pencil, "worry beads"; try doodling, or chew on paper straws or minted toothpicks.
Relaxation	You enjoy smoking; it's a reward, a time you feel good about yourself.	Consider the harm cigarettes cause you and the reward of quitting. Substitute social or physical activity; prove self-control and feel good about yourself.
Crutch	You smoke to deal with problems and negative feelings.	Prove to yourself smoking doesn't solve problems. Reduce tension other ways: Take deep breaths, call a friend, talk over feelings. Work on keeping your "cool."
Craving	You feel "hooked" and begin to think of the next cigarette before you put out present one. You're aware of the need to smoke.	Recognize that quitting will be difficult and prepare to "see it through." Plan to try to stop "cold turkey," abstaining completely. The day before quitting, smoke to the point of distaste.
Habit	You smoke automatically, often without realizing what you're doing.	Become aware of every cigarette you smoke and ask yourself why you're smoking and if you really want it. Wrap up your cigarettes or put them in a place difficult to access.

brand lower in tar and nicotine than the brand you use now, smoke fewer cigarettes each day, inhale less deeply, and put out the cigarette after you've smoked only half of it.

- Set a goal. Determine a date when you want to quit smoking. Start now to quit, and tell those around you about it.
- Use an aid such as nicotine gum or a nicotine patch, which is applied to the skin and delivers a continuous flow of nicotine to the body 24 hours a day. The patch is used in decreasing strengths for 8 to 12 weeks, gradually weaning the user from nicotine. Possible side effects include dry mouth, nervousness, insomnia, and skin irritation where the patch is applied.

- Use relaxation techniques to help you overcome the urge to smoke and also to counteract the physical withdrawal symptoms and inability to sleep.

Six-Step Smoking Cessation Approach

The following six-step plan has been developed as a guide to help you quit smoking. The total program should be completed in 4 weeks or less. Steps 1 through 4 should take no longer than 2 weeks. A maximum of 2 additional weeks are allowed for the rest of the program.

Step One. Decide positively that you want to quit. Prepare a list of the reasons you smoke and why you want to quit.

Step Two. Initiate a personal diet and exercise program. Exercise and lower body weight create more awareness of healthy living and increase motivation for giving up cigarettes.

Step Three. Decide on the approach you will use to stop smoking. You may quit cold turkey or gradually decrease the number of cigarettes you smoke daily. Many people have found that quitting cold turkey is the easiest way to do it. Although it may not work the first time, after several attempts all of a sudden smokers are able to overcome the habit without too much difficulty. Tapering off cigarettes can be done in several ways. You may start by eliminating cigarettes you do not necessarily need or switch to a brand lower in nicotine or tar every couple of days, or smoke less of each cigarette, or simply cut down the total number of cigarettes you smoke each day.

Step Four. Set the target date for quitting. In choosing the target date, a special date may add a little extra incentive. An upcoming birthday, anniversary, vacation, graduation, family reunion — all are examples of good dates to free yourself from smoking.

Step Five. Stock up on low-calorie foods — carrots, broccoli, cauliflower, celery, popcorn (butter-and salt-free), fruits, sunflower seeds (in the shell), sugarless gum, and plenty of water. Keep such food handy on the day you stop and the first few days following cessation. Replace this food for cigarettes when you want one.

Step Six. This is the day you will quit smoking. On this day and the first few days thereafter, do not keep cigarettes handy. Stay away from friends and events that trigger your desire to smoke. Drink large amounts of water and fruit juices, and eat low-calorie foods. Replace smoking time with new, positive substitutes that will make smoking difficult or impossible. When you desire a cigarette, take a few deep breaths and then occupy yourself by talking to someone else, washing your hands, brushing your teeth, eating a healthy snack, chewing on a straw, doing dishes, playing sports, going for a walk or bike ride, going swimming, and so on.

If you have been successful and stopped smoking, a lot of events can still trigger your urge to smoke. When confronted with such events, people rationalize and think, "One won't hurt." It will not work! Before you know it, you will be back to the regular nasty habit. Therefore, be prepared to take action in those situations. Find adequate substitutes for smoking. Remind yourself of how difficult it has been and how long it has taken you to get to this point. Keep in mind that it will only get easier rather than worse as time goes on.

From *Fitness & Wellness*, 2nd ed. Werner W. K. Hoeger and Sharon A. Hoeger. Englewood, CO: Morton Publishing Co., 1993. Used by permission.

- Switch progressively to brands of cigarettes that have less and less nicotine. As your body's demand for nicotine diminishes, it will be easier to stop smoking without suffering difficult withdrawal symptoms.

- Change your brand of cigarettes. Buy a brand that doesn't taste good to you.

- Each time you resist smoking, put aside the money you would have spent on that pack of cigarettes. Keep it in a separate account. When you've succeeded in quitting, take a trip, buy a new stereo, or use the money for something you've always wanted.

- As you quit, you'll struggle with common withdrawal symptoms, such as irritability, headaches, dry mouth, hunger, constipation, and trouble going to sleep. Anticipate these symptoms and compensate for them. Soak in a hot bath when you're feeling irritable or get a headache. Chew gum or sip fruit juice to moisten a dry mouth. To ease hunger, keep on hand plenty of low-fat, low-calorie snacks (such as raw fruits and vegetables or air-popped popcorn). Include plenty of fiber (such as whole-grain breads and cereals) in your diet to overcome irregularity.

- Have substitutes on hand for times you want a cigarette. Chew sugarless gum, eat raw carrot sticks, suck on hard candy, or nibble on sunflower seeds.

- Avoid situations, people, and routines that have made it easy for you to smoke. If you always smoke after you eat a meal, for example, finish with a piece of fresh fruit instead, then swish out your mouth with a great-tasting mouthwash.

PSA Support

One of the people using the airwaves to talk about the harmful effects of smoking is actor Jack Klugman, possibly best known for his TV role as Dr. Quincy. On the PSA, sponsored by the American Academy of Otolaryngology-Head and Neck Foundation, Klugman says, "The only really stupid thing I ever did in my life was to start smoking." Removal of one vocal cord saved his life but may have cost him his career. He now has a hoarse, strained voice that certainly isn't an asset. His message may be a motivator for others to begin thinking about quitting.

- Start a program of brisk exercise once a day.

- Many communities have smoking cessation programs and support groups. Consider joining a local group to get the support you need. Look in the yellow pages under "Smokers' Treatment," ask your physician to recommend a group, or call the local chapter of the American Cancer Society.

Overcoming Alcohol Addiction

Alcoholism is a complex problem that requires careful treatment by professionals. Support groups such as Alcoholics Anonymous also can be extremely helpful to people who are trying to combat alcoholism. If you think you may be alcoholic or have a serious drinking problem, see your physician.

If you do not have a drinking problem but want to make sure you use alcohol responsibly:

- Learn how much alcohol you can drink safely — how much you can enjoy without becoming impaired or intoxicated — then stick to that level. Set an actual number of drinks, and don't go over that number.

- Drink slowly. Enjoy what's going on instead of focusing on your drink. Alternate a drink with some plain mixer, soda, sparkling water, or fruit juice.

- Eat something whenever you drink. Alcohol is absorbed from the stomach more slowly if you've eaten something.

- If you're at a party, ask for a nonalcoholic beverage. Most people will be happy to provide sodas, juices, or sparkling water for those who don't want to drink.

- If you are hosting an activity, consider alcohol as a secondary aspect of the activity, not its focal point. Provide nonalcoholic alternatives for people to drink. Don't pressure people who resist alcohol, and establish firm rules about intoxication.

- If you drink any alcohol at all, *don't drive*. Ask a friend to drive you home, call a taxi, or arrange to spend the night where you are. Likewise, don't let someone else drive if that person has been drinking.

- If you are taking any kind of prescription or over-the-counter medication, do not drink alcohol.

- If you are pregnant or nursing, don't drink.

If you think you *may* have a drinking problem, here are some danger signs:

- You're preoccupied with alcohol. You think about it or plan it even when you're not drinking.
- You drink to escape your problems or relieve stress.
- You need a drink to help you go to sleep.
- You need a drink to help you get going in the morning.
- You get drunk often or stay drunk several days at a time.
- You sneak drinks or drink alone.
- You make excuses for why you drink.
- You hide the amount you drink from your mate, children, friends.
- You gulp your drinks.
- You have had blackouts, periods during which you can't remember what happened.
- You've had accidents frequently because of drinking.
- You've been ill a lot because of drinking.
- You've missed work or school because of drinking.
- You've had financial or legal problems because of drinking.
- Your personality or behavior changes after you drink.
- Once you sober up, you regret the things you did while you were drinking.
- Other people tell you that you drink too much.
- You feel guilty about your drinking.
- You've tried to stop drinking but can't.
- You don't want to talk about the negative effects of drinking.

Overcoming Drug Addiction

As with alcohol abuse, professional help usually is needed in overcoming addiction to drugs. If you think you may have a drug problem and want to quit, the following tips may be helpful.

1. Pre-understanding (thinking of stopping)
   - Note feelings and circumstances that trigger a "trip" or binge (e.g., stress, hostility, anxiety, anger).
   - List noticeable problems associated with drug-taking at school, work, home, or in public

(such as less concentration, memory lapses, reduced performance, accidents, family disputes).

2. Understanding (recognizing the problem)
   - Admit possible health and other adverse effects (possibly already evident to others).

Conclusions of the Report of the U.S. Surgeon General on Short-Term Benefits of Smoking Cessation

- Among former smokers, the decline in risk of death compared with continuing smokers begins shortly after quitting and continues for at least 10 to 15 years.

- Smoking cessation halves the risks for cancers of the oral cavity and the esophagus, compared with continued smoking, as soon as 5 years after cessation, with further reduction over a longer period of abstinence.

- The risk of cervical cancer is substantially lower among former smokers in comparison with continuing smokers, even in the first few years after cessation.

- The excess risk of coronary heart disease (CHD) caused by smoking is reduced by about half after 1 year of smoking abstinence and then declines gradually.

- After smoking cessation, the risk of stroke returns to the level of never smokers; in some studies this has occurred within 5 years, but in others as long as 15 years of abstinence were required.

- For those without overt chronic obstructive pulmonary disease (COPD), smoking cessation improves pulmonary function about 5% within a few months after cessation.

- Pregnant smokers who stop smoking at any time up to the 30th week of gestation have infants with higher birth weight than do women who smoke throughout pregnancy. Quitting in the first 3 to 4 months of pregnancy and abstaining throughout the remainder of pregnancy protects the fetus from the adverse effects of smoking on birth weight.

- Smokers with gastric or duodenal ulcers who stop smoking improve their clinical course relative to smokers who continue to smoke.

- Make a drug diary — when, with whom, how, and in what circumstances drugs are taken. When added up, the amount consumed may come as a surprise!

- Devise a balance sheet of pros and cons of drug-taking (pleasures/rewards versus negative effects).

- Determine whether drug consumption is damaging your health already (often motivates a serious attempt to quit).

- Decide that no one else is to blame. The drug-taking is your own decision and can be beaten by your own efforts.

- Ask your family doctor or other expert for advice. Medical caregivers often will explain the risks posed by specific drugs, motivate, and support quitting efforts.

- Realize that certain symptoms (such as anxiety, sleeplessness, paranoia, phobias, hostility) may have been viewed wrongly as the *cause* rather than the *consequence* of drug use.

- Check out places to get help — experts, clinics, detox centers — and how to learn new coping skills.

3. Action (making an effort to stop or cut back)

- Set realistic goals for change (such as short-term quit strategies: "a week without drugs," "not this weekend"). Cut back or abstain for a day, week, month at a time.

- Try self-help tactics using manuals, quit guides, and advice from drug addiction agencies.

- Counter temptation. List drug-taking "cues" and how to avoid or sidestep them.

- When seeking advice, adopt an open, frank approach. This is most likely to enlist the most understanding and supportive response.

- Anticipate relapses. Become wary of feelings, events, places that might trigger a relapse.

- Do not regard a relapse as a failure or loss of all that's been gained but, rather, as a learning experience — one step on the way to doing better next time.

- Be prepared for several tries before breaking a drug habit.

- Enlist cooperative support from family and friends. The families of quitters also may need counseling.

Structured treatment can help someone trying to break an addiction. The available kinds of therapy include individual therapy with a trained addiction specialist, group therapy that offers feedback from others, family therapy that addresses the needs of all family members, and formal 12-step programs (patterned after Alcoholics Anonymous) that rely on a higher power during recovery.

Consider these alternatives instead of drugs:

- If you need physical relaxation, try athletics, exercise, or outdoor hobbies.

- Stimulate your senses. Train yourself to be more aware of nature and beauty.

- If you're anxious, depressed, or uptight, turn to people — friends, professional counselors, support groups.

- Volunteer in programs where you can help others and not focus on yourself.

- If you want to escape boredom, stimulate your mind through reading, classes, creative games, discussion groups, memory training, or travel.

- Pursue training in music, art, singing, or writing. Attend more concerts, ballets, or museum shows.

- Volunteer in political campaigns, or join lobbying and political-action groups.

- Explore various philosophical theories through classes, seminars, and discussion groups.

- If you're looking for adventure, sign up for a wilderness survival outing; take up boardsailing or rock climbing.

NOTES

1. Craig Nakken, *The Addictive Personality: Understanding Compulsion in Our Lives* (San Francisco: Harper & Row, 1988).
2. Richard G. Schlaadt and Peter T. Shannon, *Drugs: Use, Misuse, and Abuse* Englewood Cliffs, NJ: Prentice Hall, Inc., 1994), p. 116.
3. Andrea LaCroix, Lucy Mead, Kung-Yee Liang, Caroline Thomas, and Thomas Pearson, "Coffee Consumption and the Incidence of Coronary Heart Disease," *The New England Journal of Medicine* 315:16 (1986), pp. 977–982.
4. P. S. Hoard, "Premenstrual Syndrome Can Trigger Relapse," *Alcoholism & Addiction* 8:6 (1988), pp. 41–42.
5. Centers for Disease Control and Prevention, 1977.
6. Data from "Health Tips," in *From Your Shouders Up*, Spring 1996, p. 3.
7. K. Liska, *Drugs and the Human Body*, 3d ed. (NY: Macmillan, 1990).
8. Charles R. Carroll, *Drugs in Modern Society*, 3d ed. (Madison, WI: Brown & Benchmark, 1993), p. 150.
9. Dorris Michael, "A Desperate Crack Legacy," *Newsweek*, June 25, 1990, p. 6.
10. 20th annual survey by University of Michigan Institute for Social Research, 1994.
11. National Institute on Drug Abuse.
12. *American Psychologist*.

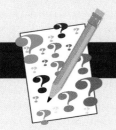

Are You An Addict?

Name _____ Date _____ Grade _____

Instructor _____ Course _____ Section _____

The following questions were written by recovering addicts in Narcotics Anonymous.

	Yes	No
1. Do you ever use alone?	☐	☐
2. Have you ever substituted one drug for another, thinking that one particular drug was the problem?	☐	☐
3. Have you ever manipulated or lied to a doctor to obtain prescription drugs?	☐	☐
4. Have you ever stolen drugs or stolen to obtain drugs?	☐	☐
5. Do you regularly use a drug when you wake up or when you go to bed?	☐	☐
6. Have you ever taken one drug to overcome the effects of another?	☐	☐
7. Do you avoid people or places that do not approve of you using drugs?	☐	☐
8. Have you ever used a drug without knowing what it was or what it would do to you?	☐	☐
9. Has your job or school performance ever suffered from the effects of your drug use?	☐	☐
10. Have you ever been arrested as a result of using drugs?	☐	☐
11. Have you ever lied about what or how much you use?	☐	☐
12. Do you put the purchase of drugs ahead of your financial responsibilities?	☐	☐
13. Have you ever tried to stop or control your using?	☐	☐
14. Have you ever been in a jail, hospital, or drug rehabilitation center because of your using?	☐	☐
15. Does using interfere with your sleeping or eating?	☐	☐
16. Does the thought of running out of drugs terrify you?	☐	☐
17. Do you feel it is impossible for you to live without drugs?	☐	☐
18. Do you ever question your own sanity?	☐	☐
19. Is your drug use making life at home unhappy?	☐	☐
20. Have you ever thought you couldn't fit in or have a good time without using drugs?	☐	☐
21. Have you ever felt defensive, guilty, or ashamed about your using?	☐	☐
22. Do you think a lot about drugs?	☐	☐
23. Have you had irrational or indefinable fears?	☐	☐
24. Has using affected your sexual relationships?	☐	☐
25. Have you ever taken drugs you didn't prefer?	☐	☐
26. Have you ever used drugs because of emotional pain or stress?	☐	☐

27. Have you ever overdosed on any drugs? ☐ ☐
28. Do you continue to use despite negative consequences? ☐ ☐
29. Do you think you might have a drug problem? ☐ ☐

Are you an addict? This is a question only you can answer. Members of Narcotics Anonymous found that they all answered different numbers of these questions "yes." The actual number of *yes* responses isn't as important as how you feel inside and how addiction has affected your life. If you are an addict, you must first admit that you have a problem with drugs before any progress can be made toward recovery.

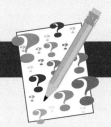

Do You Have a Problem with Alcohol?

Name _____ Date _____ Grade _____

Instructor _____ Course _____ Section _____

To determine if you have a problem with alcohol, answer yes (Y) or no (N) to the following questions about your drinking behavior. Refer to the scale at the end of the quiz for evaluation of your answers.

_____ 1. Do you occasionally drink heavily after a disappointment or a quarrel or when your parents or boss gives you a hard time?

_____ 2. When you have trouble or feel pressured at school or at work, do you always drink more heavily than usual?

_____ 3. Have you noticed that you are able to handle more liquor than you did when you were first drinking?

_____ 4. Did you ever wake up the "morning after" and discover that you could not remember part of the evening before, even though your friends tell you that you did not pass out?

_____ 5. When drinking with other people, do you try to have a few extra drinks that others don't notice?

_____ 6. Are there certain occasions when you feel uncomfortable if alcohol is not available?

_____ 7. Have you recently noticed that when you begin drinking, you are in more of a hurry to get the first drink than you used to be?

_____ 8. Do you sometimes feel a little guilty about your drinking?

_____ 9. Are you secretly irritated when your family or friends discuss your drinking?

_____ 10. Have you recently noticed an increase in the frequency of your memory blackouts?

_____ 11. Do you often find that you wish to continue drinking after your friends say they have had enough?

_____ 12. Do you usually have a reason for the occasions when you drink heavily?

_____ 13. When you are sober, do you often regret things you did or said while drinking?

_____ 14. Have you tried switching brands or following different plans for controlling your drinking?

_____ 15. Have you often failed to keep the promises you've made to yourself about controlling or cutting down on your drinking?

_____ 16. Have you ever tried to control your drinking by changing jobs or moving to a new location?

_____ 17. Do you try to avoid family or close friends while you are drinking?

_____ 18. Are you having an increasing number of financial and academic problems?

_____ 19. Do more people seem to be treating you unfairly without good reason?

_____ 20. Do you eat very little or irregularly when you are drinking?

_____ 21. Do you sometimes have the shakes in the morning and find that it helps to have a drink?

____ 22. Have you recently noticed that you cannot drink as much as you once did?

____ 23. Do you sometimes stay drunk for several days at a time?

____ 24. Do you sometimes feel very depressed and wonder whether life is worth living?

____ 25. Sometimes after a period of drinking, do you see or hear things that aren't there?

____ 26. Do you get terribly frightened after you have been drinking heavily?

If you answer *yes* to two or three of these questions, you may wish to evaluate your drinking in these areas. *Yes* answers to *several* of these questions may indicate one of the following stages of alcoholism:

■ Questions 1-8 (early stage): Drinking is a regular part of your life.

■ Questions 9-21 (middle stage): You are having trouble controlling when, where, and how much you drink.

■ Questions 22-26 (beginning of the final stage): You no longer can control your desire to drink.

ASSESSMENT 13-3

Nicotine Dependence: Are You Hooked?

Name _____ Date _____ Grade _____

Instructor _____ Course _____ Section _____

Answer each question in the list below, giving yourself the appropriate points.	**0 points**	**1 point**	**2 points**
____ 1. How soon after you wake up do you smoke your first cigarette?	After 30 minutes	Within 30 minutes	—
____ 2. Do you find it difficult to refrain from smoking in places where it is forbidden, such as the library, theater, doctor's office?	No	Yes	—
____ 3. Which of all the cigarettes you smoke in a day is the most satisfying?	Any other than the first one in the morning	The first one in the morning	—
____ 4. How many cigarettes a day do you smoke?	1-15	16-25	26+
____ 5. Do you smoke more during the morning than during the rest of the day?	No	Yes	—
____ 6. Do you smoke when you are so ill that you are in bed most of the day?	No	Yes	—
____ 7. Does the brand you smoke have a low, medium, or high nicotine content?	Low	Medium	High
____ 8. How often do you inhale the smoke?	Never	Sometimes	Always

____ **Total**

SCORING

- More than 6 points — very dependent
- Less than 6 points — low to moderate dependence.

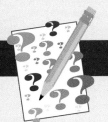

ASSESSMENT 13-4

Why Do You Smoke?

Name _____ Date _____ Grade _____

Instructor _____ Course _____ Section _____

	Always	Fre-quently	Occa-sionally	Seldom	Never
A. I smoke cigarettes in order to keep myself from slowing down.	5	4	3	2	1
B. Handling a cigarette is part of the enjoyment of smoking it.	5	4	3	2	1
C. Smoking cigarettes is pleasant and relaxing.	5	4	3	2	1
D. I light up a cigarette when I feel angry about something.	5	4	3	2	1
E. When I have run out of cigarettes I find it almost unbearable until I can get them.	5	4	3	2	1
F. I smoke cigarettes automatically without even being aware of it.	5	4	3	2	1
G. I smoke cigarettes to stimulate me, to perk myself up.	5	4	3	2	1
H. Part of the enjoyment of smoking a cigarette comes from the steps I take to light up.	5	4	3	2	1
I. I find cigarettes pleasurable.	5	4	3	2	1
J. When I feel uncomfortable or upset about something, I light up a cigarette.	5	4	3	2	1
K. I am very much aware of the fact when I am not smoking a cigarette.	5	4	3	2	1
L. I light up a cigarette without realizing I still have one burning in the ashtray.	5	4	3	2	1
M. I smoke cigarettes to give me a "lift."	5	4	3	2	1
N. When I smoke a cigarette, part of the enjoyment is watching the smoke as I exhale it.	5	4	3	2	1
O. I want a cigarette most when I am comfortable and relaxed.	5	4	3	2	1
P. When I feel "blue" or want to take my mind off cares and worries, I smoke cigarettes.	5	4	3	2	1
Q. I get a real gnawing hunger for a cigarette when I haven't smoked for a while.	5	4	3	2	1
R. I've found a cigarette in my mouth and didn't remember putting it there.	5	4	3	2	1

Scoring Your Test:

Enter the numbers you have circled on the test questions in the spaces provided below, putting the number you have circled to question A on line A, to question B on line B, etc. Add the three scores on each line to get a total for each factor. For example, the sum of your scores over lines A, G, and M gives you your score on "Stimulation," lines B, H, and N give the score on "Handling," etc. Scores can vary from 3 to 15. Any score 11 and above is high; any score 7 and below is low.

A _____ + G _____ + M _____ = _____	Stimulation
B _____ + H _____ + N _____ = _____	Handling
C _____ + I _____ + O _____ = _____	Pleasure Relaxation
D _____ + J _____ + P _____ = _____	Crutch: Tension Reduction
E _____ + K _____ + Q _____ = _____	Craving: Psychological Addiction
F _____ + L _____ + R _____ = _____	Habit

A score of 11 or above on any factor indicates that smoking is an important source of satisfaction for you. The higher you score (15 is the highest), the more important a given factor is in your smoking. See page 296 for strategies for dealing with why you smoke.

From *A Self-Test for Smokers.* U.S. Department of Health and Human Services, 1983.

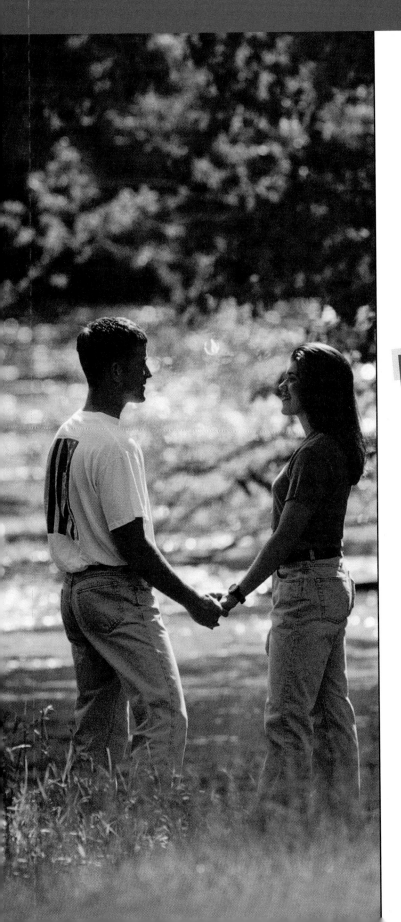

Sexually Transmitted Diseases

- Understand how sexually transmitted diseases are passed from one person to another.

- Be aware of the incidence of STDs in their various forms.

- Learn the reasons for the prevalence of STDs.

- Learn the symptoms, risks, and treatment for various STDs: chlamydia, gonorrhea, genital warts, herpes, viral hepatitis (not technically an STD), pelvic inflammatory disease, pubic lice and scabies, syphilis, and AIDS.

- Become acquainted with overall guidelines for reducing the risks of contracting STDs.

Just as their name implies, **sexually transmitted diseases** are transmitted, or passed from one person to another, through sexual contact. Several sexually transmitted diseases also can be passed in infected blood. Generally, the organisms that cause sexually transmitted diseases are fragile and can't exist outside the protective environment of the human reproductive tract. Therefore, you can't be infected by toilet seats, soap dishes, towels, or doorknobs. Some sexually transmitted diseases, formerly called venereal diseases, can be treated and cured. Others have no cure. All of them can be prevented by appropriate sexual behavior.

Sexually transmitted diseases (STDs) have been around a long time. They are mentioned in the Old Testament, and epidemics were recorded as early as the time of Columbus. Today, the more than 25 identified STDs are among the most prevalent infectious diseases in the United States. More than a million new cases are reported to the Centers for Disease Control and Prevention (CDC) every year.[1] Because many people who are infected show no symptoms, the CDC estimates that the number of Americans infected in any one year may be as high as 10 million. Only the common cold and flu are more prevalent. Most people with STDs are in the most sexually active group, between ages of 15 and 30. These diseases are no respecter of race, creed, gender, education, or socioeconomic status. Figure 14.1 lists estimated new cases of common STDs.

> *More than 25 diseases are spread through sexual contact. About one in four adults in the United States has an STD.*

Many STDs have reached epidemic proportions, even though some of them can be cured with proper medication. STDs are rampant for a number of reasons:

- Some STDs have no symptoms, so victims are unaware that they are infected. Others have only mild symptoms that can be easily confused with other ailments.
- When birth control pills became widely available, many people stopped using condoms as a form of birth control, and, though condoms prevent STDs, birth control pills do not.

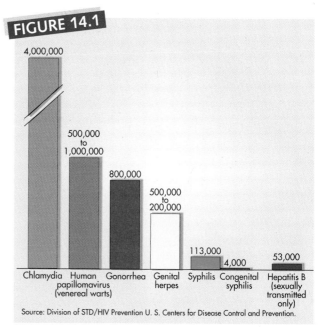

Source: Division of STD/HIV Prevention U. S. Centers for Disease Control and Prevention.

Estimated annual U. S. cases of common sexually transmitted diseases.

- As a trend, people are becoming sexually active at an earlier age and are having more than one sexual partner.
- The statistical trend toward marrying later has resulted in more sexual activity for longer periods.
- Some STDs cannot be treated and others have developed strains that resist antibiotics.

Myths About STDs

Remember the old myth about catching "something" from a toilet seat? It's just that — a myth! So are these:

- You can get an STD in a swimming pool or hot tub.
- You can get an STD from using someone else's towel or washcloth.
- If your partner doesn't have symptoms, you're safe.
- If your symptoms go away on their own, you're cured.
- You won't catch an STD if your partner is being treated.
- You can always tell if you have an STD.

- Fear of social stigma, disapproval, and condemnation stops some people from seeking treatment even when they suspect they might be infected. Others become complacent because of the past successes of penicillin and other antibiotics.

- Many victims deny the possibility of infection, believing "it can never happen to me," or they believe STDs affect only high-risk groups.

CAUSES

STDs are caused by bacteria, viruses, parasites, and fungi. Infection can recur with every new exposure. The body generally does not build up a resistance to the organisms that cause the diseases. Most affect the genitals. Left untreated, many have serious complications that affect the entire body. AIDS, which disables the immune system and leaves the body open to various opportunistic infections, leads eventually to death.

Strictly speaking, anyone who engages in sexual activity is at risk for STDs. The more sexual partners, the greater the risk. The risk also increases substantially if a person does not use condoms. Sexual behavior that tears or damages the vagina, anus, or penis increases the risk, and anal intercourse is especially dangerous. Women are at greater risk than men because they have a greater area of mucous membranes in their genital tissues. Gay and bisexual men, their sexual partners, intravenous drug users, and their partners are at highest risk. An infected mother can pass the disease to her fetus or infant during gestation and birth.

SIGNS AND SYMPTOMS

Signs and symptoms usually are slower to develop in women than in men, so women may not have as early an indication of infection. General signs and symptoms of STDs include:

- Sores on or near the genitals.
- Pain in the genitals.
- A burning sensation in the genitals.
- Discharge from the vagina or penis.
- Itching around the genitals, in the vagina, in the rectum, around the anus, or in and around the mouth.
- Abdominal pain.
- Growths or warts in the genital area; may be skin-colored or dark, flat, or raised.

Sores, warts, itching, rashes, and burning in areas of the body other than the genitals, vagina, rectum, and mouth usually don't indicate STDs. If you develop these symptoms and think you may have been exposed to an STD, however, you should see a physician.

COMMON STDS

Understanding the incidence, signs and symptoms, and risks for specific STDs can help you reduce your risk of becoming infected.

Chlamydia

The most common STD in the United States, around 4 million new cases of **chlamydia** occur each year. As many as 4 million Americans are believed to be infected at any given time. An estimated 15% of all college students in the United States are believed to be infected. As many as half a million cases in women progress to pelvic inflammatory disease (PID), which can cause sterility. An estimated 4% of all pregnant women are infected. If left untreated, chlamydia is chronic. The CDC estimates that chlamydia now is 10 times more prevalent than gonorrhea, which until recently was the most common STD in the United States.

Caused by *Chlamydia trachomatis* bacteria, chlamydia often occurs simultaneously with other STDs, most commonly gonorrhea and herpes. Unidentified for many years, the bacteria also causes non-gonococcal urethritis (NGU) and lymphogranuloma venereum (LGV).

About 90% of all men who are infected have symptoms. Only about 20% of all women who are infected have symptoms unless the infection progresses into something more serious, such as pelvic inflammatory disease. Even when women do have symptoms, these often are mild and can disappear on their own even though the woman is still infected. When symptoms occur, they usually appear 1 to 3 weeks after infection.

Chlamydia infects the mucous membranes that line the genitals, rectum, anus, mouth, and eyes. It is

Sexually transmitted disease A disease that is passed from one person to another through sexual contact.

Chlamydia STD caused by a bacteria that infects the mucous membranes that line the genitals, rectum, anus, mouth, and eyes; the most common STD in the United States.

transmitted by contact with infected mucous membranes and occurs most commonly between heterosexuals. The most common complications for newborns are pneumonia and conjunctivitis (an infection of the membranes in the eyes), found in more than 30,000 newborn babies each year in the United States.

In men, the most common symptoms are:

- Whitish or puslike discharge from the penis.
- Pain during urination; urination may be followed by a watery, clear discharge.
- Frequent urination.
- Urethral itching.
- A painful, swollen scrotum.
- Abdominal discomfort.

Women who experience symptoms may have:

- Whitish vaginal discharge.
- Itching or burning of the genitals.
- Mild pain during urination.
- Abdominal discomfort.
- Bleeding between periods.
- Symptoms of pelvic inflammatory disease (fever, painful intercourse, pelvic pain, vaginal discharge).

Complications of chlamydia in men include diseases of the urinary tract and sterility. In women,

When to Get Checked For a Possible STD

- If you are sexually active.
- If you know or suspect your sex partner is infected.
- If you change sex partners often. (Wait about 4 weeks, then get tested.)
- If there are signs of:
  - a vaginal or penile discharge ("the drip")
  - rash, warty growths, pimple, itchiness or sore on genitals
  - persistent lower abdominal pain
  - pain when urinating
  - changes in menstrual flow, unusual bleeding (in women).

Women should get regular Pap smear tests to detect early signs of cervical cancer.

chlamydia is the leading cause of pelvic inflammatory disease, which also can cause sterility. Chlamydia that is untreated can damage the arteries, heart valves, and heart muscle in men and women alike. At particular risk for chlamydia are women with more than one sexual partner, women who do not use some kind of barrier (such as condoms) during intercourse, women under age 25 who have multiple sexual partners, and women under age 20 who are pregnant.

Treatment consists of a full course of antibiotics, usually tetracycline or erythromycin. Infected and diagnosed individuals should:

1. Take all the antibiotics the doctor prescribes.
2. Have a follow-up culture 2 weeks after finishing the antibiotics to make sure the bacteria have been destroyed completely.
3. Avoid all sexual activity until the infection is gone, at least until the follow-up culture is clean.
4. Tell all sexual partners so they can get tested for chlamydia; if one of the sexual partners is infected, a person can be reinfected.

Gonorrhea

Known most commonly as "the clap," **gonorrhea** infects 800,000 or more Americans a year. The actual number of infected people in the United States may be as much as five times that high because only about 20% of all cases are believed to be reported. This STD is most common among people aged 20 to 24, and its incidence is increasing most rapidly among non-white adolescents and young adults.

Gonorrhea is caused by a bacteria that infects the cervix, rectum, urethra, or mouth. The bacteria dies rapidly when removed from the warmth and moisture of the mucous membranes, so it cannot be transmitted by inanimate objects. It is transmitted by intercourse, anal-genital sex, and oral-genital sex. Because the environment of the vagina is so conducive to growth of the bacteria that causes gonorrhea, women who are exposed to the bacteria through intercourse have an 80% chance of developing gonorrhea. The most common site of infection is the cervix. Men have only about a 20% chance. Left untreated, gonorrhea is chronic and progressive. People infected with gonorrhea do not become immune to it, so they can become infected many times.

The symptoms of gonorrhea generally develop within 2 days to 2 weeks after infection but may not appear for as long as 30 days. As with chlamydia, it may have no symptoms at all or only mild symptoms, especially in women. Gonorrhea can be transmitted even after the symptoms have disappeared.

Men generally tend to have more noticeable signs and symptoms, which include:

- A profuse, yellowish or milky, foul-smelling discharge from the penis.
- Burning, frequent urination.
- Fever.
- Abdominal pain.
- Swollen lymph glands in the groin.
- Swelling of the testicles.

An estimated 80% of women infected with gonorrhea do not have immediate symptoms. If women develop symptoms, they are usually mild and include:

- Slight burning or pain in the genital area.
- Slight foul-smelling vaginal discharge that has a different color or odor than a woman's usual discharge.
- Possible pain during urination.
- Abnormally heavy menstrual bleeding or bleeding between periods.

Gonorrhea transmitted during oral sex can cause a mild sore throat (often no more severe than the sore throat that accompanies the common cold). If gonorrhea was transmitted during anal intercourse, it can cause pain, burning, and discharge from the anus or the presence of mucous, pus, or blood in the stools.

Babies born to infected mothers may become blind. Because gonorrhea is so prevalent, the eyes of newborns are treated routinely with silver nitrate. Other complications include pneumonia and infections of the anus or rectum.

If left untreated, gonorrhea can cause permanent sterility in women and men alike. Other complications include heart damage, brain damage, liver damage, arthritis, skin lesions, and meningitis. The bacteria responsible for gonorrhea can survive in the reproductive tract for years, enabling a man or a woman without symptoms to infect multiple partners unknowingly.

Gonorrhea most often is treated with penicillin. If a chlamydia infection is present also, tetracycline is added. As many as 40% of gonorrhea infections are resistant to penicillin and must be treated with newer drugs; the number of gonorrhea infections that do not respond to penicillin has doubled since 1988.

Anyone who is infected and diagnosed with this STD should:

1. Take the full course of antibiotics prescribed by a doctor, even though the symptoms probably will ease up within 12 hours and disappear within 3 days.
2. Return for a follow-up culture a week after finishing the antibiotics.
3. Avoid sexual intercourse or other sexual contact that could spread the infection until the doctor verifies that the infection is completely gone.
4. Report the names of all sexual contacts who could have been infected; if they are not treated, reinfection could occur.

Gonorrhea is so common that some health officials recommend regular screening (usually once every 6 months) for all sexually active people.

Genital Warts

Genital warts actually are benign tumors caused by the **human papilloma virus (HPV)**. An estimated half a million to a million Americans, most of them between ages 15 and 24, develop the infection each year. It is epidemic on America's college campuses. More than 65 different strains of HPV cause genital warts and a person can be infected by more than one strain at the same time.

The most common symptom — warts on the penis (foreskin, glands, or shaft), scrotum, anus, cervix, or around the urethra — may develop as soon as 1 to 3 months following infection or as long as 8 months after infection. Outbreaks of warts are more common during pregnancy and in people who have a weak immune system. Genital warts can be transmitted by skin-to-skin contact during intercourse or by oral-genital contact during oral sex.

Gonorrhea STD caused by a bacteria that infects the cervix, rectum, urethra, or mouth.

Genital warts STD caused by the human papilloma virus (HPV) and characterized by warts around the genitals or mouth.

Human papilloma virus (HPV) The virus that causes genital warts; some strains of the virus also have been linked to cervical cancer.

Genital warts usually start with localized irritation and itching, followed by the warts. These may be soft or hard, flat, small, yellowish, and dry. In most areas of the body, they usually are larger, shaped irregularly, and may be white, pink, or gray. Genital warts have been described as looking like cauliflower. In women they often clump together, interfering with urination and sexual intercourse. If the infection was passed via oral sex, the warts may grow in and around the mouth.

Genital warts.

Only about 10% of people with HPV infection develop warts. In others, the warts are inside the vagina or rectum or on the cervix, so they may not be noticed unless a physician discovers them during an examination. Flat warts are so small that they may not be visible to the human eye.

The complications of genital warts are potentially deadly. Of the 65 strains of HPV, 12 have been linked to cervical cancer. The HPV is associated with approximately 90% of all cervical cancer, and it may play a strong role in other genital cancers as well, including cancer of the penis.

Newborns infected by their mothers can develop warts in the mouth and bronchial passages. This can interfere with breathing.

Treatment can remove the warts, but it cannot kill the virus that causes the warts. Recurrence is extremely common. The typical treatment for genital warts is the drug podophyllin, which causes the wart to slough off. It normally is applied by a physician once a week for 5 or 6 weeks until the wart has disappeared completely. Podophyllin can't be used by pregnant women or to treat warts in the cervical area.

Warts that resist treatment with podophyllin sometimes can be removed by surgery, electrocautery (burning), or cryotherapy (freezing). All these options result in scarring.

A person diagnosed and treated for genital warts should:

1. Follow the physician's instructions carefully; repeated treatment usually is necessary to remove the warts.

2. Use any antibiotic ointments the physician prescribes.

3. Avoid sexual contact during an outbreak of warts.

4. For women: Have a Pap smear every year to monitor the risk of cervical cancer.

5. Never use over-the-counter wart removers. They are useless against genital warts and can cause tissue damage if applied to the genital area.

Because treatment does not kill the virus that causes genital warts, once infected, the person always carries the virus, even though it may be dormant for months or years at a time.

Herpes

Of the different strains of herpes simplex virus, the most common is herpes simplex-1, the culprit behind the common cold sore or fever blister. Other viruses in the herpes family cause chicken pox, shingles, and infectious mononucleosis. The herpes simplex-2 virus is what causes the STD, also known as **herpes genitalis**.

Once a person gets genital herpes, it remains forever. It has no cure and no treatment. The virus always will reside in the body, even when the blistering sores characteristic of a herpes outbreak are not present. Some people have only one or two outbreaks a year; others may have them much more often. The virus can be spread even when no lesions are visible. Herpes is transmitted by contact with an active sore or with the virus-containing secretions from the vagina or penis.

Approximately half a million new cases of herpes are reported to the CDC each year. An estimated 35 million Americans have the virus. It is most common among those aged 18 to 25 years, and women are four times more likely than men to become infected. Non-whites have a greater rate of infection, but infected whites tend to develop more symptoms.

Usually within 10 days of infection, flulike symptoms arise that may include:

- Fever.
- Swollen glands, especially in the groin.
- Muscle aches and pains.
- Fatigue.
- Occasionally, shooting or stabbing pains in the abdomen and legs.

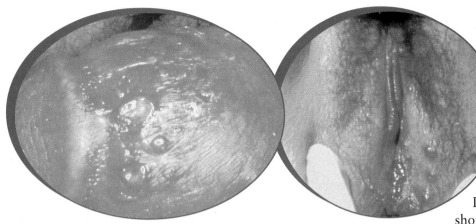

Genital herpes appears as blisters on the labia of a woman and on the male penis.

During this initial period, the infected person may feel pain during intercourse or urination. The characteristic blisters that appear on the genitals or mouth follow the flulike symptoms. These sores shed the herpes virus, and are highly contagious. Herpes sores progress through four stages:

1. At the site where the virus entered the body, the skin starts to itch or tingle, turns red, and becomes extremely sensitive. This sensation, called the **prodrome**, typically precedes all outbreaks.

2. One or more small, painful blisters or sores erupt on the glans and shaft of the penis, around the anus, at the opening of the vagina, on the clitoris, on the cervix, or on the labia. If oral-genital contact occurred, the sores may be in or around the mouth. The blisters rupture and the resulting painful, itching, open sores may weep a yellowish secretion or pus.

3. Without treatment, the sores diminish; scabs form and fall off within 1 to 2 weeks. Pain, fever, and other symptoms subside.

4. The virus lies dormant in the nerve endings for an unpredictable time. The blisters — which usually are less severe, of shorter duration, and without warning — recur in approximately two-thirds of the cases. Recurrence can be caused by unrelated illness, fever, emotional stress, lack of sleep, exposure to cold or heat, sunburn, poor nutrition, and menstruation.

The most typical complication of herpes is **autoinoculation** — in which the mouth, eyes, or other part of the body can become infected. Men don't seem to have any serious long-term complications. Women, on the other hand, run much higher risk for cervical cancer if they are infected with herpes.

Possibly the most serious complications involve babies born to mothers with herpes. If a woman with an active herpes lesion delivers a baby vaginally, the baby has a one-in-four chance of becoming infected and can be blind, have mental retardation, have damage to internal organs, and die. During active herpes, a woman should have a Caesarean section delivery to lower the risk of infecting the baby.

Herpes is caused by a virus, and it has no known cure. A topical ointment containing an antiviral drug, acyclovir, has helped relieve symptoms in some people during the initial outbreak only. Early indications are that continual use of acyclovir may help prevent recurrences, though this has not been proven. A person diagnosed with herpes should:

1. Wash the hands thoroughly after touching infected areas to avoid spreading the disease to other areas of the body.

2. Keep the infected lesions clean and dry.

3. Wear loose clothing to avoid irritating the infected areas; avoid scratching, rubbing, touching, or picking at sores.

4. Avoid sexual contact of any kind during times when lesions are active.

5. Use a latex condom to prevent spread of the infection when blisters are not present.

6. Practice good health habits to avoid getting fatigued or stressed, which can lead to recurrences.

7. For women; Have a Pap smear every 6 to 12 months to monitor the risk for cervical cancer. If pregnant, discuss the history of the infection with the doctor. Physicians usually recommend that the baby of an infected mother be delivered by cesarean section.

Herpes genitalis An infection caused by the herpes simplex-2 virus, characterized by blistering sores on the genitals.

Prodrome A sensation in which the skin starts to itch or tingle, turns red, and becomes extremely sensitive; precedes onset of the STD.

Autoinoculation The process of spreading an infection to other parts of one's own body.

Viral Hepatitis

Hepatitis, an infection that causes inflammation of the liver, is caused by one or more viruses. Of the four identified types of hepatitis, the most common is hepatitis A, more often called "infectious hepatitis." Even though hepatitis A can be transmitted sexually, it is not considered to be an STD. It is spread most often through unsanitary conditions, poor hygiene, direct exposure to the virus, or infected food and water. An estimated half of all adults in the United States have developed antibodies to hepatitis A, and it can be prevented with gamma globulin injections within 10 days of exposure.

Hepatitis B is spread through exposure to the contaminated blood or body fluids of an infected person. Besides being spread through semen, it can be transmitted through breast milk, saliva, and perspiration. People at high risk for contracting hepatitis B include intravenous drug users and their partners, as well as people with multiple sexual partners. Homosexual men are at particular risk for hepatitis B.

Signs and symptoms of hepatitis B develop within 6 months of infection and include:

- Mild fever.
- Loss of appetite.
- Nausea and vomiting.
- Diarrhea.
- Severe fatigue.
- Pain in the muscles and joints.
- Headache.
- Tenderness in the upper right section of the abdomen.

Within 2 weeks after symptoms first appear, signs of liver damage may become apparent, including:

- **Jaundice.**
- Light gray or whitish stools.
- Dark urine.
- Tender, enlarged liver.

Because the symptoms of hepatitis B are so much like those of the flu or infectious mononucleosis, a blood test is needed for proper diagnosis. Long-term complications from hepatitis B, which can be devastating, include chronic progressive hepatitis, liver cancer, liver failure, cirrhosis of the liver, and death.

Although hepatitis B has no cure, an effective vaccine is available to make uninfected people immune and prevent infection. Anyone in the high-risk group should ask for the vaccine. High-risk individuals include:

- Sexually active heterosexuals and homosexuals and their partners.
- Sexual partners of an infected person *or* a person living in the house with an infected person, even if not sexually involved.
- Intravenous drug users and their partners.
- People in the health-care professions.
- Natives of or travelers to Africa, Asia, Alaska, and the Pacific Islands.

People diagnosed with hepatitis B should:

1. Get plenty of rest. Follow the physician's guidelines for limiting activity during the acute stage of infection.
2. Avoid using drugs, including alcohol, that are metabolized by the liver, as these substances can put an excess burden an already stressed liver.
3. Avoid sexual contact.
4. If pregnant, discuss the disease with a physician. Do not breast feed the baby.
5. Have regular follow-up checkups to determine the risk of liver disease.

Pelvic Inflammatory Disease

Pelvic inflammatory disease (PID) can be caused by other sexually transmitted diseases, most commonly chlamydia and gonorrhea. The most dangerous of all STDs, it is a severe infection of the lining of the abdominal cavity that can be caused by other factors, including an intrauterine device (IUD) for birth control.

One of the factors that makes PID so dangerous is that it is difficult to diagnose, and, unless treated immediately, it can cause scar tissue to form in the fallopian tubes. A common result is sterility, because partially or completely blocked tubes prevent the egg from entering the uterus.

Signs and symptoms of PID include:

- Menstrual irregularities, including irregular cycles, profuse bleeding during menstruation, and vaginal bleeding between cycles.
- Severe menstrual cramps.
- Vaginal discharge.

■ Pain or tenderness in the abdomen or lower back.

■ Fever and chills.

■ Nausea and vomiting.

■ Loss of appetite.

■ A burning sensation during urination.

Some women who develop PID become sterile. Of those who do get pregnant, the risk of ectopic pregnancy (a fetus that attaches to the fallopian tube instead of the uterus), miscarriage, and stillbirth increases dramatically.

PID can be treated with antibiotics. Early treatment is essential. A person who is diagnosed and treated should:

1. Follow the complete course of antibiotics prescribed by a doctor, even if the symptoms disappear.

2. Stop using an IUD.

3. Avoid sexual activity until the infection has cleared.

4. Ask that any sexual partners be treated; if they are not, reinfection can occur.

5. Do not douche, as it can spread the infection.

Pubic Lice and Scabies

Commonly called "crabs," **pubic lice** are tiny parasites that move from partner to partner during sexual activity. Pubic lice actually are one of three different kinds of lice that attach to various parts of the body. Whereas pubic lice grip the pubic hair and feed on the small blood vessels of the underlying skin, other lice attach to skin or the hair of the head.

With a life cycle of approximately 2 months, pubic lice attach to the pubic hair, where females can lay as many as 10 eggs (nits) a day. The nits adhere to the pubic hair with a thick, sticky substance. Body warmth incubates the eggs until they hatch, and the new lice start feeding on the blood vessels as the old lice drop off. As they drop off, the lice are visible to the naked eye in bedding and clothing. The tiny mite that causes **scabies** has a similar life cycle, but the female mite burrows under the skin at night.

Common signs and symptoms of pubic lice include:

■ Intense itching in the pubic area.

■ Visible lice or whitish nits in the pubic hair.

■ Swollen glands in the groin.

Common signs and symptoms of scabies include:

■ Characteristic patterns of burrowing, most commonly on the buttocks, under the breasts, between the fingers and on the wrists.

■ A discharge of pus from the burrowed areas.

■ Intense itching.

Treatment options for pubic lice include Kwell, available only by prescription, and an over-the-counter preparation called A-200 Pyrinate. Both are applied to the pubic hair in a single dose; a fine-tooth comb is used to remove nits. Kwell also is used to treat scabies. Most advise against using Kwell during pregnancy, so pregnant women should check with a doctor.

Individuals diagnosed with scabies should follow the doctor's directions, as scabies also can be transmitted by close nonsexual contact. If diagnosed with pubic lice, the infected person should:

1. Follow treatment directions carefully.

2. Dip the comb in vinegar, then water, to dissolve the sticky substance holding nits to the pubic hair.

3. Wash all clothing, bedding, and linens contacted prior to treatment. This is one STD in which an innocent victim *can* be infected by towels or sheets.

4. Clean all upholstery and furniture contacted prior to treatment.

5. Avoid sexual contact, and inform all sexual partners; if they are not treated, they can be reinfected.

Hepatitis B   A form of hepatitis spread through exposure to the contaminated blood or body fluids of an infected person; can cause long-term liver damage.

Jaundice   Liver condition in which the skin and whites of the eyes appear yellow.

Pelvic inflammatory disease (PID)   A severe infection of the lining of the abdominal cavity, sometimes caused by other STDs.

Pubic lice   Commonly called "crabs," tiny parasites that feed on the small blood vessels of the skin beneath the pubic hair.

Scabies   An STD caused by tiny mites that burrow under the skin at night.

Syphilis

During the last half-decade, the incidence of **syphilis** has increased to the highest rate in 40 years. It occurs most often among urban heterosexuals between ages 20 and 29. Caused by a *spirochete* (corkscrew-shaped type of bacteria), syphilis is transmitted through direct contact with infectious sores, skin rashes, or mucous patches caused by syphilis.

Syphilis is transmitted most often through intercourse, anal-genital contact, and oral-genital contact, though it can also be transmitted by kissing a person who has a sore or mucous patches on the mouth. Syphilis also can be transmitted from a pregnant woman to her baby after the fourth month of pregnancy. (For the first four months, a special temporary membrane in the placenta protects the fetus from infectious agents in the mother's bloodstream). After the fourth month, the bacteria that causes syphilis is passed easily across the placenta from the mother's bloodstream to the baby's circulatory system.

Syphilis has four specific stages:

1. *Primary stage.* Occurring 2 to 3 weeks after the bacteria enter the body, a **chancre** develops at the site where the bacteria entered — usually on the genitals. The chancre may look like a blister or pimple but often is an open sore. It may be as large as a dime but commonly is as small as a pinhead and may go unnoticed, especially if it is in the vagina, rectum, anus, or mouth. The sore may be accompanied by painless swollen lymph nodes in the groin. Within 3 to 6 weeks, the chancre clears up without treatment, so many infected people assume it was something else. Even though the chancre has healed, infectious bacteria remain in the system.

2. *Secondary stage.* Any time from 6 weeks to a year after the chancre heals, the symptoms of secondary syphilis appear. These symptoms, which may be mild to severe and can last anywhere from a few days to a few months, include:

   ■ Low-grade fever.

   ■ Nausea and loss of appetite.

■ Whitish patches on the mouth and throat (infectious patches).

■ Sore throat.

■ Painless rash anywhere on the skin, especially on the soles of the feet and palms of the hands; though the rash does not itch, it spreads infection.

■ Headache.

■ Swollen glands.

■ Hair loss, usually patchy.

■ Arthritic-type joint pain.

■ Large sores on the genitals or around the mouth.

Even if untreated, these symptoms usually run their course, then disappear. This does not mean the infection is gone. The disease remains dormant, and symptoms can reappear at any time. The person remains infectious during this stage even though symptoms have cleared up.

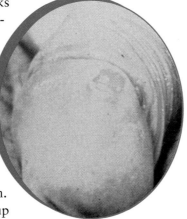
Chancre on head of penis.

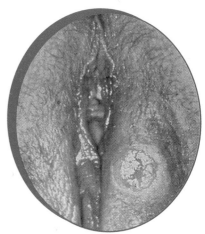
Chancre on labia of female genitalia.

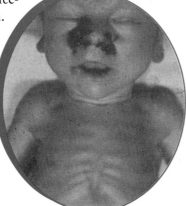
Congenital syphilis.

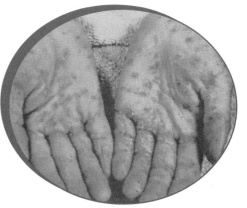
The rash of secondary syphilis.

3. *Latent stage.* No outward symptoms are present during the latent stage, which usually lasts as long as 30 years. During the latent stage, the person is no longer contagious unless moist lesions erupt. One exception is a pregnant woman, who can pass syphilis to her fetus during the latent stage. Even though nothing seems to be happening on the outside during the latent stage, the spirochetes attack the body's organs, causing substantial damage to the brain, heart, and central nervous system. Maladies characteristic of the latent stage include heart disease, senility, blindness, central nervous system deterioration, and death.

4. *Late (tertiary) stage.* The late stage of syphilis usually begins 5 to 20 years after the initial infection. Two-thirds of people with untreated infections have no further symptoms. About one-third of people with untreated infections develop blindness, deafness, central nervous system destruction, damage to the heart, paralysis, psychosis, and, finally, death during the late stage of syphilis.

A fetus infected by the mother's blood may develop mild to severe organ damage as a result. Syphilis also can result in stillbirth.

Penicillin is the drug of choice in treating syphilis. With treatment, syphilis can be cured at any stage. A person diagnosed and treated for syphilis should:

1. Follow the complete course of antibiotics as prescribed by a doctor, even if no symptoms are apparent.

2. Discuss with the doctor the possibility of simultaneous STD infections, such as gonorrhea or chlamydia. If additional infections are present, higher doses of various antibiotics are necessary.

3. Avoid sexual activity until cured.

4. Have follow-up blood tests for a year after finishing antibiotic treatment.

HIV and AIDS

A report issued by the U.S. Surgeon General estimated that one in every 250 Americans is infected with **HIV**, the virus that causes **AIDS**. Figure 14.2 shows reported cases in the United States between 1981 and 1997. More than 400,000 Americans have died of the consistently fatal disorder. The World Health Organization estimates that 17 million men,

AIDS

In the United States AIDS is increasing faster for women than for men. At last count, about 18% of all AIDS patients (14,081) are women. The rate is growing fastest among women infected by *heterosexual contact* (as opposed to injectable drug use).

Only one of the three men who have extramarital affairs wear condoms. This puts the men's girlfriends, their wives, and themselves at risk for HIV infection.

Source: Survey of 4,500 heterosexual men and women in 26 cities by Joseph Catania, University of California Medical School, San Francisco.

women, and children have been infected with HIV worldwide; approximately 4 million of them have developed AIDS. Figure 14.3 shows the number of AIDS cases, by age, reported in the United States in 1996. AIDS cases by race and ethnicity that were reported in the United States in 1996 are shown in Figure 14.4. The number of women being infected with HIV is increasing faster than any other population. Currently there is no vaccine and no cure.

Differences Between HIV and AIDS

HIV is a progressive disease. At first, people who become infected with HIV may not know they are infected. An incubation period of weeks, months, or years may go by during which no symptoms appear. The virus may live in the body 10 years or longer before symptoms develop.

As the infection progresses to the point at which certain diseases develop, the person is said to have AIDS. HIV itself doesn't kill, nor do people die of AIDS. AIDS is the term used to define the final stage of HIV infection. Death results from a weakened im-

Syphilis An STD caused by a bacteria, occurring in four stages; untreated, it is fatal.

Chancre A painless, red-rimmed sore that develops at the site where syphilis bacteria enter the body.

HIV Human immunodeficiency virus, the virus that weakens and destroys the immune system and gradually leads to AIDS.

AIDS Acquired immunodeficiency syndrome, the final stage of HIV infection, characterized by opportunistic infections that are rare or harmless in people with normal immune function.

mune system that is unable to fight off the opportunistic diseases that develop.

Earliest symptoms of the disease include unexplained weight loss, constant fatigue, mild fever, swollen lymph glands, diarrhea, and sore throats. Advanced symptoms include loss of appetite, skin diseases, night sweats, and deterioration of mucous membranes.

Though fatal to AIDS victims, most of the illnesses AIDS patients develop are harmless and rare in the general population. The two most common fatal conditions in AIDS patients are *pneumocystis carinii pneumonia* (a parasitic infection of the lungs) and *Kaposi's sarcoma* (a type of skin cancer). The AIDS virus also may attack the nervous system, causing brain and spinal cord damage.

On the average, the individual develops the symptoms that fit the case definition of AIDS about 7 to 8 years following infection. From that point on, the person may live another 2 to 3 years. In essence, from the point of infection, the individual may endure a chronic disease 8 to 10 years.

The only means to determine whether someone has HIV is through an HIV antibody test. Being HIV-positive does not necessarily mean the person has AIDS. Several years may go by before the person develops the diseases that fit the case definition of AIDS.

Upon HIV infection, the immune system's line of defense against the virus is to form antibodies that bind to the virus. On the average, the body takes 3 months to manufacture enough antibodies to show up positive in an HIV antibody test. Sometimes this may take 6 months or longer.

If HIV infection is suspected, a prudent waiting period of 3 to 6 months is suggested prior to testing. During this time, and from there on, individuals should refrain from further endangering themselves

FIGURE 14.2

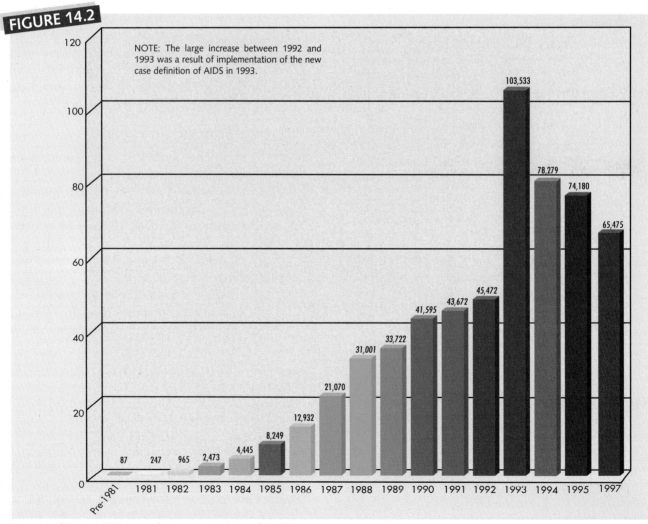

NOTE: The large increase between 1992 and 1993 was a result of implementation of the new case definition of AIDS in 1993.

Reported U.S. AIDS cases between 1981 and 1997.

and others through risky behaviors. Some people choose to be tested to be reassured that their risky behaviors are acceptable. Even if the test turns up negative for HIV, this is not a license to continue risky behaviors. Once infected with HIV, a person never will become uninfected. There is no second chance. Everyone must protect himself or herself against this chronic disease. No one should be so ignorant as to believe that it can never happen to him or her!

Although professionals disagree as to how many carriers actually will develop AIDS, sooner or later most HIV-infected individuals will be diagnosed with AIDS. Even if a person has not developed AIDS, the virus can be passed on to others who could easily develop AIDS.

HIV Transmission

Two basic conditions have to be present for HIV to be transmitted.

1. One person has to be infected.
2. The virus has to be transmitted to an area in the body where there are T-lymphocytes (specialized white blood cells the virus needs to live and multiply).

If either of these conditions does not exist, the virus will not be transmitted.

HIV is transmitted by the exchange of cellular body fluids including blood, semen, vaginal secretions, and maternal milk. These fluids may be exchanged during sexual intercourse, by using hypodermic needles used previously by infected individuals, between a pregnant woman and her developing fetus, by infection of babies from the mother during childbirth, less frequently during breastfeeding, and rarely from a blood transfusion or organ transplant.

> **Once infected with the virus, a person never will become uninfected.**

The risk of being infected with HIV from a blood transfusion today is slight. Prior to 1985, several cases of HIV infection came from blood transfusions because the blood was donated by HIV-infected individuals. Today, all individuals who donate blood are tested for HIV.

A myth regarding HIV is that it can be transmitted by donating blood. People cannot get HIV from giving blood. Health professionals use a new needle

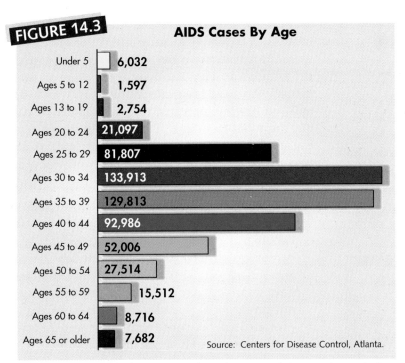

FIGURE 14.3

AIDS Cases By Age

Age	Cases
Under 5	6,032
Ages 5 to 12	1,597
Ages 13 to 19	2,754
Ages 20 to 24	21,097
Ages 25 to 29	81,807
Ages 30 to 34	133,913
Ages 35 to 39	129,813
Ages 40 to 44	92,986
Ages 45 to 49	52,006
Ages 50 to 54	27,514
Ages 55 to 59	15,512
Ages 60 to 64	8,716
Ages 65 or older	7,682

Source: Centers for Disease Control, Atlanta.

Age of AIDS patients diagnosed in the United States through December 1996.

FIGURE 14.4

AIDS Cases By Race or Ethnicity

White, not Hispanic	268,856
Black, not Hispanic	203,189
Hispanic	103,023
Asian/Pacific Islander	4,131
American Indian/ Alaska Native	1,569
Race/ ethnicity unknown	661

Source: Centers for Disease Control, Atlanta.

Race or ethnicity of persons reported with AIDS in the United States through December 1996.

every time they withdraw blood from a person. These needles are used only once and are thrown away immediately after each person has donated blood.

> *People do not get HIV because of who they are but because of what they do.*

People do not get HIV because of who they are but because of what they do. HIV and AIDS can threaten anyone, anywhere: men, women, children, teenagers, young people, older adults, whites, blacks, hispanics, orientals, homosexuals, heterosexuals, bisexuals, druggies, Americans, Africans, Europeans. Nobody is immune to HIV. HIV can be transmitted between males, between females, from male to female, or from female to male. HIV and AIDS are basically preventable. Almost all of the people who get HIV do so because they choose to engage in risky behaviors.

Risky Behaviors

You cannot tell if people are infected with HIV or have AIDS by simply looking at them or taking their word. Not you, not a nurse, not even a doctor can tell without an HIV antibody test. Although many people who have been infected with HIV look normal and healthy for years, they are capable of passing the virus to others. Therefore, every time you engage in risky behavior, you run the risk of contracting HIV. The two most basic risky behaviors are:

1. *Having unprotected vaginal, anal, or oral sex with an HIV-infected person.* Unprotected sex means having sex without the proper use of a condom. A person should select only latex (rubber or prophylactic) condoms that say "disease prevention" on the package. Although you might have unprotected sex with an infected person and not get the virus, you also can get it by having unprotected sex only once with that infected person.

   Rubbing during sexual intercourse often damages mucous membranes and causes unseen bleeding (even in the mouth). During vaginal, anal, or oral sexual contact, infected blood, semen, or vaginal fluids can penetrate the mucous membranes that line the vagina, the penis, the rectum, the mouth, or the throat. From the membrane, HIV then can travel into the previously uninfected person's blood.

   Health experts believe unprotected anal sex is the riskiest type of sex. Even though bleeding is not visible in most cases, anal sex almost always causes tiny tears and bleeding in the rectum. This happens because the rectum does not stretch easily, the mucous membrane is quite thin, and small blood vessels lie directly beneath the membrane. Condoms also are more likely to break during anal intercourse because of the greater friction produced in a smaller cavity. All of these factors greatly enhance the risk of transmitting HIV.

   Although latex condoms provide for "safer" sex if they are used correctly, they are not 100% foolproof. Abstaining from sex is the best way to protect yourself from HIV infection and other STDs.

Tips For Action — Condom Do's & Don'ts

- Use only *latex* condoms. Natural membranes have pores through which the virus can travel.

- Do use caution when opening a condom. Teeth, fingernails, or other sharp objects could tear the condom.

- Do put the condom on as soon as the penis is erect, roll it all the way to the base of the penis, and be sure it stays on until the penis is fully withdrawn. Also make sure there is no air in the tip of the condom.

- Do use plenty of water-based lubricant, not oil- or alcohol-based lubricants such as Vaseline or baby oil. These weaken latex and make condoms break more easily.

- All condoms are stamped with a date. They last for about five years, but you should look for a date within 2½ years from when you purchase them.

- Don't use a condom more than once.

- Don't continue using a condom if it breaks during sex. Stop and put on a new condom.

- Don't expose condoms to extreme light or temperature. These conditions may cause a condom to dry out and break.

- Don't stretch or inflate a condom before use.

VANESSA WAS IN A FATAL CAR ACCIDENT LAST NIGHT. ONLY SHE DOESN'T KNOW IT YET.

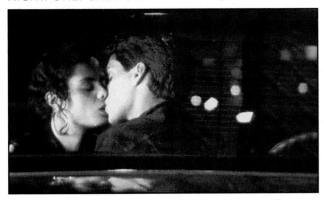

Drug and alcohol use can make people more willing to have unplanned and unprotected sex, thereby risking HIV infection.

Photo courtesy of the National Institute on Drug Abuse, U.S. Department of Health and Human Services.

2. *Sharing hypodermic needles or other drug para-phernalia with someone who is infected.* Following an injection, a small amount of blood remains in the needle and sometimes in the syringe itself. If the person who used the syringe is infected with HIV and someone else uses that same syringe, regardless of the drug used (legal or illegal), that small amount of blood is sufficient to spread the virus. All used syringes should be destroyed and disposed of immediately after they are used.

   In addition, a person must be cautious when getting acupuncture, getting a tattoo, or having the ears pierced. If the needle used was used previously on someone who is HIV-infected and was not disinfected properly, the person risks getting HIV as well.

Infrequent use of drugs, including alcohol, also heightens the risk of spreading HIV. Otherwise prudent people often act irrationally and engage in risky behaviors when they are under the influence of drugs. Getting high can make you willing to have sex when you really didn't plan to, and thereby run the risk of HIV infection.

A very small risk is present in receiving donated blood. Because of the 3- to 6-month incubation period, blood donors recently infected with HIV can test negative at the time they donate blood (or an organ). Therefore, people who are planning to have surgery should consider storing their own blood in advance so safe blood will be available if they need it.

There is no evidence of airborne transmission of the virus; HIV cannot be passed by coughing or sneezing. Small concentrations of the virus have been found in saliva and teardrops, but there is no record of anyone getting HIV through French-kissing or from someone else's tears. In principle, if both people have open cuts in the lips, mouth, or gums, HIV could be transmitted through openmouthed kissing, but such a case has never been documented.

The virus cannot be transmitted through perspiration (sweat), either. Sporting activities with no physical contact pose no risk to uninfected individuals, unless they have open wounds through which blood from an infected person can come in direct contact with the open wound of the uninfected person. The skin is an excellent line of defense against HIV. Blood from an infected person cannot penetrate the skin except through an opening in the skin. As an extra precaution, a person should use vinyl or latex gloves when performing work that requires direct contact with someone else's blood or open wound.

Some people fear getting HIV from health-care professionals. The chances of getting infected during physical or medical procedures are practically nil. Health care workers take extra care to protect themselves and their patients from HIV.

HIV is not transmitted through normal social contact. HIV cannot be caught by spending time with, shaking hands with, or hugging an infected person; from a public telephone, toilet seat, drinking fountain, swimming pool, dishes, or silverware used by an HIV patient; or by sharing a drink, food, a towel, or clothes with a person who has HIV.

Another myth regarding HIV transmission is that you can get it from insects or animals. The H in HIV stands for human. You cannot catch HIV from insects or animals, because they do not get infected with HIV. A mosquito that picks up the virus may carry the virus in its stomach, but the virus cannot reproduce in the mosquito or travel to the mosquito's saliva.

What about dating? Dating and getting to know other people is a normal part of life. Dating, however, does not mean the same thing as having sex. Sexual intercourse as a part of dating can be risky, and one of the risks is AIDS. You can't tell if someone you are dating or would like to date has been exposed to HIV. The good news is that as long as you avoid sexual activity and don't share drug needles, it doesn't matter whom you date.

A Fighting Spirit

A fighting spirit apparently can make a difference even in disease situations as serious as AIDS. The message that AIDS patients usually get is one of giving up. As one researcher put it, "All that is emphasized to AIDS patients is that it is 100% fatal. Death, death, death." When someone with a powerful fighting spirit gets infected, the prognosis may be better.

HIV Testing

A person can be tested for HIV in several ways. Testing usually is free of charge, and the results are kept confidential. Many states also conduct anonymous testing, which means the name is never recorded. Instead, a number is assigned as a link to the test.

Two types of tests are used to detect HIV.

1. The EIA or ELISA. This simple, inexpensive screening test measures whether the person has developed antibodies to the virus. If the test is negative and the person has not been exposed to HIV within the previous 3 months, he or she can be relatively certain of not being infected. Generally, no further testing is required. If the test is positive, the person is usually asked to take a second screening test to reduce the chance of a false positive result.

Hotlines

Several toll-free hotlines are available for more information on anonymous testing, treatment programs, support services, HIV and AIDS information, and STDs in general. All information discussed during a phone call to these hotlines is kept strictly confidential.

- National AIDS Hotline: 1-800-342-AIDS (La Linea Nacional de SIDA: 1-800-344-SIDA, for Spanish-speaking people)
- STD Hotline: 1-800-227-8922.
- National Institute on Drug Abuse (NIDA) Information and Treatment Referral: 1-800-622-HELP (1-800-66-AYUDA for Spanish-speaking only) (NIDA also provides information on drug abuse and addictive behavior)

2. The Western Blot Test. If the second screening test is positive, this more sophisticated, expensive test is given to confirm the positive results. If the Western Blot is positive, HIV infection is certain. If it is negative, you can be reasonably certain of not being infected, as false negative results are rare.

Neither of these tests can tell if a person has AIDS. The tests can determine only if he or she has been infected with HIV. A diagnosis of AIDS is given only if the person is infected with HIV *and*:

— the T-lymphocyte count is too low; or

— the person has one of the opportunistic infections listed by the Centers for Disease Control and Prevention.

These infections are rare or harmless in people with normal immunity.

As with any other serious illness, AIDS patients deserve respect, understanding, and support. Rejection and discrimination are traits of immature, hateful, and ignorant people. Education, knowledge, and responsible behaviors are the best ways to minimize fear and discrimination.

HIV Treatment

Even though several drugs are being tested to treat and slow down the disease process, AIDS has no known cure. At least 30 different approaches to an AIDS vaccine are being explored. The best advice at this point is to take a preventive approach.

Although HIV has no cure, medications are available that allow HIV-infected patients to live longer. The sooner treatment is initiated following infection, the better are the chances for delaying the onset of AIDS.

Developing a vaccine to prevent HIV infection or AIDS seems highly unlikely in the next few years. People should not expect a medical breakthrough. Treatment modalities, however, should continue to improve and allow HIV-infected persons and AIDS patients to live longer and more productive lives.

Presently, several AIDS clinical trials (studies) are available in the United States. These projects are co-sponsored by the Centers for Disease Control and Prevention, the Food and Drug Administration, the National Institute of Allergy and Infectious Diseases, and the National Library of Medicine. The purpose of AIDS clinical trials is to evaluate experimental drugs and various therapies for people at all stages

Myths About AIDS

You've probably heard one or more of these statements, but they're all untrue:

- You can get AIDS by donating blood.
- You can get AIDS through casual contact, such as shaking hands with or hugging an infected person.
- You can catch AIDS if an infected person coughs or sneezes on you.
- You can get AIDS from a mosquito.
- AIDS could spread rapidly through the general population.
- If you're not gay and don't shoot drugs, you're safe.
- Infected women can't transmit AIDS.
- If you don't have symptoms, you're not contagious.
- If you're HIV-positive, you'll know it from the symptoms.
- If you test positive for HIV, you have AIDS.
- Abstinence is the only way to protect yourself against AIDS.

of HIV infection.* As with all HIV testing, calls are completely confidential. Eligibility to participate in an AIDS clinical trial varies, and all applicants are evaluated individually. Those who are interested will receive information on the purpose and location of the trials that are open, eligibility requirements and exclusion criteria, and names and telephone numbers of persons to contact.

PREVENTING SEXUALLY TRANSMITTED DISEASES

With all the grim news about STDs, you can do things to prevent their spread and take precautions to keep yourself from becoming a victim. The best prevention technique is a mutually monogamous sexual relationship, one in which two people have sexual relationships only with each other. That one behavior will remove a person almost completely from any risk for developing an STD.[2]

*Interested individuals can call 1-800-TRIALS-A.

In today's society people are having difficulty knowing when to trust a person. You may be led to believe you are in a monogamous relationship when your partner actually (a) may be cheating on you and gets infected, (b) ends up having a one-night stand with someone who is infected, (c) got the virus several years ago before the present relationship and still doesn't know of the infection, (d) may not be honest with you and chooses not to tell you about the infection, or (e) is shooting up drugs and becomes infected. In any of these cases, HIV can be passed on to you.

Because your future and your life are at stake, and because you don't know if your partner is infected, you should give serious and careful consideration to postponing sex until you believe you have found a lifetime monogamous relationship. In doing so, you will not have to live with the fear of catching HIV or other STDs or deal with an unplanned pregnancy. As strange as this may seem to some, many people postpone sexual activity until they are married. This is the best guarantee against HIV. Married life will provide plenty of time for fulfilling and rewarding sex.

Some people would have you believe you are not a real man or woman if you don't have sex. Manhood and womanhood are not proven during sexual intercourse but, instead, through mature, responsible, and healthy choices. Other people lead you to believe that love doesn't exist without sex. Sex in the early stages of a relationship is not the product of love but is simply the fulfillment of a physical, and often selfish, drive. Then there are those who enjoy bragging about their sexual conquests and mock people who choose to wait. In essence, many of these conquests are only fantasies in an attempt to gain popularity with peers.

Sexual promiscuity never leads to a trusting, loving, and lasting relationship. Mature people respect others' choices. If someone does not respect your choice to wait, he or she certainly does not deserve your friendship or, for that matter, anything else. Sex lasts only a few minutes. The consequences of irresponsible sex, however, may last a lifetime. In some cases, they are fatal.

A loving relationship develops over a long time with mutual respect for each other. There is no greater sex than that between two loving and responsible individuals who mutually trust and admire each other. Contrary to many beliefs, these relationships are possible. They are built upon unselfish attitudes and behaviors.

As you look around, you will find that many believe the same way you do. Seek them out and build your friendships and future around people who respect you for what you are and what you believe. You don't have to compromise your choices or values. In the end you will reap the greater rewards of a choice and lasting relationship, free of AIDS and other STDs.

Also, be prepared so that you will know your course of action before you get into an intimate situation. Look for common interests, and work together toward them. Express your feelings openly: "I'm not ready for sex; I just want to have fun and kissing is fine with me." If your friend does not accept your answer and is not willing to stop the advances, be prepared with a strong response. Statements like "Please stop" or "Don't!" are for the most part ineffective. Use a firm statement such as:

"No, I'm not willing to do it" or "I've already thought about this and I'm not going to have sex." If this still does not work, it is effective to label the behavior as rape and say: "This is rape and I'm going to call the police."

HIV Risk Reduction

Observing the following precautions can reduce your risk for getting HIV, and subsequently AIDS:

1. Postpone sex until you and your uninfected partner are prepared to enter into a lifetime monogamous relationship. Magic Johnson stated:

   [I]f I had known what I do now when I was younger, I would have postponed sex as long as I could, and I would have tried to have it the first time with somebody that I knew I wanted to spend the rest of my life with. I certainly want my children to postpone sex. Now the rest of my life may be a

---

How to Prevent STDs

To prevent STDs, practice the following safety measures:

- Plan before you get into a sexual situation. Determine the conditions under which you will allow sex to take place. If you decide to have sex, practice safer sex.

- Discuss STDs with the person you are contemplating having sex with before you do so. Talking about STDs might be awkward, but the short-lived embarrassment of addressing intimate questions can keep you from contracting or spreading disease. If you do not know the person well enough to address this issue, or you are uncertain about the answers, do not have sex with this individual.

- Eliminate your risk of getting an STD by not having sexual contact with anyone or by having contact only with a noninfected partner who has contact only with you. Limit the number of sexual partners you have. Having one partner lowers your chance of infection.

- Unless you're sure your partner is free of an STD, protect yourself by using a latex condom every time you have sexual intercourse. For extra protection, use a spermicide with the condom. Spermicide

can kill the bacteria and viruses that cause some STDs.

- Avoid mixing alcohol or other drugs with sexual activities. They could cloud your judgment and lead you to engage in unsafe sexual practices.

- Thoroughly wash immediately after sexual activity. Washing with hot, soapy water will not guarantee safety against STDs, but it can prevent you from spreading certain germs on your fingers and may wash away bacteria and viruses that have not entered the body yet.

- If you suspect your partner is infected with an STD, ask. Also, look for signs of infection, such as sores, redness, inflammations, a rash, growths, warts, or discharge. If you are unsure, abstain.

- Consider abstaining from sexual relations if you have any kind of an illness or disease, even a common cold. Any kind of illness lowers immunity and can make you extra vulnerable to STDs.

- See a doctor. If you think you might have an STD, go to your doctor right away. Ask your partner to get tested, too, so you won't pass STDs back and forth.

Source: American Social Health Association.

Comparing Selected Sexually Transmitted Diseases

Disease	Symptoms and Outlook	Complications	Diagnosis and Treatment
Syphilis Spirochete infection. Curable in early stages. Affects mainly those in their 20s. Transmitted by oral, genital, anal contact. After a decline, case numbers rising again in North America, mainly related to drug use or exchange of sex for drugs.	Painless sore (chancre) appears 3-6 weeks after infection on genitals, mouth or rectal area, most obvious in men, hardly noticed if vaginal. Heals without scarring. About 4-10 weeks later, 2nd stage: fever, rash, which disappears but may reappear.	If untreated, chronic, occasionally fatal. Third stage appears up to 30 years later with brain and spinal cord damage, blindness, insanity. Untreated, can cause miscarriage and birth defects; infants of infected mother may be born with syphilis (congenital syphilis).	Even if no symptoms, can diagnose by simple blood test; test results usually positive by time chancre (ulcer) appears. Antibiotics, taken as prescribed, a dependable cure in early stages.
Gonorrhea ("clap") Bacterial infection, transmitted by oral, vaginal, or anal sex. Prevalent in young women, teens. Untreated, can result in pelvic inflammatory disease (PID) and infertility. Up to half of women and men have no symptoms.	Symptoms (if any) within 7 days of contact: painful urination, thick vaginal or penile discharge, bleeding between periods, sore throat (if contracted via oral sex), rectal pain or discharge (if through anal sex).	May lead to tubal scarring, PID, ectopic pregnancy (outside womb, dangerous for mother). Can cause permanent sterility in both sexes. Eye infection and possible blindness in infected newborns.	Diagnosed by smear and lab culture. Antibiotics a reliable cure, but some strains now resistant to standard antibiotics (e.g., penicillin) so require *cefixime, ceftriaxone* or other new drugs.
Herpes Viral infection due to Herpes virus types I or II. Spreads via oral, vaginal, or anal sex, kissing. Can spread silently, via asymptomatic people. Most easily transmitted by direct contact with active sores or genital secretions.	Symptoms within 10 days: slight fever, tingling, shooting pains, swollen lymph glands, then painful blisters, anywhere on genitals — mainly penis, vulva, or anal areas. Subsides without treatment, but can recur. First outbreak usually worst, but sometimes unnoticed.	Virus remains permanently in nerves, stays dormant for months or years. Newborns may get herpes during birth, resulting in central nervous system damage or death. Caesarean delivery may be advised for babies of infected mothers.	Diagnosis from blisters (scraping or culture). *Acyclovir* tablets, not a cure, ease symptoms and reduce length of attack and its severity. Herpes support groups helpful in combatting psychological problems.
Chlamydia Bacterial infection, very common, in teens, 60%–80% without symptoms. Spreads via anal, vaginal, or oral sex with infected partners. Often occurs together with gonorrhea.	Like gonorrhea: painful urination, vaginal or penile discharge, abdominal pain, genital itching. But often mild, unnoticed in carriers, can disappear without treatment.	In women, leading cause of PID, ectopic pregnancy, infertility. In men, can produce urinary tract diseases and *prostatitis*. Babies of infected mothers prone to eye infections, pneumonia.	Diagnosed by culture or other tests. Antibiotic treatment a reliable cure (if caught early).
Genital Warts Caused by human papillomavirus (HPV). Highly contagious, spread by intimate bodily contact, especially sexual activity, often accompanies other STDs.	Warts — tiny flat growths on and around genitals — usually itchy, pinkish, flat, irregularly surfaced, may increase in size. Often undetectable in women in vagina or on cervix, except by physician.	Certain HPV strains linked to cervical cancer in women (and possibly penile cancer in men). Infants born to mothers with HPV may develop warts.	Removal advised — chemically, by freezing, or with lasers. Women should have regular Pap smears to detect HPV infection and early cervical cancer changes.
Hepatitis B Virus passed on via blood, semen, vaginal secretions, saliva, needles, razors, toothbrushes. Can go from mother to infant at birth. Groups most at risk: those practicing anal sex, those with many partners, injection drug users, babies of infected mothers.	Usually subclinical with few or no symptoms. Possibly flu-like malaise, fever, fatigue typically lasting 6 weeks, perhaps jaundice/skin and eye-white yellowing. May linger in body unnoticed.	60%-90% of infected children and 10% infected as adults become lifelong carriers, at risk of cirrhosis and liver cancer. Unsuspecting carriers can infect others. Fulminant, rapidly fatal form in one per 100 cases.	Detected by blood tests for viral markers. No cure. *Effective* safe vaccine recommended for all at risk — especially healthcare workers and those living with or close to known hepatitis B carriers.

Reprinted with permission from Health News. Health News is a bimonthly publication of the University of Toronto Faculty of Medicine. Subscriptions and back issues can be obtained by writing to *Health News*, 109 Vanderhoof Ave., Suite 205, Toronto, Ontario M4G 2H7 or by calling (416) 696-8818.

lot shorter than I thought it was going to be, and I may not be around to see my son, Andre, grow up and to see what happens to the baby Cookie and I are having in the summer of '92, and, of course, I may not have the long life I want with Cookie.[3]

2. Unless you are in a monogamous relationship and you know your partner is not infected (which you may never know for sure), practice safer sex every single time you have sex. This means you should use a latex condom from start to finish (before there is any sexual contact until after the penis is withdrawn) for each sexual act, including oral sex. Put the condom on as soon as the penis is erect; pinch it to allow a little extra space at the tip, but do not let any air get trapped in the condom. Roll it all the way to the base of the penis, and keep it all the way on until the penis is fully withdrawn. When withdrawing the penis from the vagina, hold the condom tight at the base of the penis to prevent leakage. Inspect the condom for tears. If damaged in some way, insert a spermicidal agent into the vagina.

If you think your partner should use a condom but refuses to do so, say no to sex with that person.

Many experts believe greater protection can be obtained by placing a small amount of the spermicide nonoxynol–9 inside the condom at its tip and then lubricating the outside with additional spermicide. Nonoxynol–9 is used to kill the man's sperm for birth control purposes. In test tubes, it has been shown to kill STD germs and HIV. This spermicide, however, should not be used in place of a condom because it will not offer the same protection as the condom does by itself.

3. Avoid having multiple and anonymous sexual partners. Anyone you have sex with could be infected with HIV.

4. Don't have sexual contact with anyone who does not practice safer sex.

5. Avoid sexual contact with anyone who has had sex with people at risk for getting HIV, even if they are now practicing safer sex.

6. Don't have sex with prostitutes.

7. If you do have sex with someone who might be infected with HIV or whose history is unknown to you, avoid exchange of body fluids.

8. Don't share toothbrushes, razors, or other implements that could become contaminated with blood with anyone who is, or who might be, infected with HIV.

9. Be cautious regarding procedures such as acupuncture, tattooing, and ear piercing, in which needles or other nonsterile instruments may be used again and again to pierce the skin or mucous membranes. These procedures are safe if proper sterilization methods or disposable needles are used. Before undergoing the procedure, ask what precautions are being taken.

10. If you are planning to undergo artificial insemination, insist on frozen sperm obtained from a laboratory that tests all donors for infection with HIV. Donors should be tested twice before accepting the sperm — once at the time of donation and again a few months later.

11. If you know you will be having surgery in the near future, and if you are able, consider donating blood for your own use. This will eliminate completely the already small risk of contracting HIV through a blood transfusion. It also will eliminate the more substantial risk for contracting other blood-borne diseases, such as hepatitis, from a transfusion.

Avoiding risky behaviors that destroy quality of life and life itself are critical components of a healthy lifestyle. Learning the facts so you can make responsible choices can protect you and those around you from startling and unexpected conditions. Preventing sexually transmitted diseases is a key to averting both physical and psychological damage.

NOTES

1. Unless otherwise noted, all the statistics regarding STDs are from the Centers for Disease Control and Prevention, Atlanta.

2. Dr. James Mason, Director, Centers for Disease Control and Prevention.

3. In his book, *What You Can Do to Avoid AIDS* (New York: Random House, 1991).

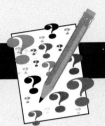

ASSESSMENT 14-1

How Much Do You Know About AIDS?

Name _____ Date _____ Grade _____

Instructor _____ Course _____ Section _____

		Yes	No
1.	AIDS is the end stage of infection caused by HIV.	_____	_____
2.	HIV is a chronic infectious disease that spreads among individuals who engage in risky behaviors such as unprotected sex or the sharing of hypodermic needles.	_____	_____
3.	AIDS now has a cure.	_____	_____
4.	Abstaining from sex is the only 100% sure way to protect yourself from HIV infection.	_____	_____
5.	Condoms are 100% effective in protecting you against HIV infection.	_____	_____
6.	If you're sexually active, latex condoms provide the best protection against HIV infection.	_____	_____
7.	Each year more and more teens are getting infected with HIV.	_____	_____
8.	You can become HIV-infected by donating blood.	_____	_____
9.	You can tell by looking at someone if he or she is HIV-infected.	_____	_____
10.	The only means to determine whether someone has HIV is through an HIV antibody test.	_____	_____
11.	HIV can completely destroy the immune system.	_____	_____
12.	The HIV virus may live in the body 10 years or longer before AIDS symptoms develop.	_____	_____
13.	People infected with HIV have AIDS.	_____	_____
14.	Once infected with HIV, a person never becomes uninfected.	_____	_____
15.	HIV infection is preventable.	_____	_____

Adapted from *Test Your Survival Smarts: Self-Quiz on Drugs and AIDS,* National Institute on Drug Abuse, U. S. Department of Health & Human Services; and *Principles and Labs for Physical Fitness and Wellness,* 3d edition, by Werner W. K. Hoeger and Sharon A. Hoeger (Englewood, CO: Morton Publishing, 1994), pp. 375–376.

Answers:

1. Yes. AIDS is the term used to define the manifestation of opportunistic diseases and cancers that occur as a result of HIV infection (also referred to as HIV disease).

2. Yes. People do not get HIV because of who they are but, rather, because of what they do. Almost all of the people who get HIV do so because they choose to engage in risky behaviors.

3. No. AIDS has no cure, and none seems likely soon.

4. No. Abstinence does protect a person from getting HIV infection from sex, but it can still be contracted by sharing hypodermic needles.

5. No. Only abstaining from sex gives you 100% protection, but condoms are effective in protecting against HIV infection if they're used correctly.

6. Yes. Proper use, however, is necessary to minimize the risk of infection.

7. Yes. In the early 1990s, the number of infected teens increased by 96% over a short span of 2 years. Probably about 20% of the AIDS patients today were infected as teenagers.

8. No. A myth regarding HIV is that it can be transmitted by donating blood. People cannot get HIV from giving blood. Health professionals use a new needle every time they draw blood. These needles are used only once and are destroyed and thrown away immediately after each individual has donated blood.

9. No. The symptoms of AIDS often are not noticeable until several years after a person has been infected with HIV.

10. Yes. Nobody can tell if an HIV infection exists unless an HIV antibody test is done. Upon HIV infection, the immune system's line of defense against the virus is to form antibodies that bind to the virus. On the average the body takes 3 months to manufacture enough antibodies to show up positive in an HIV antibody test. Sometimes it may take 6 months or longer.

11. Yes. The virus multiplies, attacks, and destroys white blood cells. These cells are part of the immune system, and their function is to fight off infections and diseases in the body. As the number of white blood cells killed increases, the body's immune system gradually breaks down and may be completely destroyed.

12. Yes. Up to 10 years may go by before the person develops AIDS.

13. No. Being HIV-positive does not necessarily mean the person has AIDS. On the average, it takes 7 to 8 years following infection before the individual develops the symptoms that fit the case definition of AIDS. From that point on, the person may live another 2 to 3 years. In essence, from the point of infection, the individual may have the chronic disease 8 to 10 years.

14. Yes. There is no second chance.

15. Yes. The best prevention technique is to abstain from sex until the time comes for a mutually monogamous sexual relationship. In the absence of sharing needles, that one behavior, according to Dr. James Mason, director of the Centers for Disease Control in Atlanta, will almost completely remove the risk of contracting HIV or developing any other sexually transmitted disease.

Nutritive Value of Selected Foods

Code	Food	Amount	Weight gm	Calories	Protein gm	Fat gm	Sat. Fat gm	Cholesterol mg	Carbohydrate gm	Calcium mg	Iron mg	Sodium mg	Vit A I.U.	Thiamin (Vit B_1) mg	Riboflavin (Vit B_2) mg	Niacin mg	Vit C mg
1.	Almond Joy, candy bar	1.5 oz.	42	227	2.5	12	10.2	0	28	3	1.2	0	0	0.00	0.00	0.0	0
2.	Almonds, shelled	1/4 c	36	213	6.6	19	1.4	0	9	83	1.7	2	0	0.09	0.33	1.3	0
3.	Apple, raw, unpared	1 med	150	80	0.3	1	0.0	0	20	10	0.4	1	120	0.04	0.03	0.1	6
4.	Apple juice, canned or bottled	1/2 c	124	59	0.1	0	0.0	0	15	8	0.7	1	0	0.01	0.03	0.1	1
5.	Apple Pie, McDonald's	1	307	260	2	15	10.0	6	30	0	0.48	240	0	0.06	0.00	0.0	12
6.	Applesauce, canned, sweetened	1/2 c	128	116	0.3	0	0.0	0	31	5	0.7	3	50	0.02	0.01	0.0	2
7.	Apricots, canned, heavy syrup	3 halves; 1¾ tbsp. liq.	85	73	0.5	0	0.0	0	19	9	0.3	1	1,480	0.02	0.02	0.3	3
8.	Apricots, dried, sulfured, uncooked	10 med halves	35	91	1.8	0	0.0	0	23	23	1.9	9	3,820	0.00	0.06	1.2	4
9.	Apricots, raw	3 (12 per lb)	114	55	1.1	0	0.0	0	14	18	0.5	1	2,890	0.06	0.04	0.6	11
10.	Arby Q, Arby's	1	190	389	18	15	5.5	29	48	84	6.1	1,268	0	0.27	0.41	9.2	0
11.	Arby Sauce, Arby's	.5 oz.	14	15	0	0	0.0	0	3	1	0.2	113	0	0.00	0.00	0.0	0
12.	Asparagus, cooked green spears	4 med	60	12	1.3	0	0.0	0	2	13	0.4	1	540	0.10	0.11	0.8	16
13.	Avocado, raw	1/2 med	120	185	2.4	19	3.2	0	7	11	0.6	4	310	0.12	0.22	1.7	15
14.	Bacon, cooked, drained	2 slices	15	86	3.8	8	2.7	30	1	2	0.5	153	0	0.08	0.05	0.8	0
15.	Bacon, lettuce, tomato sandwich	1	130	327	11.6	19	4.7	21	31	84	2.5	661	426	0.42	0.28	4.1	12
16.	Bagel	1½ in.	68	180	7.0	1	0.2	0	35	20	2.1	124	0	0.26	0.20	2.4	0
17.	Banana, raw	1 sm (7¼")	140	81	1.0	0	0.0	0	21	8	0.7	1	180	0.05	0.06	0.7	10
18.	Banana, nut bread	1 slice	50	169	3.0	8	1.5	33	22	18	0.9	172	49	0.09	0.09	0.8	0
19.	BBQ Sauce, McDonald's	1.12 oz.	32	50	1.0	0.6	0.2	0	12	0.0	0.0	350	0	0.00	0.00	0	2.4
20.	Beans, green snap, cooked	1/2 c	65	16	1.0	0	0.0	0	3	32	0.4	4	340	0.05	0.06	0.3	8
21.	Beans, lentils	1/4 c	50	53	3.9	0	0.0	0	10	12	1.0	0	10	0.03	0.04	0.4	0
22.	Beans, lima (Fordhook), froz., cooked	1/2 c	85	84	6.0	0	0.0	0	17	40	2.1	1	240	0.15	0.08	1.1	15
23.	Beans, red kidney, cooked	1 c	185	218	14.4	1	0.0	0	40	70	4.4	6	10	0.20	0.11	1.3	0
24.	Beans, refried	1/2 c	145	148	9.0	2	0.2	0	25	71	2.6	614	0	0.07	0.08	0.7	9
25.	Bean sprouts, mung, raw	1/2 c	52	18	2.0	0	0.0	0	4	11	0.7	3	10	0.07	0.07	0.4	10
26.	Beef, chuck, cooked	3 oz.	85	212	25.0	12	7.8	80	0	11	3.1	43	20	0.05	0.19	3.8	0
27.	Beef, corned, canned	3 oz.	85	163	21.0	10	8.0	70	0	22	5.0	802	0	0.02	0.27	3.9	0
28.	Beef, ground, lean	3 oz.	85	186	23.3	10	5.0	81	0	10	3.0	57	20	0.08	0.20	5.1	0
29.	Beef, lite roast deluxe, Arby's	1	182	294	18	10	3.5	42	33	156	3.0	826	200	0.27	0.52	8.4	8
30.	Beef, meatloaf	1 piece	111	246	20.0	15	6.1	125	6	37	2.4	434	181	0.08	0.23	4.1	1
491.	Beef, meatloaf, traditional Healthy Choice	1	340	320	16.0	8	4.0	35	46	40	1.8	460	750	0.00	0.00	0.0	54
31.	Beef N' Cheddar, Arby's	1	194	508	25	27	7.7	52	43	180	4.1	1,166	0	0.42	0.67	9.8	1
32.	Beef, round steak, cooked, trimmed	3 oz.	85	222	24.3	13	6.0	77	0	10	3.0	60	20	0.07	0.20	4.8	0
33.	Beef, rump roast	3 oz.	85	177	24.7	9	4.0	80	0	10	3.1	61	10	0.06	0.19	4.4	0
34.	Beef, sirloin, cooked	3 oz.	85	329	19.6	27	13.0	77	0	9	2.5	48	50	0.05	0.15	4.0	0
493.	Beef, sirloin tips, Healthy Choice	1	334	280	23.0	8	0.0	65	30	20	2.7	370	3,500	0.15	0.17	5.0	42
500.	Beef stroganoff, Weight Watchers	1	238	290	22.0	9	4.0	25	26	8	2.7	600	300	0.23	0.26	4.0	4
35.	Beef, T-bone steak	3 oz.	85	403	16.7	37	15.6	66	0	7	1.8	40	23	0.07	0.14	3.5	0
36.	Beef, thin, sliced	3 oz.	85	105	18.5	3	1.4	36	0	11	1.8	1,409	0	0.01	0.16	4.5	0
37.	Beer	12 fl. oz.	360	151	1.1	0	0.0	0	14	18	0.0	25	0	0.03	0.11	2.2	0
38.	Beer, light	12 fl. oz.	354	96	0.7	0	0.0	0	4	17	0.1	10	0	0.01	0.10	1.3	0
39.	Beets, red, canned, drained	1/2 c	80	32	0.8	0	0.0	0	8	15	0.6	164	15	0.01	0.02	0.1	2
40.	Beet greens, cooked	1/2 c	73	13	1.3	0	0.0	0	2	72	1.4	55	3,700	0.01	0.11	0.2	11
41.	Biscuits, baking powder	1 med	35	114	2.5	6	1.1	0	18	60	0.8	272	0	0.06	0.06	0.7	0
42.	Blueberries, fresh cultivated	1/2 c	73	45	0.5	0	0.0	0	11	10	0.8	1	75	0.02	0.05	0.4	10
43.	Bologna	1 slice (1 oz.)	28	86	3.4	8	3.0	15	1	7	0.5	369	0	0.05	0.06	0.7	0
44.	Bologna, turkey	2 slices	57	113	7.8	9	3.0	56	1	47	0.9	498	0	0.03	0.09	2.1	0
45.	Bouillon, broth	1 cube	4	5	0.8	0	0.0	0	0	0	0.0	960	0	0.00	0.00	0.0	0
46.	Brandy	1 oz.	28	69	0.0	0	0.0	0	0	0	0.0	1	0	0.00	0.00	0.0	0
47.	Bread, corn	1 slice	78	161	5.8	6	0.1	0	23	94	0.9	490	120	0.10	0.15	0.5	1
48.	Bread, cracked wheat	1 slice	25	65	2.3	1	0.2	0	12	16	0.7	106	0	0.10	0.10	0.8	0

Code	Food	Amount	Weight gm	Calories	Protein gm	Fat gm	Sat. Fat gm	Cholesterol mg	Carbohydrate gm	Calcium mg	Iron mg	Sodium mg	Vit A I.U.	Thiamin (Vit B₁) mg	Riboflavin (Vit B₂) mg	Niacin mg	Vit C mg
49.	Bread, French enriched	1 slice	35	102	3.2	1	0.2	0	19	15	0.8	203	0	0.10	0.08	0.9	0
50.	Bread, oatmeal	1 slice	25	65	2.1	1	0.2	0	12	15	0.7	124	0	0.12	0.07	0.9	0
51.	Bread, pita pocket	1 piece	60	165	6.2	1	0.1	0	33	49	1.5	339	0	0.27	0.13	2.3	0
52.	Bread, pumpernickel	1 slice	32	80	2.9	1	0.2	0	15	23	0.9	277	0	0.11	0.17	1.1	0
53.	Bread, rye (American)	1 slice	25	61	2.3	1	0.0	0	13	19	0.4	139	0	0.05	0.02	0.4	0
54.	Bread, white enriched	1 slice	25	68	2.2	1	0.2	0	13	21	0.6	127	0	0.06	0.05	0.6	0
55.	Bread, whole wheat	1 slice	25	61	2.6	1	0.6	0	12	25	0.8	132	0	0.06	0.03	0.7	0
56.	Broccoli, cooked drained	1 sm stalk	140	36	4.3	0	0.0	0	6	123	1.1	14	3,500	0.13	0.28	1.1	126
57.	Broccoli, raw	1 sm stalk	114	38	4.1	0	0.0	0	7	117	1.3	17	2,835	0.10	0.23	0.9	125
58.	Brownies, with nuts		20	95	1.3	6	2.3	18	11	9	0.4	51	20	0.05	0.05	0.3	0
59.	Brussels sprouts, froz., cooked, drained	1/2 c	78	28	3.2	0	0.0	0	5	25	0.8	8	405	0.06	0.11	0.5	63
60.	Bulgur, wheat	1 c	135	227	8.4	1	0.0	0	47	27	1.8	809	0	0.07	0.04	3.2	0
61.	Burrito, bean	1	166	307	12.5	9.5	3.6	14	45	173	2.4	983	283	0.15	0.22	2.3	5
62.	Burrito, combination, Taco Bell	1	175	404	21.0	16	5.9	17	43	91	3.7	300	1,666	0.34	0.31	4.6	15
482.	Burrito, 7 layer, Taco Bell	1	234	458	14.0	20	5.9	8	55	85	2.3	983	1,485	0.00	0.00	0.0	5
483.	Burrito, 7 layer light, Taco Bell	1	276	440	19.0	9	3.5	8	67	250	4.5	1,430	1,750	0.00	0.00	0.0	5
63.	Butter	1 tsp	5	36	0.0	4	0.4	12	0	1	0.0	46	160	0.00	0.00	0.0	0
64.	Buttermilk, cultured	1 c	245	88	8.8	0	1.3	5	12	296	0.1	319	10	0.10	0.44	0.2	2
65.	Cabbage, boiled, drained wedge	1/2 c	85	16	0.9	0	0.0	0	3	36	0.3	10	100	0.02	0.02	0.1	21
66.	Cabbage, raw chopped	1/2 c	45	11	0.6	0	0.0	0	3	22	0.2	9	60	0.03	0.03	0.2	21
67.	Cake, angel food, plain	1 piece	60	161	4.3	0	0.0	0	36	5	0.1	170	0	0.01	0.08	0.1	0
68.	Cake, carrot	1 piece	96	385	4.2	21	4.1	74	48	44	1.3	279	75	0.11	0.12	0.9	1
69.	Cake, cheesecake	1 piece (3½")	85	257	4.6	16	9.0	150	24	48	0.4	189	216	0.03	0.11	0.4	4
70.	Cake, chocolate, w/icing	1 piece	69	235	3.0	8	3.6	37	40	41	1.4	181	100	0.07	0.10	0.6	0
71.	Cake, coffee	1 piece	72	230	4.5	7	2.5	47	38	44	1.2	310	120	0.14	0.15	1.3	0
72.	Cake, devil's food, iced	1 piece	99	365	4.5	16	5.0	68	55	69	1.0	233	160	0.02	0.10	0.2	0
73.	Cake, pound	1 piece	30	120	2.0	5	1.0	32	15	20	0.5	98	200	0.05	0.06	0.5	0
74.	Cake, white, choc. icing	1 piece	71	268	3.5	11	3.7	2	48	35	0.3	162	40	0.19	0.14	1.6	0
75.	Candy, hard	1 oz.	28	109	0.0	0	0.0	0	28	6	0.5	9	0	0.00	0.00	0.0	0
76.	Cantaloupe	1/4 melon 5" diam.	239	35	2.0	0	0.0	0	10	20	0.8	17	4,620	0.06	0.04	0.6	45
77.	Caramel (candy, plain or choc.)	1 oz.	28	113	1.1	3	1.6	0	22	42	0.4	64	0	0.01	0.05	0.1	0
78.	Carrots, cooked, drained	1/2 c	73	23	0.7	0	0.0	0	5	24	0.5	10	7,615	0.04	0.04	0.4	5
79.	Carrots, raw	1 carrot 7½" long	81	30	0.8	0	0.0	0	7	27	0.5	34	7,930	0.04	0.04	0.4	6
80.	Cashew, roasted, unsalted	2 oz.	57	326	9.2	27	5.4	0	16	23	2.3	10	0	0.24	0.10	1.0	0
81.	Cauliflower, cooked, drained	1/2 c	63	14	1.5	0	0.0	0	3	13	0.5	6	40	0.06	0.05	0.4	35
82.	Celery, green, raw, long	1 outer stalk 8"	40	7	0.4	0	0.0	0	2	16	0.1	50	110	0.01	0.01	0.1	4
83.	Cereal, All-Bran	1/4 c	21	53	3.0	1	0.1	0	16	17	3.4	242	947	0.28	0.33	3.8	11
84.	Cereal, Alpha Bits	1/2 c	28	111	2.2	1	0.0	0	25	8	1.8	219	1,875	0.40	0.40	5.0	0
85.	Cereal, Bran	1/2 c	30	72	3.8	1	0.0	0	22	25	3.0	247	2,000	1.00	0.80	3.0	20
86.	Cereal, Cheerios	1 c	23	89	3.4	1	1.2	0	16	38	3.6	246	949	0.32	0.32	4.0	12
87.	Cereal, Corn Chex	1 c	28	111	2.0	0	0.1	0	25	3	1.8	271	75	0.40	0.07	5.0	15
88.	Cereal, Corn Flakes	1 c	25	97	2.0	0	0.0	0	21	3	0.6	251	180	0.29	0.55	2.9	9
89.	Cereal, Cream of Wheat	1 c	244	140	3.6	1	0.1	0	29	54	10.9	5	0	0.24	0.07	1.5	0
90.	Cereal, Frosted Mini-Wheats	4 biscuits	31	111	3.2	0	0.0	0	26	10	2.0	9	2,050	0.40	0.50	5.5	16
91.	Cereal, Fruit & Fibre w/dates	1 c	56	180	6.0	2	0.3	0	42	20	9.0	340	3,780	0.75	0.85	10.0	0
92.	Cereal, Granola, Nature Valley	1/2 c	57	252	5.8	10	7.0	0	38	36	1.9	116	41	0.20	0.10	0.4	0
93.	Cereal, Grape Nuts	1/2 c	57	202	6.6	0	0.0	0	47	22	2.5	394	3,815	0.80	0.80	10.0	0
94.	Cereal, Life	1 c	44	162	8.1	1	0.1	0	32	154	11.6	229	2,915	0.95	1.00	11.6	0
95.	Cereal, Nutri-Grain Wheat	1 c	44	158	3.8	1	0.1	0	37	12	1.2	299	0	0.60	0.70	7.7	23
96.	Cereal, Oatmeal, quick, cooked	1/2 c	120	66	2.4	1	0.2	0	12	11	0.7	262	0	0.10	0.03	0.1	0
97.	Cereal, Raisin Bran	1 c	49	160	4.0	1	0.2	0	40	25	24.0	293	2,500	0.51	0.57	6.7	11
98.	Cereal, Rice Krispies	3/4 c	22	85	1.4	0	0.0	0	19	3	1.4	255	971	0.30	0.30	3.8	0
99.	Cereal, Shredded Wheat	1 c	19	65	2.1	0	0.0	0	11	8	0.6	1	0	0.06	0.05	0.9	0

Code	Food	Amount	Weight gm	Calories	Protein gm	Fat gm	Sat. Fat gm	Cholesterol mg	Carbohydrate gm	Calcium mg	Iron mg	Sodium mg	Vit A I.U.	Thiamin (Vit B₁) mg	Riboflavin (Vit B₂) mg	Niacin mg	Vit C mg
100.	Cereal, Special K	1 c	21	83	4.2	0	0.0	0	16	6	3.4	199	1,430	0.30	0.30	3.8	11
101.	Cereal, Sugar Corn Pops	1 c	28	108	1.4	0	0.0	0	26	1	1.8	103	1,875	0.40	0.40	5.0	15
102.	Cereal, Sugar Frosted Flakes	1 c	35	133	1.8	0	0.0	0	32	1	2.2	284	2,315	0.50	0.50	6.2	19
103.	Cereal, Sugar Smacks	1 c	37	141	2.7	1	0.1	0	32	4	2.4	100	2,500	0.49	0.57	6.7	20
104.	Cereal, Total	1 c	33	116	3.3	1	0.1	0	26	56	21.0	409	8,845	1.70	2.00	23.3	70
105.	Cereal, Wheat Chex	1 c	46	169	4.5	1	0.2	0	38	18	7.3	308	0	0.60	0.17	8.1	24
106.	Cereal, whole wheat, cooked	1/2 c	123	55	2.2	0	0.0	0	12	9	0.06	260	0	0.08	0.03	0.8	0
107.	Cereal, whole wheat flakes, ready-to-eat	1 c	30	106	3.1	1	0.0	0	24	12	2.0	310	1,410	0.35	0.42	3.5	11
108.	Cereal, 40% Bran Flakes	1 c	39	125	4.9	1	0.1	0	31	19	11.2	363	2,610	0.51	0.59	6.9	0
109.	Cereal, 100% Bran	1/2 c	33	89	4.2	2	0.3	0	24	23	4.1	229	0	0.80	0.90	10.4	31
110.	Champagne	4 oz.	113	87	0.2	0	0.1	0	2	6	0.4	7	0	0.00	0.01	0.1	0
111.	Cheese, American	1 oz. slice	28	100	6.0	8	5.6	27	1	188	0.1	307	343	0.01	0.10	0.0	0
112.	Cheese, bleu	1 oz.	28	100	6.0	8	5.3	25	1	89	0.1	510	204	0.01	0.11	0.3	0
113.	Cheese, cheddar	1 oz.	28	114	7.0	9	6.0	30	0	204	0.2	171	300	0.01	0.11	0.0	0
114.	Cheese, cottage, 2%	1/2 c	113	103	15.5	2	1.4	10	4	78	0.2	459	79	0.03	0.21	0.2	0
115.	Cheese, cottage, creamed	1/2 c	105	112	14.0	5	6.4	15	3	99	0.3	241	180	0.03	0.26	0.1	0
116.	Cheese, creamed	1 oz.	28	99	6.0	8	3.0	31	1	167	0.3	71	320	0.02	0.14	0.0	0
117.	Cheese, feta	1 oz.	28	75	4.5	6	4.2	25	1	140	0.2	316	180	0.04	0.23	0.3	0
118.	Cheese, monterey jack	1 oz.	28	106	6.9	9	5.4	26	0	212	0.2	152	405	0.00	0.11	0.0	0
119.	Cheese, mozzarella, skim	1 oz.	28	80	7.6	5	3.1	15	1	207	0.1	150	216	0.01	0.10	0.0	0
120.	Cheese, parmesan	1 tbsp	5	23	2.1	2	1.0	4	0	69	0.1	93	45	0.00	0.02	0.0	0
121.	Cheese, ricotta, part skim	1 oz.	28	39	3.2	2	1.4	9	1	77	0.1	35	160	0.01	0.05	0.0	0
122.	Cheese, souffle	1 portion	110	240	10.9	19	9.5	189	7	221	1.1	400	880	0.06	0.26	0.2	0
123.	Cheese, swiss	1 oz.	28	107	8.0	8	5.0	26	1	272	0.1	74	360	0.01	0.10	0.0	0
124.	Cheese puffs, Cheetos	1 oz.	28	158	2.2	10	4.8	5	14	17	0.4	344	130	0.01	0.03	0.2	0
125.	Cheeseburger, McDonald's	1	115	321	15.2	16	6.7	40	29	170	2.9	736	353	0.30	0.24	4.4	2
126.	Cherries	10	75	47	0.9	0	0.0	0	12	15	0.3	8	450	0.20	0.24	1.6	41
127.	Chicken, BK Broiler sandwich, Burger King	1 sandwich	168	379	24.0	18	3.0	53	31	48	2.3	764	350	0.42	0.22	9.2	5
128.	Chicken Breast Filet, Arby's	1	204	445	22	23.0	3.0	45	52	72	1.9	958	0	0.23	0.58	9.0	5
129.	Chicken breast, roast w/skin	1	98	193	29.2	8	2.1	83	0	14	1.0	69	91	0.07	0.12	12.5	0
501.	Chicken burrito w/vegetables, Weight Watchers	1	216	330	15.0	14	4.0	65	36	56	2.3	800	190	0.52	0.39	5.9	3
484.	Chicken cacciatore, Budget Gourmet	1	312	300	20.0	13	0.0	60	27	150	1.8	810	200	0.23	0.51	5.0	21
496.	Chicken cacciatore, Lean Cuisine	1	308	280	22.0	7	2.0	45	31	40	1.4	570	500	0.22	0.17	6.0	9
130.	Chicken chow mein	1 c	250	255	31.0	11	3.6	75	10	58	2.5	718	250	0.08	0.23	4.3	10
488.	Chicken chow mein, Healthy Choice	1	241	220	18.0	3	0.8	45	31	20	1.4	440	405	0.15	0.14	4.0	4
497.	Chicken chow mein, Lean Cuisine	1	255	240	14.0	5	1.0	30	34	40	1.1	530	300	0.15	0.17	5.0	6
502.	Chicken chow mein, Weight Watchers	1	255	200	12.0	2	0.5	25	34	40	0.7	430	1,500	0.00	0.00	0.0	36
131.	Chicken club sandwich, Wendy's	1	220	520	30	25	6.0	75	44	120	9.6	980	100	0.60	0.45	16.0	9
132.	Chicken Cordon Bleu, Arby's	1	225	518	30	27	5.3	92	52	204	2.1	1,463	0	0.42	0.68	10.2	5
133.	Chicken, drumstick, Kentucky Fried	1	54	136	14.0	8	2.2	73	2	20	0.9	320	30	0.04	0.12	2.7	0
134.	Chicken, drumstick, roasted	1	52	112	14.1	6	1.6	48	0	6	0.7	47	52	0.04	0.11	3.1	0
135.	Chicken McNuggets	6	111	329	19.5	21	5.2	64	15	11	1.3	521	92	0.16	0.14	7.7	2
136.	Chicken Nuggets, Wendy's	6 pc.	94	280	14	20	5.0	50	12	48	0.48	600	0	0.09	0.11	6.0	0
137.	Chicken, patty sandwich	1	157	436	24.8	23	6.1	68	34	44	1.9	2,732	47	0.13	0.26	9.2	4
138.	Chicken, wing, Kentucky Fried	1	45	151	11.0	10	2.9	70	4	0	0.6	300	0	0.03	0.07	9.2	0
139.	Chicken, roast, light meat without skin	3 oz.	85	141	27.0	3	0.4	45	0	10	1.2	54	51	0.03	0.09	9.9	0

Code	Food	Amount	Weight gm	Calories	Protein gm	Fat gm	Sat. Fat gm	Cholesterol mg	Carbohydrate gm	Calcium mg	Iron mg	Sodium mg	Vit A I.U.	Thiamin (Vit B_1) mg	Riboflavin (Vit B_2) mg	Niacin mg	Vit C mg
140.	Chicken, roast, dark meat without skin	3 oz.	85	149	24.0	5	0.8	50	0	11	1.5	54	127	0.06	0.19	4.7	0
141.	Chicken, Roast Deluxe, Arby's	1	195	276	24	7	1.7	33	33	156	1.9	777	200	0.44	0.80	9.4	7
510.	Chicken, Rotisserie, dark w/skin, Kentucky Fried	1/4 chicken	146	333	30.0	24	6.6	163	1	10	0.2	980	75	0.00	0.00	0.0	1
511.	Chicken, Rotisserie, light w/skin, Kentucky Fried	1/4 chicken	176	335	40.0	19	5.4	157	1	10	0.2	1,100	75	0.00	0.00	0.0	1
142.	Chicken Sandwich, breaded, Wendy's	1	208	450	26	20	4.0	60	44	120	9.6	740	100	0.45	0.36	14.0	6
143.	Chicken Sandwich, Grilled, Wendy's	1	177	290	24	7	1.0	60	35	120	2.4	670	100	0.38	0.27	10.0	6
144.	Chicken Sandwich, McChicken	1	187	415	19	19	9.0	50	39	180	1.8	830	100	0.90	0.18	9.0	2.4
485.	Chicken, Teriyaki, Budget Gourmet	1	340	360	20.0	12	0.0	55	44	80	1.4	610	1,500	0.15	0.34	6.0	12
145.	Chili con carne	1 c	255	339	19.1	16	5.8	28	31	82	4.3	1,354	150	0.08	0.18	3.3	8
146.	Chocolate fudge	1 oz.	28	115	0.6	3	2.1	1	21	22	0.3	54	0	0.01	0.03	0.1	0
147.	Chocolate, milk	1 oz.	28	147	2.0	9	3.6	5	16	65	0.3	27	80	0.02	0.10	0.1	0
148.	Chocolate, milk w/almonds	1 oz.	28	150	2.9	10	4.4	5	15	61	0.6	23	30	0.03	0.13	0.3	0
149.	Clam, canned, drained	3 oz.	85	83	13.0	2	0.2	50	2	46	3.5	750	93	0.01	0.09	0.9	9
150.	Cocoa, hot, with whole milk	1 c	250	218	9.1	9	6.1	33	26	298	0.8	123	318	0.10	0.44	0.4	2
151.	Cocoa, plain, dry	1 tbsp	5	14	0.9	1	0.0	0	3	7	0.6		0	0.01	0.02	0.1	0
152.	Coconut, shredded, packed	1/2 c	65	225	2.3	23	20.0	0	6	8	1.1	165	0	0.03	0.01	0.3	2
153.	Cod, batter fried	3.5 oz.	100	199	19.6	10	3.9	55	8	80	0.5	100	2	0.02	0.02	1.8	0
154.	Cod, cooked	3 oz.	85	144	24.3	4	1.5	60	0	27	0.9	63	150	0.06	0.09	2.7	0
155.	Cod, poached	3.5 oz.	100	94	20.9	1	0.3	60	0	29	0.5	110	2	0.08	0.08	3.0	0
156.	Coffee	3/4 cup	180	1	0.0	0	0.0	0	0	1	0.2	2	0	0.00	0.00	0.1	0
157.	Coleslaw	1 c	120	173	1.6	17	1.0	5	6	53	0.5	144	190	0.06	0.06	0.4	35
158.	Collards, leaves without stems, cooked, drained	1/2 c	95	32	3.4	1	2.0	0	5	178	0.8	28	7,410	0.01	0.19	1.2	72
159.	Cookies, chocolate chip, homemade	2 2¼" diam.	20	103	1.0	6	1.7	14	12	7	0.4	70	20	0.02	0.02	0.2	0
160.	Cookies, fig bars	4 bars	56	210	2.0	4	1.0	27	42	40	1.4	180	31	0.08	0.07	0.7	0
161.	Cookies, oatmeal raisin	2 2" diam.	26	122	1.5	5	1.3	1	18	9	0.6	74	20	0.04	0.04	0.5	0
162.	Cookies, peanut butter, homemade	2 cookies	24	123	2.0	7	2.0	11	14	10	0.5	71	12	0.03	0.03	0.9	0
163.	Cookies, sandwich, all	4 cookies	40	195	2.0	8	2.0	0	29	12	1.4	189	0	0.90	0.07	0.8	0
164.	Cookies, shortbread	4 cookies	32	155	2.0	8	2.9	27	20	13	0.8	123	40	0.10	0.09	0.9	0
165.	Cookies, vanilla	5 1¾" diam.	20	93	1.0	3	0.8	10	15	8	0.1	50	25	0.00	0.01	0.0	0
166.	Cookies, vanilla wafers	10 wafers	40	185	2.0	7	1.8	25	29	16	0.8	150	70	0.07	0.10	1.0	0
167.	Corn, boiled on cob	1 ear 5" long	140	70	2.5	1	0.0	0	16	2	0.5	1	310	0.09	0.08	1.1	7
168.	Corn, canned, drained	1/2 c	83	70	2.2	1	0.0	0	16	4	0.4	195	290	0.03	0.04	0.8	4
169.	Corn chips	1 oz.	28	155	2.0	9	1.8	0	16	35	0.5	233	110	0.04	0.05	0.4	1
170.	Cornmeal, degermed, yellow, enriched, cooked	1/2 c	120	60	1.3	0	0.0	0	13	1	0.5	264	70	0.07	0.05	0.6	0
171.	Crab, canned	1 c	135	135	23.0	3	0.5	135	1	61	1.1	1,350	70	0.11	0.11	2.6	0
172.	Crackers, cheese	10 crackers	10	50	1.0	3	0.9	6	5	11	0.4	112	25	0.05	0.04	0.4	0
173.	Crackers, graham	2 squares	14	55	1.1	1	0.3	0	10	6	0.2	95	0	0.01	0.03	0.2	0
174.	Crackers, Ritz	1 cracker	3	15	0.2	1	0.2	0	2	3	0.1	30	0	0.01	0.01	0.1	0
175.	Crackers, Ryewafers, whole grain	2 crackers	14	55	1.0	1	0.3	0	10	7	0.5	115	0	0.06	0.03	0.5	0
176.	Crackers, saltines	4 squares	11	48	1.0	1	0.3	0	8	2	0.1	123	0	0.00	0.00	0.1	0
177.	Crackers, soda	1	3	13	0.3	0	0.1	0	2	1	0.1	39	0	0.02	0.01	0.1	0
178.	Crackers, Triscuits	5	5	23	0.4	1	0.3	0	3	0	0.0	0	0	0.00	0.00	0.0	0
179.	Crackers, Wheat Thins	1	2	9	0.2	0	0.1	0	1	0	0.1	17	0	0.00	0.01	0.1	0
180.	Cranberry juice	1 c	253	145	0.1	0	0.0	0	36	8	0.4	5	5	0.02	0.02	0.1	90

Code	Food	Amount	Weight gm	Calories	Protein gm	Fat gm	Sat. Fat gm	Cholesterol mg	Carbohydrate gm	Calcium mg	Iron mg	Sodium mg	Vit A I.U.	Thiamin (Vit B₁) mg	Riboflavin (Vit B₂) mg	Niacin mg	Vit C mg
181.	Cream, light coffee or table	1 tbsp	15	20	0.5	2	0.5	5	1	16	0.0	7	70	0.00	0.02	0.0	0
182.	Cream, heavy whipping	1 tbsp	15	53	0.3	6	1.3	12	1	11	0.0	5	230	0.00	0.02	0.0	0
183.	Croissant	1 roll	57	235	4.7	12	4.0	13	27	20	2.1	452	50	0.17	0.13	1.3	0
184.	Croissants (Sara Lee)	1 roll	18	59	1.6	2	0.3	0	8	22	0.6	105	0	0.14	0.09	0.8	0
185.	Croissan'wich, egg, cheese Burger King	1 sandwich	110	315	13.0	20	7.0	222	19	112	1.8	607	500	0.22	0.37	1.4	0
186.	Cucumbers, raw pared	9 sm slices	28	4	0.3	0	0.0	0	1	7	0.3	2	70	0.01	0.01	0.1	3
187.	Danish, Apple, McDonald's	1	115	390	6	17	11.0	25	51	0	1.0	370	0	0.30	0.18	2.0	15
188.	Danish, Cinnamon Raisin	1	110	440	6	21	13.0	34	58	48	0.12	430	0	0.30	0.27	3.0	4
189.	Dates hydrated	5	46	110	0.9	0	0.0	0	29	24	1.2	1	20	0.04	0.04	0.9	0
190.	Doughnut, plain	1	42	164	1.9	8	2.0	19	22	17	0.6	210	30	0.07	0.07	0.5	0
191.	Doughnut, yeast raised	1	27	235	4.0	13	5.2	21	26	17	1.4	222	2	0.28	0.12	1.8	0
192.	Dressing, Bleu cheese	1 tbsp	15	77	0.7	8	1.9	4	1	12	0.0	8	32	0.00	0.02	0.0	0
193.	Dressing, French	1 tbsp	16	83	0.1	9	1.4	0	2	2	0.1	184	0	0.00	0.00	0.0	0
194.	Dressing, French, low cal	1 tbsp.	15	24	0.0	2	0.2	0	2	6	0.1	306	0	0.00	0.00	0.0	0
195.	Dressing, Italian	1 tbsp.	15	69	0.1	9	1.3	0	2	1	0.0	73	29	0.00	0.00	0.0	0
196.	Dressing, Italian, low cal	1 tbsp.	15	10	0.0	1	0.9	0	1	1	0.0	136	1	0.00	0.00	0.0	0
197.	Dressing, Ranch style	1 tbsp.	15	54	0.4	6	1.0	6	1	15	0.0	65	36	0.01	0.02	0.0	1
198.	Dressing, Thousand island	1 tbsp.	15	60	0.2	6	0.2	4	2	2	0.1	110	75	0.00	0.01	0.0	0
199.	Dressing, Thousand island, low cal	1 tbsp.	15	25	0.1	2	1.6	2	3	2	0.1	153	70	0.00	0.00	0.0	0
200.	Egg, hard cooked	1 large	50	72	6.0	5	2.4	212	1	24	1.0	113	520	0.05	0.13	0.0	0
201.	Egg, fried with butter	1	46	95	5.4	7	5.9	240	1	28	0.9	162	320	0.04	0.13	0.0	0
202.	Egg McMuffin	1	138	327	18.5	15	3.9	259	31	226	2.9	885	591	0.47	0.44	3.8	1
203.	Egg salad sandwich	1	111	325	10.0	19	3.0	215	28	95	2.5	461	242	0.29	0.29	2.1	0
204.	Egg, scrambled, with milk, butter	1 egg	64	95	6.0	7	3.0	244	1	54	0.9	176	510	0.04	0.18	0.0	0
205.	Egg, white	1 large	33	17	3.6	0	0.0	0	0	3	0.0	48	0	0.00	0.09	0.0	0
206.	Egg, yolk, raw	1 yolk	17	63	2.8	5	1.6	212	0	26	0.9	8	390	0.04	0.07	0.0	0
207.	Enchilada, beef	1	200	487	21.8	23	8.8	63	26	425	2.9	262	595	0.02	0.27	3.5	5
208.	Enchilada, cheese	1	230	632	25.3	34	17.6	82	31	876	2.6	596	1,672	0.13	0.40	1.2	15
209.	Figs, dried	1 large	21	60	1.0	0	0.0	0	15	26	0.6	1	20	0.16	0.17	3.9	0
210.	Filet of Fish, McDonald's	1	131	402	15.0	23	7.9	43	34	105	1.8	709	152	0.28	0.28	3.9	4
489.	Fish, fillet, florentine, Healthy Choice	1	273	220	26.0	7	3.0	65	13	150	0.7	590	2,500	0.15	0.34	2.0	1
211.	Fish sandwich, Wendy's	1	182	460	16	25	5.0	55	42	120	1.8	780	0	0.60	0.45	4.0	1
494.	Fish, Sole Au Gratin, Healthy Choice	1	312	270	16.0	5	0.0	60	40	80	1.1	470	0	0.23	0.17	1.6	6
212.	Fish, sticks	2	56	140	12.0	6	1.6	52	8	22	0.6	106	40	0.06	0.10	1.2	0
213.	Flounder	3 oz.	85	171	25.5	7	1.0	55	0	21	1.2	201	0	0.06	0.06	2.1	3
214.	Flour, all purpose enriched	1 c	125	455	13.0	1	0.0	0	95	20	3.6	3	0	0.55	0.33	4.4	0
215.	Flour, whole wheat	1 c	120	400	16.0	2	0.0	0	85	49	4.0	4	0	0.66	0.14	5.2	0
216.	Frankfurter, cooked	1	57	176	7.0	16	5.6	45	1	4	1.1	627	0	0.09	0.11	1.5	0
217.	Frankfurter, turkey, cooked	1	45	102	6.4	8	2.7	39	1	58	0.8	454	60	0.04	0.08	1.7	0
218.	French Dip, Arby's	1	154	368	22	15	5.6	43	35	60	2.8	1,018	285	0.20	0.50	8.4	0
219.	French toast	1 piece	65	123	4.9	4	1.1	73	15	79	1.1	189	0	0.15	0.17	1.1	0
220.	Fries, Curly, Arby's	1 small	99	337	4	18	7.4	0	43	24	1.0	167	370	0.06	0.07	2.0	0
221.	Fruit cocktail	1 c	245	91	1.0	0	0.0	0	24	22	1.0	12	380	0.05	0.02	1.2	5
222.	Fruit cocktail, juice pack	1 c	248	115	1.1	0	0.0	0	29	20	0.5	10	10	0.03	0.04	1.0	7
223.	Grapefruit juice, raw white	1/2 med	301	56	0.6	0	0.0	0	15	11	0.5	1	10	0.05	0.03	0.3	52
224.	Grapefruit juice, unsweet. canned	1/2 c	124	50	0.3	0	0.0	0	12	11	0.2	2	50	0.05	0.03	0.3	46
225.	Grapes, seedless, European	10 grapes	50	34	0.3	0	0.0	0	9	6	0.2	3	0	0.03	0.03	0.2	2
226.	Grape juice, unsweetened bottled	1/2 c	127	84	0.3	0	0.0	0	21	14	0.4	3	0	0.05	0.03	0.3	0
227.	Gravy, beef, homemade	1 tbsp	17	19	0.3	2	1.0	1	1	1	0.1	49	0	0.01	0.01	0.2	0

Code	Food	Amount	Weight gm	Calories	Protein gm	Fat gm	Sat. Fat gm	Cholesterol mg	Carbohydrate gm	Calcium mg	Iron mg	Sodium mg	Vit A I.U.	Thiamin (Vit B₁) mg	Riboflavin (Vit B₂) mg	Niacin mg	Vit C mg
228.	Haddock, fried (dipped in egg, milk, bread crumbs)	3 oz.	85	141	17.0	5	1.0	54	5	33	0.9	150	0	0.03	0.06	2.7	3
229.	Halibut, broiled with butter or margarine	3 oz.	85	144	21.0	6	2.1	55	0	15	0.6	114	570	0.03	0.06	7.2	1
230.	Ham (cured pork)	3 oz.	85	318	20.0	26	9.4	77	0	9	2.6	48	0	0.43	0.20	3.8	0
231.	Ham, lunch meat	1 slice	28	37	5.5	1	0.5	13	.3	2	0.2	405	0	0.26	0.06	1.4	7
508.	Hamburger, Arch Deluxe, McDonalds	1	242	560	27.0	32	11.0	90	42	120	3.0	960	650	0.40	0.43	7.5	3
509.	Hamburger, Arch Deluxe w/bacon, McDonalds	1	253	610	31.0	36	13.0	105	42	120	3.7	1,190	650	0.40	0.43	7.5	3
232.	Hamburger, Big Classic, Wendy's	1	251	480	27	23	7.0	75	44	180	4.2	850	300	0.45	0.27	7.0	3
233.	Hamburger, Big Mac	1	204	581	25.1	36	12.0	85	40	207	5.0	999	388	0.49	0.39	7.3	12
234.	Hamburger bun	1 bun	40	129	3.7	2	1.0	0	23	61	1.3	271	2	0.22	0.15	1.8	0
235.	Hamburger, Jr. Bacon Cheeseburger, Wendy's	1	170	440	22	25	8.0	65	33	240	3.0	870	300	0.45	0.27	6.0	9
236.	Hamburger, McDonald's	1	99	257	13.0	9	3.7	26	30	63	3.0	526	231	0.23	0.23	5.1	2
237.	Hamburger, Mclean Deluxe	1	206	320	22	10	5.0	60	35	180	2.4	670	500	0.38	0.36	7.0	6
238.	Hamburger, Mclean Deluxe, w/cheese	1	219	370	24	14	8.0	75	35	240	2.4	890	750	0.38	0.36	7.0	6
239.	Hamburger, Quarter pounder	1 burger	160	427	24.6	24	9.1	80	29	98	4.3	718	115	0.35	0.32	7.2	3
240.	Hamburger, Quarter pounder, with cheese	1 burger	186	525	29.6	32	12.8	107	31	255	4.8	1,195	640	0.37	0.41	7.1	3
241.	Hamburger, Wendy's	1	219	440	26	23	7.0	75	36	120	3.6	850	300	0.38	0.18	7.0	9
242.	Ham N' Cheese, Arby's	1	169	355	25	14	5.1	55	35	204	1.8	1400	0	0.83	0.40	7.8	0
243.	Honey	1 tbsp	21	64	0.0	0	0.0	0	17	1	0.1	1	0	0.00	0.01	0.1	0
244.	Honeydew melon	1 slice (1/10 melon)	129	45	0.6	0	0.0	0	12	8	0.1	13	25	0.10	0.02	0.8	32
245.	Horsey Sauce, Arby's	.5 oz.	14	55	0	5	2.0	0	3	24	0.0	105	0	0.00	0.00	0.0	0
246.	Hotcakes w/Margarine & Syrup, McDonald's	1 serving	174	440	8	12	5.0	8	74	120	1.2	685	200	0.30	0.36	3.0	0
247.	Hotdog bun	1 bun	40	115	3.3	2	1.0	0	20	54	1.2	241	2	0.20	0.13	1.6	0
248.	Ice cream, vanilla	1/2 c	67	135	3.0	7	4.4	27	14	97	0.1	42	295	0.03	0.14	0.1	1
249.	Ice cream cone	1 small	115	185	4.3	5	2.2	24	30	183	0.1	109	218	0.06	0.36	0.4	1
250.	Ice cream cone, Dairy Queen	medium	142	230	6.0	7	4.6	15	35	200	0.0	150	300	0.09	0.26	0.0	0
251.	Ice cream, hot fudge sundae	1	164	357	7.0	11	5.4	27	58	215	0.6	170	233	0.07	0.31	1.1	2
252.	Ice milk, vanilla	1/2 c	61	100	3.0	3	1.8	13	15	102	0.1	45	140	0.04	0.15	0.1	1
253.	Instant breakfast, whole milk	1 c	281	280	15.0	8	5.1	33	34	301	8.0	286	2,057	0.39	0.46	5.2	29
254.	Instant breakfast, skim milk	1 c	282	216	15.4	0	0.0	4	35	312	8.0	292	1,635	0.39	0.41	5.2	29
255.	Jams or preserves	1 tbsp	7	18	0.0	0	0.0	0	5	1	0.1	1	1	0.00	0.00	0.0	0
256.	Jelly	1 tbsp	18	49	0.0	0	0.0	0	13	4	0.3	3	0	0.00	0.01	0.0	1
257.	Kale, fresh cooked, drained	1/2 c	55	22	2.5	0	0.0	0	3	103	0.9	24	4,565	0.06	0.10	0.9	51
258.	Kiwi fruit, raw	1 med	76	46	1.0	0	0.0	0	11	20	0.3	4	65	0.02	0.04	0.4	75
259.	Kool Aid, with sugar	1 c	240	100	0.0	0	0.0	0	25	0	0.0	0	0	0.00	0.00	0.0	6
260.	Lamb leg, roast, trimmed	3 oz	85	237	22.0	16	7.3	60	0	9	1.4	53	0	0.13	0.23	4.7	0
261.	Lamb loin chop, broiled, lean	3 oz	84	183	25.0	8	3.4	78	0	16	1.7	70	7	0.10	0.23	5.7	0
490.	Lasagna, Healthy Choice	1	284	260	18.0	5	0.0	20	37	100	2.7	420	750	0.30	0.26	2.0	2
262.	Lasagna, homemade	1 piece	220	357	23.6	18	8.3	50	27	413	2.8	703	1,008	0.19	0.30	3.3	6
498.	Lasagna, Lean Cuisine	1	291	260	19.0	5	2.0	25	34	150	1.8	590	500	0.15	0.25	3.0	6
263.	Lemon juice, fresh	1 tbsp	15	4	0.1	0	0.0	0	1	1	0.0	1	0	0.00	0.00	0.0	7
264.	Lemonade (concentrate)	2 oz.	340	137	0.2	0	0.1	0	36	11	0.6	11	73	0.02	0.07	0.1	13
265.	Lentils, cooked	1/2 c	100	106	8.0	0	0.0	0	19	25	2.1	0	20	0.07	0.06	0.6	0
266.	Lettuce, crisp head	1 c sm chunks	75	10	0.7	0	0.0	0	2	15	0.4	7	250	0.05	0.04	0.2	5
267.	Lettuce, cos or romaine	1 c chopped	55	10	0.7	0	0.0	0	2	37	0.8	5	1,050	0.08	0.04	0.2	10
268.	Liver, beef, fried	1 slice 3 oz.	85	195	22.0	9	2.5	345	5	9	7.5	156	45,390	0.22	3.56	14.0	23
269.	Liverwurst, fresh	1 slice 1 oz.	28	87	5.0	7	3.5	50	1	3	1.5	0	1,800	0.06	0.37	1.6	0

Code	Food	Amount	Weight gm	Calories	Protein gm	Fat gm	Sat. Fat gm	Cholesterol mg	Carbohydrate gm	Calcium mg	Iron mg	Sodium mg	Vit A I.U.	Thiamin (Vit B₁) mg	Riboflavin (Vit B₂) mg	Niacin mg	Vit C mg
270.	Lobster	1 c	145	138	27.0	2	1.0	293	0	94	1.2	305	0	0.15	0.10	0.0	0
271.	M&M's, chocolate, plain	1 oz.	28	140	1.9	6	3.3	0	19	47	0.5	24	30	0.01	0.07	0.2	0
272.	M&M's, chocolate, w/peanuts	1 oz.	28	145	3.2	7	3.2	0	17	36	0.4	17	15	0.02	0.05	0.9	0
273.	Macaroni, enriched, cooked	1/2 c	70	78	2.4	0	0.0	0	16	6	0.7	1	0	0.10	0.06	0.8	0
274.	Macaroni and cheese	1/2 c	100	215	8.2	11	4.0	21	20	181	0.9	543	430	0.10	0.20	0.9	0
275.	Margarine	1 tsp	5	34	0.0	4	0.7	2	0	1	0.0	46	160	0.00	0.00	0.0	0
276.	Mars bar	1 bar	50	240	4.0	11	4.8	0	30	85	0.6	85	1	0.02	0.16	0.5	0
277.	Matzo	1 piece	30	117	3.0	0	0.0	0	25	*	*	0	*	*	*	*	*
278.	Mayonnaise	1 tsp	5	36	0.0	4	0.7	3	0	1	0.0	28	13	0.00	0.00	0.0	0
513.	Mayonnaise, light	1 tsp.	5	17	0.0	2	0.3	2	1	0	0.0	30	0	0.00	0.00	0.0	0
507.	Milk, 1% fat	1 c	244	102	8.0	3	1.6	10	12	300	0.1	123	720	0.09	0.41	0.2	2
279.	Milk, chocolate, 2%	1 c	250	180	8.0	5	3.1	17	26	284	0.6	151	143	0.09	0.41	0.3	2
280.	Milk, evaporated whole	1/2 c	126	172	9.0	10	5.8	40	13	329	0.2	149	405	0.05	0.43	0.2	2
281.	Milk, lowfat 2% fat	1 c	244	121	8.0	5	2.9	18	12	295	0.1	121	695	0.09	0.40	0.2	2
282.	Milk shake, chocolate	1 (10 fluid oz.)	340	433	11.5	13	7.8	45	70	383	1.1	328	312	0.20	0.83	0.5	0
283.	Milk shake, Frosty, Wendy's	16 oz	324	460	13	13	7.0	55	76	480	1.0	260	500	0.15	1.08	0.8	4
284.	Milk shake, strawberry	1 (10 fluid oz.)	340	383	11.4	10	6.0	37	64	384	0.4	281	418	0.14	0.61	0.5	3
285.	Milk shake, vanilla, McDonald's	1	289	323	10	8	5.1	29	52	346	0.2	250	346	0.12	0.66	0.6	3
286.	Milk, skim	1 c	245	85	8.0	1	0.3	4	12	301	0.1	126	745	0.09	0.34	0.2	2
287.	Milk, whole 3.5% fat	1 c	244	149	8.0	8	5.1	33	11	290	0.1	119	380	0.09	0.39	0.2	2
288.	Milky Way bar	1 bar	60	260	3.2	9	5.4	14	43	86	0.5	140	125	0.03	0.15	0.2	1
289.	Molasses, medium	1 tbsp	20	50	0.0	0	0.0	0	13	33	0.9	3	0	0.01	0.01	0.0	0
290.	Muffin, apple bran, fat free, McDonald's	1	75	180	5	0	0.0	0	40	48	0.7	200	0	0.15	0.18	2.0	0
291.	Muffin, blueberry	1	45	135	3.0	5	1.5	19	20	54	0.9	198	40	0.10	0.11	0.9	1
292.	Muffin, bran	1	45	125	3.0	6	1.4	24	19	60	1.4	189	230	0.11	0.13	1.3	3
293.	Muffin, cornmeal	1	45	145	3.0	5	1.5	23	21	66	0.9	169	80	0.11	0.11	0.9	0
294.	Muffin, English, plain	1	57	140	4.5	1	0.3	0	26	96	1.7	378	0	0.26	0.18	2.1	0
295.	Muffin, English w/butter	1	63	186	5.0	5	2.3	15	30	117	1.5	310	164	0.28	0.49	2.6	1
296.	Mushrooms, fresh cultivated	1/2 c sliced	35	12	1.0	0	0.0	0	2	4	0.5	4	0	0.04	0.12	2.4	1
297.	Mustard greens, cooked drained	1/2 c	70	16	1.7	0	0.0	0	3	96	1.2	13	4,060	0.05	0.10	0.4	33
298.	Noodles, egg, enriched cooked	1/2 c	80	100	3.3	1	0.0	19	19	8	0.7	2	55	0.11	0.07	1.0	0
299.	Nuts, brazil	1 oz. (6-8 nuts)	28	185	4.1	19	4.8	0	3	53	1.0	0	0	0.27	0.03	0.5	0
300.	Nuts, pecans	1 oz.	28	195	2.6	20	1.4	0	4	21	0.7	0	40	0.24	0.04	0.3	1
301.	Nuts, walnuts	1 oz. (14 halves)	28	185	4.2	18	1.0	0	5	28	0.9	1	10	0.09	0.04	0.3	1
302.	Oil, corn	1 tbsp.	15	125	0.0	14	1.8	0	0	0	0.0	0	0	0.00	0.00	0.0	0
303.	Oil, olive	1 tbsp.	15	125	0.0	14	1.9	0	0	0	0.0	0	0	0.00	0.00	0.0	0
304.	Oil, safflower	1 tbsp.	15	125	0.0	14	1.3	0	0	0	0.0	0	0	0.00	0.00	0.0	0
305.	Oil, soybean	1 tsp.	5	44	0.0	5	2.0	0	0	0	0.0	0	0	0.00	0.00	0.0	0
306.	Okra, cooked, drained	1/2 c	80	23	1.6	0	0.0	0	5	74	0.4	2	390	0.11	0.15	0.7	16
307.	Olives, black, ripe	10 extra large	55	61	0.5	7	1.0	0	1	40	0.8	385	30	0.00	0.00	0.0	0
308.	Onions, mature	1/2 c sliced	105	31	1.3	0	0.0	0	7	25	0.4	8	40	0.03	0.03	0.2	8
309.	Onions, mature, cooked, drained																
310.	Onion rings, fried	3	30	122	1.6	8	2.3	0	11	9	0.5	113	68	0.08	0.04	1.1	0
311.	Onion rings (Brazier), Dairy Queen	1 serving	85	360	6.0	17	6.0	15	33	20	0.4	125	0	0.09	0.00	0.4	2
312.	Orange juice, froz., reconstituted	1/2 c	125	61	0.9	0	0.0	0	15	13	0.1	1	270	0.12	0.02	0.5	60
313.	Orange, raw (medium skin)	1 med	180	64	1.3	0	0.0	0	16	54	0.5	1	260	0.13	0.05	0.5	66
314.	Oysters, Eastern, breaded, fried	1 oyster	45	90	5.0	5	1.4	35	5	49	3.0	70	220	0.07	0.10	1.3	4
315.	Oysters, raw, Eastern	1/2 c (6-9 med)	120	79	10.0	2	1.3	60	4	113	6.6	145	370	0.17	0.22	3.0	0
316.	Pancakes	6" diam x 1/2" thick	73	169	5.2	5	1.0	36	25	74	0.9	310	90	0.12	0.16	0.9	0
317.	Pancakes, buckwheat	4 in. diam.	27	55	2.0	2	0.9	20	6	59	0.4	125	17	0.04	0.05	0.0	0
318.	Pancakes w/butter, syrup	1 large	100	250	4.0	5	1.9	24	47	31	1.1	535	160	0.13	0.18	1.1	2
319.	Papaya, raw	1/2 med	227	60	0.9	0	0.0	0	15	31	0.5	5	2,660	0.06	0.06	0.5	85

Code	Food	Amount	Weight gm	Calories	Protein gm	Fat gm	Sat. Fat gm	Cholesterol mg	Carbohydrate gm	Calcium mg	Iron mg	Sodium mg	Vit A I.U.	Thiamin (Vit B₁) mg	Riboflavin (Vit B₂) mg	Niacin mg	Vit C mg
320.	Parsnips, cooked	1 large 9" long	160	106	2.4	1	0.0	0	24	72	1.0	13	50	0.11	0.13	0.2	16
503.	Pasta primavera, Weight Watchers	1	238	260	15.0	11	0.8	5	22	300	1.8	800	1,750	0.23	0.26	3.0	18
321.	Peaches, canned, heavy syrup	1 half 2⅛ tbsp liq.	96	75	0.4	0	0.0	0	19	4	0.3	2	410	0.01	0.02	0.6	3
322.	Peaches, canned, juice pack	1 half	77	34	0.5	0	0.0	0	9	5	0.2	3	147	0.01	0.01	0.5	3
323.	Peaches, raw, peeled	1 2¾" diam.	175	58	0.9	0	0.0	0	15	14	0.8	2	2,030	0.03	0.08	1.5	11
324.	Peanut butter	2 tbsp	32	188	8.0	16	1.0	0	6	18	0.6	194	0	0.04	0.04	4.8	0
325.	Peanut butter, jam sandwich	1	100	340	11.4	14	2.6	0	45	87	2.3	414	0	0.32	0.22	5.3	0
326.	Peanuts, roasted	1 oz.	28	166	7.0	14	1.0	0	5	21	0.6	119	0	0.09	0.04	4.9	0
327.	Pears, canned, heavy syrup	1 half 2¼ tbsp liq.	103	78	0.2	0	0.0	0	20	5	0.2	1	0	0.01	0.02	0.1	1
328.	Pears, canned, juice pack	1 half	77	38	0.3	0	0.0	0	10	7	0.2	3	0	0.01	0.01	0.2	1
329.	Pears, raw	1 pear	180	100	1.1	1	0.0	0	25	13	0.5	1	3	0.03	0.07	0.2	7
330.	Peas, canned, drained	½ c	85	75	4.0	0	0.0	0	14	22	1.6	200	585	0.08	0.05	0.7	7
331.	Peas, frozen, cooked drained	½ c	80	55	4.1	0	0.0	0	10	15	1.5	92	480	0.22	0.07	1.4	11
332.	Peppers, sweet, raw	1 pepper 3¼" x 3" diam.	200	36	2.0	0	0.0	0	8	15	1.1	21	690	0.13	0.13	0.8	210
333.	Pickles, dill	1 large 4" long	135	15	0.9	0	0.0	0	3	35	1.4	1,928	140	0.00	0.03	0.0	8
334.	Pickles, sweet	1 large 3" long	35	51	0.2	0	0.0	0	13	4	0.4	0	30	0.00	0.01	0.0	2
335.	Pie, Apple	1 piece (3½")	118	302	2.6	13	3.5	0	45	9	0.4	355	40	0.02	0.02	0.5	1
336.	Pie, Apple, fried	1 pie	85	255	2.2	14	5.8	14	32	12	0.9	326	15	0.09	0.06	1.0	1
337.	Pie, Blueberry	1 piece (3½")	158	380	4.0	17	4.0	0	55	26	2.1	423	140	0.17	0.14	1.7	6
338.	Pie, Cherry	1 piece (3½")	118	308	3.1	13	5.0	0	45	17	0.5	355	40	0.02	0.02	0.5	1
339.	Pie, Cherry, fried	1 pie	85	250	2.0	14	5.8	137	32	11	0.7	371	95	0.06	0.06	0.6	1
340.	Pie, Chocolate cream	1 piece (1/6 pie)	175	311	7.4	13	4.5	15	42	160	1.1	427	170	0.15	0.30	1.1	1
341.	Pie, Lemon meringue	1 piece (1/6 pie)	140	355	4.7	14	3.5	137	53	25	1.4	395	330	0.10	0.14	0.8	4
342.	Pie, Pecan	1 piece (1/6 pie)	138	583	6.3	24	3.9	13	92	35	1.9	304	206	0.22	0.17	1.1	0
343.	Pie, Pumpkin	1 (3½")	114	241	4.6	13	3.0	70	28	58	0.6	244	2,810	0.03	0.11	0.6	0
344.	Pineapple, canned, heavy syrup	½ c	128	95	0.4	0	0.0	0	25	14	0.4	2	65	0.10	0.03	0.3	9
345.	Pineapple, canned, juice pack	½ c	125	75	0.5	0	0.0	0	20	17	0.3	1	24	0.12	0.24	0.3	12
346.	Pineapple, raw	½ c diced	78	41	0.3	0	0.0	0	11	13	0.4	1	55	0.07	0.03	0.2	13
347.	Pizza, cheese, thin 'n crispy, Pizza Hut	½ 10" pie	*	450	25.0	15	7.0	125	54	450	4.5	1,200	750	0.30	0.51	5.0	1
348.	Pizza, Cheese, Thick 'n Chewy, Pizza Hut	½ 10" pie	*	560	34.0	14	6.0	110	71	500	5.4	1,100	1,000	0.68	0.68	7.0	1
504.	Pizza, Cheese, Weight Watchers	1	164	300	22.0	7	3.0	35	37	450	1.4	630	1,000	0.30	0.51	3.0	12
505.	Pizza, deluxe comb. Weight Watchers	1	200	330	26.0	10	3.0	25	35	350	1.8	650	1,750	0.30	0.51	3.0	21
506.	Pizza, Pepperoni, Weight Watchers	1	171	320	26.0	10	3.0	35	31	400	1.8	710	1,000	0.23	0.51	3.0	15
480.	Pizza, pepperoni, pan, Pizza Hut	2 pieces	211	540	29.0	22	9.2	42	62	520	6.3	1,127	500	0.63	0.49	5.4	8
481.	Pizza, supreme, pan, Pizza Hut	2 pieces	255	589	32.0	30	13.8	48	53	500	5.0	1,363	600	0.81	0.80	6.0	10
349.	Plums, Japanese and hybrid, raw	1 plum 2⅛" diam.	70	32	0.3	0	0.0	0	8	8	0.3	1	160	0.02	0.02	0.3	4
350.	Popcorn, cooked, oil	1 c	11	55	0.9	3	0.5	0	6	3	0.3	86	20	0.01	0.02	0.1	0
351.	Popcorn, popped, plain, large kernel	1 c	6	12	0.8	0	0.0	0	5	1	0.2	0	0	0.00	0.01	0.1	0
352.	Pork, roast, trimmed	2 slices 3 oz.	85	179	24.0	8	2.2	65	0	11	3.1	863	0	0.55	0.22	4.3	0
353.	Pork, sausage, cooked	1 sm link	17	72	2.8	6	2.1	13	1	0	0.3	221	0	0.00	0.00	0.0	0
354.	Potato, au gratin	1 c	245	228	5.6	10	6.3	12	32	203	0.8	1,076	380	0.05	0.20	2.3	8
355.	Potato, baked in skin	1 potato 2⅓ x 4¼"	202	145	4.0	0	0.0	0	33	14	1.1	8	0	0.15	0.07	2.7	31
356.	Potato chips	10 chips	20	114	1.1	8	2.1	0	10	8	0.4	150	0	0.04	0.01	1.0	3
357.	Potato, French fried long	10 strips 3½-4"	78	214	3.4	10	1.7	4	28	12	1.0	5	6	0.10	0.06	2.4	16
358.	Potato, hashbrowns, McDonald's	1 patty	55	144	1.4	9	3.0	8	15	5	0.4	325	6	0.06	0.01	0.8	4
359.	Potato, mashed, milk added	½ c	105	69	2.2	1	0.4	8	14	25	0.4	316	20	0.09	0.06	1.1	11

Code	Food	Amount	Weight gm	Calories	Protein gm	Fat gm	Sat. Fat gm	Cholesterol mg	Carbohydrate gm	Calcium mg	Iron mg	Sodium mg	Vit A I.U.	Thiamin (Vit B₁) mg	Riboflavin (Vit B₂) mg	Niacin mg	Vit C mg
360.	Potato salad w/eggs, mayo	1/2 c	125	179	3.4	10	7.8	85	14	24	0.8	662	262	0.10	0.08	1.1	12
361.	Potato, hash brown	1/2 c	78	170	2.5	9	3.5	0	22	12	1.2	27	0	0.09	0.02	1.9	5
362.	Pretzel, thin, twists	1 oz.	28	113	2.8	1	0.3	0	23	8	0.6	456	0	0.09	0.07	1.2	0
363.	Prunes, dried "softenized" without pits	5 prunes	61	137	1.1	0	0.0	0	36	26	0.1	4	860	0.05	0.09	0.9	2
364.	Prune juice, canned or bottled	1/2 c	128	99	0.5	0	0.0	0	24	18	5.3	3	0	0.02	0.02	0.5	3
365.	Pudding, chocolate, canned	5 oz.	142	205	3	11	9.5	1	30	74	1.2	285	155	0.04	0.17	0.6	0
366.	Pudding, tapioca, canned	5 oz.	142	160	3	5	4.8	1	28	119	0.3	252	5	0.03	0.14	0.4	0
367.	Pudding, vanilla, canned	5 oz.	142	220	2	10	9.5	1	33	79	0.2	305	1	0.03	0.12	0.6	0
368.	Quiche, Lorraine	1 piece	242	825	18	66	31.9	392	40	290	1.9	898	2,250	0.15	0.44	1.7	1
369.	Raisins, unbleached, seedless	1 oz.	28	82	0.7	1	0.0	0	22	18	1.0	8	10	0.03	0.02	0.1	0
370.	Raspberries, fresh	1 c	123	60	1.1	1	0.0	0	14	27	0.7	0	80	0.04	0.11	1.1	31
371.	Raspberries, frozen	1 c	250	255	1.7	1	0.0	0	62	38	1.6	3	75	0.05	0.11	1.5	41
495.	Ravioli, baked cheese, Lean Cuisine	1	241	240	13.0	8	3.0	55	30	200	1.4	590	300	0.06	0.25	1.2	36
372.	Rice, brown, cooked	1/2 c	96	116	2.5	1	0.0	0	25	12	0.5	275	0	0.09	0.02	1.3	0
373.	Rice, white enriched, cooked	1/2 c	103	113	2.1	0	0.0	0	25	11	0.9	384	2	0.12	0.01	1.1	0
374.	Rice, wild, cooked	1/2 c	100	92	3.6	0	0.0	0	19	5	1.1	2	0	0.11	0.16	1.6	0
375.	Roast beef sand., regular, Arby's	1	155	383	22	18	7.0	43	35	72	3.2	936	0	0.28	0.50	11.0	0
376.	Roast beef sub, Arby's	1	305	623	38	32	11.5	73	47	492	5.2	1,847	500	0.56	0.76	14.2	9
377.	Roll, hard, white	1 roll	50	155	5	2	0.0	0	30	24	1.4	313	0	0.20	0.12	1.7	0
378.	Reuben sandwich	1	237	488	28.7	28	10.4	85	30	364	5.3	1,685	461	0.25	0.44	3.9	12
379.	Salad, caesar side, Wendy's	1	130	160	10	6	1.0	10	18	96	1.2	700	1,250	0.23	0.27	2.0	24
380.	Salad, chef, Burger King	1 serving	273	178	17	9	4.0	103	7	128	1.6	568	4,750	0.35	0.26	3.6	15
381.	Salad, chef, McDonald's	1	265	170	17	9	4.0	111	8	180	1.0	400	5,000	0.30	0.27	4.0	21
382.	Salad, chicken, Burger King	1 serving	258	142	20	4	1.0	49	8	32	1.3	443	4,600	0.14	0.17	8.5	20
383.	Salad, chicken w/celery	1/2 c	78	266	10.5	25	4.1	48	1	16	0.7	199	153	0.03	0.08	3.3	9
384.	Salad, deluxe Garden, Wendy's	1	271	110	7	5	1.0	0	9	240	1.0	380	3,000	0.15	0.36	1.2	36
385.	Salad, garden, Arby's	1	330	117	7	5	2.7	12	11	192	1.1	134	4,900	0.17	0.20	1.2	52
386.	Salad, grilled Chicken, Wendy's	1	338	200	25	8	1.0	55	9	240	1.8	690	3,000	0.23	0.36	8.0	36
387.	Salad, tuna	1 c	205	375	33	19	3.3	80	19	31	2.5	877	53	0.06	0.14	13.3	6
388.	Salami, dry	1 oz.	28	128	7.0	11	1.6	24	0	4	1.0	349	0	0.10	0.07	1.5	0
389.	Salmon, broiled with butter or margarine	3 oz.	85	156	23.0	6	2.2	53	0	0	0.9	99	150	0.15	0.06	8.4	0
390.	Salmon, canned Chinook	3 oz.	85	179	16.6	12	0.8	30	0	131	0.7	105	197	0.03	0.01	6.2	0
514.	Salsa	1 tbsp.	15	5	0.0	0	0.0	0	1	1	0.1	100	115	0.01	0.00	0.05	5
391.	Sardines, canned drained	1 oz.	28	58	7.0	3	1.0	20	0	124	0.8	233	60	0.01	0.06	1.5	0
392.	Sauerkraut, canned	1/2 c	118	21	1.2	0	0.0	0	5	43	0.6	878	60	0.04	0.05	0.3	17
393.	Sausage biscuit w/egg, McDonald's	1	175	505	19	33	20.0	260	33	120	2.4	1,210	300	0.45	0.36	4.0	0
394.	Sausage McMuffin, McDonald's	1	135	345	15	20	11.0	57	27	240	1.8	770	200	0.53	0.27	5.0	0
395.	Sausage McMuffin, w/Egg	1	159	430	21	25	14.0	270	27	300	2.4	920	500	0.53	0.45	5.0	0
396.	Sausage, smoked link, pork	1	68	265	15	22	7.7	46	1	20	0.8	1,020	0	1.04	0.29	5.0	14
397.	Scallops, breaded, cooked	6 pieces	90	195	15	10	2.5	70	10	39	2.0	298	105	0.11	0.11	1.6	0
398.	Sherbet	1/2 c	97	135	1.1	2	1.3	7	29	52	0.2	44	92	0.02	0.04	0.1	2
399.	Shrimp, boiled	3 oz.	85	99	18.0	1	0.1	128	1	99	2.7	0	60	0.00	0.03	1.5	0
400.	Shrimp, fried	7 medium	85	200	16.0	10	2.5	168	11	61	2.0	384	130	0.06	0.09	2.8	0
487.	Shrimp, linguini, Budget Gourmet	1	284	330	15.0	15	0.0	75	33	10	3.6	1,250	1,000	0.30	0.17	3.0	2
401.	Snickers bar	1 bar	61	290	6.6	4	5.4	0	37	70	0.5	170	25	0.03	0.11	1.8	0
402.	Soda pop, cola	12 oz.	369	144	0.0	0	0.0	0	37	27	0.0	30	0	0.00	0.00	0.0	0
403.	Soda pop, diet	12 oz.	340	2	0.1	0	0.0	0	0	13	0.1	31	0	0.00	0.00	0.0	0
404.	Soda pop, Ginger ale	12 oz.	366	113	0.0	0	0.0	0	29	8	0.0	45	0	0.00	0.00	0.0	0
405.	Soda pop, Lemon-lime	12 oz.	340	138	0.0	0	0.0	0	35	8	0.2	38	0	0.00	0.00	0.0	0

Code	Food	Amount	Weight gm	Calories	Protein gm	Fat gm	Sat. Fat gm	Cholesterol mg	Carbohydrate gm	Calcium mg	Iron mg	Sodium mg	Vit A I.U.	Thiamin (Vit B₁) mg	Riboflavin (Vit B₂) mg	Niacin mg	Vit C mg
406.	Soda pop, Root beer	12 oz	340	140	0.0	0	0.0	0	36	17	0.2	45	0	0.00	0.00	0.0	0
407.	Soup, chicken, cream	1 c	248	191	7.5	12	4.6	27	15	180	0.7	1,046	710	0.07	0.26	0.9	1
408.	Soup, chicken noodle	1 c	241	75	4.0	2	0.7	7	9	17	0.8	900	711	0.05	0.06	1.4	0
409.	Soup, clam chowder, Manhattan	1 c	244	78	4.2	2	0.4	2	12	34	1.9	1,808	460	0.06	0.05	1.3	3
410.	Soup, clam chowder, north east	1 c	248	163	9.5	7	3.0	22	16	187	1.5	992	160	0.07	0.24	1.0	4
411.	Soup, cream of mushroom condensed, prepared with equal volume of milk	1 c	245	216	7.0	14	5.4	15	16	191	0.5	955	250	0.05	0.34	0.7	1
412.	Soup, minestrone	1 c	241	80	4.3	3	0.5	2	11	34	0.9	911	1,170	0.05	0.04	0.9	1
413.	Soup, split pea, condensed, prepared with equal volume of water	1 c	245	145	9.0	3	1.1	0	21	29	1.5	941	440	0.25	0.15	1.5	1
414.	Soup, tomato, condensed, prepared with equal volume of water	1 c	245	88	2.0	3	0.5	0	16	15	0.7	970	1,000	0.05	0.05	1.2	12
415.	Soup, tomato with milk	1 c	248	160	6.0	6	2.9	17	22	159	1.8	932	850	0.13	0.25	1.5	68
416.	Soup, vegetable beef, condensed, prepared with equal volume of water	1 c	245	78	5.0	2	0.0	0	10	12	0.7	1,046	2,700	0.05	0.05	1.0	0
417.	Soup, Vegetarian vegetable	1 c	250	70	2.1	2	0.3	0	12	21	1.1	823	1,505	0.05	0.05	0.9	1
418.	Sour cream	1 tbsp	14	30	0.4	3	1.8	6	1	16	0.0	8	135	0.01	0.02	0.0	0
419.	Sour cream, imitation	1 tbsp.	14	29	0.3	3	2.5	0	1	0	0.0	14	0	0.00	0.00	0.0	0
492.	Spaghetti, Healthy Choice	1 c	284	280	14.0	6	0.0	20	42	6	3.6	480	1,250	0.38	0.26	2.0	5
420.	Spaghetti, in tomato sauce with cheese	1 c	250	260	8.8	9	2.0	10	37	80	2.3	955	1,080	0.25	0.18	2.3	13
421.	Spaghetti, plain, cooked	1 c	140	155	5.0	1	0.1	0	32	11	1.7	1	0	0.20	0.11	1.5	0
422.	Spaghetti, whole wheat, cooked	1 c	125	151	6.6	1	0.1	0	32	19	1.1	16	0	0.21	0.09	1.5	0
423.	Spaghetti, with meatballs and tomato sauce	1 c	248	332	18.6	11.7	3.0	75	39	124	3.7	1,009	1,590	0.25	0.30	4.0	22
499.	Spaghetti w/meatballs, Lean Cuisine	1	290	280	19.0	7	2.0	35	35	100	1.8	490	300	0.15	0.25	3.0	4
424.	Spareribs, cooked	3 oz.	85	377	17.8	33	12.0	73	0	8	2.2	31	0	0.37	0.18	2.9	0
425.	Spinach, canned, drained	1/2 c	103	25	2.3	1	0.0	0	4	121	2.6	242	8,200	0.02	0.12	0.3	15
426.	Spinach, frozen, cooked, drained	1/2 c	103	24	3.1	0	0.0	0	4	116	2.2	54	8,100	0.07	0.16	0.4	20
427.	Spinach, raw, chopped	1 c	55	14	1.8	0	0.0	0	2	51	1.7	39	4,460	0.06	0.11	0.3	28
428.	Squash, summer, cooked	1/2 c	90	13	0.8	0	0.0	0	3	23	0.4	1	350	0.05	0.07	0.7	9
429.	Squash, winter, baked mashed	1/2 c	103	70	1.9	0	0.0	0	18	41	1.0	1	6,560	0.05	0.14	0.7	8
430.	Strawberries, frozen, sweetened	1 c	250	245	1.4	1	0.0	0	66	28	1.5	8	31	0.04	0.13	1.0	106
431.	Strawberries, raw	1 c	149	55	1.0	1	0.0	0	13	31	1.5	1	90	0.04	0.10	0.9	88
432.	Stuffing, bread, prepared	1/2 c	70	250	4.6	15	3.1	0	25	46	1.1	627	455	0.09	0.10	1.3	0
433.	Sundae, chocolate, Dairy Queen	medium	184	300	6.0	7	4.9	79	53	200	1.1	175	300	0.06	0.26	0.0	0
434.	Sugar, brown granulated	1 tsp	5	17	0.0	0	0.0	0	5	4	0.1	0	0	0.00	0.00	0.1	0
435.	Sugar, white granulated	1 tsp	4	15	0.0	0	0.0	0	4	0	0.0	0	0	0.00	0.00	0.0	0
436.	Super roast beef, Arby's	1	254	552	24	28	7.6	43	54	108	4.3	1,174	150	0.39	0.61	12.4	9
437.	Sweet n' sour sauce, McDonald's	1.12 oz	32	60	0	0.2	0.1	0	14	0	0.0	190	300	0.00	0.00	0.0	0
438.	Sweet potato, baked	1 potato 5" long	146	161	2.4	1	0.0	0	37	46	1.0	14	9,230	0.10	0.08	0.8	25
439.	Syrup (maple)	1 tbsp	20	50	0.0	0	0.0	0	13	33	0.2	3	0	0.00	0.00	0.0	0
440.	Taco salad, Wendy's	1	510	640	34	30	12.0	80	70	540	5.4	960	1,750	0.23	0.45	3.0	27
441.	Taco shell	1 shell	10	60	1.1	3	0.3	0	9	26	0.3	62	36	0.00	0.01	0.3	0
512.	Taco, soft, Taco Bell	1	92	225	12.0	12	5.4	32	18	116	2.3	550	150	0.39	0.22	2.7	0
442.	Taco, Taco Bell	1	83	186	15.0	8	0.0	0	14	120	2.4	79	120	0.09	0.16	2.9	0
443.	Tangerine	1 med 2⅛" diam.	116	39	0.7	0	0.0	0	10	34	0.3	2	360	0.05	0.02	0.1	27
444.	Tartar sauce	1 tbsp.	14	74	0.2	8	1.2	4	1	3	0.1	182	54	0.00	0.00	0.0	0

Code	Food	Amount	Weight gm	Calories	Protein gm	Fat gm	Sat. Fat gm	Cholesterol mg	Carbohydrate gm	Calcium mg	Iron mg	Sodium mg	Vit A I.U.	Thiamin (Vit B₁) mg	Riboflavin (Vit B₂) mg	Niacin mg	Vit C mg
445.	Tea, brewed	1/4 c	180	0	0.0	0	0.0	0	0	0	0.0	0	0	0.00	0.00	0.0	0
446.	Tomato juice, canned	1 c	244	42	1.9	0	0.1	0	10	22	1.4	881	1,357	0.12	0.08	1.6	45
447.	Tomato sauce (catsup)	1 tbsp	15	16	0.3	0	0.0	0	4	3	0.1	156	105	0.01	0.01	0.2	2
448.	Tomato, canned	1/2 c	121	26	1.2	0	0.0	0	5	7	0.6	157	1,085	0.06	0.04	0.9	21
449.	Tomato, raw	1 tomato 3½ oz.	100	20	1.0	0	0.0	0	4	12	0.5	3	820	0.05	0.04	0.6	21
450.	Tortilla chips	1 oz.	28	139	2.2	8	1.1	0	17	82	1.0	140	7	0.01	0.02	0.2	0
451.	Tortilla, corn, lime	1 6" diam.	30	63	1.5	1	0.0	0	14	60	0.9	0	6	0.04	0.02	0.3	0
452.	Tortilla, flour	1	35	105	2.6	3	0.4	0	19	21	0.5	134		0.13	0.08	1.2	0
453.	Tostada	1	148	206	9.2	18	3.0	14	25	167	1.8	200	445	0.06	0.13	0.8	6
454.	Trout, broiled w/butter, lemon	3 oz.	85	175	21.0	9	4.1	71	0	26	1.0	122	300	0.07	0.07	2.3	1
455.	Tuna, canned, oil pack, drained	3 oz.	85	167	25.0	7	1.7	60	0	7	1.6	0	70	0.04	0.10	10.1	0
456.	Tuna, canned, water pack, solids and liquid	3½ oz.	99	126	27.7	1	0.0	55	0	16	1.6	161	0	0.00	0.10	13.2	0
457.	Turkey, lite roast deluxe, Arby'	1	195	260	20	6	1.6	33	33	156	2.3	1,262	200	0.29	0.43	15.4	12
458.	Turkey, roast (light and dark mixed)	3 oz.	85	162	27.0	5	1.5	73	0	7	1.5	111	0	0.04	0.15	6.5	0
459.	Turnip, cooked, drained	1/2 c cubed	78	18	0.6	0	0.0	0	4	27	0.3	27	0	0.03	0.04	0.3	17
460.	Turnip greens, cooked drained	1/2 c	73	19	2.1	0	0.0	0	3	98	1.3	14	5,695	0.04	0.08	0.4	16
461.	Veal, cooked loin	3 oz.	85	199	22.0	11	4.0	90	0	9	2.7	55	0	0.06	0.21	4.6	0
462.	Veal cutlet, braised, broiled	3 oz.	85	185	23.0	9	4.0	109	0	9	0.8	56	5	0.06	0.21	4.6	0
486.	Veal parmigiana, Budget Gourmet	1	340	440	26.0	20	0.0	165	39	30	4.5	1,160	5,000	0.45	0.60	6.0	6
463.	Vegetables, mixed, cooked	1 c	182	116	5.8	0	0.0	0	24	46	2.4	348	4,505	0.02	0.13	2.0	15
464.	Waffles	1 waffle	75	205	6.9	8	2.7	59	27	179	1.2	515	49	0.14	0.23	0.9	0
465.	Watermelon	1 c diced	160	42	0.8	0	0.0	0	10	11	0.8	2	940	0.05	0.05	0.3	11
466.	Wheat germ, plain toasted	1 tbsp	6	23	1.8	1	0.0	0	3	3	0.5	0	10	0.11	0.05	0.3	1
467.	Whiskey, gin, rum, vodka 90 proof	1/2 11 oz (jigger)	42	110	0	0	0.0	0	0	0	0.0	0	0	0.00	0.00	0.0	0
468.	Whopper, Burger King	1 sandwich	270	614	27.0	36	12.0	90	45	64	4.9	865	550	0.34	0.41	6.1	12
469.	Whopper with cheese, Burger King	1 sandwich	294	706	32.0	44	16.0	115	47	176	4.9	1,177	950	0.34	0.48	6.1	12
470.	Whopper, double, Burger King	1 sandwich	351	844	46.0	53	19.0	169	45	72	7.2	933	550	0.35	0.56	9.4	12
471.	Wine, dry table 12% alc.	3½ fl. oz.	102	87	0.1	0	0.0	0	4	9	0.4	5	0	0.00	0.01	0.1	0
472.	Wine, red dry 18.8% alc.	2 oz.	59	81	0.1	0	0.0	0	5	5	0.0	4	0	0.01	0.02	0.2	0
473.	Yeast, brewers	1 tbsp	8	23	3.1	0	0.0	0	3	17	1.4	10	0	1.25	0.34	3.0	0
474.	Yogurt, fruit	1 c	227	231	9.9	2	1.6	10	43	345	0.2	125	104	0.08	0.40	0.2	2
475.	Yogurt, nonfat, TCBY	4 oz.	113	110	4	4	0	0	23	96	0	45	0	0.03	0.14	0	2
476.	Yogurt, plain low fat	1 8-oz. container	226	113	7.7	4	2.3	15	12	271	0.1	115	150	0.09	0.41	0.2	2
477.	Yogurt, regular, TCBY	4 oz.	113	120	4	3	2.0	13	23	180	0.5	60		0.06	0.18	0	0
478.	Yogurt, sugar free, TCBY	4 oz.	113	80	4	0	0		18	96	0	40	200	0.06	0.18	0	0
479.	Yogurt, vanilla lowfat, McDonald's	3 oz.	85	105	4	1	0.3	3	22	120	0	80	100	0.03	0.18	0.4	0

"0" represents both less than 1 and 0

Sources:

Nutritive Value of American Foods in Common Units. Agriculture Handbook No. 456. U.S. Dept. of Agriculture. Washington, D.C. 1988.

Young, E. A., E. H. Brennan, and C. L. Irving, Guest Eds. Perspectives on Fast Foods. Public Health Currents, 19(1), 1979, Published by Ross Laboratories, Columbus, OH.

Dennison, D. The Dine System: the Nutrition Plan For Better Health. C. V. Mosby Company St. Louis, Missouri, 1982.

Pennington, S. A. T. and H. N. Church. Food Values of Portions Commonly Used. Harper and Row Publishers, New York, 1985.

Kullman, D. A. ABC Milligram Cholesterol Diet Guide. Merit Publications, Inc. North Miami Beach, Florida 1978.

Food Processor nutrient analysis software by Esha Corporation, P.O. Box 13028, Salem, Oregon, 97309. With permission.

Glossary

A

Abstinence To refrain completely from engaging in a particular behavior.

Accommodating resistance Strength-training program that requires the use of special equipment with mechanical devices that provide a variable resistance, with the intent of overloading the muscle group maximally through the entire range of motion.

Acquired immunodeficiency syndrome (AIDS) Virus (HIV) that destroys the immune system.

Adaptation energy stores Reserves of physical, mental, and emotional energy that give us the ability to cope with stress.

Addiction Compulsive and uncontrollable behavior(s) or use of substance(s), most frequently drugs.

Adenosine triphosphate (ATP) A high-energy chemical compound used for immediate energy by the body.

Adipose tissue Fat cells.

Aerobic capacity The maximal amount of oxygen the human body is able to utilize per minute of physical activity (usually expressed in ml/kg/min).

Aerobic exercise Exercise that requires oxygen to produce the necessary energy (ATP) to carry out the activity.

Affirmations Positive statements that help reinforce the most positive aspects of personality and experience.

AIDS *See* acquired immunodeficiency syndrome.

Alarm The first stage of the general adaptation syndrome, characterized by the release of stress hormones.

Alcohol (drinking alcohol) Known as ethyl alcohol, a depressant drug that affects the brain and slows down central nervous system activity.

Alcoholism Disease in which an individual loses control over drinking alcoholic-containing beverages.

Altruism The act of giving of oneself out of a genuine concern for other people.

Alveoli Air sacs in the lungs where gas exchange (oxygen and carbon dioxide) takes place.

Amenorrhea Cessation of regular menstrual flow.

Amino acids Chemical compounds that contain nitrogen, carbon, hydrogen, and oxygen. Amino acids are the basic building blocks that the body uses to build different types of protein.

Anabolic steroids Synthetic versions of the male sex hormone testosterone which promotes muscle development and hypertrophy.

Anabolism Process whereby simple substances are formed into more complex substances.

Anaerobic exercise Exercise which does not require oxygen to produce the necessary energy (ATP) to carry out the activity.

Aneurysm Weakness in the arterial wall allowing the formation of a balloon-like pouch.

Anger A temporary emotion that combines physiological and emotional arousal.

Angina pectoris Chest pain.

Anorexia nervosa An eating disorder characterized by self-imposed starvation to lose and maintain very low body weight.

Anthropometric measurement Measurement of body girths at different sites.

Antibodies Substances produced by the white blood cells in response to an invading agent.

Antioxidants Compounds such as the vitamins C, E, beta-carotene (a precursor to vitamin A) and the mineral selenium which prevent oxygen from combining with other substances to which it may cause damage. Antioxidants are thought to play a key role in the prevention of heart disease and cancer.

Anxiety A state of intense worry that is not grounded in reality.

Appetite Hunger for food, usually triggered by factors such as stress, habit, boredom, depression, food availability, or just the thought of food itself.

Arteries Major vessels that carry blood away from the heart to bodily tissues.

Arteriosclerosis Hardening of the arteries.

Atherosclerosis Type of arteriosclerosis characterized by plaque formation or the buildup of fatty tissue in the inner layers of the wall of the arteries.

ATP *See* adenosine triphosphate.

Atrophy A decrease in the size of a cell.

Autogenics A stress management technique. It is a form of self-suggestion where an individual is able to place him/herself in an autohypnotic state by repeating and concentrating on feelings of heaviness and warmth in the extremities.

Autoimmune disease Illness in which the body's immune system attacks the body.

Autoinoculation The process of spreading an infection to other parts of one's own body.

B

Ballistic or dynamic stretching (flexibility) Stretching exercises that are performed using jerky, rapid, and bouncy movements.

Basal cell carcinoma Type of skin cancer that occurs primarily on the face. It grows slow and rarely spreads to other parts of the body.

Basal metabolism The lowest level of oxygen consumption (uptake) necessary to sustain life.

Behavioral health The role of lifestyle in health.

Behavior modification A process to permanently change destructive or negative behaviors for positive behaviors that will lead to better health and well-being.

Benign Noncancerous.

Bereavement The process of disbonding from a person that had played an important role in one's life and is now gone.

Beta-carotene A precursor to vitamin A.

Binge drinking Imbibing at least five alcoholic beverages in one sitting for men and four for women.

Bioelectrical impedance Technique to assess body composition, including percent body fat, by running a weak electrical current (totally painless) through the body.

Biofeedback Stress management technique. A process in which a person learns to reliably influence physiological responses of two kinds: either responses which are not ordinarily under voluntary control or responses which ordinarily are easily regulated but for which regulation has broken down due to trauma or disease.

Blood pressure The pressure of the blood exerted against the walls of the arteries.

BMI *See* body mass index.

Body composition Term used in reference to the fat and nonfat components of the human body. Body composition is important in the assessment of recommended or "ideal" body weight.

Body density The weight of the body per unit volume.

Body mass index (BMI) Ratio of weight to height, usually expressed in $kg/(mts)2$.

Breathing techniques for relaxation Stress management technique where the individual concentrates on "breathing away" the tension and inhaling fresh air to the entire body.

Brown fat cells Cells that produce body heat by burning fat.

Bulimia An eating disorder characterized by a pattern of binge eating and purging to attempt to lose and maintain low body weight.

Burnout A state of physical and mental exhaustion in which few resources remain.

C

CAD Coronary artery disease. *See* coronary heart disease.

Caffeine A central nervous system stimulating drug most frequently found in coffee, tea, and colas.

Caffeinism A toxic condition resulting from chronic use of caffeine.

Calorie A unit to measure heat energy. A calorie (also referred to as small calorie) is the amount of heat necessary to raise the temperature of one gram of water one degree Centigrade. Short term for kilocalorie and it is used to measure the energy value of food and cost of physical activity.

Calorimeter Equipment used to measure the caloric value of food or heat production of animals and humans.

Calisthenics The practice or art of calisthenics exercises; the exercise of muscles for the purpose of gaining health, strength, and grace of form and movement.

Cancer Group of diseases characterized by uncontrolled growth and spread of abnormal cells into malignant tumors.

Cancer-prone personality See Type C personality.

Cannabis sativa Hemp plant from which marijuana and hashish are derived.

Capillary Smallest blood vessels carrying oxygenated blood in the body.

Carbohydrates Compounds containing carbon, hydrogen, and oxygen. Carbohydrates are the major source of energy for the human body.

Carbon monoxide The carcinogenic gas emitted in automobile exhaust.

Carcinogens Substances that contribute to the formation of cancers.

Cardiac arrhythmias Irregular heart rhythms.

Cardiac output Amount of blood ejected by the heart in one minute.

Cardiovascular diseases Diseases that affects the heart and the circulatory system (blood vessels). Examples of cardiovascular diseases are coronary heart disease, peripheral vascular disease, congenital heart disease, rheumatic heart disease, atherosclerosis, strokes, high blood pressure, and congestive heart failure.

Cardiovascular endurance The ability of the lungs, heart, and blood vessels to deliver adequate amounts of oxygen to the cells to meet the demands of prolonged (aerobic) physical activity.

Catabolism Process whereby complex substances are broken down into more simple substances.

Catecholamines Hormones, includes epinephrine and norepinephrine.

Cellulite Term frequently used in reference to fat deposits that "bulge out." These deposits are nothing but enlarged fat cells due to excessive accumulation of body fat.

CHD See coronary heart disease.

Chancre A painless, red-rimmed sore that develops at the site where syphilis bacteria enter the body.

Chlamydia A sexually transmitted disease caused by a bacterial infection that can cause significant damage to the reproductive system and may occur without symptoms.

Cholesterol A yellow, waxy substance that is technically a steroid alcohol found only in animal fats and oil.

Chronic diseases Diseases that develop over a prolonged period of time, usually associated to unhealthy lifestyle factors (hypertension, atherosclerosis, coronary disease, strokes, diabetes, and cancer).

Chronic obstructive pulmonary disease (COPD) An air flow limiting disease that includes diseases such as chronic bronchitis and emphysema.

Chronological age Actual age of the individual (also see functional age).

Chylomicrons Triglyceride-transporting molecules in the blood.

Cocaine 2-beta-carbomethoxy-3-betabenozoxytropane the primary psychoactive ingredient derived from coca plant leaves. Also referred to as coke, C, snow, blow, toot, flake, Peruvian lady, white girl, and happy dust.

Coenzyme Nonprotein molecule required in enzyme reactions.

Complete protein A protein source that contains all nine essential amino acids.

Complex carbohydrates Carbohydrates formed by three or more simple sugar molecules linked together, also referred to as polysaccharides. Commonly used to designate foods high in starch.

Compound fats A combination of simple fats with other chemicals. Examples of compound fats are phospholipids, glucolipids, and lipoproteins.

Concentric muscle contraction Shortening of fibers during muscle contraction.

Conflict The stress that results from two opposing and incompatible goals, demands, or needs.

Congenital heart disease Heart defects present at birth.

Coronary arteries Arteries that supply the myocardium or heart muscle with oxygen and nutrients.

Coronary heart disease Disease caused by the obstruction of the coronary arteries by plaque formation (also see atherosclerosis).

Coronary-prone personality See Type A personality.

Corticosteroid A hormone released during stress that affects immunity.

Crack Cocaine mixed with ammonia, baking soda, and water then heated and smoked; freebasing.

Cruciferous vegetables Plants that produce cross-shaped leaves (cauliflower, broccoli, cabbage, Brussels sprouts, and kohlrabi). These vegetables seem to have a protective effect against cancer.

D

Daily Values Standard nutrition values developed by the Food and Drug Administration (FDA) for use on food labels.

Dehydration A loss of body water below normal volume.

Delta-9-tetrahydrocannabinol The addictive psychoactive drug found in marijuana.

Deoxyribonucleic acid (DNA) Genetic material, substance of which genes are made.

Derived fats A combination of simple and compound fats.

Diabetes mellitus Condition where the blood glucose is unable to enter the cells because the pancreas either totally stops producing insulin or produces an insufficient amount for the body's needs.

Diastolic blood pressure Pressure exerted by the blood against the walls of the arteries during the relaxation phase (diastole) of the heart.

Dietary fiber Fiber in plant foods that cannot be digested by the human body.

Dietary induced thermogenesis (DIT) Extra amount of heat production caused by the metabolism of food.

Disaccharides Simple carbohydrates formed by two monosaccharide units linked together, one of which is glucose. The major disaccharides are sucrose, lactose, and maltose.

Distress Negative stress. Refers to unpleasant or harmful stress under which health and performance begin to deteriorate.

DIT See dietary induced thermogenesis.

DNA See deoxyribonucleic acid.

DRV (Daily Reference Values) Standards for nutrients and food components that do not have an established RDA (carbohydrate, fat, saturated fat, fiber, cholesterol, and sodium).

Drug Chemical substance that has the potential to alter the structure and functioning of a living organism.

Duration of exercise How long a person exercises.

Dynamic training Strength training method referring to a muscle contraction with movement.

Dysmenorrhea Painful menstruation.

E

Eccentric muscle contraction Lengthening of fibers during muscle contraction.

ECG See electrocardiogram.

EKG See electrocardiogram.

Elastic elongation (flexibility) Refers to an elastic or temporary lengthening of soft tissue (muscles, tendons, and ligaments).

Electrocardiogram (ECG or EKG) A recording of the electrical activity of the heart.

Emotional wellness The ability to understand your own feelings, accept your limitations, and achieve emotional stability.

Emphysema Pulmonary disease caused by distention (overinflation) of the alveoli.

Endorphines Morphine-like substances released from the pituitary gland in the brain during prolonged aerobic exercise. They are thought to induce feelings of euphoria and natural well-being.

Endurance See cardiovascular endurance and muscular endurance.

Energy The ability to do work.

Energy-balancing equation A principle holding that as long as caloric input equals caloric output, the person will not gain or lose weight. If caloric intake exceeds output, the person gains weight; when output exceeds input, the person loses weight.

Enzyme A catalyst that facilitates chemical reactions.

Epidemiology Science that studies the relationship between diverse factors (lifestyle and environmental) and the occurrence of disease.

Essential amino acids Amino acids that must be obtained in the diet because they cannot be produced in the body.

Essential fat Minimal amount of body fat needed for normal physiological functions. It constitutes about 3 percent of the total fat in men and 12 percent in women.

Essential hypertension Persistent high blood pressure, having no known cause.

Estrogen Female sex hormone. Essential for bone formation and bone density conservation.

Eumenorrhea Normal menstrual cycle.

Eustress Positive stress, desirable stress.

Exercise Physical activity that requires planned, structured, and repetitive bodily movement done to improve or maintain one or more components of physical fitness.

Exercise adherence Initiating and participating in an exercise program for life.

Exercise electrocardiogram An exercise test during which the workload is gradually increased (until the subject reaches maximal fatigue) with blood pressure and twelve-lead electrocardiographic monitoring throughout the test.

Exercise intolerance Exercise conducted at intensity levels well beyond a person functional capacity leading to symptoms such as very rapid or irregular heart rate, labored breathing, nausea, vomiting, light-headedness, headaches, dizziness, pale skin, flushness, excessive weakness, lack of energy, shakiness, sore muscles, cramps, and tightness in the chest.

Exercise tolerance test *See* exercise electrocardiogram.

Exhaustion stage The final stage of the general adaptation syndrome, characterized by depletion of the body's resources and loss of adaptive abilities.

Explanatory style A belief system; the way people perceive the events in their lives — i.e., optimistically or pessimistically.

External locus of control One's prevailing belief that the things that happen are unrelated to one's own behavior.

F

Faith What we perceive or believe to be real.

Family A unique cluster of people who enjoy a special relationship by reason of love, marriage, procreation, and mutual dependence.

Fatigue The inability to maintain a given workload.

Fat mass Weight of the total mount of fat in the body.

Fats Compounds made by a combination of triglycerides.

Fear A state of escalated worry and apprehension that causes distinct physical and emotional reactions.

Fetal alcohol syndrome A set of mental and physical characteristics in a newborn caused by moderate to heavy alcohol drinking during pregnancy.

Fiber A form of complex carbohydrate made up of plant material that cannot be digested by the human body.

Fight or flight mechanism Physiological response of the body to stress which prepares the individual to take action by stimulating the vital defense systems.

Fighting spirit Determination; the open expression of emotions, whether negative or positive.

Flexibility The ability of a joint to move freely through its full range of motion.

Food Guide Pyramid A configuration of daily food choices that stresses the proportion of foods needed for a healthy diet; developed by the U.S. Department of Agriculture.

Forgiveness The ability to release from the mind all past hurts and failures, all sense of guilt and loss.

Fraud *See* quackery.

Freebasing *See* Crack.

Free fatty acids (FFA) Fatty acids released by the breakdown of triglycerides.

Free radicals *See* oxygen free radicals.

Frequency of exercise How often a person engages in an exercise session.

Fructose A sugar that occurs naturally in fruits and honey.

Functional age Physiological age of the individual. Usually lower than the chronological (actual) age in fit people and vice versa in unfit people.

G

Galactose A monosaccharide produced from milk sugar in the mammary glands of lactating animals.

General adaptation syndrome A three-stage attempt of the body to react and adapt to stressors that disrupt its normal balance.

Genetics Science that studies genetic or hereditary conditions.

Genital warts A sexually transmitted disease caused by a viral infection. Genital warts increase the risk of cervical cancer. Enlargement and spread of the warts leads to obstruction of the urethra, vagina, and anus.

Girth measurements technique Technique to assess body composition, including percent body fat, by measuring circumferences at various body sites.

Glucose Blood sugar, type of carbohydrate (monosaccharide), a primary source of energy for the human body.

Glucose intolerance Inability to properly metabolize glucose.

Glycogen Form of carbohydrate (polysaccharide) storage in muscle.

Glycolysis Breakdown of glucose to pyruvic or lactic acid.

Gonorrhea A sexually transmitted disease caused by a bacterial infection that can lead to pelvic inflammation in women, infertility, widespread bacterial infection, heart damage, arthritis in men and women, and blindness in children born to infected women.

Grief The overwhelming sorrow that follows a loss.

H

Hardiness A set of personality traits marked by commitment, control, and challenge.

Hassles Seemingly minor, irritating, everyday annoyances that increase the level of stress.

Hatha Yoga An ancient exercise technique involving stretching, used today to relieve stress and induce calm.

HDL *See* high density lipoprotein.

Health The balance of the physical, emotional, social, and spiritual aspects of personality that is conducive to optimal well-being.

Health promotion Programs aimed at helping people develop healthy lifestyle behaviors that will lead to a higher state of wellness.

Health-related fitness Refers to fitness components that when enhanced lead to better health (cardiovascular endurance, body composition, muscular strength and endurance, and muscular flexibility).

Heart attack *See* myocardial infarct

Heart rate reserve The difference between the maximal heart rate and the resting heart rate.

Heat cramps Muscle cramps caused by heat-induced changes in electrolyte balance in muscle cells.

Heat exhaustion Heat-related condition; symptoms include fainting, dizziness, profuse sweating, cold clammy skin, headaches and a rapid, weak pulse.

Heat stroke Heat-related emergency; symptoms include serious disorientation, warm dry skin, no sweating, rapid full pulse, vomiting, diarrhea, unconsciousness, and high body temperature.

Hemoglobin Protein-iron compound in red blood cells that transports oxygen in the blood.

Hepatitis B A form of hepatitis spread through exposure to the contaminated blood or body fluids of an infected person; can cause long-term liver damage.

Herpes A sexually transmitted disease caused by a viral infection (herpes simplex virus types I and II). No known cure is available for the disease. The disease is characterized by the appearance of sores on the mouth, genitals, rectum, or other parts of the body.

Hidden fat Fat in food that cannot be readily observed (lean meats contain about 30 to 40 percent fat calories).

High density lipoprotein (HDL) Cholesterol-transporting molecules in the blood. High HDL-cholesterol (good cholesterol) seems to offer protection against some forms of cardiovascular disease.

HIV *See* human immunodeficiency virus.

Homeostasis State of balance within body systems that allows a person to react to stressors in a healthful manner.

Hope Optimism in the absence of fear; positive expectation.

Hopelessness A mental state marked by negative expectations about the future.

Hostility An ongoing accumulation of anger and irritation; a permanent, deep-seated type of anger that hovers quietly until some trivial incident causes it to erupt.

Human immunodeficiency virus (HIV) Virus that causes acquired immunodeficiency syndrome (AIDS).

Human papilloma virus (HPV) The virus that causes genital warts; some strains of the virus also have been linked to cervical cancer.

Hunger The actual physical need for food.

Hydrogenated Hydrogen added to fats to increase shelf life and make the product more spreadable; increases saturation of the fat.

Hydrostatic weighing Underwater weighing technique to assess body composition, including percent body fat.

Hyperglycemia Elevated blood sugar (glucose).

Hyperlipidemia Elevated blood fats or lipids.

Hyperplasia An increase in the number of cells.

Hypertension Chronically elevated blood pressure.

Hypertrophy An increase in the size of the cell (for example, muscle hypertrophy).

Hypoglycemia Low blood sugar (glucose).

Hypokinetic disease Diseases associated with a lack of physical activity (for example, hypertension, coronary heart disease, obesity, and diabetes).

I

Imagery Vivid mental visualization.

Immunity The body function that guards the body from invaders, both internal and external.

Incomplete proteins Proteins that do not contain all the essential amino acids.

Insoluble fiber Fiber that can't be dissolved in water or digested.

Insulin Hormone secreted by the pancreas that increases the absorption and utilization of glucose by the body.

Intensity of exercise In cardiorespiratory exercise, how hard a person has to exercise to improve or maintain fitness.

Internal locus of control One's prevailing belief that negative events are a consequence of one's own actions and, thus, potentially can be controlled.

Interval training Training method with repeated bouts of exercise with rest intervals between each exercise bout.

Irradiation Exposing foods to gamma radiation to prolong shelf-life.

Ischemia Lack of blood flow.

Isokinetic contraction Muscular contraction at a constant velocity.

Isokinetic training Strength-training method where the speed of the muscle contraction is kept constant because the equipment (machine) provides an accommodating resistance to match the user's force (maximal) through the range of motion.

Isometric training Strength-training method that refers to a muscle contraction producing little or no movement, such as pushing or pulling against immovable objects.

Isotonic training Strength-training method that refers to a muscle contraction with movement, such as lifting an object over the head.

J

Jaundice Liver condition in which the skin and whites of the eyes appear yellow.

K

Kilocalorie A unit to measure heat energy. A kilocalorie (kcal) or large calorie is the amount of heat necessary to raise the temperature of one kilogram of water one degree Centigrade. One kcal equals 1,000 calories.

L

Lactic acid Strong acid, end product of anaerobic glycolysis (metabolism).

Lactose A disaccharide consisting of glucose plus galactose.

Lactovegetarians Vegetarians who also eat foods from the milk group.

LDL *See* low density lipoprotein.

Lean body mass Body weight without body fat.

Life experiences survey Questionnaire used to assess sources of stress in life.

Locus of control A person's perception of how much influence he or she has over life events; at extreme ends of the continuum are *external* and *internal*.

Loneliness The result of a breakdown of a person's network of social relationships.

Low density lipoprotein (LDL) Cholesterol-transporting molecules in the blood. High LDL-cholesterol (bad cholesterol) seems to increase the risk for some forms of cardiovascular disease.

Lymphocytes Specialized immune system cells.

M

Macrominerals Seven minerals the body needs in relatively large amounts.

Malignant Cancerous.

Malignant melanoma Deadliest of all types of skin cancer. Tumors grow at a rapid rate and readily spread to other parts of the body if not treated at an early stage.

Maltose A disaccharide consisting of two units of maltose.

Marijuana A psychoactive drug prepared from a mixture of crushed leaves, flowers, small branches, stems, and seeds from the hemp plant cannabis sativa. Also referred to as pot and grass.

Maximal exercise test Any test that requires the participant's all-out or nearly all-out effort.

Maximal heart rate (MHR) Highest heart rate for a person, primarily related to age.

Maximal oxygen uptake (VO$_{2max}$) The maximal amount of oxygen that the body is able to utilize per minute of physical activity, commonly expressed in ml/kg/min. The best indicator of cardiovascular or aerobic fitness.

Meditation Stress management technique used to gain control over one's attention, clearing the mind and blocking out the stressor(s) responsible for the increased tension.

Megadose (of vitamins) Large amount of vitamin(s) intake. For most vitamins, a megadose is ten times the RDA or more.

Mental wellness A state in which your mind is engaged in lively interaction with the world around you.

Metabolism All energy and material transformations that occur within living cells necessary to sustain life.

Metastasis The spread of cancer that occurs when cancer cells from a growth breaks off and enter other parts of the body through the blood or lymph system.

METS (metabolic equivalents) A measurement unit of resting energy expenditure. One MET is the equivalent of 3.5 ml/kg/min.

Minerals Inorganic elements found in the body and in food which are essential for normal body functions.

Mitochondria Structures within the cells where energy transformations take place.

Mode of exercise Form of exercise.

Modes of training Form of training used to improve strength.

Moderate intensity physical activity Physical activity that uses 150 calories of energy per day, or 1,000 calories per week.

Monosaccharides The simplest carbohydrates (sugars) formed by five- or six-carbon skeletons. The three most common monosaccharides are glucose, fructose, and galactose.

Monounsaturated fat Fatty acids with only one double bond found along the carbon atom chain.

Motor skill-related fitness Refers to fitness components that when improved lead to enhanced athletic performance (agility, balance, coordination, power, reaction time, and speed).

Motor unit The combination of a motor neuron and the muscle fibers that it innervates.

Muscle fiber A muscle cell.

Muscular endurance (localized muscular endurance) The ability of a muscle to exert submaximal force repeatedly over a period of time (for example, 30 repetitions on a bench press exercise). It usually implies a specific muscle group (chest, thighs, abdominals).

Muscular strength The ability of a muscle to exert maximum force against resistance (for example, 1 repetition maximum or 1 RM on the bench press exercise).

Myocardial infarct Death of part of the myocardium.

Myocardium Heart muscle.

Myoglobin Iron-containing compound that holds oxygen in muscle tissue.

N

Neuron A nerve cell.

Nicotine Poisonous, addictive component of tobacco, inhaled when smoking or absorbed through the lining of the mouth when chewing it.

Nonessential amino acids Amino acids that can be manufactured in the body, therefore, the do not have to be obtained in the diet.

Nulliparity Never having had a child.

Nutrient density Ratio of nutrients to calories in food.

Nutrient Substance found in food that provide energy, regulate metabolism, and help with growth and repair of body tissues.

Nutrition Science that studies the relationship of foods to optimal health and performance.

O

Obesity Refers to an excessive accumulation of body fat, usually about 30 percent above recommended body weight according to body size.

Olestra Fat substitute made from sugar and fatty acids; provides no calories to the body because it passes through the digestive system without being absorbed.

Oligomenorrhea Irregular menstrual cycles.

Omega-3 fatty acids Polyunsaturated fatty acids found primarily in cold water seafood and are thought to be effective in lowering blood cholesterol and triglycerides.

Oncogenes Pieces of genetic material that serve as markers to predict later mutation and development of certain cancers, probably by encouraging mutation of related cells.

One repetition maximum (1 RM) The maximal amount of resistance (weight) that an individual is able to lift in a single effort.

Open circuit indirect calorimetry (direct gas analysis) The most precise way to determine VO_{2max} using a metabolic cart to measure the amount of oxygen consumed by the body.

Osteoporosis Softening, deterioration, or loss of total body bone.

Overload principle Key training concept stating that the demands placed on a system (cardiovascular, muscular) must be systematically and progressively increased over time to cause physiologic adaptation (development or improvement).

Overweight Indicates an excess amount of weight against a given standard such as height or recommended percent body fat.

Ovolactovegetarians Vegetarians who include egg and milk products in their diet.

Ovovegetarians Vegetarians who allow eggs in their diet.

Oxygen free radicals Substances formed during metabolism which attack and damage proteins and lipids, in particular the cell membrane and DNA; leading to the development of diseases such as heart disease, cancer, and emphysema. Antioxidants are believed to exert a protective effect by absorbing free radicals before they can cause damage and also by interrupting the sequence of reactions once damage has begun.

P

Pelvic inflammatory disease (PID) Severe infection of the lining of the abdominal cavity most commonly caused by chlamydia and gonorrhea.

Percent body fat Term used in body composition assessment. It represents the total amount of fat in the body based on the person's weight. It includes both essential and storage fat.

Peripheral vascular disease Narrowing of the peripheral blood vessels (it excludes the cerebral and coronary arteries).

Personality The whole of one's personal characteristics; the pattern of behavior that distinguishes a person.

Physical activity Bodily movement produced by skeletal muscles that requires energy expenditure and produces progressive health benefits.

Physical fitness (health-related) The general capacity to adapt and respond favorably to physical effort, implying that individuals are physically fit when they can meet the ordinary as well as the unusual demands of daily life safely and effectively without being overly fatigued, and still have energy left for leisure and recreational activities.

Physical wellness Flexibility, endurance, strength, and optimism about your ability to take care of health problems.

Plastic elongation (flexibility) Refers to a permanent lengthening of soft tissue (capsules, tendons, and ligaments).

PNF *See* proprioceptive neuromuscular facilitation.

Polyunsaturated fat Fatty acids with two or more double bonds along the carbon atom chain.

Precancerous A condition in which a benign (noncancerous) condition has the potential to become cancerous.

Prevention index An annual measure of the effort Americans are making to prevent disease and accidents and to promote good health and longevity. The index is based on the 21 most significant health-promoting behaviors in the United States.

Prodrome A sensation in which the skin starts to itch or tingle, turns red, and becomes extremely sensitive; precedes onset of an STD.

Progressive muscle relaxation Stress management technique. It involves progressive contraction and relaxation of muscle groups throughout the body.

Proprioceptive neuromuscular facilitation (PNF for flexibility development) Stretching technique in which muscles are progressively stretched out with intermittent isometric contractions.

Protein Complex organic compounds containing nitrogen and formed by combinations of amino acids. Proteins are the main substances used in the body to build and repair tissues such as muscles, blood, internal organs, skin, hair, nails, and bones. They are also part of hormones, antibodies, and enzymes.

Psychoneuroimmunology (PNI) The scientific investigation of how the brain affects the body's immune cells and how the immune system can be affected by behavior.

PSA test Protein-specific antigen blood test used to help diagnose prostate cancer.

Pubic lice Commonly called "crabs," tiny parasites that feed on the small blood vessels of the skin beneath the pubic hair.

Q

Quackery (fraud) The conscious promotion of unproven claims for profit.

R

Rate of perceived exertion (RPE) A perception scale to monitor or interpret the intensity of aerobic exercise.

RDA *See* recommended dietary allowances.

RDI (Reference Daily Intakes) Reference values and minerals for protein, vitamins.

Recommended dietary allowances (RDA) Daily recommended intakes of nutrients for normal, healthy people in the United States.

Recommended weight Body weight at which there seems to be no harm to human health.

Red muscle fibers (slow-twitch or type I) Muscle fibers with greater aerobic potential and slow speed of contraction.

Reframing Changing the way one looks at the world.

Relaxation response The body's ability to enter a scientifically defined state of relaxation.

Religion The science of how to know God.

Repetition (in strength training) The number of times that a given resistance is performed (for example, 12 repetitions on the bench press exercise).

Repetition maximum (in strength training) The maximum number of repetitions (RM) that can be performed with a specific resistance or weight (for example, 10 RM with 150 pounds).

Residual volume Volume of air left in the lungs following complete exhalation.

Resistance (in strength training) The amount of weight that is lifted.

Resistance stage The second stage of the general adaptation syndrome, characterized by meeting the perceived challenge.

Resting heart rate Rate after a person has been sitting quietly for 15–20 minutes.

Resting metabolism The amount of energy (expressed in milliliters of oxygen per minute or total calories per day) an individual requires during resting conditions to sustain proper body function.

Retroviruses Viruses that invade a cell's genetic structure and are passed on to each succeeding generation of cells as the cells divide.

Reverse cholesterol transport A process in which HDL molecules attract cholesterol and carry it to the liver, where it is changed to bile and eventually excreted in the stool.

Ribonucleic acid (RNA) Genetic material involved in the formation of cell proteins.

Risk factors Lifestyle and genetic factors that may lead to disease.

RNA *See* ribonucleic acid.

RPE *See* rate of perceived exertion.

S

Saturated fat Fatty acids with carbon atoms fully saturated with hydrogens, therefore only single bonds link the carbon atoms on the chain. High intake of saturated fats increases the risk for coronary heart disease.

Scabies An STD caused by tiny mites that burrow under the skin at night.

Secondhand smoke A mixture of smoke exhaled by smokers and smoke from the burning end of a cigarette, pipe, or cigar.

Self-esteem A sense of positive self-regard.

Self-efficacy One's perception of his or her ability to do specific things.

Serum cholesterol Blood cholesterol level.

Set (in strength training) Number of repetitions (1 set of 12 repetitions).

Setpoint theory The weight control theory that indicates that the body has an established weight and strongly attempts to maintain that weight.

Sexually transmitted diseases (STDs) Diseases spread through sexual contact.

Shin splints Injury to the lower leg characterized by pain and irritation in the shin region or front of the leg.

Simple carbohydrates Carbohydrates formed by simple or double sugar units with little nutritive value (for example, candy, pop, cakes, etc.), frequently denoted as sugars. Simple carbohydrates are divided into monosaccharides and disaccharides.

Simple fats A glyceride molecule linked to one, two, or three units of fatty acids (monoglycerides, diglycerides, and triglycerides).

Skinfold thickness Technique to assess body composition, including percent body fat, by measuring the thickness of a double fold of skin at different body sites.

Slow-sustained or static stretching (flexibility) Stretching technique where the muscles are gradually lengthened through a joint's complete range of motion and the final position is held for a few seconds.

Social support The human resources that people provide to each other.

Social wellness The ability to relate well to others, both within and outside the family unit.

Soluble fiber Fiber that dissolves in water, forming a thick, gel-like substance.

Specificity of training Training programs must be specifically aimed at the desired outcome. This is accomplished by training with the specific activity that the person is attempting to improve (aerobic, anaerobic, strength, flexibility).

Sphygmomanometer Equipment used to measure blood pressure. Consists of an inflatable bladder contained within a cuff and a mercury gravity manometer or an aneroid manometer from which the pressure is read.

Spiritual health The ability to develop our spiritual nature to its fullest potential.

Spiritual wellness The sense that life is meaningful, that life has purpose, and that some power brings all humanity together; the ethics, values, and morals that guide us and give meaning and direction to life.

Spontaneous remission Inexplicable recovery from incurable illness.

Spot reducing Theory that claims that exercising a specific body part (for example, abdominal or midsection of the body) will result in significant fat reduction in that area. It does not work!

Squamous cell carcinoma Type of skin cancer that grows at a faster rate that basal cell carcinomas and seems to grow on sun-damaged areas. Squamous cell tumors spread to other parts of the body if not treated at an early stage.

STDs *See* sexually transmitted diseases

Storage fat Body fat in excess of the essential fat. It is stored in adipose tissue.

Strength *See* muscular strength.

Strength training A conditioning program that requires the use of weights to help increase muscular strength, endurance, power, and/or body size.

Stress An automatic biological response to demands made on an individual; the result of any event or condition that causes us to adapt.

Stress buffers Factors that alleviate the deleterious effects of stress such as social support, a sense of control, physical fitness, a sense of humor, self-esteem, optimism, advantageous coping styles, and hardiness.

Stress test *See* exercise electrocardiogram.

Stressor Any situation or event that makes us adapt or adjust.

Stroke volume Amount of blood ejected by the heart in one beat.

Structured Interview Assessment tool used in determining behavioral patterns (Type A and B personality).

Sucrose Table sugar (glucose plus fructose).

Suppressor genes Pieces of genetic material that are part of a cell's normal protective mechanism against development of cancer.

Synergistic effect A phenomenon in which the effects of using more than one drug simultaneously are different and greater than using any of the drugs alone.

Syphilis A sexually transmitted disease caused by a bacterial infection. During the last stage of the disease, some people will suffer from paralysis, crippling, blindness, heart disease, brain damage, insanity, and even death.

Systolic blood pressure Pressure exerted by the blood against the walls of the arteries during the forceful contraction (systole) of the heart.

T

Tar Chemical compound that forms during the burning of tobacco leaves.

Testosterone Male sex hormone.

THC The psychoactive ingredient in marijuana.

Toxic core Type A personality traits most detrimental to health; anger, cynicism, suspiciousness, and excessive self-involvement.

Trace minerals Fourteen minerals that the body needs in very small amounts.

Triglycerides Fats formed by glycerol and three fatty acids.

Type A (personality) Sometimes referred to as "hurry sickness," a classification that describes a person who is hard-driving and competitive and also is hostile, angry, and suspicious; sometimes referred to as coronary-prone behavior.

Type B (personality) A classification that describes a person who is easy-going and generally free of hostility, anger, and suspicion.

Type C (personality) A classification that describes an emotionally nonexpressive person who demonstrates ambivalence and is at increased risk for cancer; sometimes referred to as cancer-prone personality.

Type I diabetes Found primarily in young people. A condition in which the pancreas produces little or no insulin. Also called juvenile diabetes.

Type II diabetes A condition in which the body is unable to use insulin properly.

U

U.S. RDA The United States recommended daily allowances used between the late 1960s and the early 1990s. Derived from the RDA and developed as a standard for nutrition labeling.

V

Vasoconstriction Narrowing or clamping down of blood vessels.

Vasodilation Widening or opening up of blood vessels.

Vegans Vegetarians who eat no animal products at all.

Vegetarian Individuals whose diet is of vegetable or plant origin.

Veins Major vessels that carry blood back to the heart.

Very low density lipoprotein (VLDL) Triglyceride, cholesterol and phospholipid-transporting molecules in the blood. Only a small amount of cholesterol is carried by the VLDL molecules.

Vigorous activity Any activity that requires a MET level equal to or greater than 6 METs (21 ml/kg/min).

Viral hepatitis An infection that causes inflammation of the liver; has four identified types.

Vitamins Organic substances essential for normal metabolism, growth, and development of the body.

VLDL *See* very low density lipoprotein.

VO$_{2max}$ *See* maximal oxygen uptake.

W

Waist-to-Hip Ratio Test designed by a panel of scientists appointed by the National Academy of Sciences and the Dietary Guidelines Advisory Council for the U. S. Departments of Agriculture and Health and Human Services to assess potential risk for diseases associated with obesity.

Warm-up Starting a workout slowly.

Weight training A conditioning program that requires the use of weights to help increase muscular strength, endurance, power, and/or body size.

Weight-regulating mechanism (WRM) Physiologic mechanism located in the hypothalamus of the brain that regulates how much the body should weigh (*also see* setpoint theory).

Wellness The complete integration of physical, mental, emotional, social, and spiritual well-being — a complex interaction of the factors that lead to a quality life.

White muscle fibers (fast-twitch or type II) Muscle fibers with greater anaerobic potential and fast speed of contraction.

Work The ability to utilize energy.

Workload A given level of exercise intensity or physical performance.

Worry A state in which we dwell on something so much that we become apprehensive.

Y

Yellow fat cells Cells used for fat storage (stores of energy in the form of fat).

Yo-yo dieting Constantly losing and gaining weight.

Index